RECENT DEVELOPMENTS IN

ALCOHOLISM

VOLUME 4

RECENT DEVELOPMENTS IN

Edited by

MARC GALANTER

Albert Einstein College of Medicine
Bronx, New York

Associate Editors

HENRI BEGLEITER, RICHARD DEITRICH,
DONALD GOODWIN, EDWARD GOTTHEIL,
ALFONSO PAREDES, MARCUS ROTHSCHILD,
and DAVID VAN THIEL

Editorial Assistant

VIRGINIA PRIVITAR

An Official Publication of the American Medical Society on Alcoholism and Other Drug Dependencies and the Research Society on Alcoholism. This series was founded by the National Council on Alcoholism.

ALCOHOLISM

VOLUME 4

Combined Alcohol and Drug Abuse
Typologies of Alcoholics
The Withdrawal Syndrome
Renal and Electrolyte Consequences

PLENUM PRESS • NEW YORK AND LONDON

The Library of Congress has cataloged this work as follows:

Recent developments in alcoholism: an official publication of the American Medical Society on Alcoholism, and the Research Society on Alcoholism, and the National Council on Alcoholism—Vol. 1- —New York: Plenum Press, c1983-
v.: ill.; 25 cm.
Cataloging in publication.
Editor: Marc Galanter.
ISSN 0738-422X = Recent developments in alcoholism.

1. Alcoholism—Periodicals. I. Galanter, Marc. II. American Medical Society on Alcoholism. III. Research Society on Alcohol (U.S.) IV. National Council on Alcoholism. [DNLM: 1. Alcoholism—periodicals. W1 RE106AH(P)]

HV5001.R4	616.86′1′05—dc19	83-643791
Library of Congress	[8311]	AACR 2 MARC-S

ISBN 0-306-42170-4

A Division of Plenum Publishing Corporation
233 Spring Street, New York, N.Y. 10013

Printed in the United States of America

Contributors

Arthur I. Alterman, Veterans Administration Medical Center, Philadelphia, Pennsylvania 19104; and University of Pennsylvania School of Medicine, Philadelphia, Pennsylvania 19104

Thomas F. Babor, Alcohol Research Center, Department of Psychiatry, University of Connecticut Health Center, Farmington, Connecticut 06032

Jerome F.X. Carroll, Continuum Program, Eagleville Hospital, Eagleville, Pennsylvania 19408

Richard R. Clayton, Department of Sociology, University of Kentucky, Lexington, Kentucky 40506

Paul Cushman, Jr., Drug Dependency Treatment Program, McGuire Veterans Hospital, Richmond, Virginia 23249; and Departments of Medicine, Psychiatry, Pharmacology and Toxicology, Medical College of Virginia, Richmond, Virginia 23298

Dennis M. Donovan, Department of Psychiatry and Behavioral Sciences, University of Washington, Seattle, Washington 98195; and Alcohol Dependence Treatment Program, Veterans Administration Medical Center, Seattle, Washington 98108

Dora B. Goldstein, Department of Pharmacology, Stanford University School of Medicine, Stanford, California 94305

David A. Gorelick, Alcohol and Drug Treatment Program, Behavioral Pharmacology Laboratory, Brentwood Division, West Los Angeles Veterans Administration Medical Center, Los Angeles, California 90073; and Department of Psychiatry, School of Medicine, University of California, Los Angeles, California 90024

Edward Gottheil, Department of Psychiatry and Human Behavior, Jefferson Medical College, Thomas Jefferson University, Philadelphia, Pennsylvania 19107

Michie N. Hesselbrock, Department of Psychiatry, University of Connecticut Health Center, Farmington, Connecticut 06032

Daniel R. Kivlahan, Department of Psychiatry and Behavioral Sciences, University of Washington, Seattle, Washington 98195; and Alcohol Dependence Treatment Program, Veterans Administration Medical Center, Seattle, Washington 98108

Richard J. Lauerman, Alcohol Research Center, Department of Psychiatry, University of Connecticut Health Center, Farmington, Connecticut 06032

Roger E. Meyer, Alcohol Research Center, Department of Psychiatry, University of Connecticut Health Center, Farmington, Connecticut 06032

Leslie C. Morey, Department of Psychology, Vanderbilt University, Nashville, Tennessee 37240

Claudio A. Naranjo, Clinical Pharmacology Program, Addiction Research Foundation Clinical Institute, and Departments of Pharmacology and Medicine, University of Toronto, Ontario M5S 2S1, Canada

Alfonso Paredes, Department of Psychiatry, The Neuropsychiatric Institute, Alcohol Research Center, University of California, Los Angeles, California 90024

Thomas O. Pitts, Renal–Electrolyte Division, Department of Medicine, Pittsburgh, University of Pittsburgh School of Medicine, Pittsburgh, Pennsylvania 15261

Eugene P. Schoener, Department of Pharmacology, Wayne State University School of Medicine, Detroit, Michigan 48201

Edward M. Sellers, Clinical Institute, Addiction Research Foundation, and Departments of Pharmacology and Medicine, University of Toronto, Ontario M5S 2S1, Canada

Harvey A. Skinner, Addiction Research Foundation, Toronto, Ontario M5S 2S1, Canada

Ralph E. Tarter, Department of Psychology, University of Pittsburgh School of Medicine, Pittsburgh, Pennsylvania 15213

David H. Van Thiel, Division of Gastroenterology, Department of Medicine, University of Pittsburgh School of Medicine, Pittsburgh, Pennsylvania 15261

R. Dale Walker, Department of Psychiatry and Behavioral Sciences, University of Washington, Seattle, Washington 98195; and Alcohol Dependence Treatment Program, Veterans Administration Medical Center, Seattle, Washington 98108

Jeffery N. Wilkins, Crisis Oriented Psychiatric Evaluation Service, Clinical Psychopharmacology Unit, Brentwood Division, West Los Angeles Veterans Administration Medical Center, Los Angeles, California 90073; and Department of Psychiatry, School of Medicine, University of California, Los Angeles, California 90024

Preface

From the President of the Research Society on Alcoholism

In recent years the alcohol research field has matured and is attracting a substantial number of eager and technically sophisticated researchers. There is a feeling of excitement and premonitions of breakthroughs as more and more of alcohol's actions are being detailed. I, however, have at times been sobered by the perception that the lure of parsimonious explanations and the appeal of studying easily demonstrable effects obscure the critical issues regarding alcohol abuse and alcoholism. Central questions regarding (1) the reinforcing properties of ethanol and other factors responsible for inappropriate consumption of alcohol, (2) the heterogenous characteristics (both biologic and sociologic) of the alcoholic population, and (3) the differential predisposition of individuals to alcohol-induced medical problems needed to be vigorously pursued. Researchers who used animals as models for the human condition needed to become more intimately aware of the variety of factors that are of importance in the development of alcoholism in an individual. On the other hand, researchers studying humans needed to attempt to more clearly define and categorize diagnostic criteria and characteristics of various alcoholic populations. Such categorization and continued characterization of alcoholism allows not only for a framework of concepts within which proper animal models for studies of biologic mechanisms can be developed but also allows for consideration of the most apt treatment approaches.

I have been most heartened during the last two years by the increased attention being paid to the development of appropriate concepts for studies of alcoholism. This increase in attention to concepts has certainly been evidenced in the presentations at the annual meeting of the Research Society on Alcoholism (RSA) and in the published material appearing in the AMSAODD/RSA journal and in this book series. I would hope that continued insight will be displayed by the experienced researchers in the alcoholism field and that this insight will be used to guide those newly entering alcohol research. Science is the testing of hypothesis, but hypothesis should be firmly grounded. Progress toward the solution of the major problems in the alcoholism field will be swift with adherence to proper concepts and good scientific methods.

Boris Tabakoff, Ph.D.

From the President of the American Medical Society on Alcoholism and Other Drug Dependencies

As our basic and clinical scientific knowledge of chemical dependency expands, so does our recognition that mood-altering chemicals have similar yet different effects at the cellular, tissue, organ and behavioral levels. This fourth volume of *Recent Developments in Alcoholism* reflects the increasing acceptance of the commonalities of alcoholism and other drug dependencies. The concepts of multiple drug use—either collectively ("polydrug") or in series—have caused the inclusion of a broader selection of topics, at once attractive to both clinician and scientist.

These same concepts prompted the American Medical Society on Alcoholism (AMSA) to expand its name to the American Medical Society on Alcoholism and Other Drug Dependencies (AMSAODD). Its annual Scientific Forum, the Ruth Fox Course, other educational and professional activities (including the forthcoming certification of physicians in chemical dependency), as well as the journal *Alcoholism* (published jointly with the Research Society on Alcoholism) have likewise broadened their scope.

The membership in AMSAODD is soaring—reflecting the interest of increasing numbers of physicians in this field. This will mean better care for the victims of alcoholism and other drug dependencies. It is to that end that this Society and this annual volume are dedicated.

Max A. Schneider, M.D.

From the Editor

With the publication of this fourth volume, the series *Recent Developments in Alcoholism* now encompasses a perspective on much of the terrain of the current alcoholism field. The summary contents, including those planned for the next volume, are as follows:

Volume 1: Genetics
Behavioral Treatment
Social Mediators and Prevention
Current Concepts and Diagnosis

Volume 2: Learning and Social Models
Alcohol and the Liver
Aging and Alcoholism
Anthropology

Volume 3: High-Risk Studies
Prostaglandins and Leukotrienes
Cardiovascular Effects
Cerebral Function in Social Drinkers

Volume 4: Combined Alcohol and Drug Abuse Problems
Typologies of Alcoholics

	The Alcohol Withdrawal Syndrome
	Renal and Electrolyte Consequences of Alcohol Abuse
Volume 5:	Memory Deficits
	Sociology of Treatment
	Ion Channels
	Early Problem Drinking

The current volume highlights some issues which will complement those in previous volumes, extending the scope of the series as a comprehensive review of the field. The first section, Combined Alcohol and Drug Abuse Problems, edited by Dr. Edward Gottheil, reflects an important clinical area for pharmacology and treatment in alcoholism. It also offers the reader entry into issues which will be increasingly highlighted by the American Medical Society on Alcoholism and Other Drug Dependencies, in light of the extension of the work of that society into the field of substance abuse. As usual, this section reflects the format of our series, namely one which spans the breadth of research from epidemiologic and preclinical issues to ones of clinical management.

The second section of the volume was prepared by Dr. Thomas Babor and Dr. Roger Meyer, who were invited to serve as guest editors, because of the valuable work being done in their research center on the developing typologies of alcoholics. Drs. Babor and Meyer invited a number of investigators, both from their own research group and from other research settings, to provide a background for this issue, which stands at the interface between the research laboratory and clinical application. It is anticipated that both the researcher and the clinician will be able to turn to this material for insight into underlying mechanisms and clinical options.

A third section of the book dedicated to the Alcohol Withdrawal Syndrome is edited by Dr. Alfonso Paredes. Valuable new work has become available since the original studies which defined the physiologic concomitants of this syndrome in the middle decades of this century. These findings range from changes in membrane chemistry through observations on derangement in neuroendocrinology, and are allied with a more sophisticated understanding of the treatment options available in the management of the syndrome.

Finally, we chose to include in this volume a section on Renal and Electrolyte Consequences of Alcohol Abuse, edited by Dr. David Van Thiel. This offered an opportunity to highlight an important issue in the metabolic derangements associated with alcoholism but one which has not been widely addressed in the clinical literature. The inclusion of the section provided the opportunity to review important abnormalities in electrolytes and acid–base balance as well as problems associated with urinary tract infection. These observations also shed light on interesting possibilities regarding an association between renal sodium retention and ascites formation in cirrhosis.

Marc Galanter, M.D.

Contents

I. Combined Alcohol and Drug Abuse Problems

Edward Gottheil, Section Editor

Chapter 4

Treating Multiple Substance Abuse Clients
Jerome F.X. Carroll

II. Typologies of Alcoholics

Thomas F. Babor and Roger E. Meyer, Section Editors

Chapter 5

Classification and Forms of Inebriety: Historical Antecedents of Alcoholic Typologies
Thomas F. Babor and Richard J. Lauerman

Chapter 6

Empirically Derived Classifications of Alcohol-Related Problems
Leslie C. Morey and Harvey A. Skinner

Chapter 7

An Examination of Selected Typologies: Hyperactivity, Familial, and Antisocial Alcoholism
Arthur I. Alterman and Ralph E. Tarter

III. The Alcohol Withdrawal Syndrome

Alfonso Paredes, Section Editor

Chapter 12

Clinical Assessment and Pharmacotherapy of the Alcohol Withdrawal Syndrome

Claudio A. Naranjo and Edward M. Sellers

Chapter 13

Special Aspects of Human Alcohol Withdrawal

David A. Gorelick and Jeffery N. Wilkins

IV. Renal and Electrolyte Consequences of Alcohol Abuse

David H. Van Thiel, Section Editor

I

Combined Alcohol and Drug Abuse Problems

Edward Gottheil, Section Editor

Overview

Edward Gottheil

Although people have been using and abusing many substances for many centuries, the field of addiction is relatively new. It probably had its origins in the 1940s when it gained public and scientific attention mainly through the efforts of Alcoholics Anonymous and the National Council on Alcoholism. There was further recognition in the 1950s, with acceptance by the American Medical Association and inclusion in the Diagnostic and Statistical Manual (DSM) of the American Psychiatric Association. It was firmly established with the creation of the National Institute on Alcohol Abuse and Alcoholism (NIAAA).

Prior to the 1960s, the field was not very complicated. To be sure, there was much to be learned, but the main research and clinical problems, by far, were those relating to alcoholism. The field expanded markedly with the drug abuse epidemic of the 1960s and the establishment of the National Institute on Drug Abuse (NIDA). Currently, the field may be undergoing another expansion with the emergence of cocaine use and abuse and becoming more complicated with the steadily increasing numbers of polydrug abusers.

Since the field is as young as it is and there are so many gaps in our knowledge regarding the epidemiology, etiology, pharmacology, diagnosis, and treatment of alcoholism and narcotic addiction, to say nothing of cocaine abuse and the many other substance abuse disorders, it is not surprising that research and clinical programs have tended to focus either on alcoholism or on drug abuse and to avoid studying and treating combined disorders. Indeed, there are still many problems regarding definition and classification and whether there should be a unified field of addiction. We thought it would be worthwhile, therefore, to bring together reviews of what was known about the epidemiology, interactive mechanisms, pharmacologic management, and psychosocial treatment of combined substance use disorders.

Any attempt to study the prevalence of polydrug use must begin by specifying what is to be counted. What constitutes abuse and what qualifies as combined or multiple abuse? In the case of illicit drugs, any use may be considered abuse even though we know that some individuals are able to

Edward Gottheil • Department of Psychiatry and Human Behavior, Jefferson Medical College, Thomas Jefferson University, Philadelphia, Pennsylvania 19107.

use some of these drugs recreationally without any escalation of use and without any apparent adverse consequences. If occasional use of marijuana is not to be counted, or if DSM III criteria for abuse are to be employed, this must be explicitly stated. For licit drugs such as alcohol, tobacco, or prescribed substances, it is clear that abuse must be defined and distinguished from use. It is also necesssary to indicate whether abuse of one substance along with use, but not abuse, of other substances is to be included or excluded; i.e., do we count an alcoholic who smokes one package of cigarettes per day and occasionally uses marijuana and cocaine in social situations? Moreover, should we include multiple sequential users as well as multiple concurrent users, i.e., does an individual who sniffed glue as a child, was an amphetamine abuser during his teens, and who recently began taking heroin qualify?

Once the data are collected and tabulated, the next issue is how to classify the possible combinations. There are 362,880 combinations of ten drugs taken two at a time. The possibilities increase markedly if we consider more than ten drugs which may also be taken three, four, or five at a time; and we have not yet considered the amount ingested of each drug in the combination, the frequency of use, and the route of administration. In Chapter 1 Clayton discusses such issues and critically reviews the various ways that have been used to describe patterns of multiple drug use: developmental patterns of onset, drug clusters, typologies of drug users, and the construction of composite indices intended to reflect the seriousness of drug use.

Clayton then goes on to examine the information available in several national data sets to ascertain the extent of multiple drug use and comes to the straightforward conclusion that multiple drug use is pervasive. In view of this reality, he suggests we rethink some of our ideas and reexamine some of our studies that almost automatically attribute automobile accidents to alcohol and overdose deaths to heroin and that we inquire whether and to what extent specific combinations of multiple drugs may play a role in the occurrence of these adverse consequences. Similarly, he discusses policy issues relevant to prevention and treatment that may require reevaluation. For example, current concerns about health care costs are resulting in policies that focus on lengths of stay for specific treatments of specific conditions, while, at the same time, the increasing prevalence of multiple drug use is resulting in patients entering treatment who often do not come in the sizes and shapes that fit the particular slots specified by our treatment system.

Multiple drugs may be used for enhancement (e.g., alcohol and valium) or counteraction (e.g., cocaine and heroin). These interactions, or at least some of them, have been learned on the "street" and are not new to the pharmacologist. However, the number of studies needing to be done to determine the effects of so many different combinations of drugs that vary in their acute and chronic patterns of use and in their dosage, frequency, and route of administration is staggering. Schoerner in Chapter 2 notes that when we take into account the dynamic and kinetic processes of the individual drugs, as well as their interactions in combinations, and also factor in the different time frames and drug use histories that occur in real life, we are faced with a situation of virtually infinite complexity because of the ever-changing blood/brain levels of free drug and the functional tolerance and dependence that are engendered to varying degrees over time. He emphasizes the need for subjecting these interactions to sophisticated multivariate analyses, which at present are only in their infancy.

Nevertheless, much is known about the basic principles of drug interactions. Schoerner illustrates these principles with respect to the depressant group of drugs. He reviews the pharmacodynamic and pharmacokinetic properties of ethanol, the benzodiazepines, and the sedative hypnotics and discusses the various types of mechanisms involved in their depressant actions and interactions.

Cushman (Chapter 3) also comments about the increasing use of combinations of drugs and the gaps in our knowledge about interactions among them. He gives examples that emphasize the importance of recognition and diagnosis for the appropriate medical management of these conditions. The acute and chronic actions of these drugs, alone and in combination, are reviewed in relation to the development of appropriate principles of treatment. Throughout the chapter, practical issues related to clinical management are considered, such as the effects of adulterants when street drugs have been used, indications for inpatient detoxification, and the special problems for the anesthesiologist of tolerance and cross-tolerance.

In the final chapter of this section, Carroll (Chapter 4) contends that to continue to maintain the current segregation of alcohol dependence and drug dependence programs in the face of mounting clinical and scientific evidence of the preeminence of multiple substance abuse makes no sense. It may lead to inadequate diagnoses, a failure to admit many cases with multiple substance abuse, incomplete treatment, a lack of understanding of the epidemiology of substance abuse, and, worst of all, relapse to addiction subsequent to treatment.

He proposes the adoption of a "generic" perspective of addictions or substance abuse problems, according to which the choice of a particular substance and its particular manifestations is less important than the fact that one is abusing some substance capable of leading to dependence and addiction. Although there are differences that are important for detoxification and medical management, the etiology, defenses, dynamics, and therapeutic principles are seen as essentially similar regardless of the substance or substances abused. From this perspective, varieties of combined treatment methodologies are described in detail, as well as implications for staffing and training.

It seems apparent that multiple substance abuse is a real and pervasive public, clinical, and scientific problem. As a research area it should be extremely attractive to investigators of many disciplines. It is an important problem; there is a need to know; and the area is not uncharted. Many of the principles and techniques are available and gaps in our knowledge are clearly identified. Yet, there are effective barriers to such research resulting from the segregation of our alcohol and drug research and treatment institutions.

Earlier in this century, the psychoanalysts searching for broad psychodynamic explanations of behavior were impressed by the many similarities they found in the histories of alcoholics and drug addicts. Together with smokers, gamblers, and the obese, they were seen as deriving from difficulties encountered during the oral stage of psychosexual development and considered as varieties of impulse disorders. In recent decades, however, alcoholism and drug addiction reappeared as separate entities. NIAAA was established in response to the pressure of Alcoholics Anonymous and the National Council on Alcoholism, and, later, NIDA was created almost overnight in response to the drug abuse epidemic of the 1960s. Representing different constituencies, their research and treatment programs, not surprisingly, were not integrated but underwent separate developments with little overlap. While the psychoanalysts had emphasized similarities among individuals, the programs funded by separate institutes emphasized differences between substances.

Although there are notable exceptions, by and large, NIAAA funds research on alcoholism and NIDA funds research on drug abuse; the alcoholic goes to an alcoholism treatment program, and the drug abuser goes to a drug abuse treatment program. Where, then, is the researcher interested in studying combined alcohol and drug abuse problems to go for funds or subjects? The institutionalized separation of alcoholism and drug addiction has become ingrained in our thought and language patterns. It seems perfectly natural to talk about alcohol and drug abuse even though alcohol is a drug. We would not talk about cows and animals, since the class of animals includes cows. We would refer to cows and *other* animals. Interestingly, to our programmed ears, alcohol and *other* drug abuse sounds stilted though correct, and we prefer alcohol and drug abuse though incorrect.

There has been some movement toward reintegration. Combined alcohol and other drug abuse research, prevention, teaching, and clinical programs have been developed and have been funded. Journals and national societies are reflecting this movement. Yet, much remains to be done and much remains to be learned about combined or multiple substance abuse. In the meantime, whether our researchers, administrators, and program planners are ready or not, our clinicians are continuing to see steadily increasing numbers of polydrug abusers.

1

Multiple Drug Use
Epidemiology, Correlates, and Consequences

Richard R. Clayton

Abstract. The initial focus is on the conceptual issues essential to the understanding of multiple drug use. This is followed by a discussion of the developmental nature of multiple drug use and the various strategies that have been designed to measure multiple use. The third section of the paper contains a review of the extent of multiple drug use in various segments of society with data from the Monitoring-the-Future surveys of high school seniors, the National Survey on Drug Abuse, and the Treatment Outcome Prospective Study of drug abuse treatment clients. The conclusion is that multiple drug use is pervasive. The next section deals with several consequences associated with multiple drug use: automobile accidents, delinquency, and emergency room visits. The final section outlines some of the prevention and treatment implications of multiple drug use from a public policy perspective.

1. Introduction

In a study of the effects of a single drug upon behavior, the implications are manifold. Dosage levels, modes of administration, baseline states, the expectations of the subjects and of the investigators, the environment in which the drug is taken—all these variables, and others as well, make human psychochemical studies difficult and complex. When two or more drugs are used together or in sequence, the problems become magnified. Add to this analysis the vagaries of street drugs with their contaminants, adulterants, diluents, and haphazard quality and quantity control, and the situation almost defies scientific scrutiny. Nevertheless, since polydrug use is notably prevalent and shows no signs of becoming less so, an effort must be made to estimate the impact of multiple drug abuse.

Of all polydrug patterns, those involving alcohol are the most frequently encountered and, perhaps, the most dangerous. The days when substance abusers were categorically labelled—as alcoholic, cokehead, hophead, pothead, and pillhead—seem to be rapidly disappearing. Instead, we are seeing people overinvolved with a primary substance of

Richard R. Clayton • Department of Sociology, University of Kentucky, Lexington, Kentucky 40506.

choice, but also using a variety of others depending on availability, price, social situation, peer group usage, and the latest wisdom from the so-called underground press.

This 1979 statement by Sidney Cohen[1] of the difficulties and complexities inherent in studying the impact of one drug upon the human organism, and the multipliers that must be employed when multiple substances are involved, was a realistic appraisal of some of the more formidable challenges facing scientists in the drug abuse field in the 1980s.

There is an understandable tendency in this field to link research studies and findings to pharmacologically defined categories of drugs. After all, each substance has certain known chemical properties and fits into a particular class of substances with known effects on various systems of the human body. Given the difficulties inherent in studying drug effect, it is not surprising that most laboratory work with drug effects focuses on what happens when specific drugs are ingested in specific regimens by specific routes of administration. This kind of basic research is at the cutting edge of methodology in the drug abuse field. However, human ingestion of drugs, as Cohen notes, is not particulary consonant with the milieu of research laboratories. There is substantial evidence that multiple drug use has been around for quite awhile, and that its incidence and prevalence has been increasing in the past 10 or 15 years.[2–5] Furthermore, it is known that some multiple drug use is indiscriminant and that it is not unusual for drugs such as marijuana to be "laced" with other drugs such as PCP.

The purposes of this chapter are: (1) to identify some of the conceptual elements that must be addressed in discussing multiple drug use; (2) to discuss some of the measurement issues and confounding variables that may make the study of multiple drug use difficult; (3) to review some of the existing epidemiological data concerning multiple drug use; (4) to discuss some of the problems inherent in untangling the causes of consequences that may be attributable to multiple drug use; and (5) to examine, albeit briefly, some of the policy implications of multiple drug use.

2. Conceptual Issues in Multiple Drug Use/Abuse

2.1. Use versus Abuse

There is at least one generic conceptual issue that emerges in any discussion of drugs—the distinction between "use" and "abuse." In recognition of the illegal status of some drugs, defining any use of these drugs as abuse is not without logical foundation. However, the drugs lumped together under the rubric of "illegal" differ from each other on many dimensions, including addictive potential and the potential health and other hazards that may result from ingestion of the substance. For these and other reasons, the binary categorization (use versus no use) is inadequate. Instead, it is necessary to conceptualize and operationalize differing levels of involvement with each drug and subsequently to represent the levels of involvement with multiple substances for each individual being studied. The difficulty here is to identify the criteria that will be used to determine what is and what is not abuse (see section on measuring the developmental nature of multiple drug use).

2.2. Sequential versus Concurrent Use/Abuse

Much of the writing to date on multiple drug use is based on cross-sectional samples and retrospective life-history interviews. Separate questions are asked for each drug class, usually with regard to lifetime extent of use defined as number of times or number of occasions and then age at onset. It is thus possible to determine the "temporal order" in which various drugs were used on a pairwise basis (alcohol and cigarettes, alcohol and marijuana, alcohol and cocaine, cigarettes and marijuana, cigarettes and cocaine, etc.) by cross-tabulating the age at onset of use of one drug with the age at onset of use of the other drugs. This provides an assessment of the sequential order of onset of use for those persons who have "ever" used various pairs of drugs (i.e., sequential use of multiple drugs). While potentially useful, analyses of sequential order of onset are usually employed to confirm the developmental nature of involvement with drugs rather than multiple drug use.

In retrospective life-history interviews the investigators are often interested in drug usage during a particular period of time (i.e., a specific year). If the respondents are asked if they used each of several drugs during that time period, it would be possible to differentiate the concurrent multiple users from those who have used only one substance. This comes closer to the nominal definition of multiple drug use: simultaneous use of various substances or use of multiple substances during the same drug-using episode or occasion. It should be noted that acceptance of this definition does not mean the definition of sequential involvement with drugs as multiple drug use is inappropriate.

2.3. Reasons for Simultaneous Multiple Drug Use

There are at least four primary reasons for simultaneous multiple drug use: (1) to enhance the effects of another drug; (2) to counteract the effects of another drug; (3) as a substitute for preferred drugs that are not available; and (4) to conform to normative ways of using drugs. While it is clear that some people engage in what has been called the "garbage head" syndrome, they are a small proportion of the overall population of drug users. The most common reason for simultaneous multiple use of drugs is to enhance effects. For example, use of other classes of depressants (narcotics, sedatives, minor tranquilizers, or volatile solvents) along with alcohol will add to or enhance the depressant action. There are some drugs that are supraadditive (e.g., the effect is greater than the sum of their doses) that are used for enhancement purposes in multiple drug use. Examples of this kind of potentiating effect are alcohol and barbiturates (only for the nontolerant person or for the chronic user of alcohol who is actively drinking), alcohol and methaqualone, and alcohol and sedatives. Multiple drug use also occurs commonly in the context of counteracting effects. For example, a person who is "wired" because of use of amphetamines may use alcohol to reduce the jittery feeling, just as the cocaine user may "speedball" with heroin to counteract or balance the effects. The third reason for simultaneous use of multiple substances is substitution. Given the vagaries of the supply of drugs, there may be times when the preferred drug is simply not available. At that point a heavy user of a drug such as heroin may substitute codeine-based cough syrup, propoxyphene (Darvon), alcohol, and marijuana—alone or in combinations to carry him over until the supply and/or the quality of heroin available increases. The fourth reason for multiple drug use is normative influences. For example, the prevalence of alcohol and marijuana is so high that it is common practice for the two drugs to be used together—combined use is "normative."

3. Measuring the Developmental Nature of Multiple Drug Use

There have been a number of studies in which attempts have been made to measure or assess multiple drug use. Some of these are from general populations while others are focused on specific subpopulations of users. The studies are grouped more on the basis of the approach taken to assessing multiple drug use than on the patterns uncovered. There are at least four different groupings of studies and some studies fit into more than one grouping.

3.1. Developmental Patterns of Onset of Use

One of the most influential attempts to describe patterns of multiple drug use is the "stages of drug use" model developed by Kandel.[6] Kandel posited that persons proceed from licit to illicit drugs and from use of less to more serious drugs. The stages of drug use involvement that she identified were: (1) no use of any drugs; (2) use of beer or wine; (3) use of cigarettes and/or hard liquor; (4) use of marijuana; and (5) use of illicit drugs other than marijuana. Although it is not made explicit by Kandel, there is an implication that the drugs from the earlier stages of development are "carried forward" into the later stages of drug involvement. Thus, a marijuana user is likely to continue his or her use of cigarettes/hard liquor and beer or wine.

Kandel and her colleagues[7] utilized unidimensional Guttman scaling techniques and assumptions to assess the fit of data to the stages of development model. These analyses allowed her to state that use of marijuana is a "necessary" condition for use of other illicit drugs such as heroin and cocaine. This interpretation has been confirmed independently in a number of other studies.[1,8,9] Recently, Donovan and Jessor[10] suggested that problem drinking is a stage that exists subsequent to marijuana use and prior to use of heroin and cocaine. Although their point is to add another sequential marker to the "unidimensional" conceptual defintion of drug use, Donovan and Jessor's claim underscores the reality of multiple drug use that is implied by the developmental stages model. Yamaguchi and Kandel conducted a follow-up interview of persons 24–25 years old who were initially interviewed 9 years earlier in a study of a representative sample of 10–11th graders in New York state. They found the following:[11]

> For men, the pattern of progression is one in which the use of alcohol precedes marijuana; alcohol and marijuana precede other illicit drugs; and alcohol, marijuana and cigarettes precede the use of prescribed psychoactive drugs. Eighty-seven percent of men (82 percent not by chance) are characterized by this pattern. For women, the pattern of progression is one in which either alcohol or cigarettes precedes marijuana; alcohol, cigarettes, and marijuana precede other illicit drugs; alcohol and either cigarettes or marijuana precede prescribed psychoactive drugs. Eighty-six percent of women (77 percent not by chance) share this pattern.

There are at least two things to note about the relatively invariant stages of drug involvement. First, the stages are invariant at this point in history. The order could change at some future point for a number of reasons, especially changes in the sociolegal aspects of drugs or new knowledge about negative effects. Second, it should be remembered that the stages-of-development model "implies" use of multiple substances, not just a sequence in which drugs at later stages are "substituted" for drugs used at prior stages. Drug users carry forward their use of substances appearing at earlier stages, often at higher or more intensive levels of frequency and quantity consumed.

3.2. Clusters of Drugs

The development in recent years of more sophisticated statistical techniques for uncovering the "latent" constructs for measured variables (i.e., frequency and extent of use of various drugs) has provided a different window or perspective on multiple drug use. Huba *et al.*[12] used data from 1634 students in the 7th through the 11th grades in Los Angeles to compare their "common factor" model with Kandel's "simplex" model. The respondents were asked the number of times they had used 13 different classes of drugs. Using maximum likelihood confirmatory factor analysis techniques, Huba and his colleagues[12] found three latent constructs:

> There are positive loadings for beer, wine, liquor, cigarette, and inhalant use on the first latent variable of alcohol use. The second latent variable of cannabis use has positive loadings for marijuana, hashish, and cigarettes, and a significant negative loading for wine. The third latent variable of hard drug use has significant positive loadings for cocaine, tranquilizers, drugstore medication, heroin, hashish, inhalants, hallucinogenics, amphetamines, and liquor.

The essential conclusions of this study were that drug use among adolescents is unidimensional even at the first-order latent factor level and that the fit of the data to the common factor model is not significantly better than the fit to the simplex model. Examination of the drugs clustered in each of the three latent variables illustrates the reality of multiple drug use only implied in discussions of sequential conceptualizations of the stages of development in drug use. However, neither the Kandel nor the Huba *et al.* approaches tell us anything about when the various drugs are/were used or whether use of one drug had anything to do with use of the other drugs. These two models merely allow the researcher to locate respondents on a crude scale of drug involvement; they do not provide a very good basis for substantive conclusions about levels of multiple drug use in society.

3.3. Typologies of Drug Users

There is a longstanding tradition in the drug abuse field to attempt to place individuals into descriptive categories or types based on (1) their use of various drugs and (2) their psychosocial characteristics.

Bachman, O'Malley, and Johnston[13,14] have developed a fairly simple index of multiple "illicit" drug use for the annual survey of high school seniors. The principal assumption underlying the index is that there is a developmental pattern to use of drugs. The index consists of five types: (1) none, (2) marijuana only, (3) few pills, (4) more pills, and (5) any heroin. Types 1, 2, and 5 are quite clear. Types 3 and 4 are defined according to no use of heroin and differences in the level of use of the following drugs: LSD, other psychedelics, cocaine, amphetamines, tranquilizers, methaqualone, barbiturates, and other narcotics. To qualify for inclusion in Type 3 (few pills), the respondent would have used one or more of the above drug classes one or two times and would never have used heroin. Persons in Type 4 would have used one or more of the above drug classes on three or more occasions and no heroin. It is clear that a substantial proportion of persons in the types beyond "marijuana only" had used marijuana as well as alcohol and cigarettes.[15] Therefore, although the labels given the types of drug use do not explicitly mention multiple drug use, the persons in the types are increasingly "multiple" moving from Type 1 to Type 5. The index of illicit drug use developed for the high school senior study is similar to one developed by Miller and her colleagues[5] for data from the 1982 National Survey on Drug Abuse. This index had three categories or types: (1) never used any illicit drug; (2) used marijuana only; (3) used cocaine, hallucinogens, or heroin. This index does not explicitly acknowledge but implies and allows for the possibility that those in Type 3 could also be using marijuana as well as cigarettes and alcohol.

The typological approach to multiple drug use is fairly common among researchers studying clients in drug treatment programs. Simpson and his colleagues[16] identified 28 different patterns of use for a set of eight drug classes (heroin, other opiates, barbiturates, cocaine, amphetamines, hallucinogens, marijuana, and other drugs) in their study of over 11,000 clients in the Drug Abuse Reporting Program (DARP). Frequency of use in the 2 months prior to treatment was recorded along the scale from daily use, weekly use, less than weekly use, to no use. The modal pattern was heroin only (28.3%). Heroin in combination with marijuana (7.8%), with cocaine (8.8%), and with both marijuana and cocaine (7.3%) constituted the other prevalent types of multiple drug use. Alcohol use was not considered in the DARP study of mutiple drug use.

Bray and his colleagues[17] used data from the 3389 clients in the Treatment Outcome Prospective Study (TOPS) to replicate the pattern of multiple drug use found in the DARP study. There were major differences. Heroin only, the modal pattern (28.3%) for the DARP study, constituted only 3.2% of the TOPS clients. TOPS had a much larger percentage in the marijuana-only type (10.3 versus 0.6%), fewer heroin–cocaine users (4.5 versus 8.8%), more heroin–cocaine–marijuana users (15.2 versus 7.3%), more polydrug users defined as heroin and other opiates less than weekly plus any use of three or more nonopiates (9.7 verus 4.9%), and fewer polydrug and opiate users defined as heroin or other opiates more than weekly plus any use of three or more nonopiates (5.5 versus 13.3%). One of the biggest differences between the TOPS and the DARP studies was the percentage of clients who did not fit into the 28 categories identified in the DARP study (1.0 versus 17.9%). One thing is clear from these two studies: the percentage of multiple drug users in the 1979 TOPS sample of drug treatment clients was considerably higher than that found in the DARP sample from the early 1970s.

Braucht *et al.*[18] studied patterns of drug use among 440 clients in four drug and alcohol treatment programs. Using responses concerning 15 drug classes and cluster analysis techniques, they were able to identify six clusters of drugs and empirically identify eight types of drug abusers. The distribution of the sample into the eight types is quite skewed. However, these investigators asked each respondent "how often they had used drugs in combinations to achieve an effect." The first type, "infrequent experimenters," constituted 55% of the total sample of 440 clients, and 42% of this group indicated they had "never" used drugs in combinations to achieve an effect. The second type was "alcoholics," 16% of the sample (65% had never used combinations to achieve an effect). The third type, "barbiturate and minor tranquilizer users," was only 4.1% of the sample. However, over 30% of these users reported "always" using combinations of drugs to achieve an effect. "Narcotics users" were only 3.8% of the sample and 30% "always" used drugs in combination. The fifth type consisted of persons who are users of "amphetamines, marijuana, and major tranquilizers." Although they constitute only 2.8% of the sample of clients, 73% reported "always" using drugs in combination, and none of the clients in this category reported "never" using drugs in combination. The sixth type (methaqualone, minor tranquilizers, and barbiturates) and the seventh type (codeine, inhalants, analgesics, and methaqualone) of users each represented less than 2% of the sample. The eighth type (hallucinogenic users) included almost 15% of the sample. This group was primarily involved with marijuana and other hallucinogenic drugs and heavily involved with using various combinations of drugs simultaneously.

The Braucht *et al.* study demonstrates that among persons who have used several drugs, a large proportion "always" use the drugs in combinations. Although they did not ask the respondents to specify the motivations for multiple use (e.g., to enhance the effects or to counteract the effects), it is likely that those who said they "always" used drugs in combination would list one or both of these reasons for simultaneous multiple drug use.

3.4. Composite Indices of Drug Use

The fourth way that researchers have attempted to deal with the "problem of multiple drug use" is to create composite indices or scales of use. This is a very tricky and formidable task. Among the issues that must be dealt with are: (1) the drugs to be included in a composite index; (2) the dimensions of use (e.g., frequency, volume, extent, quantity, and other factors); (3) the procedures to be used in creating the weights for the drugs and the categories of each dimension; and (4) the sample on which the index is to be normed.

Why create a composite index in the first place? The answer to this question is simple. Most researchers would rather conduct statistical analyses once with one score than many times with each drug class treated separately in the analyses. The disadvantage of a composite index is that it makes more difficult the linkage of specific consequences to patterns of use of specific drugs. However, the researcher can always rely on the patterns of use of each drug from which the index is constructed if specific linkages are needed. A more formidable disadvantage is the implication that index scores reflect the relative "seriousness" of use of various drug classes.

How does one assess the relative seriousness of various classes of drugs? One way is to use "expert" judges. Bucky and his colleagues[19] had a panel of judges assign a weight to the following drugs: marijuana, LSD, amphetamines, barbiturates, and heroin. Hoffman and his associates[20] had four experts rate eight drugs with respect to their "hazard for users." The drugs rated were marijuana, cigarettes, alcohol, stimulants, depressants, methamphetamines, hallucinogens, and narcotics in that order, from least to most serious. The obvious limitation of this approach is the lack of reliability. The weights assigned by the judges reflect arbitrary evaluations and different panels might produce different weights. What is needed are weights for various drug classes that are derived objectively and normed on a representative sample of the population.

Two other attempts to create composite indices of multiple drug use rely on the distributions of use in a sample. Douglass and Khavari[21] obtained information on use of 19 drugs or drug classes. For each, a score of 0 to 7 was assigned to the responses of having never used it, using none now, using it less than monthly, and so on to using it several times a day. The responses were treated as if they constituted an interval level scale of measurement. The mean and standard deviation were computed for each drug and a normal score was computed for each level of use. The difference between levels for each drug is a constant, and it is used as a weight for that drug. For each drug a person had used, the level was multiplied by the weight, and the sum of these products formed the drug use index. There are several problems with this approach. The first and most obvious is that the scores for levels of use are treated as if the intervals between them are equal. This assumption, which is central to the Douglass and Khavari index, is faulty. For example, if one were to estimate the number of times a drug had been used in a month on the basis of response categories such as about once a month, about once a week, several times a week, daily, and several times a day, the result would probably be 1, 4, 10, 30, and 75 or more. The numbers in the Douglass and Khavari index were 1 through 7. With a wider range and more realistic numbers, the means and the standard deviations would have been quite different. The weights for the drugs would have been substantially different. However, the most serious limitation of this index is that it is useful only with the sample on which it is constructed. The weights are not transferable from study to study. They must be constructed anew for each study.

Lu[22] attempted to construct a composite index of multiple drug use by assigning weights to the categories of extent of use of each drug. The weights are determined by the proportion of cases in the total sample that are found in the various categories. The weights reflect the frequency or rarity of a given level of drug use in a sample. Herein lies a major limitation of the Lu index. For example, O'Donnell and his colleagues[2] found in their nationwide sample of young men the following weights for marijuana: no use (.225); experimental use (.534); light use (.664); moderate use (.755); and heavy use (.900). There is a nice and even progression with this more frequently used drug. However, they found the following weights for heroin: no use (.471); under ten times (.955); under 100 times (.978); under 1000 times (.989); and 1000 times or more (.996). As one can see, nonuse of heroin gets almost as high a score as experimental use of marijuana. Furthermore, there is little difference in the scores between use of heroin under ten times and use of heroin 1000 times or more. The Lu indexing approach to multiple drug would therefore be useless for samples drawn from drug treatment centers or heavy-using street populations because everyone would be getting a high score. The Lu index score is obtained by adding the scores for each drug class. Pandina *et al.*[23] used the Lu index computational scheme by creating scores for each of three dimensions (extent, frequency, recency) for each of ten drugs. O'Donnell *et al.*[2] found that the correlation between the Lu index score for multiple drug use and a simple count of the number of separate drugs ever used was .971. In simple terms, this approach represents an improvement in the attempt to measure multiple drug use but fails in that attempt because of problems with the ways the weights are obtained and the fact that the scores are based entirely on the distribution of use in each sample.

Clayton and Voss[24] were responsible for developing the most comprehensive composite index of multiple drug use to date. They used data from: (1) the 1977 National Household Survey on Drug Abuse; (2) the 1977 Client Oriented Data Acquisition Process (CODAP) admission file; (3) emergency room mentions from the Drug Abuse Warning Network (DAWN); (4) drug mentions from the DAWN Medical Examiner data; (5) the Drug Enforcement Administration data on illicit prices; (6) data from the Supported Work study of ex-addicts, ex-offenders, unemployed minority youth, and AFDC mothers; and (7) data from the nationwide study of young men.[2,24] After extensive preliminary analyses, the following weights were derived: marijuana (1); psychedelics (2); opiates other than heroin (3); stimulants (5); sedatives (6); cocaine (7); and heroin (24). Using these weights for the drugs, a researcher can then develop reasonable weights for various dimensions of use such as frequency or extent and multiply for a composite index. For example, in testing this multiple drug use indexing scheme, Clayton and Voss[24] applied the drug use weights listed above to a sample of 20- to 30-year-old men (125 blacks, 98 white, and 78 men from other race/ethnic groups) drawn randomly from high drug use areas in Manhattan. The figures below indicate how the response categories were used to derive multipliers for the drug classes.

Interview response categories	Assumed mean no. of times for response	Weight
Never used	0	0
Less than 10 times	5	1
Under 100 times	40	4
Under 1000 times	200	40
1000 times or more	600	120

The range of possible scores on this index is from zero or no use of any drug to the sum of the products obtained by multiplying the drug class weight by 120. Thus, the total possible score is marijuana (120) + psychedelics (240) + opiates other than heroin (360) + stimulants (600) + sedatives (720) + cocaine (840) + heroin (2880), or 5760. The higher the score the higher multiple drug use.

The utility as well as the disadvantages of measuring multiple drug use in this manner can be seen in the data in Table I. The primary advantage is that the "dependent variable," drug use, is captured in a single, interval level score. This allows the researcher to use more robust parametric level statistical techniques such as analysis of variance. Expected relationships such as the one between educational attainment and drug use can be readily examined within categories of race/ethnicity. In addition, if one has longitudinal measures on the same sample or repeated cross-sectional data on similar samples, it is possible to use a single score to measure change. However, a limitation of this approach to assessing multiple drug use is that one cannot know readily *which* drugs go into making up the score. Further, the Clayton and Voss index is most useful with samples from the "normal" population. It is not very

Table I. Analysis of Variance: Lifetime Drug Use Index by Race and Educational Attainment for the Manhattan Young Men Sample[a]

Independent variables		N	Lifetime drug use index: Mean	Lifetime drug use index: S.D.
Total sample		294	469.90	1036.77
Black		125	737.21	1188.43
Less than high school		40	1176.80	1304.44
High school graduate		40	806.58	1325.09
Some college		34	352.03	823.32
College graduate		11	77.00	127.97
White		98	223.20	789.46
Less than high school		9	1282.44	2342.60
High school graduate		12	249.00	480.58
Some college		31	151.16	231.57
College graduate		46	57.78	139.65
Other		71	339.80	950.61
Less than high school		18	418.11	908.82
High school graduate		25	234.40	964.34
Some college		22	477.09	1102.75
College graduate		6	40.67	62.84
F for race	3.477	p .032		
F for education	7.548	p .001		
F for race–education interaction	1.593	p .149		

[a] Source: Clayton and Voss[24]

useful for samples of treatment clients where use of illicit drugs is extensive and intensive.[17]

3.5. Measurement of Multiple Drug Use: Preliminary Conclusions

Clinicians and survey researchers agree that multiple drug use is a major problem, both in terms of measurement and treatment. Ask them how to measure this phenomenon and they will throw up their hands in despair. Drugs differ in their pharmacological composition, the biochemical effects they have on the human organism, in their abuse liability, and in the way they are used and abused in this society. Drugs are often used in combinations to enhance effects, to counteract effects, to substitute for drugs that are not available, or because combined use is normative. However, the problem of how to measure and treat multiple drug use is as elusive as the Loch Ness monster.

From the foregoing discussion the following can be assumed. First, persons go through relatively invariant stages of involvement with drugs. Second, drugs begun at earlier stages are continued into subsequent stages, often with higher frequency and quantity of ingestion. Third, because of their abuse liability and possible physical and medical consequences, some drugs are considered more serious to use than others. Fourth, some drugs are often used in combination with each other for various purposes. Fifth, the long-term health and other consequences associated with use of licit drugs such as alcohol and tobacco may be substantially higher, given the extent to which they are used, than those associated with the illicit drugs. Sixth, persons who use drugs at latter stages of development usually smoke cigarettes and drink alcoholic beverages, often in conjunction with their use of illicit drugs.

At this time, emphasis on developing adequate measures of multiple drug use is relatively new. The attempts that have been made along this line are at best crude and limited. The goal of such research should be to create a composite index of multiple drug use that is comprehensive, sensitive to differences between drug classes yet sensitive as well to patterns of use within classes, objectively and empirically sound, easy to construct and use, and able to discriminate between groups known to differ on this phenomenon. The ultimate goal of epidemiology and etiologic research on multiple drug use should be the development of a diagnostic tool that would allow clinicians to assess the problem of multiple drug use and use that information to link clients to appropriate treatment.

4. The Epidemiology of Multiple Drug Use

How much multiple drug use is there? What proportion of the population at any one point in time is using/abusing multiple substances? Has use of multiple substances become more normative in the recent past as opposed to exclusive use of a favorite drug? What are the principal consequences of multiple drug use? Do these consequences differ according to pharmacological parameters for interactive potential or are there other parameters of almost equal predictive value? To what extent are the consequences attributed to single drugs (traffic accidents labeled as alcohol related) really the result of impaired judgment and performance from ingestion of multiple substances? These are just a few of the questions that need to be addressed within the scientific and public policy communities. In the following section some epidemiological data pertinent to understanding the "extent" of multiple drug use are presented.

4.1. Monitoring-the-Future Studies

Each year since 1975, researchers at the Institute for Social Research at the University of Michigan have administered questionnaires to about 17,000 high school seniors attending schools randomly chosen to be representative of all high schools in the continental United States. These seniors are asked to provide detailed information on their use of various drugs in addition to attitudes/opinions/beliefs/observations on a host of topics. There are five separate forms of the questionnaire with some core content shared by all. The study does not include persons who dropped out of school prior to their senior year or persons who are absent on the day the questionnaries are administered. It is estimated that the dropout rate in the United States may average 20–25% of a birth cohort. It is also known that drug use among dropouts is higher and more extensive than among their peers who continue in school.[25] However, in an analysis of how noncoverage of these populations would affect the prevalence and incidence rates for drug use, Clayton and Voss[26] concluded that the effect would be relatively small. A high rate of use in a small proportion of the population has only minimal effects on overall rates for most drugs. Data from the Monitoring-the-Future studies are therefore conservative estimates of the "true" scope of the problem. Stated differently, because the same measures have been used on similar populations every year, the configuration of the slope for drug use is very reliable, and only the height of the slope for each year is off because of the populations not covered.

Has multiple drug use among high school seniors increased? One way to answer this question is to examine changes in the percentage of youth who have used "only marijuana" during the past year compared to those who have used other illicit drugs. As noted earlier, use of marijuana seems to be a prerequisite for use of other illicit drugs.[27] Furthermore, Akers[28] notes that ". . . while a great many young people drink without using marijuana, drinkers are more likely than non-drinkers to smoke marijuana, and almost all marijuana users drink." Therefore, even the "marijuana-only" users (defined solely in terms of use of illicit drugs) are usually multiple drug users because of their use of alcohol. With this caveat in mind, the data in Table II show

Table II. Multiple Drug Use in Past 12 Months: Ratio of Use of Marijuana Only to Use of Other Illicit Drugs by High School Seniors

					Ratio by sex and by college plans			
					Sex		College plans	
Class of	Any use of illicit drugs (%)	Marijuana only (%)	Other illicit drugs (%)	Ratio: marijuana only divided into other illicit drugs	Male	Female	No	Yes
1976	48	23	25	1.08	96	1.26	1.32	.91
1977	51	25	26	1.04	.90	1.14	1.25	.81
1978	54	27	27	1.00	.90	1.13	1.15	.82
1979	54	26	28	1.08	1.00	1.08	1.28	.89
1980	53	23	50	1.30	1.15	1.50	1.71	1.08
1981	52	18	34	1.89	1.57	2.00	2.11	1.58
1982	51	17	34	2.00	1.60	2.50	2.24	1.61
1983	49	16	33	2.06	1.78	2.20	2.31	1.65

the "annual" prevalence rates of any use of an illicit drug, use of only marijuana, and use of other illicit drugs (the implication is that these youth have used or also use marijuana) for each high school senior class from 1976 through 1983. Simple visual inspection reveals that any use of illicit drugs increased from 48% in 1976 to 54% in 1978 and 1979 and since then has dropped to 49%. The range of increase–decrease is not large. The figures for marijuana only went from 23% in 1976 to a high of 27% in 1978. Since then, the percentage of high school seniors who used only marijuana during the preceding year has dropped steadily until it was 16% in 1983. In contrast, the column for other illicit drugs (e.g., any use of hallucinogens, cocaine, heroin, or any use not under a physician's order of other opiates, stimulants, sedatives, or tranquilizers during the preceding 12 months) reveals an increase from 25% in 1976 to 34% in 1981 and 1982. In 1983, this figure was 33%. Simply put, at least 33% of the class of 1983 could be classified as multiple illicit drug users.

Perhaps a better way to illustrate the changes in multiple drug use with this sample would be to create a score for multiple illicit drug use compared to use of only marijuana. This can be accomplished by dividing the marijuana-only percentage into the percentage reporting use of other illicit drugs, the implication being that they were also using marijuana. The resulting ratio score reflects multiple illicit drug use during that year.

The ratio of "marijuana-only" users to those who had used "other illicit drugs" during the preceding 12 months was 1.0 in 1978. As one reads down the columns of ratio values in Table II, it is clear that multiple illicit drug use has increased. For the class of 1983, the percent who reported use of "other illicit drugs" (and by implication, marijuana as well) was more than twice as large as the percent reporting "marijuana only" during the preceding year. This pattern of increase in the proportion of high school seniors who are multiple illicit drug users appears also to have occurred for both men and women and among those who plan to go on to college and those who will not go on.

Although somewhat crude, and limited to just the past 12 months, this ratio measure suggests that there has been an increase in multiple illicit drug use among high school seniors since 1978 or 1979. The slope of the increase curve seems to be rather steep and seems to have basically the same configuration for both sexes and for college bound as well as non-college-bound seniors. However, the ratio assesses multiple drug use in macrolevel terms and does not seems to address the questions of simultaneous use of multiple substances or the number of persons at risk for problems because of combined use of multiple drugs.

The Monitoring-the-Future surveys contain essentially the same questions each year. Some of these questions require the respondents who have used a drug during the preceding year to estimate the number of times their use of that drug coincided with use of other drugs so that the effects would have overlapped. The exact question is: How many of the times when you used (*drug*) during the last year did you use it along with (*drug*)—that is, so that their effects overlapped? The response alternatives are: not at all, a few of the times, some of the times, most of the times, every time. Clearly, those who claim simultaneous use "most of the time" or "every time" are multiple drug users in the most rigorous definition of the term. From a prevalence/incidence epidemiological perspective, it should be remembered that the subset of persons reporting combined use of a pair of drugs on most or all occasions during the past year are really a part of a part of the overall sample. This will be illustrated in the description of the data found in Table III taken from the classes of 1976, 1978, 1980, and 1982.

Reading across the first row of Table III, 41% of the Class of 1978 reported having used marijuana or hashish during the preceding 12 months. Another

Table III. Number of High School Seniors per 100 Who Reported Combined Use Most of the Times or Every Time They Used a Particular Drug[a]

Drug combinations	Class	Number per 100 who used marijuana/hashish in past 12 months	Percent using alcohol most of times or every time they used marijuana	Number per 100 seniors who used in combination most of times or every time
Alcohol with marijuana	1976	41	21	8.61
	1978	48	19	9.12
	1980	45	21	9.45
	1982	43	20	8.60
		Number per 100 who used cocaine in the past 12 months	Percent using marijuana most of times or every time they used cocaine	Number per 100 seniors who used in combination most of time or every time
Marijuana with cocaine	1976	6	40	2.40
	1978	9	41	3.69
	1980	11	36	3.96
	1982	12	31	3.72
		Number per 100 who used cocaine in the past 12 months	Percent using alcohol most of times or every time they used cocaine	Number per 100 seniors who used in combination most of times or every time
Alcohol with cocaine	1976	6	16	.96
	1978	9	22	1.98
	1980	11	29	3.19
	1982	12	26	3.12

[a] Monitoring-the-future studies.

way of saying this is that 41 out of 100 high school seniors in 1978 reported having used marijuana during the prior year. Twenty-one percent of that part of the class of 1978 reported using alcohol most of the times or every time they used marijuana. Therefore, 8.61 out of 100 seniors in the class of 1978 (41 × .21) used marijuana and alcohol in combination almost every time they used marijuana. A quick perusal of the other figures for the marijuana–alcohol combination reveals very little difference across the four classes—about 9 out of 100 seniors in each class reported use of alcohol on virtually all of the occasions when marijuana was used.

The interpretation given these data depends upon one's orientation and interests. Someone concerned about changes that reflect an increase might say that the number of high school seniors reporting simultaneous combined use of alcohol and marijuana most or every time they used marijuana has not changed much since 1976. Someone concerned about highway traffic safety and the magnitude of the problem of automobile accidents among youth would be very alarmed. All or almost all of the youth in this study are old enough to have a driver's license. Close to 9 out of every 100 said they used alcohol and marijuana in combination most of the times or every time they used marijuana during the past 12 months. These are therefore conservative estimates of the number of high school seniors "at risk" to have accidents resulting from impaired judgment and motor performance because of multiple drug use. It is certainly clear from these data that multiple drug use (alcohol with marijuana) may be normative for a sizable minority of the high school senior population.

The data for combined use of marijuana with cocaine and alcohol with cocaine are presented to illustrate the problem of continued use of drugs begun earlier in the developmental process, often in combination with drugs that appear at later developmental stages of drug involvement. Among those who used cocaine in the past 12 months, use of marijuana with cocaine is normative for a relatively large percentage. It is likely that those falling in the combined cocaine–marijuana or cocaine–alcohol categories of multiple drug use are a subset of those who reported combined use of alcohol with marijuana. In analyzing data from the class of 1980, Clayton and Ritter[15] found that 86% of those classified as "daily" marijuana users (used on 20 or more occasions in the past 30 days) had used illicit drugs other than marijuana (e.g., cocaine, amphetamines, tranquilizers) during the past 12 months, in addition to use of cigarettes and alcohol. Daily marijuana users are usually multiple drug users. However, there is a tendency to direct attention to specific, pharmacologically defined classes of drugs with which youth are overinvolved. This tendency sometimes leads us to infer that the correlates, causes, and consequences of drug use are attributable to the class with which persons are overinvolved, such as marijuana. If daily marijuana users are more likely than those who use marijuana less frequently to have automobile accidents, be absent from school or work, or exhibit characteristics of the amotivational syndrome, we are prone to attribute these consequences to their use of marijuana. As Clayton and Ritter[15] note: "A more plausible inference is that these behavioral characteristics may be emergent from the ingestion of multiple substances which may be interacting pharmacologically to produce the effects/consequences."

4.2. National Survey on Drug Abuse

The National Survey on Drug Abuse has been conducted seven times, the most recent being 1982. It is a study of drug use in a representative sample of the household population. In 1982 there were 5624 respondents distributed

Table IV. Extent of Use of Other Illicit Drugs within Categories of Extent of Use of Marijuana by Age Group[a,b]

	Lifetime extent of use of marijuana										
	No use		1–2 times		3–10 times		11–99 times		100+ times		
Age groups	*N*	%	*N*	%	*N*	%	*N*	%	*N*	%	Total (*N*)
Youth	1190	75	122	8	109	7	85	5	75	5	1581
Young adults	491	38	121	9	164	13	210	16	297	23	1283
Mid-adults	775	49	186	12	185	11	211	13	264	16	1621
Older adults	1009	89	55	5	31	3	18	2	26	2	1139
Stimulants											
Youth		1		6		12		26		47	6
Young adults		1		2		7		26		49	17
Mid-adults		2		4		9		19		50	13
Older adults		1		4		10		0		38	2
Cocaine											
Youth		[c]		3		9		21		59	5
Young adults		2		7		17		41		76	28
Mid-adults		1		2		15		38		69	19
Older adults		[c]		0		19		39		73	3
Tranquilizers											
Youth		1		2		5		27		43	4
Young adults		1		4		6		20		42	14
Mid-adults		1		2		3		11		36	9
Older adults		[c]		0		0		6		15	1
Analgesics											
Youth		[c]		3		5		16		29	3
Young adults		1		1		7		14		35	12
Mid-adults		1		3		4		11		29	7
Older adults		0		0		0		6		19	1

[a] National Survey on Drug Abuse, 1982.
[b] Youth, 12 to 17 years old; young adults, 18–25 years old; mid-adults, 26–34 years old; older adults, 35 and over.
[c] Less than 0.5%.

as indicated in Table IV. The data shown in Table IV reflect the increasing probability of using multiple substances as one moves from less to more extensive use of marijuana, regardless of one's age group. These data do not refer to simultaneous combined use of multiple drugs. However, the 1982 National Survey interview does contain questions about the frequency (e.g., usually, about half the time, occasionally, rarely, never) with which various pairs of drugs have been used with marijuana.

The data in Table V show the lifetime patterns of extent of use of marijuana and cocaine (1–2 times, 3–10 times, 11–99 times, 100 times or more) for those who have ever used both drugs along with the reported frequency with which the two drugs have been used together, presumably to either enhance the effects or as part of a normative pattern of use. Several things are clear from these data. First, multiple use of these two drugs is clustered primarily among those who have used marijuana 100 or more times, the highest category of use identified in the interview instrument. Second, among those who have used marijuana 100 times or more, the percentage reporting combined use with cocaine usually or about half the time goes up linearly with extent of use of cocaine. Seventy-one percent of those who have used marijuana and cocaine 100 times or more report combined use is a frequent

Table V. Frequency with Which Marijuana and Cocaine Are Used in Combination for Those Who Have Ever Used Both Drugs by Lifetime Extent of Use of Both Drugs[a]

Lifetime extent of use (times)		Usually or about half the times		Occasionally or rarely		Never		
Marijuana	Cocaine	*N*	%	*N*	%	*N*	%	Total (*N*)
1–2	1–2	2	20	0		8	80	10
1–2	3–10	1	33	2	67	0		3
1–2	11–99	0		1	50	1	50	2
1–2	100+	0		0		0		0
3–10	1–2	4	10	5	13	30	77	39
3–10	3–10	3	14	7	32	12	55	22
3–10	11–99	0		2	29	5	71	7
3–10	100+	0		0		2	100	2
11–99	1–2	29	35	14	17	41	49	84
11–99	3–10	14	21	27	40	27	40	68
11–99	11–99	9	24	18	47	11	29	38
11–99	100+	0		1	100	0		1
100+	1–2	39	41	16	17	41	43	96
100+	3–10	95	57	52	31	19	11	166
100+	11–99	99	64	48	31	8	5	155
100+	100+	37	71	9	17	6	12	52
	Totals	332	45	202	27	211	28	745

[a] National Survey of Drug Abuse, 1982.

occurrence. Third, only 28% of the persons in this nationally representative sample of households who had ever used marijuana and cocaine report having "never" used these drugs in combination. Finally, it is important to put these figures into epidemiological perspective. The 745 people who have ever used both drugs constitute 13.25% of the total sample of 5624. The 45% who report combined use usually or about half the time represent 5.96 persons per 100 in the total population (13.25 persons × .45 = 5.96). It should be noted that this is a rather conservative estimate because the denominator initially contained the entire sample of 5624, including youth as young as 12 and 13 and older adults in their fifties, sixties, and seventies. The data from this survey indicate that the preponderance of use of marijuana and cocaine occurs in the 18–34 age range. The number of persons per 100 in this shortened age range who usually or about half the time use marijuana and cocaine in combination is bound to be considerably higher.

It should be noted again that the data from the Monitoring-the-Future surveys and the National Survey on Drug Abuse come from the "normal" population. The respondents in these studies have not been filtered through the institutional or community service agencies where persons with alcohol and drug problems would be clustered. For this reason, the data presented above on multiple drug use are extremely important. They suggest first that multiple drug use may be more prevalent in the general population than previously suspected. They also suggest the need for a new terminology and classification system for drug users. If "heavy" marijuana users are highly at risk for combined use of multiple substances, then attribution of effects/consequences based on classification of them according to the substance with which they are overinvolved may be inaccurate. The problems and troubles experienced by heavy marijuana users in particular may actually reflect interactions among the drugs being ingested rather than the impact of marijuana. Stated differently, perhaps it is time for attention to be directed toward overall consumption patterns in addition to queries about use of particular drug classes.

4.3. Treatment Outcome Prospective Study (TOPS)

If multiple drug use is found so readily in the general population, the prevalence of multiple use should be substantially higher among persons in treatment for drug abuse. Evidence from the 3389 drug abuse clients in the 1979 TOPS[17] cohort confirms this expectation. The data in Table VI show the percentage of clients reporting weekly or more frequent use of various drugs by the "primary" drug with which they are having problems. For example, 1439 or 42.5% of the sample is classified with heroin as the primary problem. Among the primary heroin problem clients, the drugs and the percentage using them on a weekly or more frequent basis are: alcohol (53%); marijuana (64%); cocaine (42%); heroin (88%); illegal methadone (16%); minor tranquil-

Table VI. Weekly or Greater Use of Drugs by Primary Drug Problem: Treatment Outcome Prospective Study (TOPS)[a]

Primary drug problem	*N*	Drugs used weekly or more often (%) Alcohol	Marijuana	Inhalant	Hallucinogen	Cocaine	Heroin
Alcohol	188	89.7	63.1	1.6	7.5	5.9	2.7
Marijuana	239	64.7	94.9	0.4	8.1	10.9	4.2
Inhalants	8	50.0	75.0	62.5	12.5	12.5	0.0
Hallucinogens	54	77.8	85.2	3.7	66.7	20.4	7.4
PCP[b]	18	100	94.4	0.0	44.4	16.7	0.0
Cocaine	125	68.6	71.5	3.2	9.8	81.5	27.2
Heroin	1439	52.6	64.2	0.4	1.5	42.2	87.8
Illegal methadone	163	50.6	55.0	0.0	1.9	17.3	20.9
Other narcotics	317	50.2	52.1	1.0	1.0	11.9	29.5
Minor tranquilizers[b]	88	54.1	59.8	0.0	6.9	9.2	8.0
Librium/Valium	8	62.5	37.5	0.0	0.0	12.5	12.5
Major tranquilizers	6	66.7	83.3	0.0	0.0	16.7	0.0
Barbiturates	39	76.9	73.7	2.6	13.2	23.1	10.3
Sedatives	25	72.0	70.8	4.0	16.7	8.3	4.4
Amphetamines	125	66.4	75.2	2.4	8.8	12.9	6.4
Preludin[b]	17	23.5	76.5	0.0	0.0	17.7	35.3
Other	24	66.7	54.2	4.2	8.3	20.8	25.0
No problem	442	51.4	54.4	1.4	3.5	6.0	8.9
Missing	64	66.7	75.0	9.7	19.7	15.0	11.5
All respondents	3389	57.4	64.9	1.2	5.2	26.9	45.1

[a] Source: Bray *et al.*
[b] Data for clients mentioning a specific drug (phencyclidine-PCP, Librium/Valium, Preludin) as the primary problem are not included in the data for the more general drug types (hallucinogens, minor tranquilizers, amphetamines).

izers (21%); and amphetamines (11%). While these figures are not from questions specifically about simulatneous combined use, the percentages reflect weekly or more frequent use of all of these substances by a group of heroin addicts in treatment across the United States. Multiple drug use is certainly the norm among those most heavily involved in the use of illegal drugs.

4.4. National Drug/Alcohol Collaborative Project (NDACP)

This study was conducted from 1974 through 1978 and involved 1544 clients in alcohol and drug treatment programs around the country. Those who were "regular" users of various substances were asked if they used another substance to "boost, balance, counteract, or sustain" the effects of that drug. If the response was yes, they were asked to specifically identify which substances were used for that purpose for each drug.

Illegal methadone	Other narcotics	Minor tranquilizers	Major tranquilizers	Barbiturates	Sedatives	Amphetamines
0.0	7.0	18.3	7.0	5.9	4.3	27.3
2.1	11.1	16.7	3.4	9.4	8.9	21.0
0.0	0.0	25.0	12.5	12.5	37.5	37.5
0.0	16.7	31.5	3.7	16.7	11.1	46.3
0.0	0.0	11.8	11.1	16.7	0.0	38.9
6.6	13.6	23.2	1.6	8.9	5.7	22.7
15.6	17.6	20.9	0.8	6.4	3.5	10.6
66.3	7.0	34.2	2.5	12.6	5.1	5.1
5.1	78.0	37.5	3.8	11.2	7.6	19.9
3.5	25.6	75.3	5.8	20.0	13.8	17.7
0.0	37.5	87.5	0.0	25.0	12.5	12.5
0.0	33.3	50.0	66.7	50.0	33.3	60.0
5.1	29.0	60.5	15.4	73.7	34.2	38.5
8.0	29.2	52.2	8.0	37.5	60.0	28.0
0.8	17.7	28.0	2.4	13.8	9.6	83.2
6.3	41.2	56.3	0.0	29.4	11.8	88.2
8.7	50.0	26.1	4.2	20.8	8.3	20.8
1.2	6.7	12.3	1.2	3.5	2.1	7.7
3.3	37.7	29.5	8.2	16.4	16.4	53.2
11.2	21.2	24.7	2.6	9.4	6.1	18.4

Listed below are the drugs included in the analyses and the percentage of regular users reporting use of other substances to enhance the effects of that drug.

Alcohol	53%	Illegal methadone	72%
Heroin	71%	Cocaine	77%
Other opiates	66%	Hallucinogens	72%
Amphetamines	72%	Inhalants	36%
Barbiturates	76%	OTC drugs	54%
Minor tranquilizers	55%	Antidepressants	80%
Marijuana/hashish	76%	Major tranquilizers	57%

For alcohol and the hallucinogens, the major altering substance is marijuana. For heroin, cocaine and marijuana are the primary enhancement drugs, while heroin provides a buffering effect for cocaine among these clients. Heroin and alcohol are used to alter the effects of taking illegal methadone. For the remainder of the drugs, alcohol is the drug used most often to alter, enhance, or counteract the effects of the drug.

4.5. Preliminary Conclusions

There are at least two conclusions concerning multiple drug use that seem virtually beyond refutation. First, multiple drug use is not limited to those most heavily involved in the drug culture, although the heavier the involvement the more likely the occurrence of multiple drug use. The evidence for this conclusion is that multiple drug use seems to be part of a developmental process of drug involvement in the general population and seems to be rather prevalent in those segments of the population clearly identifiable because of their problems with drugs. Second, there is a relatively small proportion of the population that meets the most rigorous definition of multiple drug use (i.e., simultaneous use of multiple substances to either enhance or counteract the effects of the other drug). However, the simultaneous multiple drug users constitute a large enough percentage of the population to justify serious concern.

There are still a number of questions to be answered about multiple drug use from an epidemiological perspective. First, what is the extent of multiple drug use and has it increased over the past decade or so? Second, has the age at which onset of multiple drug use (i.e., particularly simultaneous use to enhance or counteract effects) increased, decreased, or remained the same? Third, what is the "normative" hiatus between using drugs separately for their individual effects and together for their multiple effects? Fourth, what are the predictors that differentiate those who become multiple users from those whose use is essentially exclusive? These are not new questions. They are the same questions that are raised whenever a "new" epidemic of drug use occurs in society. However, the questions take on added significance when there may be a multiplier effect present for consequences associated with the drugs being mixed on multiple use occasions. This last point is discussed in the next section.

5. The Consequences of Multiple Drug Use: Untangling the Causes

What are the consequences of drug use and abuse? Even a brief perusal of the literature reveals that virtually every discussion of drug consequences is limited to specific consequences for specific drugs. More often than not, these discussions reify the common sense types of causal attributions that would be made by laypersons. For example, it is often assumed that alcohol is *the* causal factor in a motor vehicle accident if the driver has a blood alcohol content score above the "minimum" level. Likewise, it is often assumed that marijuana is *the* causal factor in the lack of motivation shown by students who are "stoned" in the classroom. Our commonsense notions about the consequences of drug use and abuse often contain substantial truth. However, attribution of consequences to the drug "most likely" to be involved is different from attempting to determine the proportion of the consequence attributable to one drug and the proporion attributable to other drugs being used simultaneously. Multiple drugs may mean multiple causes of impairment or exacerbated impairment over and above the level of impairment that would result had only one drug been used. Thus, when one is trying to explain decrements in pulmonary functions, it is important to ask what proportion of the decrement is due to long-term regular use of cigarettes, to chronic marijuana use, to the smoking of free base of cocaine, to environmental hazards, and to genetic propensities.

It is not unusual in the drug and alcohol fields to devote more attention to identifying the consequences than to specifying the independent or causal variable(s). As noted above, *the* causal variable is often determined *a priori* because of the dependent variable and its assumed cause.

With what is now known about multiple drug use, perhaps far more attention should be devoted to identifying, measuring, and incorporating multiple drug use patterns into the nexus of predictor variables that are drug related. Measurement of patterns of use of individual drugs is still important. However, the point being made here is for greater emphasis on the fact of multiple use as well as on patterns of multiple use. Our understanding of the consequences of drug use and abuse will increase substantially when we begin to untangle the drug-based causes.

6. Consequences of Multiple Drug Use: Specifying the Causes

In order to illustrate these points, three specific consequences of drug use will be discussed in some detail below. These three consequences are traffic accidents, involvement in delinquent/criminal acts by youth and young adults, and emergency room visits related to drug abuse.

6.1. Traffic Accidents

The Monitoring-the-Future surveys contain several questions concerning traffic accidents. The seniors are first asked how many accidents (i.e., a collision involving property damage or personal injury—not bumps or scratches in parking lots) they had while they were driving in the past 12 months. If the answer is one or more, the senior is asked how many occurred after he/she was drinking alcoholic beverages and then how many occurred after he/she was smoking marijuana or hashish. By piecing together the information from these separate questions, it is possible to estimate the proportion that would be due to alcohol, to marijuana, and to alcohol and marijuana. The data in Table VII are for seniors in the class of 1980 classified according to the extent

Table VII. Motor Vehicle Accidents and Their Connection to Use of Alcohol, Use of Marijuana, and Use of Both Alcohol and Marijuana[a,b]

				Motor vehicle accidents							
				Not drug related		After use of alcohol		After marijuana		After alcohol and marijuana	
Marijuana (1980)	Alcohol (1980)	*N*	No accidents *N*	*N*	%	*N*	%	*N*	%	*N*	%
None	None	344	298	46	14	0		0		0	
None	<40	1015	827	182	18	6	1	0		0	
None	40+	110	75	29	26	6	5	0		0	
<40	None	18	15	2	11	0		1	6	0	
<40	<40	786	570	189	24	19	2	5	1	3	*
<40	40+	297	194	69	23	30	10	0		4	1
40+	None	1	1	0		0		0		0	
40+	<40	165	126	29	18	0		7	4	3	2
40+	40+	353	224	74	21	14	4	7	2	34	10
	Totals	3089	2330	620	20	75	2	20	1	44	1

[a] Monitoring-the-future studies.
[b] The marijuana and alcohol patterns are for the past 12 months and are categorized by none, use on less than 40 occasions during the past year, and use on 40 or more occasions during the past year. The *N*'s in this table are unweighted and come from the part of the class of 1980 that completed Questionnaire Form 2.

of alcohol and marijuana use reported during the preceding 12 months (e.g., none, use on less that 40 occasions, and use of 40 or more occasions).

Altogether, 25% or 759 of these 3089 seniors reported having at least one automobile accident during the past 12 months. Some 139 or 18% of the total sample reported the accidents occurred after use of alcohol, marijuana, or both. The largest number was the 75 who reported having an accident after they were drinking. This is only 1.7 times as many as reported an accident occurring after drinking and smoking marijuana ($n = 44$). These 44 individuals represent automobile accidents related to multiple drug use to traffic accidents among adolescents, it would seem important to differentiate or specify the substances, singular and multiple, that are causally related to the accident.

6.2. Delinquency

One of the most widely replicated findings in the drug abuse field is a correlation between involvement in drug use and involvement in delinquent or criminal acts. It is traditional to report the association on a drug-by-drug basis and to emphasize the so-called "criminogenic" potential of drugs such as heroin. However, it is quite possible, given what is known about multiple drug use among addicts,[17] that much of the criminality attributed to the use of "heroin" by addicts is actually a function of chronic heavy use of many drugs, particularly alcohol. The following statement from an intensive study of 61 heroin addicts illustrates this point.[30]

> Our findings suggest that alcohol plays an important role in the commission of crime among these heroin abusers; a role much greater than generally believed . . . These men report a physical and psychological dependence on alcohol as well as on heroin and state that this motivates them to commit crimes. . . . They [the addicts] were more likely to report being under the influence of alcohol when they committed a crime than any other drug.

From a multiple drug use perspective, the important point here is that persons who would traditionally be classified according to the "most serious" drug with which they are overinvolved are heavily involved on a daily basis with other drugs, particularly alcohol. This finding is replicated in the preliminary findings of a study of arrestees being conducted in Central Harlem.[31] Out of 455 male arrestees who provided urine for testing by EMIT (78% of those eligible), 250 or 55% tested positive within 36 hr after booking for the presence of cocaine, opiates, methadone, and/or PCP. Of the 250 who tested positive for at least one of these drugs, 42% had the metabolites of cocaine in their system. A total of 48 or 19% of those who tested positive had 2 or more drugs present. These data would seem to suggest that multiple drug use is normative among those who have made it into the deepest regions of the drug culture.

The prevalence of multiple drug use among heroin addicts is not a new finding.[32] However, most of the studies in this genre have dealt with heroin addicts. The significance of multiple drug use in relation to involvement in crime would be more apparent if the data were from youth in the "general" population.

Such data exist in the National Youth Survey, a prospective longitudinal study being conducted by Elliott and his colleagues. The sample was drawn initially in late 1976 and consisted of 2360 eligible youth aged 11–17. Of these, 73% or 1725 agreed to participate. The fifth wave of data was collected in 1980 when the respondents were 15–21 and will be used here to illustrate the relationship between multiple drug use and delinquency. The data in Table VIII contain the percent of the sample in each of four developmental "types" or "categories" of drug use. The no use and alcohol use categories do not require comment. The alcohol–marijuana use category invoves use of alcohol and use of marijauna on at least four or more occasions during the preceding year, but no use of other drugs. The multiple illicit drugs category involves use of alcohol, marijuana, and other drugs (amphetamines, barbiturates, hallucinogens, cocaine, or heroin) four or more times each in the preceding 12 months.

Even a brief perusal of the data in Table VIII reveals a linear type of relationship of drug use type to the prevalence of these types of criminality; the multiple illicit users are more likely than the alcohol–marijuana users to report crimes, and they are more likely than the alcohol or the nonusers to

Table VIII. The Prevalence of Delinquent Behavior by Types of Drug Use among Youth in 1980 (Aged 15–21): National Youth Survey[a]

Delinquent behavior	Multiple illicit[b]	Alcohol–marijuana[c]	Alcohol[d]	No drugs[e]
Felony assaults				
Percent prevalence	24	14	5	4
Percent of all offenses	47	27	17	9
Felony thefts				
Percent prevalence	27	14	4	2
Percent of all offenses	70	21	7	3
Robberies				
Percent prevalence	6	3	[f]	1
Percent of all offenses	44	16	5	36
Minor assaults				
Percent prevalence	30	23	19	17
Percent of all offenses	52	18	16	15
Minor thefts				
Percent prevalence	36	23	11	5
Percent of all offenses	49	40	9	3
Illegal services				
Percent prevalence	50	19	1	1
Percent of all offenses	94	6	[f]	[f]
Public disorder				
Percent prevalence	88	69	50	16
Percent of all offenses	56	26	16	3
Vandalism				
Percent prevalence	31	20	12	10
Percent of all offenses	30	33	21	16

[a] Source: Elliott and Huizinga[32].
[b] N = 187 (13%).
[c] N = 319 (21%).
[d] N = 504 (34%).
[e] N = 483 (32%).
[f] Less than 0.5%.

report them. The only exception is for robberies. Another clear finding is that the multiple illicit users, who constitute only 13% of this sample of persons 15–21 years old, account for a disproportionate share of all of the criminal acts reported by the sample. Given the rather crude and conservative criteria for inclusion in the multiple illicit drug user group, the direction and magnitude of these differences are in reported criminality are even more impressive. Simply put, multiple illicit drug use is a rather potent predictor of the probability of invovlement in criminality, even in a sample from the "normal population."

6.3. Emergency Room Episodes

The third area where specification of the causes might help us to better understand the importance of multiple drug use is drug-related emergency room visits. Data from emergency rooms participating in the Drug Abuse

Warning Network (DAWN) during 1982 provide support for this conclusion. The data in Table IX show that of 199,093 drug mentions in the 1982 reporting year, only 32.1% involved a single substance. In 38.4% of the emergency room episodes containing a drug mention, one other drug was involved; in 23.1%, two other drugs were mentioned; and in 6.4% of the cases, three or more drugs were involved in the episode. Stated differently, two thirds of the drug-related emergency room episodes in 1982 involved multiple drug abuse.

At least two findings are of particular importance from the multiple drug use perspective. First, the largest category of drug mentions is the "alcohol-in-combination." By definition, this category involves multiple drug use. The fact that it is the largest suggests the important role alcohol plays in the lives of Americans who seem to mix it with both licit and illicit drugs, often with serious negative consequences. Second, multiple drug use is quite often found in the mainstream of American society and may be tied, at least in terms of medical consequences, to prescription practices and the availability of over-the-counter (OTC) types of drugs. The basis for this conclusion can be seen in the rows of Table IX that deal with tranquilizers and narcotic and non-narcotic analgesics. These types of drugs used with other drugs account for a large percentage of emergency room episodes each year.

Table IX. Percent Distribution of Drug Mentions by Number of Other Drugs Used in Combination According to Drug Group[a]

Primary drugs	Number of other drugs used in the episode				Number of mentions
	None	One	Two	Three or more	
Tranquilizers	29.9	39.1	24.5	6.6	21,968
Narcotic analgesics	46.7	3019	17.1	5.3	22,503
Nonnarcotic analgesics	39.4	33.0	20.2	7.4	17,557
Nonbarbiturate sedatives	35.5	33.7	25.2	5.5	14,499
Antidepressants	39.8	32.0	21.4	6.8	8,346
Antipsychotics	45.8	29.5	20.0	4.7	8,336
Barbiturate sedatives	25.2	39.2	28.9	6.7	7,256
Amphetamines	35.3	29.6	29.6	5.5	5,081
Hallucinogens	51.4	28.0	16.8	3.6	7,163
Other drugs					
Alcohol-in-combination	.2	68.9	26.6	4.4	29,348
Cocaine	29.3	40.3	25.7	4.7	6,190
Marijuana	21.5	38.0	36.0	4.5	5,295
All other drugs	30.1	30.7	27.0	12.2	25,906
Total drug mentions	32.1	38.4	23.1	6.4	199,093

[a]DAWN emergency room data, 1982.

6.4. Preliminary Conclusions

There is an understandable tendency in the drug and alcohol fields to be substance specific. After all, our laws and the scheduling of drugs are specific. However, there is substantial and growing evidence that a large minority, perhaps a majority of drug abusers, regularly ingest multiple substances simultaneously in order to enhance the effects of the drugs they are taking, to counteract the effects of one drug with another, or to use one or more drugs as substitute for drugs not available. Simply put, multiple drug use and abuse are a reality that must be recognized and dealt with realistically by anyone and everyone involved in the drug and alcohol field. This will not be easy for researchers and clinicians who have enough difficulty dealing with the use and abuse and measurement of single substances, but we can't mold reality to fit our wishful perception of reality.

It is time for a rethinking of the way "consequences" of drug abuse have been conceptualized. The automatic attribution of certain consequences/effects to particular drugs (i.e., traffic accidents to alcohol, overdose deaths to heroin among heroin addicts) will have to be scrutinized by researchers and clinicians. The first step is to begin to untangle the causes of different types of consequences, to sort out which drugs are most often involved in which consequences. The second step is more difficult. It requires an attempt to specify the percentage of variance in the occurrence of various consequences that may be attributed to single drugs and to specific combinations of multiple drugs. Both of these steps require a substantially revised paradigm of the consequences of drug use and abuse, a paradigm that allows for and explicitly takes into consideration the impact of single as well as multiple drug use. It is not possible to untangle and specify the "causes" of consequences until a better understanding of what the consequences are is attained.

7. Policy Implications of Multiple Drug Use

Public policies that deal with the use and abuse of alcohol and drugs are very fragmented, reflecting in many ways the history of various substances as well as the role played by the substances in this society. Alcohol is a good example. Because the impact of alcohol on traffic fatalities is so painfully obvious, public interest in the control of alcohol has increased in the recent past. There have been a number of initiatives at Federal, state, and local levels concerning enforcement of minimum age drinking and dram shop liability laws and a push in some areas for raising the driving age.[33,34,35] However, very little public policy attention has been directed toward the other control strategies that might have a larger impact on alcohol consumption and its relationship to traffic accidents and fatalities (i.e., changes in laws that would eliminate tax deductions for advertising, restriction of advertising of various types of alcoholic beverages, or substantial increases in the tax placed on alcoholic beverages and thus on the price). After all, when the economics of alcohol is examined it is easy to see how thoroughly interwoven alcohol is in society. The value of alcohol in the advertising, trucking, and agricultural sectors of society is massive. If public policies concerning one substance such as alcohol are this fragmented, it should not be surprising that no public policies exist concerning multiple drug use, even though alcohol plays an integral role in most patterns of multiple drug use and abuse. Tobacco provides another good example. While few deny the impact of cigarette smoking on the morbidity and mortality statistics in this society, public policies on tobacco have perhaps as much to do with agriculture and family farms as they do with public health. In an open society, one of the negative aspects of dealing with any social problem is that it must compete with other social problems for a priority score on an already full agenda. Suffice it to say that public policies on drug use and abuse, including alcohol and tobacco, will probably never be monolithic or coherent and integrated. Because multiple drug use is so varied and difficult to conceptualize, existing public policies concerned with specific substances or with alcohol and drug abuse in general will have to serve as the mechanisms through which the problem of multiple drug use is attacked.

7.1. Policy Implication 1: Recognition of Developmental Aspects of Multiple Drug Use for Prevention Purposes

"Prevention" is a powerful and attractive word in the Federal dictionary these days. This is particularly so in the public health arena. The genesis of such an intense interest in prevention can probably be traced back to antiquity. A more proximate stimulus is the 1979 publication entitled *Promoting Health, Preventing Disease: Objectives for the Nation*. In this influential volume, specific objectives were targeted for cigarette, alcohol, and drug abuse as well as topics such as physical fitness and exercise. The recommended prevention strategies ranged from traditional educational and informational campaigns to regulatory and economic incentives/disincentives.[36]

Given what is known about the developmental nature of use of specific drugs and, as noted earlier in this chapter, of multiple drug use and abuse, the health promotion and disease prevention approach to reducing use of cigarettes, alcohol, and other drugs may be the most efficacious prevention policy. The most effective way to reduce use of illicit drugs other than marijuana is to reduce use of marijuana. The most effective way to reduce use of marijuana is to reduce the percentage of the population that uses cigarettes and alcohol. Drug use or multiple drug use is developmental. Effective early intervention will reduce the need for secondary and tertiary prevention efforts. Significant progress has been made in the past few years concerning the prevention of cigarette, alcohol, and marijuana use. However, policies based on the health promotion and disease prevention model are, developmentally speaking, still in infancy. There is room for optimism though as a result of the success of the various community-based heart disease prevention programs.[37,38]

However, there has been a tendency in the prevention field to cast a "broad net," to use generic prevention messages for children primarily at risk because of their young age and the fact that they are children. Most of these studies are located within the schools and are adjuncts to the health curriculum. These efforts must clearly be continued. Equally clear is the need to direct more prevention resources toward early detection of risk for multiple drug use and early intensive intervention for this relatively small percentage of the youth population. It could be argued, appropriately, that any attempt at early detection/identification/intervention incurs a high risk of false positives. It could also be argued that the knowledge base concerning the predictors of multiple drug use and the phenomenon itself is very sparse. However, these are facts of life in practically every social problem arena. It would be better to detect/identify/intervene with less than the best possible instruments than to wait until such are available. A failure to act has significant negative consequences that are more severe than known risk of false positives.

7.2. Policy Implication 2: Recognition of Multiple Drug Use for Treatment Purposes

The basic human need for identifying and solving social problems is nowhere clearer than in the alcohol and drug abuse fields. Ambiguity is the enemy. Complexity is the enemy. In order for public policies to be accepted, articulated, and implemented, they must be simplified and homogenized so that competing interest groups can't sabotage the entire process. This is certainly true in the treatment arena. Every data set available suggests that exclusivity is not a prevalent characteristic among substance users and abusers. There are few alcoholics, heroin addicts, heavy marijuana users, speed freaks cocaine users, or users of any other drug class whose use is limited to just one drug. We all know that the persons entering treatment programs across this country are, for the most part, multiple drug users. It simply doesn't make a great deal of sense to put persons through a 21-day detoxification program for one drug when they have been abusing a number of drugs, using them simultaneously to enhance effects, to counteract effects, or as substitutes for preferred drugs temporarily not available. The tendency in this society to pigeonhole everything into one slot and then to assign numerical values to the slots is counterproductive in the alcohol and drug treatment areas. The symptoms simply don't fit neatly into one slot. As the prevalence of multiple drug use is increasing, at the same time concerns about containing health care costs and redefining DRGs are pushing the treatment fields toward greater differentiation and more explicit classification. A major public policy issue related to multiple drug use is how to reconcile this push toward greater differentiation and specificty with the reality that treatment clients simply don't come in those sizes and shapes. This is one issue where scientists and clinicians must effectively translate the complexity of the real world into clear and persuasive language that will preserve the quality of health care for alcohol and drug abusers without diluting the commitment of government to deal with this societal problem.

In conclusion, there is no doubt that multiple drug use is a large, complex, and growing problem in all segments of American society. No sector of society is immune from the deleterious effects of simultaneous use of multiple drugs. If multiple drug use is to be dealt with effectively, more creative and realistic approaches to prevention and treatment must be devised. The costs to society of alcohol and drug abuse are large and getting larger.[39] The best place to start anything is at the beginning. The potential for multiple drug use begins with use of any drug. The best way never to begin "other drugs" is never to begin using the so-called "gateway" drugs. Multiple drug use can be stopped at the beginning.

ACKNOWLEDGMENTS. This paper was written with support from Grant DA-03584 from the National Institute on Drug Abuse and a University Research Professor award to the author from the Graduate School of the University of Kentucky.

References

1. Cohen S: The effects of combined alcohol/drug abuse on human behavior, in Gardner SE (ed): *Drug and Alcohol Abuse: Implications for Treatment.* Rockville, Maryland, National Institute on Drug Abuse, 1981, pp 5–20.
2. O'Donnell JA, Voss HL, Clayton RR, et al: *Young Men and Drugs—A Nationwide Survey.* Rockville, Maryland, National Institute on Drug Abuse, 1976.
3. Carroll JFX, Malloy TE, Kendrick FM: Multiple substance abuse: A review of the literature, in Gardner SE (ed): *National Drug/Alcohol Collaborative Project: Issues in Multiple Substance Use.* Rockville, Maryland, National Institute on Drug Abuse, 1980, pp 9–24.
4. Johnston LD, O'Malley PM, Bachman JG: *Highlights from Drugs and American High School Students 1975–1983.* Rockville, Maryland, National Institute on Drug Abuse, 1984.
5. Miller JD, Cisin IH, Gardner-Keaton H, et al: *Highlights from the National Survey on Drug Abuse: 1982.* Rockville, Maryland, National Institute on Drug Abuse, 1983.
6. Kandel DB: Stages in adolescent involvement in drug use. *Science* 190:912–914, 1975.
7. Kandel DB, Marguilies RZ, Davies M: Analytical strategies for studying transitions into developmental stages. *Soc of Educa* 51:162–176, 1978.
8. O'Donnell JA, Clayton RR: The stepping-stone hypothesis—marijuana, heroin, and causality. *Chem Depend* 4:229–241, 1982.
9. Clayton RR, Voss HL: Marijuana and cocaine: The causal nexus. Unpublished manuscript.
10. Donovan JE, Jessor R: Problem drinking and the dimension of involvement with drugs: A Guttman scalogram analysis. *Am J Public Health* 73:543–552, 1983.
11. Yamaguchi K, Kandel DB: Patterns of drug use from adolescence to young adulthood: II. Sequences of progression. *Am J Public Health* 74:668–672, 1984.
12. Huba GJ, Wingard JA, Bentler PM: A comparison of two latent variable causal models for adolescent drug use. *J Pers Soc Psychol* 40:180–193, 1981.
13. Bachman JG, O'Malley PM, Johnston LD: Developing composite measures of drug use: Comparisons among lifetime, annual and monthly reports for thirteen classes of drugs. Ann Arbor, Michigan, Institute for Social Research, Monitoring the Future Occasional Paper Series, paper 5, 1979.

14. O'Malley PM, Bachman JG, Johnston LD: Period, age, and cohort effects on substance use among American youth. *Am J Public Health* 74:682–688, 1984.
15. Clayton RR, Ritter CJ: The epidemiology of alcohol and drug abuse among adolescents. *Adv Alcohol Substance Abuse* 4:33–51, 1985.
16. Simpson DD: Patterns of multiple drug abuse, in Sells SB (ed): *The Effectiveness of Drug Abuse Treatment,* Vol 1. Cambridge, Massachusetts, Ballinger, 1974.
17. Bray RM, Schlenger WE, Craddock SG, et al: Approaches to the assessment of drug use in the Treatment Outcome Prospective Study. Research Triangle Park, North Carolina, Research Triangle Institute, 1982.
18. Braucht GN, Kirby MW, Berry GJ: Psychosocial correlates of empirical types of multiple drug abusers. *J Consult Clin Psychol* 45:1463–1475, 1978.
19. Bucky SJ, Edwards D, Thomas ED: Intensity: The description of a realistic measure of drug use. *J. Clin Psychology* 30:161–163, 1974.
20. Hoffman AM, Hudson GR, Warner RW Jr.: Alienation and drug use among college students. *J College Student Personnel* 16:277–281, 1975.
21. Douglass F, Khavari K: The drug use index: A measure of the extent of polydrug usage. *Int J Addict* 13:981–983, 1978.
22. Lu KH: The indexing and analysis of drug indulgence. *Int J Addict* 9:785–804, 1974.
23. Pandina RJ, White HR, Yorke J: Estimation of substance use involvement: Theoretical considerations and empirical findings. *Int J Addict* 16:1–24, 1981.
24. Clayton RR, Voss HL: *Young Men and Drugs in Manhattan: A Causal Analysis.* Rockville, Maryland, National Institute on Drug Abuse, 1981.
25. Kandel DB, Raveis VH, Kandel PI: Continuity in discontinuities: Adjustment in young adulthood of former school absentees. *Youth Soc* 15:325–352, 1984.
26. Clayton RR, Voss HL: *Technical Report on Drug Abuse and Dropouts.* Rockville, Maryland, National Institute on Drug Abuse, 1982.
27. Yamaguchi K, Kandel DB: Patterns of drug use from adolescence to young adulthood: III. Predictors of progression. *Am J Public Health* 74:673–681, 1984.
28. Akers R: Delinquent behavior, drugs, and alcohol: What is the relationship? *Today's Delinquent* 3:19–47, 1984.
29. Strug D, Wish E, Johnson B, et al: The role of alcohol in the crimes of heroin abusers: preliminary findings. New York, New York State Division of Substance Abuse Services, March, 1983.
30. Wish ED, Brady E, Cuadrado M, et al: Preliminary findings from the drug use as a predictor of pretrial behavior in arrestees project. New York, Narcotic and Drug Research, Inc., November 5, 1984.
31. Kaufman E: The relationship of alcoholism and alcohol abuse to the abuse of other drugs. *Am J Drug Alcohol Abuse* 9:1–17, 1982.
32. Elliott DS, Huizinga D: The relationship between delinquent behavior and ADM problems. Boulder, Colorado, Behavioral Research Institute, April, 1984.
33. Dooley D, Mosher JF: Alcohol and legal negligence. *Contemp Drug Probl* 7:145–179, 1978.
34. Moore M, Gerstein D: *Alcohol and Public Policy: Beyond the Shadow of Prohibition.* Washington, D.C., National Academy Press, 1981.
35. Clayton RR: Multiple problem youth: Defining the problem and searching for solutions. Unpublished manuscript.
36. Johnson CA, Solis J: Comprehensive community programs for drug abuse prevention: Implications of the community heart disease prevention programs for future research, in Glynn TJ, Leukefeld CG, Ludford JP (eds): *Preventing Adolescent Drug Abuse: Prevention Strategies.* Rockville, Maryland, National Institute on Drug Abuse, 1983, pp 76–114.
37. Perry CL, Jessor R: Doing the cube: Preventing drug abuse through adolescent health promotion, in Glynn TJ, Leukefeld CG, Ludford JP: *Preventing Adolescent Drug Abuse: Prevention Strategies.* Rockville, Maryland, National Institute on Drug Abuse, 1983, pp 51–75.
38. Harwood JH, Napolitano DM, Kristiansen PL, Collins JJ: *Economic Costs to Society of Alcohol and Drug Abuse and Mental Illness: 1980.* Research Triangle Park, North Carolina, Research Triangle Institute, 1984.

2

Mechanisms of Depressant Drug Action/Interaction

Eugene P. Schoener

Abstract. Whereas the effects of individual psychotropic drugs depend upon drug type, route of administration, dose, and frequency of use, as well as unique subject (patient) variables, the actions achieved by two or more psychotropics taken concurrently are complicated by their influence upon each other. Interactions may be antagonistic, additive, or synergistic and are frequently predictable, given a basic understanding of the kinetic and dynamic characteristics for each drug. This knowledge should enable rational interpretation, therapeutic intervention, and possible prevention of polydrug toxicity.

Classically, pharmacodynamic drug interaction is described in terms of common receptor activation or antagonism. This limited view is inadequate in the present context and should be broadened to encompass all of the mechanistic elements that initiate, transduce, and amplify neuronal membrane action. Thus, although psychotropic drugs may compete for a limited number of specific binding sites, as the opiates do, they may also interact through allosteric mechanisms and nonspecific modulation of the receptor environment or subsequent effector cell mechanisms. Drugs in the depressant class often act synergistically in these ways. Through consideration of nonreceptor mediated interaction, we can more fully appreciate the potentiation that occurs between seemingly unrelated substances (e.g., antihistamines and ethanol) and the ability or lack thereof to medically treat such interactions specifically.

The pharmacokinetic determinants of drug action provide many opportunities for synergy between psychotropic drugs. Each process is a fertile substrate. Absorption from the gastrointestinal tract is sensitive to drugs that alter peristaltic motility and glandular secretion. Those that inhibit motility tend to delay the rate, if not the extent, of absorption and consequently reduce peak intensity and prolong duration of the psychotropic effect. Serum albumin binding can be a vital point of interaction for drugs with high intrinsic binding affinity (e.g., 98% for methadone); displacement of a small amount of bound drug by a competing substance may increase the free drug concentration severalfold and thereby potentiate its actions(s). Psychotropic drug effects would last for days and even weeks, were it not for the body's ability to synthetically alter drug molecule configuration. This process takes place primarily in the liver where oxidative reactions are frequently catalyzed by the mixed function oxidase system. Competition between drugs for reactive sites on these and other hepatic enzymes can result in reduced metabolic rates, increased half lives, and thus prolonged effects of the acutely interacting agents. Sedatives and tranquilizers are notable examples of this type of kinetic potentiation—beyond their additive dynamic effects.

The other primary means by which drug actions are terminated is urinary excretion of the native, pharmacologically active substance. Although glomerular filtration is not subject to significant drug–drug interference, the active process of tubular secretion is subject to such interference due to competition of like substances (e.g., organic bases) for a finite number of carrier

Eugene P. Schoener • Department of Pharmacology, Wayne State University School of Medicine, Detroit, Michigan 48201.

sites. Clearly, such circumstances could lead to enhanced and enduring drug action, unless otherwise limited by metabolism. Most of the depressant psychotropics are cleared to a great extent by metabolic means.

1. Introduction

With the advent of technological progress, the pharmacopoeia of psychotropic agents available to us has grown in both number and legitimacy. Whether or not total per capita consumption of mood-altering drugs may have changed, the variety and complexity of abused substances certainly has. Polypharmacy is now the rule, rather than the exception, and recreational users are more sophisticated than ever. Western society's tacit validation of psychotropic drug use has permitted and even encouraged this trend.

To contend with the burgeoning problems emerging from recreational psychotropic polypharmacy, physicians must possess a solid understanding of the actions and interactions of these drugs. Knowledge of the basic mechanisms underlying adverse interactions provides the clinician with a rational basis for diagnosing, interpreting, treating and, at times, preventing the medical consequences of combined drug abuse. For purposes of both clarity and brevity, this review will focus on abused drugs with primary depressant actions, including ethanol, anxiolytics, and sedative hypnotics. A number of pertinent reviews have been published previously on different facets of drug interaction[1–14] and, indeed, several books have been written on the general subject.

2. General Considerations

Chemical substances are imbued with psychotropic activity for two fundamental reasons: (1) they can modify brain function through a specific effect on neuronal conduction or transmission, and (2) they have ready access to the CNS and their specific sites(s) of action. We refer to these as the pharmacodynamic and pharmacokinetic properties of the drugs, respectively. Together, they are responsible for expression of the latency, intensity, and duration, as well as the character and quality, of drug effects. Interactions may result from the dynamic and/or kinetic influence of one drug upon another and vice versa, producing greater or lesser net effects. Complex interactions of recreationally used psychotropics reportedly produce novel experiences of mind. In actuality, the interactions of multiple depressant drugs are responsible for the most pernicious and devastating of drug complications today.

2.1. Pharmacodynamic Aspects of Drug Action

Psychotropics exert their actions either specifically or nonspecifically to modulate neuronal excitability and communication. Agents that operate in a specific mode do so by combining with and activating unique macromolecular drug recognition sites in synaptic membranes. Subsequent to this selective binding, the flux and/or distribution of ions essential to electrogenic functions of excitable membranes are altered, and neurons become more or less receptive to ongoing processes of conduction and transmission. Drugs that operate nonspecifically may achieve similar ends through interaction with lipid membrane components that structurally support the ion transport machinery.

CNS excitability is generated at the molecular level by electrochemical gradients across neuronal membranes due to the semipermeable nature of these ionic barriers and an energy-dependent ionic pump that sustains large gradients of potassium, sodium, and chloride. Potassium concentration is high in the internal cytoplasmic compartment, while sodium and chloride are low. A potential difference of 70–90 mV (inside negative) is maintained under resting conditions. Stimulation provokes a selective increase in sodium conductance that subsequently causes depolarization to a critical threshold and propagation of this excitable state as an action potential down the length of the continuous neuronal membrane. The absolute value of the resting membrane potential and relative potential difference to threshold regulate excitability with some degree of finesse. A prime mediator of this control is the negatively charged chloride ion that, though normally excluded from the intracellular milieu, can elevate the resting potential—hyperpolarize the cell—upon entering and make it more difficult to achieve threshold with usual levels of stimulation. Drugs that produce primary CNS depression may therefore act directly upon the excitable cell membrane by enhancing chloride conductance. Less likely, they may also depress CNS excitability through inhibition of sodium conductance that is responsible for initiating depolarization.

Synaptic transmission is an important site of pharmacodynamic modulation by psychotropic agents. Restricted to chemically sensitive regions of interneuronal communication, the process depends upon ionic mechanisms that are different from those responsible for conduction. Here, the divalent cation calcium bears an essential role, for it is not only associated with the process of membrane depolarization, but perhaps more importantly with the exocytotic secretion of neurotransmitter substances. Transmitter release is specifically dependent upon and promoted by increased free intracellular calcium; thus drugs that reduce calcium mobility inhibit neurotransmission. The net effect of this action is determined by the fundamental character of the transmitter(s) involved, i.e., whether their postsynaptic actions are excitatory or inhibitory.

2.2. Pharmacokinetic Aspects of Drug Action

In order to express their dynamic effect(s), psychotropic agents must achieve adequate interstitial concentrations at their sites of action within the brain. Consideration of this lies in the province of pharmacokinetics—absorption, distribution, metabolism, and excretion of the drugs. These processes of transport and elimination are, in many cases, critical to the character and intensity of drug action. Thus, a given substance may produce an orgasmic rush or only a mild euphoria, depending on its rapidity of action. In addition, they may be responsible for a wide variety of positive and negative interactions. The net pharmacokinetic equation for any given drug or combination of drugs frequently reflects a complex interplay of kinetic processes.

Psychotropics are taken in myriad forms by many different routes; tablets are consumed by mouth, powders may be snorted, leaves are smoked, and solutions injected. Route largely determines latency to onset of the desired effects and, as a general rule, the *rate* of absorption is directly correlated with the intensity of the pleasurable psychotropic experience. Certain drugs can be taken by several routes. It is generally acknowledged that inhalation produces the most rapid onset and oral consumption the slowest. Intravenous injection results in a latency only slightly longer than inhalation, while insufflation (snorting), which requires absorption across the nasal mucosa, is slower.

The absorptive process may be conceived of as a translocation of drug molecules across lipid barriers (single and multiple membranes). Thus, a drug is best prepared for permeation in its uncharged, molecular state. Processes that encourage or impede dissolution and protonation may be expected to alter the rate of transit. Interestingly, a given set of circumstances will at times facilitate dissolution, but yield a hydrophilic molecule, i.e., one which crosses membranes with greater difficulty. The oral consumption of a basic compound like morphine provides a clear example of this: in the acidic environment of the stomach, this drug dissolves readily; however, it also takes on a positive charge that retards its ability to cross the gastric mucosa. When the substance is passed into the alkaline compartment of the intestine, it loses much of its charge (depending on its specific pK_a) and so becomes more amenable to absorption.

Because the intestinal mucosa is specialized for absorption, it is here that the rate and degree of drug uptake are largely determined. Access to this compartment therefore controls absorption and the rate of gastric emptying regulates the process. Drugs that affect gastrointestinal motility (e.g., vagolytics) can alter the rate of gastric emptying significantly. So too can alcohol, barbiturates, and the opiates. With their unique antiperistaltic action, the latter drugs specifically delay movement of gastric contents, including other psychoactive substances that may have been ingested. The actual *extent* of drug absorption under these circumstances may not be changed considerably, but the *rate* of absorption might be reduced significantly, thereby delaying and diminishing actual peak brain levels and intensity of action.

Once a drug is in the vascular compartment, it may have access to all well-perfused tissues. Distribution of psychotropics to the brain is not generally limited by blood flow, for it is one of the most highly perfused organs in the body. However, it is dependent on the affinity of ligand binding to the target tissue, as well as albumin and other body tissues (e.g., adipose or muscle). If a drug is bound with high affinity to plasma proteins, then a greater dose may be required to elevate the free drug concentration—that available for passage into the brain—to pharmacologically active levels. Drugs in the opiate class provide examples of this. Morphine is bound to albumin only moderately (~35%), whereas methadone binds to the same plasma proteins to a much greater extent (~85%). These differences are responsible, in part, for their differential latencies, potencies, and durations of action. One consequence of extensive, tight albumin binding would be a small volume of distribution, but this is not the case for methadone, due to its concurrently large uptake in muscle and adipose tissue.

Ease of permeation, the property so intimately dependent on lipid solubility, also promotes tissue distribution of psychotropics. Because a blood–brain barrier exists for substances of moderate to large molecular size, agents with CNS activity are generally lipophilic. Their latencies and potencies are highly correlated with this property. However, some of the volatile anesthetics and barbiturate sedatives are so lipophilic that their CNS actions are terminated rapidly by redistribution to more attractive lipid depots.

Biotransformation is an important determinant of psychotropic drug efficacy and duration of action. Rate of drug inactivation depends upon the capacity of the metabolic machinery, located predominantly in the liver. Metabolic processing may be oxidative or reductive and products are frequently prepared for facile excretion (polarized) by conjugation, e.g., with glucuronic acid. Most drugs are processed by enzymatic stores that are adequate to support first-order (proportional) kinetics; thus, the more drug present, the faster it is eliminated. However, ethanol is consumed in such large quantities that its unique catabolic system is inundated immediately, resulting in zero-order kinetic behavior. Thus, ethanol inactivation is linear with time. Under certain circumstances, the metabolic influence may be complicated by the fact that one or more drug metabolites express significant biologic activity, e.g., drugs in the benzodiazepine series. The half-life of a parent compound in this case would not accurately predict the functional duration of drug action. Many psychotropics also have the ability to accelerate their own disposition after repeated administration. This is accomplished by inducing a greater synthesis of metabolic enzymes, particularly those of the mixed-function oxidase (MFO) systems residing in the liver. The inductive effect of barbiturates is legion and thought to be responsible, in part, for tolerance and cross tolerance to the entire group of sedative-hypnotics. However, other sedatives, tranquilizers, and even ethanol, which does not depend primarily on the MFO enzymes for inactivation, induce new enzyme synthesis to some extent.

Age must be considered an important variable when dealing with drug metabolism. Although rate of hepatic biotransformation varies between individuals, it has been clearly demonstrated that catabolism is less efficacious in the very young and old. For this reason, psychotropic drug action may be quite exaggerated in the peri- or neonatal recipient who gets the drug secondhand by a placental or mammary route. Problems are further compounded by the fact that a functional blood–brain barrier, which could delay onset or reduce intensity of CNS action, does not exist in the immature fetus or neonate. The elderly frequently respond to psychotropic drugs with enhanced sensitivity, much as the very young do. This is largely attributable to their diminished hepatic capacity for protein synthesis and biotransformation of drugs. Active drug levels can remain high in these patients for long periods of time. The same result should be expected in younger adults with specific hepatic lesions, e.g., viral hepatitis or cirrhosis.

Excretory processes remove pharmacologically active as well as inactive substances from the body. In some cases, they are major determinants of the drug's duration of action, because the active material can be removed by the kidney more rapidly than it can be metabolized in the liver. Although psychoactive drugs can be excreted via expired air, bile, and sweat, the most common route is urinary. The two fundamental renal processes involved are glomerular filtration and tubular secretion. The former is simply size-limited passage of soluble drug molecules through the glomerular apparatus of the kidney. Most psychoactive substances are small enough to pass the limiting barrier unless they are bound to plasma proteins. Because a dynamic equilibrium exists between bound and free drug in the plasma, loss by filtration leads to further release of the protein-bound substance. Several common endogenous and exogenous substances also adhere to albumin binding sites and can displace albumin bound drug, e.g., thyroid hormone and aspirin, increasing its elimination by filtration and possibly its central nervous system effects.

Free drug that has escaped glomerular filtration may also be subject to removal by renal tubular secretion. This active process can transport substances into the urine against a concentration gradient. In order to qualify for the carrier-mediated, energy-dependent mechanism, drugs must be either weak acids or bases, and many psychotropics are so formulated. Because the number of carrier sites is finite, the possibility exists for competition between chemically similar agents (e.g., organic acids) and consequent potentiation of their actions on the body.

Drugs commuted to the tubular urine cannot be considered successfully excreted from the body, for they may reenter the vascular compartment via tubular reabsorption. In fact, lipophilic substances do so with alacrity by passive diffusion down their concentration gradients. More polar (charged) compounds tend to accumulate in the tubular urine, and it is possible to promote their excretion (limit reabsorption) by employing a pH-dependent ion trapping process. The hallucinogen phencyclidine provides a relevant example, for it is a basic compound with a pK_a of 5.5. A well-acidified urine drives the drug into its protonated (charged, ionized) form, and it cannot pass through the lipid membrane barrier as easily as it does when it is not charged. Other basic compounds, such as methamphetamine or meperidine, and acids, such as the barbiturates, are subject to the same manipulation.

2.3. Implications of Chronic Drug Use for Interaction

Chronic consumption of psychotropic agents, especially the depressants, frequently yields a chemically dependent condition—a physiologically compensated equilibrium state where normalcy requires regular drug administration. The degree of dependence bears a direct relationship with intensity of drug use, (i.e., frequency times dose) and is often accompanied by a similar degree of tolerance. The chronic user exists in a perpetual, precarious state of need, where drugs have become less effective due to enhanced rates of disposition and decreased tissue sensitivity. An individual who has grown tolerant to one of the depressants would appear relatively resistant to the action of others in the class. It can be anticipated, for example, that an alcoholic patient would require inordinately high doses of general anesthetic in preparation for surgery. Such cross tolerance does not extend to drugs in other classes, and so this same alcoholic patient may be normally responsive to the effects of opiates, including those of sedation and respiratory depression elicited by specific receptor activation.

3. Specific Mechanisms of Depressant Action

3.1. Ethanol

Although it is one of the oldest and most enduring psychotropic agents used, ethyl alcohol has tenaciously resisted attempts to reveal its precise mode(s) of action. Over the past decade, our understanding of its molecular mechanism(s) has been illuminated to some extent through the use of sophisticated physicochemical techniques. Because the drug has relatively low potency compared with that of other psychotropics and rather wide-ranging effects on afferent neurotransmitter systems at normally inebriating dosage, it is believed to produce behavioral depression through a nonspecific, anestheticlike effect on neural membranes. In other words, the drug renders excitable membranes incapable of sustaining the necessary electrochemical gradients and ionic means to achieve propagated neuronal conduction and transmission. Seeman and his colleagues[15] originally demonstrated that nerve-blocking concentrations in a series of alcohols and general anesthetics closely correlated with their membrane solubility and advanced the concept that membrane lipid displacement was fundamental to their depressant effects. Experiments with model membranes from erythrocytes and synaptosomes[16] showed that ethanol, like the other substances, was incorporated into the lipid phase and significantly reduced membrane density. Since ethanol itself is not highly lipid soluble, it probably locates in the more hydrophilic regions of the membrane, at surfaces and near protein constituents (e.g., receptors, ion channels).

Employing nuclear magnetic resonance technology, Goldstein and her colleagues[17] provided further direct evidence that ethanol could enter the lipid membrane and disorder normal structural relationships betwen fatty acid chains. This decrease in the order parameter of spin-labeled membranes has been interpreted as representing "fluidization," a loss of rigid structural integrity that supports necessary transport processes. Chin and Goldstein[18] have since shown that cholesterol, which invests itself in superficial membrane regions, exerts a rigidifying influence and thus something of a physiological ethanol antagonism. Indeed, Goldstein has theorized that cholesterol is implicated in the mechanism of tolerance to ethanol after chronic consumption and has recently shown that the drug does accelerate cholesterol movement among membranes.[19,20] A second rigidifying mechanism has been proposed by Littleton and his colleagues[21] to account for pharmacodynamic tolerance to ethanol. They have argued that adaptation is due to altered phospholipid composition in synaptic membranes and that the proportion of polyunsaturated to saturated fatty acids is lowered by selective turnover of fatty acid constituents. Indeed, it has been reported that turnover increases acutely with intoxication and decreases upon withdrawal.[22]

Although it is still controversial, a discussion of ethanol pharmacodynamics would be incomplete today without attention to the putative role(s) of tetrahydroisoquinolines (TIQ) and other pharmacologically active "alkaloids" that may be formed *in vivo* after ethanol consumption. The issue was first raised in 1970, when two independent reports[23,24] suggested that acetaldehyde undergoes condensation with catecholamine neurotransmitters to produce these pharmacologically novel substances. Upon isolating the TIQs (e.g., salsolinol from dopamine and acetaldehyde), Cohen and his colleagues proposed a multifaceted interaction with catecholamine transmission, including blockade of presynaptic uptake, activation of α- and β-adrenergic receptors and inhibition of both MAO and COMT enzyme activities. Indeed, some of these functions had already been well established (for review, see ref. 25). Davis and her co-workers generated support for a similar thesis but extrapolated their findings to complex TIQs that might be synthesized by the same condensation process due to secondary competition for aldehyde dehydrogenase between acetaldehyde and DOPAldehyde.[26] The products of such a reaction would closely resemble synthetic precursors of opioids, they noted, and so they went on to propose that TIQs could potentially act through opiate mechanisms. The idea was most imaginative, but immediately drew a negative reaction.[27] In subsequent years, with discovery of the endorphins, harsh criticism has given way to skepticism rooted in concerns about the inability to demonstrate *in vivo* synthesis of TIQs in the brain after normal ethanol consumption. Actually, as those on both sides of the controversy agree, this synthetic process may bear little or no responsibility for the *acute* depressant actions of alcohol. Perhaps it should not be judged in this light. It could, however, participate in some other aspect of the addictive process. Melchior and Myers[28] tested this possibility in the laboratory and discovered that direct infusion of TIQs into the rat's cerebroventricular space for 15 days did, in fact, create a sustained preference for consumption of alcohol over water in the free choice setting. Whether or not this animal model accurately reflects the human condition of alcoholism has been debated. However, the basic findings have been corroborated by another laboratory[29] and bolster the contention that alcoholism may be an acquired neurochemical disorder. Specific molecular mechanisms of action have not been delineated, but they are the subject of much current investigation.

Its chemical simplicity and small molecular size imply that ethanol enjoys a broad, relatively unfettered distribution in the body after normal oral consumption. This has been demonstrated repeatedly over the years.[30] Because of its hydroxyl substituent, the drug is infinitely soluble in the aqueous milieu, but, unlike longer-chain aliphatic alcohols, it is not highly lipophilic. Consequently, ethanol does not accumulate in adipose tissues. Its movement across membranes of the gastrointestinal tract is governed by principles of passive diffusion; i.e., larger concentration differences generate more rapid transport. Thus, absorption into the vascular compartment is largely a function of ethanol concentration, mucosal blood flow, and available surface area. Little transport actually occurs in the oral cavity, although it is possible. Systemically meaningful absorption usually begins in the stomach and continues to a greater extent in the duodenum and jejunum, declining somewhat in the colon.[31] The significance of these differential absorptive capacities lies in the fact that the rate of gastric emptying literally controls the velocity with which ethanol achieves pharmacologically effective levels in the brain. Agents that retard this process extend the latency and reduce the intensity of ethanol effects, e.g., opiates, anticholinergics, sympathomimetics, aspirin, and even high concentrations (>15%) of ethanol itself. Ethanol absorption is impeded by the presence of food in the stomach[32]; however, specific composition of the meal has been a source of controversy. Some believe that a simple mixed meal is optimal,[33] while others feel that fats more effectively inhibit gastric motility.[34] The latter thesis was discredited on the basis of experiments with exceedingly large amounts of oil, which actually accelerates gastric emptying by direct mechanical action.

Ethanol does not exhibit special partitioning in the blood. It distributes rather homogeneously among cellular and noncellular constituents, and most of that present is readily available for transport into the aqueous compartments of perfused tissues. Single pass extraction of 90% or more occurs in the cerebral bed[35]; systemic distribution in all tissues is similarly perfusion dependent. Ethanol has no particular affinity for certain tissues or organs, as receptor-specific or highly lipophilic agents do, and because of its relatively low potency psychoactivity, many diverse tissues are exposed to high, often toxic concentrations of the drug.

Much has been written about the metabolic implications of ethanol. As a result, we now have a rather clear picture of the relevant processes entailed. Lieber has recently reviewed the important work from his laboratory and others on this subject.[36] Simply put, we can expect from 90 to 98% of ethanol imbibed to be oxidized in the body, primarily in the liver. Three enzyme systems seem to participate in the process, but the most important by far is the reaction catalyzed by alcohol dehydrogenase (ADH). The other pathways employ a mixed function oxidase referred to as the microsomal ethanol-oxidizing system (MEOS) and catalase, which requires participation of peroxide. Several isozymes of ADH have been identified. Distinguished by their velocities, they are critical to the overall metabolic rate[37] and, possibly, the predilection for abusive behavior.[38]

ADH participates in a variety of oxidative reactions. However, it does not take part in the metabolism of sedative hypnotics and other depressant drugs. The MEOS pathway, employing cytochrome P450, is far more important for these. Whether the same enzymes or only shared cofactors are employed in both ethanol and sedative-hypnotic metabolism, the net result is some degree of cross-reactivity, with consequences for both acute and chronic use. Acutely, a competition occurs that is responsible for prolonging the half-life of the active compounds and, chronically, dispositional cross-tolerance develops, i.e., the alcoholic subject oxidizes barbiturates more rapidly than a nonalcoholic one. Enzymes of the MEOS system proliferate in response to the continuous presence of ethanol.

Further pharmacokinetic significance derives from the dual involvement of ADH and MEOS in biotransformation of ethanol. Because the more sensitive ADH is relatively slow (K_M approximately 2 mM) and in limited supply, we generally characterize metabolism of ethanol at or above blood levels of 15 mg/100 ml, as a zero-order process with a fixed rate of 150 mg/kg/h.[39] However, it is entirely possible, as demonstrated in laboratory experiments, that the less sensitive, but faster (K_M approximately 10 mM) MEOS pathway is enjoined as blood alcohol level rises. This would produce a turn toward first-order kinetics and *partial* dependency of rate on blood ethanol level.

Native ethanol can leave the body unchanged, but only a very small portion of that consumed actually does. Once again, this is a consequence of the molecule's small size and electrical neutrality. Although easily filtered by the glomerular apparatus of the kidney, ethanol is reabsorbed from the renal tubules to recirculate in the body. Special transport mechanisms are not required, and other substances in the urine do not directly promote or compete with its permeation.

3.2. Anxiolytics

For many years, clinicians prescribed barbiturates and propanediols (meprobamate) for relief of anxiety with limited enthusiasm, for although these agents could produce sedation they seemed to lack the necessary specificity of action. True anxiolytic drugs made their appearance in the late 1950s, with the serendipitous discovery of the first benzodiazepine, chlordiazepoxide.[40] Three years after its clinical debut, a more potent analog, diazepam, was introduced. Together, they rose to heights of unbridled success and gave birth to a family of drugs whose pharmacokinetic differences have enabled their use in a variety of clinical situations. It was appreciated early on that, although the benzodiazepines exhibited a significant degree of specificity for anxiolysis, they were also rather effective anticonvulsants, sedatives, and muscle relaxants. Their wide spectrum of action, as well as apparent safety (low toxicity relative to anxiolytic dose), promoted their clinical usage to such an extent that they became the largest selling class of drugs in the western world. The social implications of this phenomenon are intriguing, but beyond the scope of this chapter. With such wide clinical exposure, a great deal has been learned about benzodiazepines that perhaps was not evident at the outset. For example, although the sedative-hypnotic property is usually manifested at doses greater than those needed for anxiolysis, it occurs quite frequently in many patients on chronic regimens. It has also been found that both psychological and physical dependence of the depressant type (akin to alcohol and barbiturates) may occur with chronic *moderate* use.

As is so often the case, empiricism led to the discovery and use of anxiolytics, and it has taken nearly two decades of concerted research effort to identify the likely mechanisms of action for these drugs. Direct membrane interactions like those of ethanol have been ruled out, based on the high potency of benzodiazepines and the fact that electrical properties of excitable membranes are not altered by clinically relevant drug concentrations. First attempts to describe the mechanisms focused on a number of diverse neurotransmitter systems, including the monoamines norepinephrine, dopamine and serotonin, whose turnovers and reuptake processes were found to be diminished by benzodiazepines.[41,42] A reported inhibition of cyclic AMP phosphodiesterase[43] suggested the possibility of an adenylate cyclase mechanism. Glycine receptor activation was explored in other early work.[44] All of these possibilities suffered the weight of limited specificity and/or reproducibility. The high doses required to elicit these actions implied secondary rather than primary relationships. Ultimately, the inhibitory synaptic process mediated by γ-amino butyric acid (GABA) clearly emerged as the preeminent locus of action.[45,46] We now know that benzodiazepines do not bind to or directly interact with GABA receptors, yet they operate by facilitating their performance through a primary and specific receptor interaction, which accounts for the relatively high potency of the class. Discrete benzodiazepine receptors were first identified and characterized in 1977,[47,48] and, although they were initially thought to be a single, homogeneous group, there is now reason to believe that at least two types exist.[49,50] These binding sites generally meet the criteria by which receptors are measured[51]; i.e., they exhibit binding affinity in the nanomolar range (consistent with the fact that an intravenous dose of diazepam at 30–50 μg/kg provides effective clinical anxiolysis); they are saturated at high dosage; their affinity for drugs is highly specific as demonstrated through competitive displacement by other anxiolytic or anxiogenic compounds; their affinity is stereoselective for the (+) enantiomer of specific drugs; they are distributed heterogeneously throughout the brain and spinal cord; and they are highly concentrated in the synaptic regions where neurotransmission occurs. Functional implications of benzodiazepine receptor multiplicity are, as yet, undetermined. However, the relationship of certain high-affinity benzodiazepine receptors with GABA receptors is well established. GABA receptors themselves are not unimodal in character,[52] and it appears that distributions of benzodiazepine and GABA receptors in the central nervous system are only partially concordant. Thus, both transmitter systems may perform a variety of functions together and individually. Both pre- and postsynaptic inhibition produced by benzodiazepines, however, seem to be mediated by the joint receptor complex.

As earlier noted, primary mechanisms of synaptic inhibition involve control of chloride ion flux. It is not surprising, therefore, to discover that GABA receptors associated with benzodiazepine recognition sites are also intimately linked with chloride channels in the excitable membrane.[53] Activation of these GABA receptors opens the channels to permit increased chloride flux. In most cases, the postsynaptic cell membrane responds with an electrogenic influx of the negatively charged ion, causing hyperpolarization and functional inhibition. Electrophysiologic experiments have shown that benzodiazepines amplify GABA action, specifically, by increasing the frequency of chloride channel opening.[54]

Like the transmitter receptor elements in this macromolecular complex, the ionophore is a unique protein whose operation may be influenced directly or indirectly (via GABA activation). Studies have revealed the existence of drug recognition sites directly on the ionophore.[55] The convulsive agent picrotoxin binds to these receptors and apparently promotes closure of the anion channel.

An interesting feature of this complex structure is the high degree of integration that seems to exist between its constituents. In fact, it has been demonstrated that benzodiazepines enhance the affinity of GABA for its receptors,[56,57] while GABA agonists do the same for benzodiazepines.[58,59] The picrotoxin binding site on the chloride ionophore may bear similar interrelationships with these other two.[60] It has been argued that the integrative nature of this supramolecular complex requires the participation of another element, a coupling protein that Costa and his colleagues have termed GABA-modulin.[61] Although experimental support for this is credible, the concept of a separate coupling element is not yet generally accepted.

Given the conclusive evidence that benzodiazepine receptors exist and function in tandum with the chloride channel-modulating GABA transmitter system, pharmacologists have turned their attention to the problem of isolating and characterizing the natural, endogenous ligand(s) that certainly must exist. A number have been suggested, including inosine, hypoxanthine, and nicotinamide, based on their ability to mimic benzodiazepine effects, specific binding characteristics, and displacement of benzodiazepines.[62–64] However, it appears that these and most of the others are either too weak or lack sufficient specificity to be considered seriously. Costa and his colleagues[65] have recently obtained and purified a putative endogenous effector from brain tissue in the form of a basic protein (104 amino acids; 11,000 daltons molecular weight). While its binding affinity is only in the micromolar range, the material does have biologic activity. It is possible that a more potent (and specific) peptide resides within this ligand they have called diazepam binding inhibitor. Indeed, his group[66] has just reported isolation of a peptide (18 amino acids) from the parent chain that retains its biologic activity. Work continues on this and other possible candidates for the natural benzodiazepine receptor ligand(s).

Research in the pharmaceutical laboratory has generated a multitude of benzodiazepine and similar compounds. Some of these simply mimic the familiar anxiolytic effects of the prototypes. However, others have been characterized as antagonists (i.e., able to bind without initiating biologic activity) or "inverse agonists."[67–71] The latter produce anxiety and convulsions in a dose-related manner and seem to operate through the very same benzodiazepine receptor sites of action. The antagonists and "inverse agonists" are all experimental, synthetic compounds at the present time, but it is entirely possible that some endogenous benzodiazepine receptor ligands possess anxiogenic rather than anxiolytic actions. Apparently, this is the case for the peptide derivative recently isolated from DBI.[66] Bidirectional receptor efficacy is unique in pharmacology, and the potential that exists for multiple pharmacodynamic action and interaction with benzodiazepines has yet to be fully appreciated.

A minority opinion on the mechanism of anxiolytic drug action holds that these agents cause depression through inhibition of adenosine reuptake.[72] This purine is reportedly endowed with neuronal depressant properties,[73,74] and benzodiazepine–adenosine synergy has been demonstrated in the laboratory.[75] Indeed, the adenosine receptor antagonist caffeine is known to inhibit various neural/behavioral effects of benzodiazepines, although no specific receptor interaction has been postulated for the endpoint of anxiety. In general, the drug concentrations required to demonstrate putative purinergic phenomena are higher than those found to facilitate the GABA-mediated inhibitory mechanism. Yet it is conceivable that enhanced adenosine action contributes to the CNS depression (hypnosis) induced by larger doses of benzodiazepines.

The specific anxiolytic agents in use today operate via common pharmacodynamic mechanisms of action. Therefore, functional differences (latency, duration of action, etc.) between the drugs relate largely to pharmacokinetic factors.[76–78] When taken orally for their sedative or hypnotic effects, some are distinguished by more rapid rates of absorption than others. The highly lipid soluble diazepam moves quickly across the gut, achieving peak plasma levels within 30–90 min, while oxazepam may require 4 hr and prazepam as much as 6 hr to reach peak levels. Lipid solubility is primarily responsible for the rate of permeation, although pharmaceutical properties (e.g., tablet dissolution rate) may determine the amount of drug available for transport. As weak bases, the benzodiazepines tend to remain impassive in the gastric environment but readily cross the intestinal mucosa. One drug in common use, clorazepate, is both inactive and relatively impermeable in its native form, but the acidic environment of the stomach enables its hydrolytic conversion to the highly permeant and pharmacologically active configuration of nordiazepam.

Most benzodiazepines are extensively bound to plasma proteins (albumin) generally on the order of 86–89%. Flurazepam and diazepam are exceptions to this rule in that the former is very poorly bound and the latter is almost entirely (98–99%) bound. A strong correlation seems to exist between drug lipophilicity and extent of plasma protein binding, and this is certainly true for diazepam. Drugs like this are prime candidates for competitive interaction, because a relatively small displacement can increase the free drug concentration two- and even threefold. Brain uptake is rapid for most of the benzodiazepines, but the more lipophilic ones are subject to redistribution; i.e., they leave the brain's gray matter for the white and other fatty tissues throughout the body. The elimination pattern for such drugs is clearly multiphasic as a result of the delayed release from these depots.

Biotransformation of the benzodiazepines represents a complex and somewhat unique circumstance, for many of the metabolites retain pharmacologic activity. Some even exhibit greater potency than their parent compounds. In a number of cases, second- and third-generation metabolites are also active. Obviously, limited pharmacokinetic consideration of the blood levels for a given agent may bear little relevance to its actual pharmacodynamic performance. The picture is further complicated when the drug is repeatedly administered, resulting in accumulation of multiple active compounds that have their own pharmacokinetic and dynamic profiles.

Although some presystemic metabolism of benzodiazepines may occur, hepatic mechanisms bear prime responsibility for their biotransformation. Typically, the drugs undergo three reactions: (1) dealkylation of substituents on the diazepine nucleus, (2) hydroxylation on the same ring, and (3) conjugation at the hydroxyl substituent. Some nitro-substituted compounds (e.g., nitrazepam) undergo reduction to amino metabolites. Only the conjugation reaction (which usually employs glucuronic acid) produces truly inactive products. However, we find that under certain conditions even this appears to be a reversible process. For example, conjugated benzodiazepines that are excreted in the bile are subject to intestinal cleavage and subsequent reabsorption.[79] This enterohepatic recirculation may well explain the observation of a "resurgence" in diazepam blood levels 6 hr after administration.[80]

Dealkylation seems to be preferential to hydroxylation, and so it occurs first. Compounds with large substituents are processed faster than those with small ones; e.g., flurazepam (triethylamine sidechain) has a half-life of 2.3 hr, while diazepam (methyl group) has a 20- to 30-hr half-life. Because hydroxylation is a slower reaction, active dealkylated metabolites have longer half-lives than the parent compounds, indeed, nordiazepam (or desmethyldiazepam) exhibits a half-life of 40–100 hr. The conjugation process is typically much faster than either of the others. For oxazepam (the hydroxylated product of nordiazepam), the half-life is approximately 6–12 hr. This hierarchy is not absolute. Consequently, a variety of products, each with its own kinetic properties, is possible.

The clinical significance of this metabolic array resides in the potential for excessive accumulation of several active compounds and detrimental interaction with other depressants. Clearly, the safest drugs in the group are those which are already hydroxylated and thus amenable to conjugation (e.g., oxazepam and lorazepam.)

3.3. Sedative-Hypnotic Drugs

Clinical discussions frequently suggest that sedative and hypnotic drugs act in much the same manner as anxiolytic agents. They are simply more potent, according to this rubric. Indeed, the superficial appearance of barbiturate action lends credence to such thinking. However, subtle differences between CNS depression induced by barbiturates and benzodiazepines belies their commonality. Although they share functions (e.g., anxiolysis, antiseizure, sedation, and hypnosis), their spectral overlap is incomplete and their specificities for various endpoints are distinctly different. Pharmacodynamic mechanisms seem to account for both similarities and differences. It now appears that sedative-hypnotic drugs produce their inhibition, in part, through modulation of GABA-mediated chloride flux, much as the anxiolytics do. The specific means by which barbiturates influence this process differ from those employed by benzodiazepines. Barbiturates themselves do not bind to, or directly activate, benzodiazepine receptors. Discrete, specific binding sites for barbiturates appear to exist either alone or in a contiguous relationship with receptors for both GABA and benzodiazepines.[81,82] Indeed, barbiturates are capable of selectively and competitively displacing the convulsant drug picrotoxin from its receptors, which are located on, or in close proximity to, chloride ion channels. Consistent with these observations, we attribute much of the pro and anticonvulsant character of these drugs to their respective inhibition and facilitation of chloride flux across the excitable membrane. Neurophysiological studies have provided some corroboration for the notion that barbiturates depress the CNS by enhancing indigenous inhibitory mechanisms.[83–88] They appear to accomplish this by prolonging the time during which chloride channels remain open,[54] thus allowing for greater influx of the negatively charged ion and hyperpolarization of the excitable membrane. Unlike the anxiolytics, these true sedative-hypnotics are capable of producing neuronal depression through a number of other mechanisms.[89] For example, they can enter the lipid membrane and fluidize it much like ethanol[90]; they can restrict calcium flux and binding required for synaptic transmission as well as sodium and potassium conductance[91–93]; and they can inhibit the release of excitatory transmitters.[94,95] In some cases, higher concentrations have been employed to elicit these additional actions.

Receptors for barbiturates that colocate with the GABA–benzodiazepine complex enjoy some interplay with these other binding sites, presumably through steric or other conformational influence. Recent studies have shown that both GABA and benzodiazepines bind to their receptors with greater affinity in the presence of barbiturates.[96–99] Consequently, the sedative-hypnotics can indirectly reinforce their primary action and, when administered together with benzodiazepines, may result in synergistic depression.

The class of sedative-hypnotics and their prototypes, the barbiturates, present a picture of considerable pharmacokinetic diversity.[100] Some of these drugs are capable of inducing sleep within seconds of administration, while others require hours. Durations of action are similarly variable. These phenomena are directly attributable to the extent of lipid solubility for the different compounds. Liability for their abuse seems to bear a relationship with kinetic properties; agents that exhibit the most rapid and briefest effects, as well as those at the other end of the spectrum with the slowest and most enduring effects, are not favored. Nonbarbiturate sedatives (e.g., glutethimide, methaqualone) that manifest midrange kinetic behavior have been introduced at various times with the expressed promise of lower abuse liability. None has yet fulfilled this promise.

Drugs of this class are usually taken orally for their sedative, hypnotic, or euphorigenic effects, although other routes may be employed for specific therapeutic purposes (e.g., intravenous infusion for seizure or anesthesia). As weak acids, the barbiturates enjoy an excellent opportunity for gastric absorption. However, the rate-limiting process here seems to be chemical dissolution and so most absorption actually occurs in the small intestine. Presence of food in the stomach retards drug dissolution and dispersal, thereby slowing the rate (though not extent) of absorption. Glutethimide is absorbed more erratically from the gut than the barbiturates, although it is highly lipophilic.[101] Methaqualone, which is even more lipid soluble, is so permeant that its absorption is virtually complete within 2 hr.[102] In this regard, it resembles the thiobarbiturates, which have one sulfur substituent in place of an oxygen in their molecular structure (e.g. thiopental, thiamylal), making them far more lipid soluble than their oxybarbiturate analogs. For such drugs, it is important to realize that functional impact correlates poorly with kinetic behavior; i.e., half life does not predict duration of action. They undergo a multiphasic, multicompartmental distribution—at first determined by the extent of tissue perfusion, but later dependent upon the avidity with which they partition in fatty tissues. These same drugs show significant plasma protein binding (on the order of 60–70%), but the dynamics of equilibration seem to favor their removal from, rather than reentry to, CNS gray matter. Distribution of the more hydrophilic agents (e.g., barbital, phenobarbital) is largely flow dependent and so their kinetic properties relate more accurately to drug-induced depression. Because of their longer half-lives, these compounds are usually employed at subhypnotic dosage to inhibit focal irritability in the CNS, but they can certainly potentiate the activity of other depressants taken concomitantly.

The fate of barbiturates in the body and, indeed, that of most hypnosedatives, is determined by hepatic biotransformation. Only the hydrophilic members of this class are excreted unchanged in the urine to any significant extent, because they are polar in their native state and less extensively bound to plasma proteins (25–50%). Unlike the anxiolytic benzodiazepines, most of the hypnosedative metabolites are pharmacologically inactive. The process of N-dealkylation, however, can result in active products with certain drugs (e.g., mephobarbital, which produces phenobarbital by this route).[103] Oxidation is probably the most common metabolic transformation (via mixed function oxidase enzymes), but various other reactions are possible. Following biotransformation, the metabolites generally undergo conjugation (glucuronide) prior to renal excretion. Half lives of the sedative-hypnotics range from about 3 hr for the thiobarbiturates (e.g., hexobarbital) to 48 hr or more (e.g., phenobarbital). Most fall within the 18- to 32-hr range and so it can be expected that repeated use will produce cumulative sedation, characterized by hangover and zombielike dysfunction.

Chronic administration of sedative hypnotics and particularly the oxybarbiturates that utilize the hepatic MFO (P450) enzyme systems most heavily, has profound implications for their action and interaction with other drugs. Pharmacokinetic as well as dynamic tolerance obtain with continuous use. The latter presumably occurs via membrane and/or receptor-specific compensatory mechanisms, the details of which remain veiled for the present. Kinetic tolerance, on the other hand, is characterized by the abbreviation of plasma half life due to accelerated hepatic metabolism.[100] These changes are accompanied by and dependent upon enhanced protein synthesis in the liver; i.e., metabolic enzymes proliferate when challenged with excess barbiturate. Because these enzymes have wide applicability, the ramifications of this induced synthesis may be extensive. Biotransformation of other depressants, as well as many unrelated drugs (e.g., phenytoin, tricyclic antidepressants, anticogulants, steroids, and certain antibiotics), is accelerated, resulting in reduced blood levels and thus efficacy of these compounds. This consideration must be tempered, however, by the knowledge that acute, concurrent administration of two drugs with similar dispositional patterns will competitively inhibit each other's transformation, even with the expanded hepatic capacity.

4. Comment

For the sake of clarity and comprehension, the interaction of depressant drugs is often portrayed in a static context. Thus, we state glibly that any two of these that operate via distinct dynamic or kinetic processes will produce additive or synergistic depression. Carefully controlled laboratory studies have established this behavior as fact.[11,12] However, real world experience demands that time and drug use history be considered as essential variables in the equation. When these are factored into consideration, we are faced with a situation of virtually infinite complexity because of the ever-changing blood–brain levels of free drug and the functional tolerance and dependence that are engendered to varying degrees over time. Seldom are two drugs of the same half-life, latency, and duration of action administered by the same route simultaneously, as in a laboratory experiment. Thus, at any given point in time, drugs of diverse nature may show blood levels (and effects) that are waxing, waning, or at their zenith and that, for reasons of repeated use, have provoked systemic changes in drug efficacy. Indeed, the complexity is further magnified by consideration of the dependent system itself under drug-free conditions, i.e., the presence and intensity of an abstinence syndrome.

Sophisticated multivariate analysis of depressant drug interactions is truly in its infancy. The nature of the problem is understood,[5] but explicit and definitive research is lacking. Thus, for purposes of clinical direction, we must presently rely upon our understanding of general drug action/interaction concepts.

References

1. Anonymous: *Drug Interactions: General Mechanisms,* in *Evaluations of Drug Interactions.* Washington, American Phamaceutical Association, 1976.
2. Kock-Weser J, Greenblatt DJ: Drug interactions in clinical perspective. *Eur J Clin Pharmacol* 11:405–408, 1977.
3. Ariens EJ, Simonis AM: Pharmacodynamic aspects of drug interactions. *Naunyn-Schmiedebergs Arch Pharmacol* 297:37–41, 1977.
4. Sellers EM, Holloway MR: Drug kinetics and alcohol ingestion. *Clin Pharmacokin* 3:440–452, 1978.
5. Sellers EM: Mechanisms of alcohol interactions with drugs, in Avogaro P, Sirotori CR, Tremoli E: *Metabolic Effects of Alcohol.* Amsterdam, Elsevier, 1979, pp 113–118.
6. Prescott LF: Clinically important drug interactions, in Avery GS (ed): *Drug Treatment, Principles and Practice of Clinical Pharmacology and Therapeutics,* ed 2. Sydney, ADIS, 1980, pp 236–262.
7. Mezey E: Actions and interactions of ethanol with drugs on intermediary metabolism. *Pharmacol Ther* 14:411–430, 1981.
8. Hoyumpa AM, Schenker S: Major drug interactions: Effect of liver disease, alcohol and malnutrition. *Annu Rev Med* 33:113–149, 1982.
9. Sellers EM, Busto U: Benzodiazepines and ethanol: Assessment of the effects and consequences of psychotropic drug interactions. *J Clin Psychopharmacol* 2:249–262, 1982.
10. Lieber CS: Interaction of ethanol and drug metabolism, in Lieber CS (ed): *Medical Disorders of Alcoholism.* Philadelphia, Saunders, 1982, pp 237–258.
11. D'Arey PF, McElnay JC: Drug interactions involving the displacement of drugs from plasma protein and tissue binding sites. *Pharmacol Ther* 17:214–220, 1982.
12. Schou JS: Drug interactions at pharmacologically active receptor sites. *Pharmacol Ther* 17:199–210, 1982.
13. Pippenger CE: An overview of antiepileptic drug interactions. *Epilepsia* 23:581–586, 1982.
14. Deitrich RA, Petersen DR: Interaction of ethanol with other drugs, in Tabakoff B, Sutker

P, Randall CL: *Medical and Social Aspects of Alcohol Abuse*. New York, Plenum Press, 1983, p 247–272.
15. Seeman P: The membrane actions of anesthetics and tranquilizers. *Pharmacol Rev* 24:583–655, 1972.
16. Roth S, Seeman P: The membrane concentrations of neutral and positive anesthetics fit the Meyer-Overton rule of anesthesia: Negative narcotics do not. *Biochem Biophys Acta* 255:207–219, 1972.
17. Chin JH, Goldstein DB: Effects of low concentrations of ethanol on the fluidity of spin-labeled erythrocyte and brain membranes. *Mol Pharmacol* 13:435–441, 1977.
18. Chin JH, Goldstein DB: Membrane-disordering action of ethanol: Variation with membrane cholesterol content and depth of the spin label probe. *Mol Pharmacol* 19:425–431, 1981.
19. Chin JH, Parsons LM, Goldstein DB: Increased cholesterol content of Erythrocyte and brain membranes in ethanol tolerant mice. *Biochem Biophys Acta* 513:358–363, 1978.
20. Daniels CK, Goldstein DB: Movement of free cholesterol from lipoproteins or lipid vesicles into erythrocytes. Acceleration by ethanol in vitro. *Mol Pharmacol* 21:694–700, 1982.
21. Littleton JM, John GR, Grieve SJ: Alterations in phospholipid composition in ethanol tolerance and dependence. *Alcoholism: Clin Exp Res* 3:50–56, 1979.
22. Lee NM, Friedman HJ, Loh HH: Effect of acute and chronic ethanol treatment on rat brain phospholipid. *Biochem Pharmacol* 29:2815–2818, 1980.
23. Davis VE, Walsh MJ: Alcohol, amines and alkaloids: A possible biochemial basis for alcohol addiction. *Science* 167:1005–1007, 1970.
24. Cohen G, Collins M: Alkaloids from catecholamines in adrenal tissue. Possible role in alcoholism. *Science* 167:1749–51, 1970.
25. Hirst M, Hamilton MG, Marshall AM: Pharmacology of isoquinoline alkaloids and ethanol interactions, in Blum K (ed): *Alcohol and Opiates: Neurochemical and Behavioral Mechanisms*. New York, Academic Press, 1977, pp 167–187.
26. Davis VE, Walsh MJ, Yamanaka Y: Augmentation of alkaloid formation from dopamine by alcohol and acetaldehyde in vitro. *J Pharmacol Exp Ther* 174:401–412, 1970.
27. Seevers MH: Morphine and ethanol physical dependence: A critique of a hypothesis. *Science* 170:1113–1114, 1970.
28. Melchior CL, Myers RD: Preference for alcohol evoked by tetrahydropapaveroline (THP) chronically infused in the cerebral ventricle of the rat. *Pharmacol Biochem Behav* 7:19–35, 1977.
29. Duncan C, Dietrich RA: A critical evaluation of tetrahydroisoquinoline induced ethanol preference in rats. *Pharmacol Biochem Behav* 13:265–281, 1980.
30. Kalant H: Absorption, diffusion, distribution and elimination of ethanol, in Kissin B, Begleiter H (eds): *The Biology of Alcoholism*. Plenum Press, New York, 1971, vol 1, pp 1–62.
31. Elbel H, Schleyer F: *Blutalkalkohol. Die Wissenschaflichen Grundlugen der Beurteilung von Blutalkoholbefinden bei Strassen verkehrsdelikten*, ed 2. Stuhtgart, George Thieme, 1956.
32. Tuovinen PI: Uber den Alkoholgehalt des Blutes unter verscheidenen Bedingungen. *Skand. Arch. Physiol.* 60:1–134, 1930.
33. Rauschke J: Uber die Blutalkoholkurve in Stadium der Resorption. *Deut Z Ges Gericht Med* 41:474–479, 1952.
34. Berggren SM, Goldberg L: The absorption of ethyl alcohol from the gastrointestinal tract as a diffusion process. *Acta Physiol Scand* 1:246–270, 1940.
35. Crone C: The permeability of brain capillaries to non-electrolytes. *Acta Physiol Scand* 64:407–417, 1965.
36. Lieber CS: Metabolism of ethanol, in Lieber CS: *Medical Disorders of Alcoholism*. Philadelphia, Saunders, 1981, pp 1–42.
37. Crow KE, Cornell NW, Veech RL: The rate of ethanol metabolism in isolated rat hepatocytes. *Alcoholism: Clin Exp Res* 1:43–47, 1977.
38. Schuckit MA, Haglund RMJ: An overview of the etiological theories on alcoholism, in Estes NJ, Heinemann ME (eds): *Alcoholism: Development, consequences and interventions*. St. Louis, CV Mosby, 1977.

39. Coldwell BB, Smith HW: Alcohol levels in body fluids after ingestion of distilled spirits. *Can J Biochem* 37:43–52, 1959.
40. Sternbach LH: The discovery of CNS active 1,4-benzodiazepines, in Costa E (ed): *The benzodiazepines, from Molecular Biology to Clinical Practice.* New York, Raven Press, 1983, pp 1–6.
41. Taylor KM, Laverty R: The effect of chlordiazepoxide, diazepam and nitrazepam on catecholamine metabolism in regions of the rat brain. *Eur J Pharmacol* 8:296–301, 1969.
42. Weise CD, Berger BD, Stein L: Benzodiazepines: Antianxiety reducing activity by reduction of serotonin turnover in the brain. *Science* 177:180–183, 1972.
43. Beer B, Chasin M, Clody DE, et al: Cyclic adenosine monophosphate phosphodiesterase in brain: Effect on anxiety. *Science* 176:428–430, 1972.
44. Snyder SH, Enna SJ: The role of central glycine receptors in the pharmacological actions of benzodiazepines, in Costa E, Greengard P (eds): *Mechanism of Action of Benzodiazepines.* New York, Raven Press, 1975, pp 81–91.
45. Costa E, Guidotti A, Mao CC, et al: New concepts on the mechanism of action of benzodiazepines. *Life Sci* 17:167–186, 1975.
46. Haefely W, Kulcsar A, Mohler H, et al: Possible involvement of GABA in the central actions of benzodiazepines, in Costa E, Greengard P (eds): *Mechanism of Action of Benzodiazepines.* New York, Raven Press, 1975, pp 131–151.
47. Squires RF, Braestrup C: Benzodiazepine receptors in the brain. *Nature* 266:732–734, 1977.
48. Mohler H, Okada T: Benzodiazepine receptors: Demonstration in the central nervous system. *Science* 198:849–851, 1977.
49. Squires RF: Benzodiazepine receptor multiplicity. *Neuropharmacology* 22:1443–1450, 1983.
50. Richards JG, Mohler H: Benzodiazepine receptors. *Neuropharmacology* 23:233–242, 1984.
51. Speth RC, Guidotti A, Yamamura HY: The pharmacology of benzodiazepines, in Palmer GC (ed): *Neuropharmacology of Central Nervous System and Behavioral Disorders.* New York, Academic Press, 1980, pp 244–283.
52. Bowery NG, Price GW, Hudson AL, et al: GABA receptor multiplicity. Visualization of different receptor types in the mammalian CNS. *Neuropharmacology* 23:219–231, 1984.
53. Paul SM, Marangos PJ, Skolnick P: The benzodiazepine-GABA-chloride ionophore receptor complex: Common site of minor tranquilizer action. *Biol Psychiatry* 16:213–229, 1981.
54. Study RE, Barker JL: Diazepam and pentobarbital: Fluctuation analysis reveals different mechanisms for potentiation of GABA responses in cultured control neurons. *Proc Natl Acad Sci USA* 78:7180–7184, 1981.
55. Ticku MK, Ban M, Olsen RW: Binding of [^{3}H]-dihydropicrotoxinin, a gamma-aminobutyric acid synaptic antagonist, to rat brain membranes. *Mol Pharmacol* 14:391–402, 1978.
56. Costa E, Guidotti A: Molecular mechanisms in the receptor action of benzodiazepines. *Annu Rev Pharmacol Toxicol* 19:531–545, 1979.
57. Matsumoto K, Fukuda H: Stimulation and protective effects of benzodiazepines on GABA receptors labeled with [^{3}H] muscimol. *Life Sci* 30:935–943, 1982.
58. Wastek GJ, Speth RC, Reisine TD, et al: The effect of gamma-aminobutyric acid on [^{3}H] flunitrazepam binding in the rat brain. *Eur J Pharmacol* 50:445–447, 1978.
59. Gallager DW, Thomas JW, Tallman JP: Effect of GABAergic drugs on benzodiazepine binding site sensitivity in rat cerebral cortex. *Biochem Pharmacol* 27:2745–2749, 1978.
60. Supavilai P, Karobath M: Stimulation of benzodiazepine receptor by SQ 20009 is chloride dependent and piorotoxin-sensitive. *Eur J Pharmacol* 60:111–113, 1979.
61. Guidotti A, Konkel DR, Ebstein B, et al: Isolation, characterization and purification to homogeneity of a rat brain protein (GABA-modulin). *Proc Natl Acad Sci USA* 79:6084–6088, 1982.
62. Skolnick P, Marangos PJ, Goodwin FK: Identification of inosine and hypoxanthine as endogenous inhibitors of [^{3}H] diazepam binding in the central nervous system. *Life Sci* 23:1473–1480, 1978.
63. Asano T, Spector S: Identification of inosine and hypoxanthine as endogenous ligands for the brain benzodiazepine binding sites. *Proc Natl Acad Sci USA* 76:977–981, 1979.

64. Mohler H, Polc P, Cumin R, et al: Nicotinamide is a brain constituent with benzodiazepine-like action. *Nature* 278:563–565, 1979.
65. Costa E, Corda MG, Guidotti A: On a brain polypeptide functioning as a putative effector for the recognition sites of benzodiazepine and beta carboline derivatives. *Neuropharmacology* 22:1481–1492, 1983.
66. Ferrero P, Guidotti A, Conti-Tronconi B, et al: A brain octadecaneuropeptide generated by tryptic digestion of DBI (diazepam binding inhibitor) functions as a proconflict ligand of benzodiazepine recognition sites. *Neuropharmacology* 23:1359–1362, 1984.
67. Boast CA, Bernard PS, Barbaz BS, et al: The neuropharmacology of various diazepam antagonists. Neuropharmacology 22:1511–1521, 1983.
68. Paul S, Marangos P, Brownstein M, et al: Demonstration and characterization of an endogenous inhibitor of GABA-enhanced [^{3}H]-diazepam binding from bovine cerebral cortex, in Costa E, Dichiara G, Gessa GL (eds): *GABA and Benzodiazepine Receptors.* New York, Raven Press, 1981, pp 103–110.
69. Haefely W, Bonetti EP, Burkard WP, et al: Benzodiazepine antagonists, in Costa E (ed): *The Benzodiazepines, from Molecular Biology to Clinical Practice.* New York, Raven Press, 1983, pp 137–146.
70. Braestrup C, Nielsen M, Honore T, et al: Benzodiazepine receptor ligands with positive and negative efficacy. *Neuropharmacology* 22:1451–1457, 1983.
71. Weissman BA, Cott J, Hommer D, et al: Pharmacological, electrophysiological and neurochemical actions of the convulsant benzodiazepine RO-5-4864 (4′-Chlordiazepam), in Biggio G, Costa E (eds): *Benzodiazepine Recognition Site Ligands: Biochemistry and Pharmacology.* New York, Raven Press, 1983, pp 139–151.
72. Phillis JW, Bender AS, Wu PH: Benzodiazepines inhibit adenosine uptake into rat brain synaptosomes. *Brain Res* 195:494–498, 1980.
73. Phillis JW: A potent depressant action of adenine derivatives on cerebral cortical neurons. *Eur J Pharmacol* 30:125–129, 1975.
74. Siggins GR, Schubert P: Adenosine depression of hippocampal neurons in vitro: An intracellular study of dose dependent actions on synaptic and membrane potentials. *Neurosci Lett* 23:55–60, 1981.
75. Phillis JW: Diazepam potentiation of purinergic depression of central neurons. *Can J Physiol Pharmacol* 57:432–435, 1979.
76. Schwartz MA: Pathways of metabolism of the benzodiazepines, in Garattini S, Mussini E, Randall LO (eds): *The Benzodiazepines.* New York, Raven Press, 1973, p 53.
77. Kaplan SA, Jack ML: Metabolism of the benzodiazepines: Pharmacokinetic and pharmacodynamic considerations, in Costa E (ed): *The Benzodiazepines, from Molecular Biology to Clinical Practice.* New York, Raven Press, 1983, pp 173–199.
78. Greenblatt DJ, Shader RI, Divoll M, et al: Benzodiazepines: A summary of pharmacokinetic properties. Br J Clin Pharmacol 11:115–165, 1981.
79. Alvan G, Jonsson M, Sundwall A, et al: First pass conjugation and enterohepatic recycling of oxazepam in dogs: Intravenous tolerance of oxazepam in propylene glycol. *Acta Pharmacol Toxicol* 40 (suppl l):16–27, 1977.
80. Baird ES, Hailey DM: Delayed recovery from a sedative: Correlation of the plasma levels of diazepam with clinical effects after oral and intravenous administration. *Br J Anaesth* 44:803–808, 1972.
81. Ticku MK, Ban M, Olsen RW: Binding of [^{3}H]-dihydropicrotoxinin, a gamma aminobutyric acid synaptic antagonist, to rat brain membranes. *Mol Pharmacol* 14:391–402, 1978.
82. Olsen RW, Ticku MK, Greenlee D, et al: GABA receptor and ionophore binding sites: Interactions with various drugs, in Krogsgaard-Larsen P, Scheel-Kruger J, Kotod M (eds): *GABA Neurotransmitters.* Copenhagen, Munksgaard, 1979, p 165.
83. Barker JL: CNS depressants: Effects on postsynaptic pharmacology. *Brain Res* 92:35–55, 1975.
84. Nicoll RA, Eccles JC, Oshima T, et al: Prolongation of hippocampal inhibitor post-synaptic potentials by barbiturates. *Nature* 258:625–627, 1975.

85. Ransom BR, Barker JL: Pentobarbital selectively enhances GABA-mediated post-synaptic inhibition in tissue cultured mouse spinal neurons. *Brain Res* 114:530–535, 1976.
86. MacDonald RL, Barker JL: Enhancement of GABA-mediated postsynaptic inhibition in cultured mammalian spinal cord neurons: A common mode of anticonvulsant action. *Brain Res* 167:323–336, 1979.
87. Schulz DW, MacDonald RL: Barbiturate enhancement of GABA-mediated inhibition and activation of chloride ion conductance: Correlation with anticonvulsant and anesthetic actions. *Brain Res* 209:177–188, 1981.
88. MacDonald RL, McLean MJ: Cellular bases of barbiturate and phenytoin anticonvulsant drug action. *Epilepsia* 23:S7–S81, 1982.
89. Ho IK, Harris RA: Mechanism of action of barbiturates. *Annu Rev Pharmacol Toxicol* 21:83–111, 1981.
90. Goldstein DB: Th effects of drugs on membrane fluidity. *Annu Rev Pharmacol Toxicol 24:43–64, 1984.*
91. Blaustein MP, Ector AC: Barbiturate inhibition of calcium uptake by depolarized nerve terminals in vitro. *Mol Pharmacol* 11:369–378, 1975.
92. Hood WF, Harris RA: Effects of pentobarbital, ethanol and morphine on subcellular localization of calcium and magnesium in brain. *Biochem Pharmacol* 28:3075–3080, 1979.
93. Blaustein MP: Barbiturates block sodium and potassium conductance increases in voltage clamped lobster axons. *J Gen Physiol* 51:293–307, 1968.
94. Cutler RWP, Young J: Effect of barbiturates on release of endogenous amino acids from rat cortex slices. *Neurochem Res* 4:319–329, 1979.
95. Friedman MB, Coleman R, Leslie SW: Barbiturate depression of calcium-mediated stimulus secretion coupling in synaptosomes: A species and strain comparison. *Life Sci* 25:735–738, 1979.
96. Willow M, Johnston GAR: Enhancement of GABA binding by pentobarbitone. *Neurosci Lett* 18:323–327, 1980.
97. Willow M, Johnston GAR: Enhancement by anesthetic and convulsant barbiturates of GABA binding to rat brain synaptosomal membranes. *J Neurosci* 1:364–367, 1981.
98. Leeb-Lundberg F, Snowman A, Olsen RW: Barbiturate receptors are coupled to benzodiazepine receptors. *Proc Natl Acad Sci USA* 77:7468–7472, 1980.
99. Ticku MK: Interaction of depressant, convulsant and anticonvulsants barbiturates with [^{3}H]-diazepam binding site at benzodiazepine–GABA receptor–ionophore complex. *Biochem Pharmacol* 30:1573–1579, 1981.
100. Breimer DD: Clinical pharmacokinetics of hypnotics. *Clin Pharmacokinet* 2:93–109, 1977.
101. Curry SH, Riddall D, Gordon JJ, et al: Disposition of glutethimide in man. *Clin Pharmacol Ther* 12:849–857, 1971.
102. Delong AF, Smyth RD, Polk A, Nayak RK, Reavey-Cantwell NH: Blood levels of methaqualone in man following chronic therapeutic doses. *Arch Int Pharmacodyn Ther* 222:322–331, 1976.
103. Tang BK, Inaba T, Kalow W: N-Hydroxylation of Pentobarbital in man. *Drug Metab Dispos* 5:71–74, 1977.

3

Sedative Drug Interactions of Clinical Importance

Paul Cushman, Jr.

Abstract. In an age of widespread availability of psychoactive drugs, use of multiple sedatives is very common. Why such multiple drug use prevails is poorly understood. Sequential drug use may leave sequential problems. Concomitant use of several drugs can produce a host of interactions. Increasingly, the metabolic basis of sedative interactions are becoming known. Cross-tolerance between sedatives permit substitution of one for another and reduced sedation when combined. Metabolic interactions at the hepatic oxidation enzyme level may greatly affect drug disposal rates. Recognition of polysubstance abuse can assist in management. Treatment ranges from urgent life support to abrupt or slow withdrawal, to substitution long-term treatment usually requiring specialized care, with abstinence the preferred goal. However, polysubstance abusers seem to have low probabilities of achieving lasting abstinence.

1. Introduction

Use of sedative drugs by Americans both singly and in combination, has soared in recent years.[1] One major trend is for polydrug use to continue after the initial drug experimentation phase. Thus drug users are mixing and varying their drugs in numerous ways. Therefore, interactions between sedating drugs have increased in frequency and clinical importance. It is timely to review the clinical aspects of these interactions. It is envisioned that better recognition, diagnosis, and clinical management of these patient problems will ensue.

While our knowledge of the clinical effects of single drugs of abuse is extensive, a number of major gaps remain. Far less solid information exists about the effects of drug combinations. Major considerations hindering accumulation of such data involve the need to control not only bioavailability, dose, pharmacokinetics, and effects of both drugs simultaneously but also their pharmacoactive metabolites. All these problems need evaluation under varying but controlled circumstances. Thus, it is not surprising that the rel-

Paul Cushman, Jr. • Drug Dependency Treatment Program, McGuire Veterans Hospital, Richmond, Virginia 23249; and Department of Medicine, Psychiatry, Pharmacology and Toxicology, Medical College of Virginia, Richmond, Virginia 23298.

evant clinical, metabolic, and pharmacological data, carefully collected and appropriately controlled, are sparse.[2]

When drugs are mixed, untoward effects not anticipated from the actions of either drug alone can arise from many possible sources.[3,4] One possibility is an idiosyncratic reaction to one drug, with other effects being merely coincidental. These problems lie outside the scope of this study. The vast majority of unexpected drug reactions can be attributed to some sort of biological interaction between the drugs. The most common and simplest is the augmented sedation observed when two sedatives are combined, as with the simultaneous use of the benzodiazepines (BD) and alcohol.[5] Their additive sedation is usually attributed to some combined central nervous system (CNS) actions. Other locations of possible sedative drug–drug interactions lie at the level of gut binding, intestinal wall absorption, or blood transport mechanisms. Changes in the number of drug receptors or their binding affinities could also be implicated in drug interactions.[6,7] More importantly, drug disposal mechanisms can be readily altered by other drugs. A prime example is the changes in enzyme activities in the mixed enzyme-oxidizing system (MEOS) in the liver microsomes after exposure to various drugs. Finally, medical disorders associated with one drug may modify conditions by which other sedatives are metabolized. The best example of the latter is in patients with major alcoholic liver disease. Impressive retardation of metabolism and disposal of a variety of sedating drugs usually occur.[8]

Some drug–drug interactions become important only after long-term use, while others are more immediately apparent. This review will encompass both acute and chronic interactions.

2. Why Persons Consume Drug Combinations

The precise motives behind human mind-altering drug consumption are still not well understood. We usually do not know why some persons start, continue, cease, or relapse to the use of a single drug. We are even less sure of why polydrug use is carried out. Some subjects seem to be using several drugs in the same category, sometimes together or in tandem, as if to obtain a modicum of sedation by whatever means are available. Some may experiment with various combinations and others may seek augmented effects. Some may use drugs that have opposing effects, such as the "speedball" addict, who shoots a mixture of the stimulant cocaine together with the sedative heroin. In this combination some of the less desirable effects of each drug are attenuated by the other. However, many polydrug users do not seem to have a discernable logic or pattern to their hodge-podge of drug use.[9]

An intriguing theory attempts to link some of the mind-altering drugs into a unified action.[10,11] No matter what their structure or initial site of action, they are hypothesized to produce eventually a similar, psychic reward in the CNS. Some circumstantial substantiation for this view comes from the recent discovery of CNS reward centers that can be activated by direct electrical stimulation.[12,13] Possibly such rewards may be achievable by chemical messengers either directly by the drug itself or indirectly by some interpolated CNS circuits.[13] The leading candidates for such putative neuromodulators or neurotransmitters which may mediate these exogenous chemically induced effects are the endogenous opiate peptides (EOP; endorphins, dynorphins, and enkephalins).[14,15]

3. Recognition and Diagnosis

With increasing use of several types of drugs, selected from the large menu of possible sedatives, recognition of the precise causes of chemically induced sedation can be difficult at first encounter. Of course, the history of recent drug use is of greatest help. Patients usually know what they have taken and usually are able to produce an adequate history. Nevertheless, street transactions involving drugs have many uncertainties. Buyers are often deceived about doses, diluents, and even the presence of the major drug. For example, many purchasers, seeking potent cannabis experiences, obtained the more costly "THC" powders from street vendors. Whatever they used, it is certain that they could not have obtained THC, which is a liquid oil at room temperature.[16]

Sometimes the history is unobtainable. In some cases the diagnosis can be readily inferred from the clinical picture: constricted pupils strongly suggest opioids; dilated ones hint at glutethimide; nystagmus, doll-eye stare, hypertension, and tachycardia in an anesthetized, heavily sedated person indicate phencyclidine (PCP). Needle puncture marks, suspicious tattoos, and cutaneous scars are all helpful signs of past injections. But for precision in diagnosis, it is most important to turn to the clinical chemistry laboratory. With the widespread availability of thin-layer chromatographic screening and rapid immunoassay procedures in biological fluids, speedy detections of most sedatives (or metabolites) are possible. Such information can be of great help in clinical management. For example, the early detection of glutethimide is especially important. It is very slowly excreted and its lipid solubility is such that the clinical management of the severely overdosed patient may require hemodialysis, including substitution of a lipid for the usual aqueous dialysate.[17] Recognition of serious PCP intoxification should engender efforts to produce acidosis and lower the urine pH, thereby to enhance renal excretion of the alkaloid.[18]

4. Treatment Principles

1. Acutely intoxicated patients may require more than just passage of time to excrete or metabolize their drug(s). When first seen, it is often uncertain whether they are at their most depressed state or will develop further obtundation. Therefore, it is important immediately to remove any residual

drug that has not yet been absorbed. Gastric lavage or instillation of activated charcoal are preferred to induction of emesis.[19] Some patients may need major life-support procedures, including fluids, assisted respiration, and chemically supported blood pressure. Others may require efforts to enhance drug excretion. Rates of renal excretion can be augmented by acidification of the urine with NH_4Cl or ascorbic acid (some alkaloids) or saline infusions (some barbiturates that use a renal pathway for excretion, such as barbital and phenobarbital).

2. Some specific antidotes should be tried. If any possibility of an opioid component in the total sedation exists, parenteral naloxone is administered, up to three doses 5 min apart. Naloxone, an opioid antagonist, exerts only minor effects in the normal subject and at only very high doses.[20,21] Therefore, it can be given safely to all persons suspected of being opioid users; its use is routine in most emergency rooms in the management of nontraumatic coma. The RO-15,1788 or similar BD antagonist will probably also become a routine therapeutic agent.[22] It has little or no effect in the normal subject, is free of toxicity, and may depend on the continuing presence of a BD agonist effect.[23]

3. In nonemergency situations combined-sedative abusers are approached in much the same way as abusers of single sedative drugs. After the recognition or suspicion that drug abuse has occurred, confirmation by urinary drug screening should be done. Direct confrontation of the patient with the clinical findings and formulation of an agreed treatment plan ensues.

4. If the history and/or physical examination suggest that physical dependency, i.e., a withdrawal syndrome, is likely, then most persons should be referred for inpatient detoxification. This is mandatory for abusers of glutethimide, barbiturates, some other sedatives, many heavy alcohol abusers, and almost all patients with extensive combined-sedative dependency.

While ambulatory detoxification with or without pharmacological support can be a cheap, effective alternative to hospital care, although readily acceptable by many patients, some cautions are urged. The patient should be screened for medical, nutritional, psychiatric, or environmental factors precluding outpatient initial management. Large sedative tolerances are indicative of significant withdrawal symptoms.[24] Some indication of the level of the patient's tolerance can come from the blood alcohol concentration (BAC) or sedative or barbiturate concentrations. If the blood levels are much higher than what would be expected from the clinical level of intoxification, then the presumption of a significant tolerance to sedatives can be made. The ambulatory detoxification is best reserved for those with small degrees of physical dependence.

5. Referral to a specialized drug treatment center should be made after (or for) detoxification. Every effort should be made to encourage the patient to enter and remain in substance abuse aftercare treatment.

6. After detoxification, abstinence should be the goal. Maintenance of abstinence, often difficult in drug abusers, may be more difficult in the poly-

drug abuser.[25,26] Many patients will need extensive services after initial care. Remedial education programs, substance abuse educational programs, counseling, group or individual therapy, behavior modification, and vocational counseling are frequently helpful. Introduction to Alcoholics Anonymous or Narcotics Anonymous should be strongly encouraged. Family therapy may assist the substance abuser directly or indirectly as families become more aware of the substance abuse problems that affect the total family. Some alcoholic subjects seem to be sustained in their abstinence with disulfiram.[27] Some chronic opioid abusers do better than controls taking oral methadone regularly as a maintenance opioid in a structured program.[28]

Polydrug abusers are usually refractory to the cognitive processes of psychotherapy as long as their drug use continues. Accordingly, the initial step requires cessation of activities associated with drug dependency. Once this has been achieved, then an individualized treatment process can be initiated. Insight-oriented psychoanalytic therapy is generally unhelpful as the process is often too lengthy for many persons accustomed to much faster, rapid rewards. Thus encounter, Gestalt, transactional analysis, or simple supportive pragmatic therapy are more acceptable to many patients.[29]

The regular use of psychotropic drugs is of little positive use in the rehabilitation of most polysubstance abusers. Benzodiazepines, although chemically effective, tend to be abused no matter how skillfully they are prescribed, and most phenothiazines are not well accepted by the patients. Antidepressants can be useful in the occasional patient, especially those with vegetative signs of depression. Their routine use can not be encouraged, as they offer little over the routine compared to placebo if the nonsedating ones are used.[30] Lithium has been helpful in bipolar and manic patients but of uncertain value in others.

Frequent examinations for drugs or alcohol in urine or breath under careful collection procedures are invaluable. They provide objective verification of use, or nonuse, of abused drugs. They also tend to strengthen the patient–treatment interactions by a layer of objective measurements in addition to the verbal interchange. Since these procedures are widely available, swift in execution, and small cost, their routine use should be obligatory in follow-up care.

5. Tolerance

5.1. Mechanisms of Tolerance

Tolerance is a central nervous system (CNS) cellular adaptation to repeated exposure to sedatives. The precise mechanisms by which this process develops are unknown. With alcohol, the changes appear to reside in the cellular membrane.[31,32] Alcohol's initial cellular effect is likely a physicochemical change in membrane structure, resulting in greater plasticity. With sustained alcohol exposure, the cell membrane adapts such that much larger doses of alcohol are needed to produce the same degree of fluidization that small doses produce in the normal cell. These conclusions are well supported by pharmacological data.[33,34] It is probable that these findings could underly the well-known clinical observations of tolerance: The chronic drunk can consume large volumes of alcohol, carry blood alcohol concentrations much beyond the legal limits of sobriety, and yet show only modest signs of alcohol intoxification.

Mechanisms of opiate tolerance have had some recent clarification.[35–38] They may involve postreceptor events, such as calcium ion fluxes and cyclic AMP production and require the synthesis of new protein.

Evidence for the latter came from the effects of antibiotics such as cyclohexamide or antinomycin D, which inhibit new protein synthesis. The extrapolation of these promising data to human opioid physiology is tentative at present.

Benzodiazepines act on its receptors to augment the effects of γ-aminobutyric acid (GABA).[39] A possible mechanism of BD tolerance could involve some alterations or reductions in GABA such that larger doses of BD are required to produce the same effects.[40–42] The cessation of BD therapy could lead to a relative GABA deficiency. The clinical effects of such GABA deficiency would be anxiety, tremors, seizures, agitation, etc., or the opposite of GABA inhibitory actions. The BD receptors are widely distributed in the CNS, mainly in the limbic system, the cortex, thalamus, hypothalamus, etc.[43]; the location of human antianxiety or physical dependency effects is still unknown.

The barbiturate actions are even less clear. Some recent evidence points to an involvement with GABA–GABA receptor complex.[44,45] Conceivably tolerance caused by barbiturates could be similar to that of BD. Barbiturates are believed to act in the reticular activating system primarily to suppress arousal. The mechanisms of action of chloral hydrate, methaqualone, and the other hypnotics are still obscure, as are their CNS loci of action.[45]

5.2. Clinical Consequences of Cross-Tolerance

Clinical experience over the years has repeatedly established that tolerance to one drug can be readily crossed over to many other sedatives.[46] With such diversity of receptors, target tissue, and cellular effects emerging from the pharmacological studies of abused drugs, it is impossible at present to account for cross-tolerance. Whatever its mechanisms, many subjects have been able to substitute one sedative for another. Physicians have made use of this fact to supply a more desired sedative to persons who had been abusing others. The acute pharmacological management of sedative dependency supplies a quantum of sedation sufficient to suppress the stigma of withdrawal but not high enough to exceed the tolerance. Regularized dose reductions follow and ultimately stop. In Table I are listed equivalent doses of the commonly used sedatives.[47]

Table I. Withdrawal Equivalents for Common Sedative-Hypnotics

Drug	mg
Barbiturates	
Amobarbital	100
Pentobarbital	100
Phenobarbital	30
Secobarbital	100
Other sedative-hypnotics	
Chloral hydrate	500
Ethchlorvynol	350
Glutethimide	250
Meprobamate	400–600
Methaqualone	250–300
Methyprylon	300
Benzodiazepines	
Chlordiazapoxide	100
Diazepam	50
Flurazepam	60
Oxazepam	100

5.3. Substances used in Detoxification of Sedative Dependency

The extensive list of substances used in their detoxification is largely composed of sedatives (Table II).[48,49] The most popular sedative drug over the years to modify withdrawal is, of course, ethyl alcohol. Myriads of persons do this daily. However, its medical use has fallen into disfavor because it is difficult to control, has a short duration of action, and leaves the person with a continuing exposure to toxic effects of alcohol or its major metabolite acetaldehyde. Despite extensive experiences over the decades, paraldehyde has been bypassed in recent years. As a liquid, it needs to be given orally or rectally, is burdened with a characteristic and disconcerting odor, and has a potential for hepatotoxicity per se.[50] Barbiturates, extensively used for withdrawal over the years are effective.[46] The benzodiazepines are the most commonly prescribed sedative in the United States for detoxification because of superior efficacy and safety.

Clinical experiences with sedative substitution indicate that some drugs may affect some of the symptom complex of sedative withdrawal, leaving others relatively unaffected. The α-adrenergic agonist drugs, which attenuate the catecholamine symptoms associated with alcohol (or opiate) withdrawal, may not modify other withdrawal manifestations as craving or sleep disturbances.[51,52] Similarly phenytoin may or may not prevent sedative withdrawal seizures,[53,54] which carbamazepine does,[46] but neither one is notably effective in attenuating other features of alcohol withdrawal. The antipsychotics also have a limited pharmacological role, perhaps to control hallucination or delirium.[48]

Table II. Drugs Used in Sedative (Alcohol) Withdrawal

Drugs showing cross-tolerance across categories of sedatives
Sedatives
Barbiturates
Chloral hydrate
Chlormethiazole[a]
Ethyl Alcohol
Meprobamate
Methaqualone[b]
Paraldehyde
Anxiolytics
Benzodiazepines
Drugs not showing cross-tolerance
Anticonvulsants
Carbamazepine
Phenytoin
Valproate sodium
Neuroleptics
Butyrophenones
Phenothiazines
Antihistamines

[a] Used in Europe.
[b] No longer used for this purpose.

Cross-tolerance to sedatives presents a major challenge to the anesthesiologist when the occasion arises to anesthetize the sedative abuser.[55] If the emergency mandates immediate anesthesia, the standard sedating drugs are generally used in lower amounts, with very close monitoring, if the patient is already somewhat asleep at the outset. However, most anesthesia and surgery can be delayed until the acute effects of the sedatives wear off. The alcoholic or sedative abuser may have important metabolic problems, i.e., disturbances in fluid or acid–base balance, electrolytes, and phosphates, head trauma, subdural hematomas, serious liver disease, and encephalopathy. Therefore, it is prudent to correct or rule out these possibilities before anesthesia is administered. The sedative abuser will likely have a major increase in his MEOS activity, which together with probable increased CNS tolerance, will require much larger doses of hypnotics. Thus it is not unusual to use two to three times usual amounts of thiopental for induction of anesthesia in the alcoholic.[56]

6. Benzodiazepines: Alone and in Combination

6.1. Introduction

The benzodiazepines are antianxiety, anticonvulsant tranquilizers. Their actions start after stereospecific binding to the BD receptor.[57,58] The anxietolytic actions, which seem to have a different mechanism from the anticonvulsant ones,[58] involve augmentation of GABA effects. Since GABA is viewed as an inhibitory but common neurotransmitter, the actions of BD are also inhibitory. A newly discovered BD, RO-15,1788, binds to the BD receptor and attenuates specifically the agonist BD actions. Of great theoretical interest are some newly discovered compounds, which bind to the BD receptor, but whose effects are exactly opposite to those of the standard BD drugs. These drugs, which include the β carbolines, produce anxiety, and are attenuated by the BD agonists and RO-15,1788.[59–61]

It is appropriate to classify the BD drugs into two major subgroups based on their elimination kinetics. The slowly eliminated drugs, which include diazepam (DZP), chlordiazepoxide (CDP), and flurazepam (FZP), are initially dealkylated in liver MEOS to produce active derivatives also having slow elimination rates. Thus, enduring effects may appear long after the last or only drug use. These derivatives are further metabolized into other active derivatives; ultimately they evolve into end products which are swiftly conjugated in liver and excreted in the urine. Thus, with repeated dosing of the slowly eliminated drugs both parent and active derivative compounds accumulate in plasma. Abrupt discontinuation usually results in a slowly disappearing tail of pharmacological activity. In contrast, the rapidly excreted drugs, e.g. lorazepam, temazepam, and oxazepam, enter at the final stage,[62] are conjugated, rapidly excreted, and do not accumulate. (See Table III) for classification of BD drugs).

6.2. Clinical Consequences of Sustained BD Use

Studies regarding such clinically significant problems of chronic long-acting BD drugs as balance, alertness, psychomotor activity, or memory are generally (but not always) negative.[63] Tolerance may have been protective from these undesirable effects.

The elderly warrant special attention, as they are vulnerable to untoward sedation after relatively small doses of sedatives.[64] The pharmacological bases of this vulnerability in advanced age are numerous and include delayed drug

Table III. Benzodiazepines: A Classification Based on Pharmacokinetics

Administered drug	Active ingredient	Metabolized by mixed oxidases	Conjugated	Elimination kinetics
Alprazolam	Alprazolam	Yes	Yes	Intermediate
Chlordiazepoxide	Same	Yes	Yes	Slow
(CPD)	Desmethyl CPD	Yes	Yes	Slow
	Demoxepam	Yes	Yes	Slow
Diazepam	Same	Yes	Yes	Slow
(DZP)	Desmethyl DZP	Yes	Yes	Slow
Flurazepam	Desalkyl flurazepam	Yes	Yes	Slow
Lorazepam	Lorazepam	No	Yes	Swift
Oxazepam	Oxazepam	No	Yes	Swift

disposal.[65] Ordinary doses of BD are usually too toxic. Hence, it is frequently recommended that the elderly receive one half or less of the usual doses of DZP, FZP, CDP, or the short-acting BD drugs, which do not seem to have major changes in elimination rates.[63]

The high rates of citations of BD from drug treatment centers, hospitals, police jurisdictions, and medical examiners' offices attest to widespread abuse of BD.[66] Many of these citations include other drugs simultaneously. Accordingly, in both acute and chronic drug problems BD alone or in combination are well represented. It is frequently difficult to determine what each of the various individual drugs contributed to the clinical findings.

6.3. Acute Drug Reactions Involving the Benzodiazepines

When two BD drugs are combined, their agonist effects are additive in the therapeutic range. When doses moderately exceed the therapeutic ones, then additive effects may be difficult to demonstrate. For example, 30 mg of flurazepam is only marginally more hypnotic than 15 mg.[67] With larger doses a large margin of safety is present, although very large doses produce excessive sedation and coma, but rarely death.[68]

Acute combinations of BD with alcohol, barbiturates, sedatives, and opioids produce additive effects greater than what would occur from comparable doses of either drug alone. The list of such drugs also includes methaqualone, chloral hydrate, sedating antidepressants, and methypryplon. It may also include some cold preparations and over-the-counter sleep preparation, especially those containing antihistamines or scopolamine. Many physicians routinely forewarn their patients about such interactions, especially to emphasize their vulnerability even long after their last dose.

BD metabolism by the MEOS is retarded by drugs such as estrogens, disulfiram, and cimetidine, and also by liver disease and old age. Therefore, persons with these drugs or clinical states are particularly vulnerable to excessive BD sedative effects.

6.4. Chronic Drug Reactions Involving the Benzodiazepines

Common and increasingly important, the BD–sedative interactions are complex because of not only the variety of BD or metabolites but also the variety of sedatives available.

Alcohol and BD combinations can be especially deleterious in tasks requiring coordination, motor skills, or speedy reactions to stimuli. Even relatively small amounts of alcohol may be hazardous in users of long-acting BD because of the lengthy BD psychoactivity effect. Driving of motor vehicles was significantly worse when BD and alcohol are taken together than when either drug is used alone.[69] Highway traffic data obtained in persons stopped by police because of suspected drunk driving have also shown that sedatives, usually BD, are commonly used in addition to alcohol upon laboratory analysis.[70] Thus the magnitude of the combined sedative problem is large and probably much greater than is generally realized.

Chronic BD treatment, not an important influence on MEOS, does not alter significantly the disposal kinetics of other MEOS metabolized drugs.[71] Thus in acute alcohol and chronic BD use, the clinical consequences are most likely shaped by doses, timing, and the extent of the CNS tolerance to sedatives, rather than rates of metabolism. On the other hand, MEOS induction by many other drugs, including barbiturates, phenytoin, or chronic alcohol, speeds up the elimination kinetics of slowly eliminated BD drugs. When these combinations are used clinically, faster rates of BD disposal occurs. However, this phenomenon is not usually clinically important, and no adjustment in BD dosage is required. But when the inducing drug is taken simultaneously with long-acting BD, the competition for drug disposal in the MEOS may arise. Thus, a delay in elimination kinetics of both drugs can follow and may account for the much-enhanced sedation resulting from combined BD and alcohol. Detailed study of alcohol–benzodiazepine interactions by Vesell extensively clarified their interaction.[72]

6.5. Management of BD in Combination with Other Sedatives

Users who combine BD and other sedatives are advised that their drug use is hazardous, ill advised, and tantamount to drug abuse. Unless compelling reasons exist for the contrary, they are managed as any sedative abuser. Initially, withdrawal of all sedatives is carried out, followed by aftercare to maintain abstinence.

Some BD users are physically dependent, and need careful, supportive withdrawal. These patients usually have been taking long-acting BD drugs for many months, usually in doses above the recommended ranges, and frequently have had past histories of dependence on other illicit or addicting drugs.[73] Many BD users do not seem physically dependent. However, some who are taking only the recommended amounts of BD will show an abstinence syndrome and thereby reveal a subtle physical dependency on BD.[74]

All BD–sedative-dependent persons or patients with medical or other complicating factors should undergo withdrawal in the hospital where special attention can be directed to the appearance of delayed withdrawal syndromes.[74] Patients using BD plus alcohol in combination had similar delayed withdrawal reactions as those using BD alone.[75] Cessation of BD alone may produce three clusters of symptoms. First, some patients show anxieties over the perceived loss of their medication. Those who believed their BD was being discontinued, but who had not as yet actually started BD reduction, showed these anxieties immediately after starting the study.[76] A second symptom cluster is the sedative withdrawal syndrome. These symptoms include autonomic nervous system hyperactivity, insomnia, neuromuscular irritability, seizures, and psychomotor disturbances.[75] It is especially noteworthy that the timing of these symptoms may be clinically delayed. They may be swift ($\frac{1}{2}$–2 days) after the short-acting BD or long (2–12 days) after the slowly eliminated BD. Thus clinicians should be alert for a relatively late appearance of BD withdrawal and warn their patients accordingly. Gradual cessation with tapered doses of BD are recommended. The third cluster of symptoms represent the return of those problems for which the BD were prescribed in the first place.[77]

Management of BD withdrawal depends on which category of symptom is encountered. Reassurance is helpful for those anticipating problems. A tapering of sedatives may prevent the more serious withdrawal symptoms. Substitution of a barbiturate or a short-acting BD are often recommended. The long-acting BD drugs are also useful as they have a self-tapering effect; their psychoactivity slowly abates even after abrupt cessation.

The return of anxieties or insomnia present a challenge for the patient and physician adviser. Most patients are best counseled to cope with these feelings without chemical intervention. While situational reactions are often well handled by a short course of benzodiazepine, treatment of long-term anxiety with drugs is not generally recommended.

Abstinence maintenance by former abusers of BD alone or in combination with other sedatives is especially difficult. Treatment programs, psychological therapy, or Alcoholics or Narcotics Anonymous can be helpful. However, the widespread availability of BD, the absence of societal disapproval, low risks, low cost, and the widespread notion by patients that a return to BD is likely to produce a rewarding experience are strong factors in recidivism.

7. Alcohol Alone and in Combination

7.1. Introduction

Alcohol is used by about 70% and abused by about 10% of adult Americans. Heavy alcohol use is a major health and safety problem. It is hardly surprising that extensive recognition of problems involving alcohol and other sedatives has arisen in hospitals, emergency treatment facilities, medical examiners' offices, industrial medical departments, highway safety enforcement agencies, and drug treatment programs.[78] It is often uncertain what precise contribution each component may have played in the total clinical picture.[79]

Patients, physicians, the general public, and emergency room personnel should be vigilant about the possibility of alcohol combined with other sedatives. In sedative intoxification the blood or breatholyzer alcohol (BAC) determinations are especially useful. If the BAC is lower than expected, a search for additional factors, including mixed drug abuse, is warranted.

While adverse reactions after large quantities of combined sedatives are well recognized, some oversedations arise after relatively modest amounts of alcohol in combination with the sedating antihistamines, the sedating antidepressants, or benzodiazepines.[80] The sedative properties of even some over-the-counter cold or sleep remedies can be excessive in association with alcohol. Thus, social drinkers may realize greater intoxification after their usual alcohol doses when these sedatives are also consumed. The impairment to performance of complex, skilled tasks requiring coordination, such as operating machines or automobiles, is significant.

7.2. Acute Drug Reactions Involving Alcohol

Acute combinations of alcohol and other sedatives produce added sedative effects. Other pharmacological drug interactions such as tolerance or change in drug disposal kinetics are lacking. One special example of combined alcohol and sedative use is the Mickey Finn, where chloral hydrate and alcohol produce an exaggerated sedation. The locus of this metabolic interaction is in the dehydrogenase in the hepatocyte.[81]

The degree of combined sedation of alcohol and other drugs ranges from a somewhat greater intoxification than expected with either drug alone to extreme sedation and death.

7.3. Drug Reaction Involving Chronic Alcohol

Chronic alcohol–sedative reactions are also very common. The clinical findings depend on what drugs were used, what the level of CNS tolerance was, and whether any metabolic changes have occurred because of drug use. Chronic alcohol use stimulates the MEOS to produce swifter rates of alcohol and other substrate metabolism.[82] Substrates included are various drugs, barbiturates, meprobamate, and to a lesser extent, long-acting BD. Another mechanism of alcohol–BD interactions might result from an alcohol effect on BD receptors.[83,84] Accordingly, the sedation expected from these drugs in the sober alcoholic may be somewhat dampened by this mechanism. If the alcoholic is also drinking actively, then competition in the MEOS arises, leading to slower[85] plasma disappearance rates of drugs. However, the degree of clinical sedation much more depends on the level of CNS sedative tolerance than the blood levels.[86,87]

Major alcoholic liver disease may greatly affect the rates of sedative disposal, especially by injuring the MEOS system. Accordingly, the magnitude of sedation that may arise may be much greater than generally expected from the sedative doses employed. This has important consequences in the acute management of alcoholic with manifest liver disease. Disappearance rates from plasma of chlordiazepoxide, a drug widely used to attenuate alcohol withdrawal, can be very slow.[88] Since the disappearance rates of desmethyl CPD are also retarded, CPD should be very carefully monitored. Once given, the effects of CPD may endure protractedly; therefore, repeat doses should be very cautiously given, with attention to quantity and dose intervals. Since hepatic conjugation rates are much more resistant to injury, many physicians prefer to use the short-acting BD in alcoholic liver disease. However, when major clinical manifestations of of alcohol liver disease appear as ascites or jaundice, impairment of hepatic conjugation mechanisms may also arise in these patients.[89] Plasma disappearance curves of diazepam can be greatly slowed, as were those of lorazepam. These subjects are unusually sensitive to all sedatives and easily develop oversedation or hepatic encephalopathy.

7.4. Management of Alcohol–Sedative Reactions

Deeply depressed patients need emergency life-support measures. Those with lesser degrees of impairment may require corrections of fluid, electrolyte, pH, or other medical complications as clinically warranted. Subjects with prolonged use of sedative may need supported detoxification, with or without pharmacological assistance, as the level of physical dependency dictates.

In all cases after the major effects of drug use have abated, rehabilitation therapy should follow. Abstinence should be strongly recommended and aftercare stressed. Treatment for mixed sedative use generally includes the same mix of educational, psychological, and group support that alcoholics usually receive, together with emphasis on abuse of other drugs. Polydrug abuse is usually more refractory to abstinence-oriented treatment than alcoholism alone. This is well documented in the opioid using alcoholic.[90] However, treatment providers cite numerous instances where polydrug abusers have adopted the abstinent approach, renounced all their psychoactive drugs, and achieved impressive remissions. Often the motivation of the patient seems a more important determinant of outcome than the specific drug(s) that the patient happened to be using at time of entry into treatment.

8. Opioids and Other Sedatives

8.1. Introduction

While opioids are generally classified as narcotics, they do possess impressive sedative properties. They are agonists, with morphine as the prototype, or antagonists, as naloxone, or mixed agonist-antagonists, with nalbuphine or pentazocine as major examples. They bind to the opiate receptors, which are not only widespread but also heterogeneous.[91] Multiple ligands bind to opiate receptors. The precise roles that the endogenous opioid peptides may in normal and diseased subjects remain unclear.[92,93] Abundant data support an important role of EOP in analgesia, sedation, tolerance, physical dependence, and some endocrine effects.[91] However, it is far from settled what happens to the EOP systems during and after exogenous opiate exposure, as in the heroin addict or the methadone treated patient.[94] Furthermore, any clinically significant EOP changes that may arise after sedatives, alcohol, or cocaine, remain to be established.

Alcohol can produce some changes in the opiate receptor,[95–98] but the clinical significance of these observations is uncertain. Possibly, the euphoria or depression that results from sedative or alcohol use may involve these peptides.[99,100] These notions underlie the experimental and therapeutic use of naloxone to detect whatever morphine-like effects could be attributed to sedatives or alcohol.[101] The results of various studies indicate conflicting results.[102–105] At present the data do not support the routine use of naloxone in the clinical management of non-opioid-induced intoxification.

8.2. Acute Sedative Drug Reactions Involving Opioids

The use of opioids and sedatives together generally results in a summation of the effects of each drug alone.[106,107] Dose and routes of administration are the principle determinants of the clinical effects. Opioid actions on the benzodiazepine receptor–ligand complexes are incompletely evaluated,[108] and may be of more than theoretical interest. A special combination of opioid–sedative use has arisen in the Midwest recently. The intravenous mixture of illicit pentazocine plus tripenylamine (T's and blues) have been used by chronic street opiate addicts as a substitute for heroin.[109] The antihistamine appears to have some opioidlike properties as well as some sedative properties.[110] Acutely, alcohol may interfere with hepatic methadone metabolism and augment sedation, while the chronic pharmacological effects of combined ethanol and methadone are enhanced excretion second to cytochrome P450 interaction.[111]

8.3. Chronic Opioid and Sedative Use

Clinical findings in these subjects are also related to the specific drugs used, route of administration, and the degree of metabolic interaction, and, most importantly, the extent of central nervous system tolerance. Chronic opioids produce extensive tolerance to the sedative, antinociceptive, and other effects of a variety of opioids, but cross tolerance to other sedatives or alcohol has not been established. Both methadone[112] and morphine[113] are partially metabolized by the MEOS. Since they are poor inducers, their sedative reactions are relatively free of hepatic drug–drug effects.

Alcohol abuse by narcotic addicts has been extensively reported.[114,115] The alcohol abuse may precede, coincide with, or follow opiate addiction. Most of the carefully controlled observations have been made in methadone-maintained patients. The important clinical question regarding the significance of alcoholism in the methadone treated addict is still unsettled. Recent data disclose no important alcohol–methadone interaction of both drugs in plasma levels in the social-drinking, stable, chronic methadone recipient.[116] Sedative use by opiate addicts is also common. This combination is best managed by the abstinence approach, although the results of abstinence oriented therapy are poor. The opioid addict's propensity to use sedatives also includes the benzodiazepines; since the preponderance of data demonstrate a greater hazard from their combined use. The general recommendation is against this combination. In methadone programs, BD, sedating antidepressants, and antihistamines are widely believed to complicate standard methadone therapy. These combinations should be discontinued.

8.4. Treatment of Combined Opioid–Sedative Abuse

In acute intoxification, general principles prevail: life support, naloxone, removal of residual drugs, and correction of metabolic or other medical problems as clinically warranted. Of special note is the relatively long half-life of methadone. The methadone-intoxicated patient requires hospital care and vigilance for a return of the opioid depression after the naloxone effects wear off.[117] After the acute intoxification has subsided, patients should be referred for further care. The chronic combined opioid–sedative abuser merits careful, usually inpatient care for initial treatment. Detoxification customarily involves administration of oral opioids, which are tapered off over a few days. An alternative approach uses clonidine or lofexidine,[118,119] which greatly modifies the opiate withdrawal syndrome. While they appear to shorten the detoxification process, they do not produce any significant long-term abstinence by themselves.[119]

The conventional management of the nonopioid component of combined opioid–sedative abuse proceeds with the sedative detoxification first.[9] The opioid dependency can be managed with a stabilizing methadone dose of 15–30 mg/day. Then, when the sedative withdrawal is complete, the opioid detoxification can proceed. However, both dependencies can be managed simultaneously in cases where small quantities of drug withdrawal symptoms are expected.[120]

Opioid addicts on methadone programs who also abuse other sedatives present major clinical challenges. Often refractory to treatment, which should address both components simultaneously, these patients usually leave treatment prematurely. They may need repeated hospital-based detoxification, extensive counseling, referral to Narcotics Anonymous, and psychotherapy. Many are better referred to drug-free groups, therapeutic communities, or other self-help groups to encourage total abstinence.

Many methadone programs report alcoholism among their patients before or during treatment (20–40%).[121] One carefully conducted prospective program study at Mt. Sinai Hospital in New York City followed a group of methadone recipients at the start and prospectively for two years. The prevalence of alcoholism was about the same at the onset as it was for 2 years later. The number of patients achieving remission and losing this label equaled the number of new patients developing alcoholism. These data imply that there is not a major pathway toward alcoholism for patients in the methadone maintenance programs. These data are at variance with the view that many addicts turn excessively to alcohol to get "high" if the cross-tolerance conferred by methadone blocks the highs formerly obtained through other narcotics.

The alcoholic methadone recipient generally can have the opioid component managed with methadone. However, the alcohol component can be more refractory. Cessation of methadone has not been a useful clinical step per se, as the alcohol abuse is usually not favorably affected. Treatment for mixed methadone–alcohol addictions can also include disulfiram, as there is no pharmacologic reason precluding this combination.[122] They should not be dispensed in one container for take-home purposes. However, even if well labeled, as unexpected toxicity may arise by alcohol consumption in an uninformed opiate user.

9. Barbiturates and Other Sedatives

9.1. Introduction

Use of barbiturates by Americans in recent years has been largely replaced by better alternatives. Thus, the incidence of barbiturate abuse has sharply decreased.[123] Occasionally, they are a primary drug of abuse per se, but more often they are used as one of many components in polydrug abuse. Mainly metabolized by the MEOS, the barbiturates can also be potent MEOS inducers. Accordingly, as with other MEOS-inducer drugs, they are more rapidly metabolized when used singly and compete when combined with most MEOS-metabolized drugs.[124] Recent studies of receptor interaction and discrimination between barbiturates and other sedatives are suggestive of some similarities and differences.[125,126] Other formerly popular sedatives such as methaqualone have also become much less involved in drug abuse recently.

9.2. Acute and Chronic Sedative Reactions

Acutely, barbiturates or other sedatives in combination produce added sedation. Chronically, the effects depend on doses, magnitude of tolerance, and the specific pharmacodynamics of the sedatives used.

9.3. Management

Management of acute barbiturate overdose with or without additional sedatives has become well standardized in emergency rooms and intensive care units. The chronic barbiturate abuser should be immediately hospitalized for a regularized, closely supervised withdrawal of drugs. The withdrawal syndrome usually begins about 12–36 hr after the last dose and include signs of catecholamine hyperactivity, such as tachycardia, tremulousness, insomnia, diaphoresis, hyperreflexia, and grand mal convulsions. When very severe, it may progress to fever, confusion, cardiovascular collapse, and death. The general principles include a phenobarbital or pentobarbital substitution and then gradual tapering of the dose.[47] The initial stabilizing dose may be estimated from the patient's history, although its reliability may be questionable. An alternative procedure consists of a pentobarbital sedative tolerance test. Initially 200 mg of oral pentobarbital is given followed by 100 mg every hour until signs of sedative excess occur, such as ataxia, slurred speech, somnolence, or nystagmus. The total dose is then the initial stabilization dose and is given in divided aliquots for 1–2 days. Then, daily tapering of 50–100 mg of pentobarbital follows. Referral to substance abuse treatment centers should ensue for chronic care.

9.4. Cannabis

The psychoactive cannabinoids have sedative properties. They are frequently consumed together with alcohol, probably for reasons that may be more associative or resultant from learned behavior than pharmacological.[127,128] Moreover, there do not seem to be important interactions between cannabis, alcohol, or other sedatives other than enhanced depression.[129] The detection of recent cannabis use was not a factor in the retention in substance abuse treatment of patients with alcoholism.[130] Their use, with or without other sedatives, may be hazardous in operating machinery, such as motor cars.

Conclusions

1. In this age of widespread availability of psychoactive drugs, use of multiple sedatives is very common.
2. Recognition of mixed-sedative abuse explains some otherwise perplexing clinical findings.
3. The metabolic bases of sedative interactions are increasingly well understood.
4. Recognition of mixed-sedative abuse can result in better overall clinical management.
5. Mixed-sedative abuse may have different prognostic significance than abuse of single drugs.

References

1. Chambers CD, Hunt LG: Epidemiology of drug abuse, in Pradhan SN, Dutta SN (eds): *Drug Abuse: Clinical and Basic Aspects*. St. Louis, CV Mosby, 1977, pp 11–39.
2. Hoyumpa AM: Alcohol interactions with benzodiazepines and cocaine. *Adv Alcohol Substance Abuse* 3:21–33, 1984.
3. Mayer JM: Mechanisms of drug interactions with alcohol. *Adv Alcohol Substance Abuse* 3:7–20, 1984.
4. Stockley I: *Drug Interactions*. Oxford, Blackwell Scientific Publications, 1981.
5. Greenblatt DJ, Shader RI: Benzodiazepines. *New Engl J Med* 23:1239–1245, 1974.

6. Charness ME, Gordon AS, Diamond I: Ethanol modulation of opiate receptor in cultured neural cells. *Science* 222:1246–1248, 1984.
7. Freund G: Benzodiazepine receptor loss in brains of mice after chronic alcohol consumption. *Life Sci* 27:987–992, 1980.
8. Lieber CS, Leo MA: Alcohol and the liver, in Lieber CS (ed): *Medical Disorders of Alcoholism: Pathogenesis and Treatment. Major Problems in Internal Medicine.* Philadelphia, WB Saunders, 1982, vol 22, pp 250–350.
9. Cohen, S: *The Substance Abuse Problem.* New York, Hayworth Press, 1981, pp 96–135.
10. Routtenberg A: Drugs of abuse and the endogenous reinforcement system: The resistance of intracranial self stimulation behavior to the inebriating effects of ethanol. *Ann NY Acad Sci* 362:60–66, 1981.
11. Lorens SA, Savinati SM: Naloxone blocks the excitatory effects of ethanol on chlordiazepoxide in the lateral hypothalamus self stimulation behavior. *Life Sci* 25:1359–1364, 1978.
12. Boxarth MA, Gerber GJ, Wise RA: Intracranial self stimulation as a technique to study the reward properties of drug abuse. *Pharmacol Biochem Behav* 13:245–247, 1980.
13. Clavier RM, Routtenberg A: In search of reinforcement pathways: A neuroanatomical odyssey, in Routtenberg A (ed): *Biology of Reinforcement: Facet of Brain Stimulation Rewards.* New York, Academic Press, 1980, pp 81–105.
14. Bermudez-Rattonu F, Cruz-Morales S, Reid LD: Addictive agents and intracranial stimulation (ICS): Novel antagonists and agonists of morphine and pressing for ICS. *Pharmacol Biochem Behav* 18:77–78, 1983.
15. Weibel SL, Wolf HH: Opiate modification of intracranial self stimulation in the rat. *Pharmacol Biochem Behav* 10:71–78, 1979.
16. Nahas GC: *Marijuana: Chemistry, Biochemistry, and Cellular Effects.* New York, Springer Verlag, 1976.
17. Morelli HF: Rational therapy of poisoning, in Melmon KL, Morelli HF (eds): *Clinical Pharmacology: Basic Principles of Therapeutics.* New York, Macmillan, 1978, pp 1044–1045.
18. Sioris LJ, Krenzelak EP: Phencyclidine intoxification: A literature review. *Am J Hosp Pharm* 35:1362–1367, 1978.
19. Morrelli HF: Rational therapy of poisoning, in Melmon KL, Morelli HF (eds): *Clinical Pharmacology: Basic Principles of Therapeutics.* New York, Macmillan, 1978, pp 1040–1057.
20. Cohen MR, Cohen RM, Pickar D, et al: High dose naloxone infusion in normals. *Arch Gen Psychiatry* 45:613–619, 1982.
21. Martin WR: Naloxone, *Ann Intern Med* 85:765–768, 1976.
22. Darragh A, Lambe R, Kenny M, et al: Tolerance of healthy volunteers to intravenous administration of the benzodiazepine antagonist RO 15,1788. *Eur J Clin Pharmacol* 24:569–70, 1982.
23. Darragh A, Lambe R, Kenny M: RO-15,1788 antagonizes the central effects of diazepam without altering diazepam bioavailability. *Br J Clin Pharmacol* 677–682, 1982.
24. Pristach CA, Smith CM, Whitney RB: Alcohol withdrawal syndromes—prediction from detailed medical and drinking histories. *Drug Alcohol Depend* 11:177–199, 1983.
25. Maddox JF, Elliott B: Problem drinkers among patients on methadone. *Am J Drug Alcohol Abuse* 2:245–254, 1975.
26. Dutta SN, Kaufman E: Multiple drug abuse, in Pradhan SN, Dutta SN (eds): *Drug Abuse: Clinical and Basic Aspects.* St. Louis, CV Mosby, 1977.
27. Fuller RH, Roth HP: Disulfiram for treatment of alcoholism. *Ann Intern Med* 90:901–904, 1979.
28. Dole VP, Nyswander ME, DesJarlais D, et al: Performance-based rating of methadone maintenance programs. *New Engl J Med* 306:169 170, 1982.
29. Kaufman E: The abuse of multiple drugs. *Am J Drug Alcohol Abuse* 3:279–301, 1976.
30. Kleber HD, Weissman MM, Rounsaville BJ, et al: Imipramine as treatment for depression in addicts. *Arch Gen Psychiatry* 40:649–653, 1983.
31. Kalant H: Observations on a decade of alcohol and drug research. *Drug Alcohol Depend* 11:3–8, 1983.

32. Tabakoff B: Current trends in biological research in alcoholism. *Drug Alcohol Depend* 11:33–37, 1983.
33. Chin JH, Goldstein DB: Drug tolerance in biomembranes. *Science* 196:684–685, 1976.
34. Droitte Y, Lamboeuf Y, de Saint Blanquat G: Membrane fatty acid changes and ethanol tolerance in rat and mouse. *Life Sci* 35:1221–1229, 1984.
35. Klemm WR: Opiate mechanisms: Evaluation of research involving neuromal action potentials. *Prog Neuropsychol Pharmacol* 5:1–33, 1981.
36. Nicholl RA: Responses of central nerves to opiates and opioid peptides. *Adv Biochem Psychopharmacol* 33:337–346, 1982.
37. West RE: Opiates, second messengers and cell response. *Br Med Bull* 39:53–58, 1983.
38. Way EL: Some thoughts about opiopeptins, peptides with opiate like activity. *Drug Alcohol Depend* 111:23–32, 1983.
39. Lippa AS, Meyerson LR, Beer B: Molecular substrates of anxiety: Clues from the heterogeneity of benzodiazepine receptors. *Life Sci* 31:1409–1417, 1982.
40. Skolnick P, Paul SM: Molecular pharmacology of the benzodiazepines. *Int Rev Neurobiol* 23:103–140, 1982.
41. Geller HM, Hotter BJ, Taylor DD: Electrophysiological actions of benzodiazepines. *Fed Proc* 39:3016–3023, 1982.
42. Study RE, Barker JL: Cellular mechanisms of benzodiazepine action. *JAMA* 247:2147–2152, 1982.
43. Young WS, Kuhar M: Radiohistochemical localization of benzodiazepine receptors in rat brains. *J Pharmacol Exp Ther* 212:337–346, 1980.
44. Yamada KA, Moerschbaecher JM, Hamosh P, et al: Pentobarbital causes cardiorespiratory depression by interacting with GABAergic system at the ventral surface of the medulla. *J Pharmacol Exp Ther* 226:349–352, 1983.
45. Wilder BJ, Bruni J: Mechanism of action of antiepileptic drugs. *Clinical Neuropharmacol* 5:23–43, 1982.
46. Sillanpaa ML: Alcoholism: Treatment of alcohol withdrawal symptoms: *Br J Hosp Med* 27:343–350, 1982.
47. Czechowicz D: *Detoxification Treatment Manual.* National Institute of Drug Abuse. Rockville, Maryland, 1981.
48. Sellars EM, Kalant H: Alcohol intoxification and withdrawal. *New Engl J Med* 294:757–762, 1976.
49. Greenblatt DJ, Greenblatt M: Which drug for alcohol withdrawal? *J Clin Pharmacol* 12:429–431, 1972.
50. Thompson WL, Johnson AD, Maddrey WL: Diazepam and paraldehyde for treatment of serious delirium tremens: A controlled trial. *Ann Intern Med* 82:175–180, 1975.
51. Washton AM, Resnick RB, Geyer G: Opiate withdrawal using lofexidine, a clonidine analogue with fewer side effects. *J Clin Psychiatry* 44:335–337, 1983.
52. Wilkins AJ, Jenkins WJ, Steiner JA: Efficacy of clonidine in treatment of alcohol state. *Psychopharmacology* 81:78–80, 1983.
53. Gessner PK: Failure of phenytoin to prevent alcohol withdrawal convulsions in mice. *Eur J Pharmacol* 27:120–129, 1974.
54. Sampliner R, Iber FL: Diphenylhydantoin control of alcohol withdrawal seizure. *JAMA* 230:1431–1432, 1974.
55. Keilty SR: Anesthesia for the alcoholic patient. *Anesthesia Analgesia* 48:649–664, 1969.
56. Caton DG: *The Anesthesiologist Handbook,* ed 3. Baltimore, University Park Press, 1983, p 47.
57. Greenblatt DJ, Shader RI: Dependence, tolerance, and addiction to benzodiazepines; clinical and pharmacokinetic considerations. *Drug Metab Rev* 8:13–28, 1978.
58. Costa E, Guidsh A: Molecular mechanism in the receptor action of benzodiazepines. *Annu Rev Pharmacol Toxicol* 19:531–545, 1979.
59. Dorow R, Hosowski R, Paschelke G, Amin M, Braestrop C: Severe anxiety induced by FG 142, a B carboline ligand for benzodiazepine receptors. *Lancet* 2:98–99, 1983.
60. Nivan PT, Insel TM, Cohen RM, et al: Benzodiazepine receptor-mediated experimental anxiety in primates. *Science* 218:1332–1334, 1982.

61. Mendelson WB, Cain M, Cook JM, et al: A benzodiazepine receptor antagonist decreases sleep and reverses the hypnotic action of flurazepam. *Science* 219:414–416, 1983.
62. Greenblatt DJ, Divoll M, Abernathy DR, et al: Benzodiazepine kinetics: Implication for therapeutics and pharmacogeriatrics. *Drug Metab Rev* 14:251–292, 1983.
63. Greenblatt DJ, Shader RI: Caution in the use of benzodiazepines in the elderly. *New Engl J Med* 300:1054–1055, 1979.
64. Kenny AD: Designing therapy for the aged. *Drug Therapy* 9:49–64, 1979.
65. Atkinson RM, Kofoed LL: Substance abuse in the elderly. *Substance Abuse* 5:1–14, 1984.
66. Project DAWN. V. National Institutes on Drug Abuse, Rockville, Maryland, 1977.
67. Solomon F, White CC, Parron DL, et al: Sleeping pills, insomnia and medical practice. *New Engl J Med* 300:803–804, 1979.
68. Finkle BS, McCloskey KL, Goodman LS: Diazepam and drug-associated deaths. *JAMA* 242:429–431, 1979.
69. Oswald I, Adam K, Borrow E, et al: The effects of two hypnotics on sleep, subjective feelings and skilled performances, in Passouant P, Oswald I (eds): *Pharmacology of the States of Alertness*. London, Pergamon Press, 1979.
70. Neuteboom W, Zweipfenning PGM: Driving and the combined use of drugs and alcohol in the Netherlands. *Forensic Sci Int* 25:93–104, 1984.
71. Ruffalo RL, Thompson JF: Effect of cimetidine on the clearance of benzodiazepines. *New Engl J Med* 303:753, 1980.
72. Vesell ES: Elucidation of the pharmacokinetic interaction between acutely administered ethanol and benzodiazepines. *Clin Pharmacol Ther* 95:305–309, 1980.
73. Woody GE, O'Brien CP, Greenstein R: Use and misuse of diazepam. *Int J Addict* 10:843–845, 1975.
74. Winokur A, Rickels K, Greenblatt DJ, et al: Withdrawal reaction from long term, low dosage administration of diazepam. *Arch Gen Psychiatry* 37:101–105, 1980.
75. Benzer D, Cushman P: Benzodiazepines and alcohol: Withdrawal syndromes. *Alcoholism: Clin Exp Res* 4:243–251, 1980.
76. Tyrer P, Owen R, Dawling S: Gradual withdrawal of diazepam after long-term therapy. *Lancet* 1:1402–1404, 1983.
77. Fontaine R, Chouvinard G, Annable L: Rebound anxiety in anxious patients after abrupt discontinuation of benzodiazepines. *Am J Psychiatry* 141:848–857, 1984.
78. Comfort A: Alcohol as a social drug and health hazard. *Lancet* 1:443–444, 1984.
79. Ruttenberg, AJ, Luke J: Heroin-related deaths: New epidemiologic insights. *Science* 226:14–19, 1984.
80. Pirola RC: *Drug Metabolism and Alcohol: A Survey of Alcohol–Drug Reactions—Mechanisms, Clinical Aspects, Experimental Studies*. Baltimore, University Park Press, 1978.
81. Sellars EM, Lang M, Koch-Weser J, et al: Interaction of chloral hydrate and alcohol in man. *Clin Pharmacol Ther* 13:37–49, 1972.
82. Lieber CS, DeCarli LM: Ethanol oxidation by hepatic microsomes. *Science* 162:917–918, 1968.
83. Schoemaker H, Smith TL, Yamamura MI: Effect of chronic ethanol consumption on central and peripheral type benzodiazepine binding sites in the mouse brain. *Brain Res* 258:347–350, 1983.
84. Melchior CL, Tabakoff B: Interaction between ethanol and compounds which act at the benzodiazepine receptor. *Alcoholism Clin Exp Res* 8:107, 1984.
85. Lieber CS, Pirola RC: Clinical relevance of alcohol–drug reactions *Adv Alcohol Substance Abuse* 1:41–66, 1981.
86. Chan AWK: Cross tolerance between ethanol and chlordiazepoxide in mice. *Alcoholism Clin Exp Res* 8:84, 1984.
87. Hoyumpa AM, Desmond PV, Roberts RK, et al: Effect of ethanol on benzodiazepine disposition. *J Lab Clin Med* 95:310–317, 1980.
88. Roberts R, Wilkinson GR, Branch RA, et al: Effect of age and cirrhosis on the disposition and elimination of chlordiazepoxide. *Gastroenterology* 75:479–485, 1978.

89. Sellars EM, Greenblatt DJ, Giles HG, et al: Chlordiazepoxide and oxazepam disposition in cirrhosis. *Clin Pharmacol Ther* 26:240–246, 1979.
90. Gordis E, Sereny G: Effect of prior narcotic addition on response to treatment in alcoholism. *Alcoholism Clin Exp Res* 4:35–39, 1980.
91. Simon EJ: Recent studies on opioid receptors: Heterogeneity and isolation problems of drug dependence, National Institutes on Drug Abuse Monograph #48, Rockville Maryland, 1983, pp 5–13.
92. Goldstein A: Some thoughts about endogenous opioids and addiction. *Drug Alcohol Depend* 11:11–15, 1983.
93. Malickm JB, Bell RMS: *Endorphins: Chemistry, Physiology, Pharmacology and Clinical Relevance.* New York, Marcel Dekker, 1982.
94. Simon EJ: Recent studies on opioid receptors: Heterogeneity and isolation. NIDA Research monograph #49, Rockville, Maryland, 1983.
95. Tabakoff B, Borg S, Valvenus P, et al: Neuronal receptors and transmitter enzymes in brain and platelets of alcoholics. *Alcoholism Clin Exp Res* 81:250, 1984.
96. Schultz R, Wuster M, Duka J, et al: Acute and chronic ethanol treatment changes endorphin levels in brain and pituitary. *Psychopharmacology* 68:221–227, 1980.
97. Charness ME, Gordon AS, Diamond I: Ethanol modulation of opiate receptors in cultured neural cells. *Science* 222:1246–1248, 1983.
98. Seizinger BR, Bovermann K, Maysinger D, et al: Differential effects of acute and chronic ethanol treatment on particular opioid peptide systems in discrete regions of rat brain and pituitary. *Pharmacol Biochem Behav* 18(suppl 1):361–369, 1981.
99. Ewing JA, McCarthy D: Are the endorphins involved in mediating the mood effects of ethanol? *Alcoholism Clin Exp Res* 7:271–276, 1983.
100. Eidelberg E: On the possibility that opiate and ethanol actions are mediated by similar mechanism. *Adv Exp Biol Med* 85:87–94, 1977.
101. Berman RF, Lee JA, Olson KL: Effects of naloxone on ethanol dependence in rats. *Drug Alcohol Depend* 13:245–254, 1984.
102. Malarkey HG, Mezey E: Induction of alcohol withdrawal symptoms by nalorphine in chronic alcoholic patients. *Int J Addict* 13:395–402, 1978.
103. Hemmingsen R, Sorenson SC: Absence of an effect of naloxone on ethanol intoxification and withdrawal reactions. *Acta Pharmacol Toxicol* 46:62–65, 1980.
104. Bass MD, Friedman HJ, Lester D: Antagonism of naloxone hyperalgesia by ethanol. *Life Sci* 22:1939–1946, 1978.
105. Sorenson SC, Mattisson K: Naloxone as an antagonist in severe alcohol intoxification. *Lancet* 2:688–689, 1978.
106. Kreek MJ: Opioid interactions with alcohol. *Adv Alcohol Substance Abuse* 3:35–46, 1984.
107. McCormick GY, White WJ, Zagon IS, et al: Effects of diazepam on arterial blood gas concentrations and pH of adult rats acutely and chronically exposed to methadone. *J Pharmacol Exp Ther* 230:353–361, 1984.
108. Cooper SJ: Benzodiazepines—opiate antagonist interactions in relation to feeding and drinking behavior. *Life Sci* 32:1043–1051, 1983.
109. True WR, Pevnick JS: Abuse of pentazocine combined with tripelennamine: An interaction of pharmacological and demographic characteristics. *Int J Addict* 18:1063–1071, 1983.
110. Jasinski DR, Boren JJ, Henningfield JE, et al: Progress report from the NIDA Addiction Research Center. National Institutes of Drug Abuse monograph #49. Rockville, Maryland, 1983, pp 69–76.
111. Borowsky SA, Lieber CS: Interaction of alcohol and methadone. *J Pharmacol Exp Ther* 207:124–129, 1978.
112. Inturrisi CE, Verebely K: Disposition of methadone after a single dose. *Clin Pharmacol Ther* 13:923–929, 1972.
113. Brunk SF, Delle MD: Morphine metabolism in man. *Clin Pharmacol Ther* 16:51–58, 1974.
114. Jackson GW, Richmond A: Alcohol use among narcotic addicts. *Alcohol World* 1:25–28, 1973.
115. Kreek MJ: Medical complications in methadone patients. *Ann NY Acad Sci* 311:110–134, 1978.

116. Cushman P, Kreek MJ, Gordis E: Ethanol and methadone in man: A possible interaction. *Drug Alcohol Depend* 3:35–40, 1978.
117. O'Brien CP, Greenstein R, Ternes J, et al: Clinical pharmacology of narcotic antagonists. *Ann NY Acad Sci* 311:222–239, 1978.
118. Gold MS, Pottash AC, Sweeney DR, et al: Opiate withdrawal using clonidine. *JAMA* 243:343–345, 1980.
119. Gold MS, Pottash ALC, Annito WL, et al: Lofexidine in opiate withdrawal. *Lancet* 1:992–993, 1981.
120. Novick DM: Major medical porblems and detoxifying treatment of parenteral drug-using alcoholics. *Adv Alcohol Substance Abuse* 3:87–105, 1984.
121. Stimmel B, Hanbury R, Sturiano V, et al: Alcoholism as a risk factor in methadone maintenance. *Am J Med* 73:631–636, 1980.
122. Liebson I, Biegelow G, Flamer R: Alcoholism among methadone patients: A specific treatment method. *Am J Pyschiatry* 130:483–491, 1973.
123. Nicholson AN: The use of short- and long-acting hypnotics in clinical medicine. *Br J Clin Pharmacol* 11:16s, 1981.
124. Rickels K: Clinical trials of hypnotics. *J Clin Psychopharmacol* 3:133–139, 1983.
125. Skolnick P, Moncada V, Barker JL, et al: Pentobarbital: Dual actions to increase brain benzodiazepine receptor affinity. *Science* 211:1446–1450, 1980.
126. Ator NA, Griffiths RR: Lorazepam and pentobarbital drug discrimination in baboons: Cross drug generalization and interactions with RO 15-1788. *J Pharmacol Exp Ther* 226:776–781, 1983.
127. Barbor TF, Mendelson JH, Gallant D, et al: Interpersonal behavior in group discussion during marijuana intoxification. *Int J Addict* 31:89–102, 1978.
128. Mello NK, Mendelson JH, Sellars ML, et al: Effect of alcohol and marijuana and tobacco smoking. *Clin Pharmacol Ther* 27:202–209, 1980.
129. Siemens AJ, Khanna JM: Acute metabolic interactions between ethanol and cannabis. *Alcoholism Clin Exp Res* 1:343–349, 1977.
130. Benzer D, Cushman P: Marijuana and alcoholism: Demographic characteristics and effects on early therapy. *Adv Alcohol Substance Abuse* 2:53–60, 1982.

4

Treating Multiple Substance Abuse Clients

Jerome F. X. Carroll

Abstract. The traditional separation of alcohol-dependent from drug-dependent persons no longer accords with contemporary patterns of substance abuse, especially for people below the age of 40. In ever-increasing numbers, the pattern of abuse is one of multiple substance abuse (MSA). Overwhelmingly, MSA involves the sequential or concurrent abuse of alcohol and one or more other drugs. Treatment centers need to be cognizant of this development, especially in taking accurate substance abuse histories and providing effective inpatient and aftercare services. A generic perspective of etiology, defenses, and treatment is provided, as well as a discussion of three varieties of combined treatment (conscious, overt; conscious, covert; and unconscious). Specific treatment interventions are suggested, as well as strategies for staffing and staff training. Finally, the need to provide a suitable therapeutic and living environment for the heterogeneity of clients likely to present with MSA is stressed.

1. Introduction

By now, most people in the substance abuse field are quite familiar with the phenomenon of multiple substance abuse (MSA). Examples of MSA would include: the 18-year-old who gets high on PCP, marijuana, and alcohol at parties; the 65-year-old women who drinks five or six shots of whiskey each day while also taking some of her sister's Valiums and Seconals to "quiet her nerves"; the methadone maintenance patient who "stays straight" from heroin but who gets "a little high" on weekends from alcohol and marijuana; and the "speed" addict who uses alcohol and/or Quaaludes to ease his/her withdrawal.

Some important questions posed by the phenomenon of MSA are these: To what extent should MSA be a matter of concern to those who provide rehabilitative services to substance abusers? Do the multiple substance abuser's (MSAer) treatment needs differ sufficiently from the single substance abuser's (SSAer) treatment needs? Who can best treat the MSAer and with what treatment modalities?

Jerome F.X. Carroll • Continuum Program, Eagleville Hospital, Eagleville, Pennsylvania 19408.

2. Scope and Significance of the Problem

More and more, the trend in substance abuse in the United States[1] and other nations[2] is toward MSA. MSA involves the abuse of two or more psychoactive substances, either in some sequence wherein a person begins abusing one substance and then moves on to another or the individual abuses several substances in an interrelated manner during the same time frame (e.g., to boost, balance, counteract, or sustain the effects of the "high").

In one of the earliest survey studies designed specifically to investigate MSA, the National Drug/Alcohol Collaborative Project (NDACP)[3] obtained detailed substance abuse data on 1544 subjects from ten federally funded treatment centers. Subjects were asked about their use/abuse of the following substances over their entire life history ("ever") and during the last 3 months prior to their admission to treatment: alcohol, heroin, other opiates, amphetamines, barbiturates, minor tranquilizers, marijuana/hashish, illegal methadone, cocaine, hallucinogens, inhalants, over-the-counter drugs, antidepressants, and major tranquilizers.

The principal finding of the NDACP was that the majority of substance abusers (80%) reported they had abused two or more substances, either sequentially and/or concurrently, at some time during their history of substance abuse ("ever"). With few exceptions, the MSA involved alcohol and one or more other psychoactive substances, such as marijuana, amphetamines, or "minor tranquilizers."[3,4] Only 20% reported single substance abuse (SSA) during the "ever" period. When only the 3-month period prior to admission to treatment was considered, 56% reported MSA, while 34% reported SSA (10% reported no substance abuse for that period, due almost exclusively to incarceration).

SSA for the "ever" period always involved alcohol. For the 3-month period, alcohol still accounted for most of the SSA (81% of all SSA). SSA patterns for marijuana/hashish (8%) and heroin (4%) were also reported for the 3-month period. Nearly half (49%) of all SSAers were 40 years or older, which suggests that MSA is the pattern that most treatment centers will be encountering in future years.[3,4]

The findings of the NDACP have been corroborated by a number of other studies and clinical observations reported in the literature.[5–19]

2.1. Segregation by Substance of Abuse Persists

Despite mounting clinical and scientific evidence that clearly demonstrates the preeminence of MSA (especially of alcohol and one or more other psychoactive substances), the substance abuse field remains relatively steadfast in its segregation of "alcoholics" from "addicts" with respect to treatment. This form of segregation gives rise to a number of significant negative consequences, including the following:

1. A client's complete substance abuse history typically will not be accurately obtained and/or evaluated; therefore the problem will only be partially addressed in treatment.

2. Staff usually are not fully trained and/or encouraged to treat those aspects of the client's addiction that are not the primary focus of the treatment center (e.g., a methadone maintenance program may give little attention to past or present instances of alcohol abuse).

3. Clients with MSA problems will be turned away from certain treatment centers and self-help groups who will not work with anyone who has abused one or more of the substances in the MSA pattern. In many cases, this rejection can be a life-threatening situation.

4. Clients assume that certain substances they have occasionally used in some "minor" way are "safe" to use after completing treatment. This assumption leads to the attempted "social use" of the "safe" substance which often precipitates a total relapse.

5. Research data on substance abuse patterns reported from these treatment centers to NIDA and NIAAA are inaccurate to the extent they are incomplete, which, in turn, distorts the entire field's understanding of the epidemiology of substance abuse patterns within the United States.

6. The general public, including legislators, takes its lead from the professionals; therefore if the professionals act as if contemporary substance abusers are either "alcoholics" or "addicts," the general public will continue to view these two groups as very different (the drug addict usually being viewed and treated less well).

2.2. Identifying Overt and Covert MSA

With respect to overt MSA, where the client is willing and able to honestly provide a complete history of his/her substance abuse, the attitudes and experience of the staff member taking the substance abuse history becomes the critical variable. Since some institutions (e.g., a private hospital treating middle- to upper-class alcoholics) will not admit clients who have abused certain substances (e.g., heroin), a staff member desiring to admit a particular client may do one of two things. S/he may simply not inquire about any involvement with substances that would preclude admission, or s/he may inquire, but not record the information. In the latter instance, staff will often minimize the significance of that involvement.

In other instances (e.g., a drug treatment center), staff may not ask any questions about alcohol abuse and/or ask only the most superficial of questions about the client's drinking. Often drawing upon their own experience with a substance (e.g., heroin), staff members may incorrectly assume that the "primary" cause of most, if not all, of the client's problems is his/her abuse of heroin; therefore, there seems to be no real need to ask in-depth questions about alcohol.

2.3. Covert Forms of MSA

If this problem were not enough of an impediment, consider what happens in the case of covert MSA. Covert MSA may take one of two forms. One form involves those cases wherein a client is unaware of the significant role played by a particular substance in his/her substance abuse problem. A classic example would be the individual who identifies him/herself as a "drug addict" and gives little attention to his/her past and/or present abuse of alcohol. Another would be the older "alcoholic" who never thought much about his/her misuse of prescriptive medications, because "The doctor told me to take 'em." In such cases, the initial line of inquiry concerning abuse may meet with a genuine "No," and unless the staff person taking the substance abuse history persists with some collateral questions, the whole issue will go undetected and unreported.

The second form of covert MSA involves those cases wherein the client does know that his/her abuse of some "secondary" substance of abuse is significantly related to the addiction. The client in this instance simply does not want to commit him/herself to total abstinence (e.g., a heroin or amphetamine addict who does not want to stop using marijuana or alcohol). When asked about the use and/or significance of these "secondary" substances by a staff member, the client will either deny such use or greatly minimize its significance.

Four strong recommendations to guard against obtaining inaccurate data are:

1. Take a complete substance abuse history, starting with any use at any age; ask about all categories of substances, using both the pharmaceutical and street names (having pictures of substances aids the inquiry); even "experimental use" should be recorded (i.e., "tried it a few times [5 or less] to see what it was like").
2. Ask the client what substance(s) s/he used when s/he could not get the substance they normally used and/or when circumstances prevented such use.
3. Ask if s/he ever used any other substance(s) to boost, balance, counteract, or sustain the effects of the substance s/he normally used.
4. Update the substance use history at regular intervals as new information is obtained by staff instructed to inquire about MSA throughout the entire course of treatment.

Some specific questions which can be asked are these:

For alcoholics:

Have you ever taken any medication for problems associated with your drinking? If so, what medications did you use and for how long?

Did you ever use these medications in a manner different from that prescribed by your doctor (e.g., taking more than the prescribed amount and/or using them longer than your doctor had indicated?)

Did you ever use medication prescribed by a doctor for a relative or friend to help you calm your nerves or get to sleep at night?

Did you ever take any medication or pills just to see what it was like and how it would work?

Did you ever take any medication or pills just to enjoy the feeling they give you?

Did you ever take any medication or pills for some other nonmedical reason, and not because you needed it?

Have you ever taken medication or pills to help you get ready for some big event, or to help you accomplish something?

Have you ever taken any medication or pills before going out, so that you could enjoy yourself more with other people?

Did you ever take any medication or pills when drinking to get a better "buzz" or a different kind of high?

Did you ever take any medication or pills to help you counteract the effects of hangovers?

Did you ever smoke any "grass," marijuana? If so, how often and for how long? Did you ever smoke grass while you were drinking?

For drug-dependent persons:

Do you still attend social gatherings/parties where you do some social drinking? If yes, what do you typically drink? How much? How often?

At these gatherings did you typically make contact with others who were using drugs or could supply them to you? Did you ever use drugs while attending such parties?

What did you typically use when you couldn't get your drug of choice? Did you ever use alcohol as a substitute? (If client names marijuana, inquire whether it was used along with alcohol). Have you ever gotten "high" on drugs and alcohol? Was it a pleasant "high"?[20]

3. Treatment Issues

3.1. The Generic Perspective

If one assumes a generic perspective on substance abuse, the treatment of a MSA problem involving alcohol *and* drugs becomes less imposing a task than if one perceives the abuse of alcohol and the abuse of drugs as very different phenomenon. The generic concept of addictions or substance abuse problems has been used to convey the idea that all substance abuse problems are part of the same problem, even though the choice of substance varies from person to person and the manifestations resulting from substance abuse differ from substance to substance. That one person is addicted to heroin and another to alcohol is less important from the generic perspective than the fact that both are abusing some chemical substance capable of leading to dependence and addiction.

The choice of a particular substance and consequent development of dependence to that substance (or group of substances) is in large part accidental. Who becomes an alcoholic and who is a narcotic addict or psychedelic substance abuser appear to depend on chance factors of time, place, and circumstance, as much as on individual constitutional or psychological factors. Where and when one was born, into what race, and which substances were available and being used by family members and/or one's peers are factors that together play a primary role in determining whether or not one will become substance dependent and to which substance(s).

This does not deny that some persons experiment with a variety of substances until they find what they like best, or that others practice self-medication, switching back and forth among several types of substances. The point being stressed is that social, cultural, and family variables are powerful determinants of substance abuse in contemporary life, and these factors are not specific to particular substances.

That there are special characteristics of various addictions or substance dependencies that makes them distinguishable from one another is not denied by those espousing the generic perspective. Thus, among the various substance dependencies, withdrawal states differ, if they occur at all. Tolerance develops at different rates and to different degrees, if at all. These differences, which some observers point to as evidence of specificity of various addictions, result from the specific pharmacologic and toxic properties of various chemicals. The existence of different qualities and effects of different drugs, however, does not negate the rationale for considering all types of substance abuse and dependence as varieties within a single class or genus.

3.2. Differences Most Critical in Detoxification

These "specific" differences that at certain times separate the alcoholic from the LSD abuser and the heroin addict from the glue sniffer are of utmost importance for the prompt and proper treatment of acute syndromes that occur in substance-abusing persons. In this phase of treatment (detoxification), one is dealing with specific effects of drugs, calling for specific treatments. Typically, this is a medical phase of treatment, which occurs in hospitals, medical clinics, emergency rooms, and physicians' offices where persons go for help or are taken when suffering from acute withdrawal symptoms or from the toxic or complicating effects of drugs. Once the acute, medically supervised phase of treatment is over, however, these specific, distinguishing variables dissipate and henceforth have relatively little importance in the treatment of the underlying addiction or substance dependence.

With respect to the detoxification of multiple substance-abusing patients, it is essential that the physician understand the relationship between various groups of substances that the patient may have abused. For example, any drugs that demonstrate cross-tolerance and cross-dependence with one another have a similar mechanism for the development of dependence. It is possible, therefore, to use a single medication to withdraw patients from one or more drugs in that class.[21,22]

Table I lists all of the drugs in the depressant or sedative-hypnotic class. Withdrawing patients from any of these drugs can be performed safely with phenobarbital.[23,24] Drugs that fall into the opiate class (Table I) all display cross-tolerance and cross-dependence with methadone, which is the drug of choice for withdrawal. For patients dependent on stimulant drugs, there are no specific drugs effective in treating the withdrawal symptoms.

When patients present with a mixed dependence that crosses drug classes, the treatment of choice is to place the patient on a medication that specifically blocks the withdrawal for each class of drug he or she has abused. Once stabilized, the patient should be withdrawn from one drug at a time. This tends to prolong the withdrawal process but makes it easier for the patient.

As the use of increasing numbers of drugs continues, the treatment of withdrawal and other medical aspects of drug abuse becomes more complicated. For example, patients may report having taken various drugs that they bought on the street; however, what they received may have been quite different from what they intended to purchase.[21,26] Thus, it is possible that patients may be dependent on drugs they never knew they were taking, or they may become dependent, because they were unaware of the close relationship between two or more drugs they were taking.

Any program involved in treating the multiple substance-abusing patient should have a member on the staff or a consultant who is familiar with this problem and the pharmacology of MSA.

A generic concept has no difficulty accommodating variations that result from the interaction of an individual person and a specific substance or substances. These are specific differences that do tend to distinguish various

Table I. Drug Classification by Substances Abused[a]

Sedative-hypnotics
Alcohol
Barbiturates: Seconal (secobarbital); Nembutal (pentobarbital); Amytal (amobarbital); Tuinal (secobarbital and amobarbital); Luminal (phenobarbital)
Sleeping pills: Noctec (chloral and/or hydrate); Quaalude, Parest, and Sopor (methaqualone); Placidyl (ethclorvynol); Doriden (glutethimide); Nodular (methyprylon); Dalmane (flurazepam)
Minor tranquilizers and anxiolytics: Equanil and Miltown (meprobamate); Valium (diazepam); Librium (chlordiazepoxide); Serax (oxazepam); Ativan (lorazepam); Tranxene (clorazepate); Verstran (prazepam)
Opiates: Opium; Heroin (diacetylimorphine); Morphine; Dilaudid (hydromorphinone); Numorphan (oxymorphone); Codeine; Talwin (pentazocine); Dolophine (methadone); Darvon (meperidine)
Stimulants: Benzedrine (amphetamine); Methedrine (methamphetamine); Dexedrine (dextroamphetamine); Preludin (phenmetrazine); Plegine (phendimetrazine); Ritalin (methyiphenidate); Cocaine

[a] Source: Carroll and Schnoll.[25]

types of substance dependence from one another at certain times. What is not acceptable to those adhering to a generic perspective are popularly held perceptions that imply either absolute difference or more differences than similarities between alcoholics and other substance-abusing groups. Little valid scientific evidence exists to support such claims.

Most of the perceived differences that distinguish one type of substance abuser from another have to do with such factors as age, race, generational lifestyle and values, language, degree of conformity to conventional modes of behavior, and so forth. None of these variables, however, is specific to any substance of abuse. Moreover, when researchers either "match" or statistically control for the effects of these variables in making comparisons of alcoholics and other substance abusers, far more similarities than differences are noted.[27–30]

3.3. Etiology, Defenses, Dynamics, and the Therapeutic Process

When one considers the etiology of alcoholism and drug addiction, the following factors are generally cited by researchers and clinicians as being the root cause(s) of the addiction: disturbed family relationships; parental modeling of substance abuse; social alienation; loneliness; feelings of powerlessness and inadequacy; normlessness; depression and anxiety; poverty; social prejudice; sexual frustration; guilt; repressed feelings of anger and rage; and acts of violence and crime. It should be obvious that these "causative factors" are commonly found in the backgrounds of both alcoholics and drug addicts, as well as MSAers.

With respect to defenses, alcoholics, addicts, and MSAers employ essentially the same defenses: denial, rationalization, and projection. Both manipulate while in treatment in order to avoid making meaningful changes in their addictive lifestyles. Examples of some of the more commonly encountered manipulative "games" of substance dependent persons include the "gorilla" game of intimidation; the perpetual jokester or entertainer who claims to have no serious problems; exaggerating depression; acting "crazy"; projecting an image of extreme fragility, weakness, inadequacy, helplessness, befuddlement, and indecisiveness; acting the part of the perfect patient; compulsively challenging all rules and authority in order to get discharged from treatment; acting as an assistant therapist for others' problems; totally absorbing one's self with music or sports while in treatment; and using sex to allay anxieties and/or get discharged from treatment.

Finally, the therapeutic process of substance abuse rehabilitation, regardless of the substance(s) abused, is essentially the same, which is to say that it is generic in character. The process involves:

1. Detoxification* and Continuing Detoxification
2. Restoration of Physical Health

* This goal, as previously stated, does necessitate specific forms of medical intervention depending on what substances were abused.

3. Restoration of Emotional Stability
4. Motivation to Accept Treatment
5. Aftercare Planning I: Establishing the Need for Post-Inpatient Treatment/Support
6. Challenging Destructive Defenses
7. Facilitation of Catharsis and Development of Insight
8. Establishing a Chemically Free Sense of Identity
9. Aftercare Planning II: Developing a Post-Inpatient Treatment/Support Plan
10. Aftercare Planning III: Implementing a Post-Inpatient Treatment/Support Plan

Each of the above generic goals can be evaluated in terms of very specific behavioral criteria.[31] For example, goal 4, Motivation to Accept Treatment, can be described in terms of four dimensions or elements. Progress in treatment, regardless of what substance(s) the person has abused, can be described in behavioral terms, for example, by using a five-point scale, from "very much in need of inpatient treatment" (Level 1) through "able to autonomously sustain sobriety and satisfy psychosocial needs" (Level 5) as follows:

Goal 4; Motivation to Accept Treatment
Element A: Acceptance of Problem
Element B: Level of Trust
Element C: Cooperation with Therapeutic Program
Element D: Personal Appearance and Mannerisms

Level 1
Element A: Denies or seriously doubts s/he is addicted, rejects information designed to heighten awareness of addiction.

Element B: Evidences extreme distrust of staff and/or peers; holds values in opposition to community's concern for honesty, responsible concern, and sharing thoughts and feelings.

Element C: Refuses to attend scheduled appointments and/or is frequently late; refuses to cooperate in therapeutic activities (e.g., will not share feelings in therapy sessions) and/or complete assigned tasks.

Element D: Patient's dress and grooming is disheveled, flamboyant, or projects a "street," addictive image; manner of speech and/or behavior reflects a hostile, threatening, or very guarded attitude toward treatment and members of the therapeutic community; very resistive to confrontations and suggestions to change.

Level 2
Element A: Patient beginning to consider that s/he may have an addiction or substance abuse problem, but only as a result of considerable staff and/or peer pressure; beginning to absorb selective addiction information, but only as a result of staff and/or peer pressure.

Element B: Shows minimal trust of selected staff and/or peers; begrudgingly will admit, when pressed, that there may be some value to therapeutic values of program; beginning to question former "street" addictive values, but only when pressed by staff and/or peers.

Element C: Patient will keep appointments and be on time, provided staff and/or peer pressure and support is applied; cooperation in therapeutic activities improving, but only as a result of staff and/or peer insistence to do so (e.g., will speak up in group when asked); will complete therapeutic tasks and assignments, but only under close supervision and with insistence to do so.

Element D: Patient's dress and grooming, as well as manner of speaking and behaving, still reflective of addictive lifestyle; however s/he will make minor changes when strongly confronted by staff and/or peers.

Level 3

Element A: Patient showing more acceptance of addictive/substance abuse problem(s), but regresses from time to time—needs staff and/or peer confrontation and support to sustain goals; s/he listening more carefully and accepting more addiction information, but still evidencing some denial and selective hearing (defending against) on selected occasions.

Element B: Trust level increasing, but still unstable and defensively selective in trusting staff and/or peers; evidences more acceptance and incorporation of therapeutic values, although still subject to sudden reversals to addictive values when staff and/or peer supports lessen.

Element C: Patient is on time and completes appointments, but does not yet exercise personal initiative in resolving schedule conflicts and/or adjusting to unanticipated schedule changes; client taking some initiative in sharing personal thoughts and feelings, but is inconsistent—will occasionally regress to closed, defensive behaviors when threatened or stressed; completes most assigned tasks—only occasionally needs staff and/or peer pressure support.

Element D: Patient's dress and grooming, as well as manner of speaking and behaving, show modest improvement, but gains are very much dependent on staff and/or peer pressure. Left alone, patient likely to regress to former addictive appearance and mannerisms.

Level 4

Element A: Patient generally acknowledges s/he is addicted—only occasionally needs confrontation or feedback in accepting personal significance of this fact; open to most addiction information provided him/her; occasionally helps others to acknowledge their addiction; will share with others, when asked, that s/he is addicted.

Element B: Trust level now extends to nearly all staff and to peers seriously making changes for sobriety—only occasionally needs staff and/or peer support to sustain gains during stressful periods; incorporation of program's therapeutic values is fairly strong and consistent, only occasionally needs support to prevent regression during stressful periods.

Element C: Patient keeps appointments and is on time—able to exercise limited initiative in revising schedules and insuring s/he gets what s/he needs therapeutically; patient's behavior in therapeutic setting is generally open, honest, and relevant—except for very stressful or threatening sessions, little regression noted; completes nearly all assigned therapeutic tasks in constructive and enthusiastic manner, with only limited staff and/or peer pressure needed to sustain this behavior.

Element D: Patient's dress and grooming, as well as manner of speaking and behaving, show modest improvement; only occasionally needs feedback from staff and/or peers to sustain gains.

Level 5

Element A: Patient sincerely acknowledges addiction and has an accurate, comprehensive grasp of the meaning of the term for him/her; s/he actively seeks out information on addiction; helps new patients and others to understand meaning of addiction; readily acknowledges s/he is a recovering person in appropriate situations.

Element B: Evidences appropriate trust in the therapeutic process; discriminates accurately among staff and clients regarding who should or should not be trusted; has internalized the therapeutic values of honesty, responsible concern, and sharing; attempts to help others understand and accept these values.

Element C: Patient exercises initiative and good time management in keeping appointments and resolving scheduling conflicts; seeks out therapeutic, self-development experiences on own; actively and constructively works in therapeutic settings; assists and urges others to work and take advantage of program; completes all therapeutic tasks on own and urges and assists others to do the same.

Element D: Patient's dress and grooming is clean, neat, and appropriate to the community's standards; manner of speech and behavior reflects an open, responsive, and positive attitude toward treatment and members of the therapeutic community. S/he exercises self-control and self-monitoring of these behaviors.

3.4. Combined Treatment

The discussion of treating the MSA client and the generic perspective naturally leads to a consideration of how these concepts relate to the concept of combined treatment.[25,32,33] Combined treatment consists of treating persons considered to be alcoholics and others considered to be drug addicts or drug abusers, as well as persons who have abused both drugs and alcohol in the same program. All types of substance abusers are treated together by the same staff using the same treatment procedures. Stated otherwise, although treatment regimens may vary to meet differing individual clinical problems, treatment does not differ simply on the basis of which substances have been abused, with the exception of how detoxification is medically managed.

The essential feature of combined treatment is that persons with different substance abuse histories and preferences are fully integrated into a single treatment program and process. Even though a treatment agency provides services to both drug addicts and alcoholics, it is not conducting combined treatment unless these two types of clients are treated in the same place, at the same time, by the same methods, and by the same staff.

The concept of combined treatment is most meaningful when applied in residential treatment settings, where persons of various backgrounds and substance abuse experience mingle in everyday living situations as well as during therapy per se. Combined treatment also is applicable in outpatient locations, although the impact on clients and staff and the issues that arise are different from the experience in the live-in environment.

3.5. Varieties of Combined Treatment

For purposes of elucidation, one can distinguish three varieties of combined treatment: (1) conscious, overt combined treatment; (2) conscious, covert combined treatment; and (3) unconscious combined treatment. In the first instance, programs, such as Eagleville Hospital's, publicly declare their intention to treat together clients presenting with all forms of addiction, within the same therapeutic program, using the same staff.

In the second case, a program that has publicly declared its intention to treat one particular variety of addiction (e.g., alcoholics or heroin addicts) recognizes that one or more "secondary" substances have been abused by its clientele, but for economic-political purposes it chooses not to publicize that such abuse has occurred and/or that these forms of abuse are being confronted and dealt with in treatment.

Lastly, there are programs that publicly declare they are in existence to treat one and only one variety of substance abuse. They deny other forms of

Table II. Eagleville Hospital Inpatient Discharges: January–December 1983

	Phase complete[a]			Phase incomplete[b]			AMA, AWOL, disciplinary[c]			Total	
	No.	%	Days in treatment	No.	%	Days in treatment	No.	%	Days in treatment	No.	Days in treatment
Alcohol only	266	55	38.9	74	15	19.9	143	30	14.5	483	28.8
Alcohol with secondary drug	169	53	40.0	55	17	19.8	94	30	15.0	318	29.1
Drug only	229	49	38.1	81	17	18.9	156	33	13.1	466	26.4
Drug with secondary alcohol	174	56	40.4	43	14	18.6	93	30	13.7	310	29.4

[a] Patient successfully completed treatment program.
[b] Patient failed to complete treatment program for other than disciplinary reasons.
[c] AMA, against medical advice; AWOL, absent without leave; disciplinary, for violence, use or possession of unauthorized substances or egregious and/or repeated violations of program rules.
[d] Average length of stay.

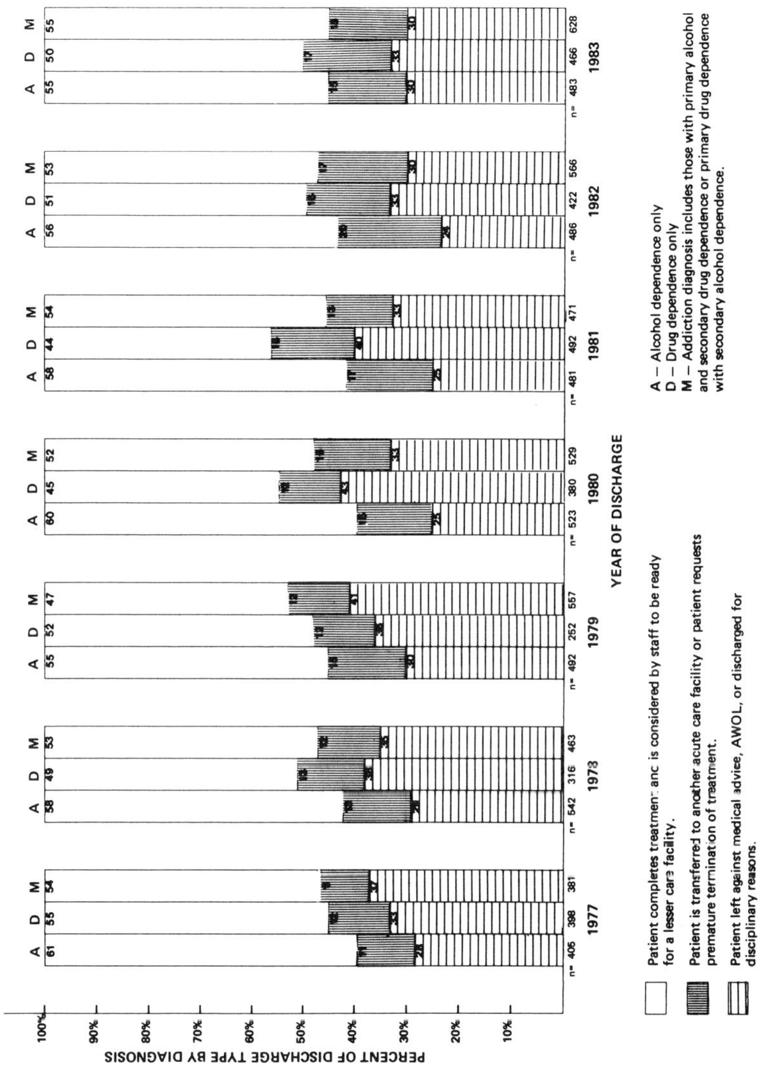

Figure 1. Eagleville Hospital inpatient discharges. Type of discharge by addiction diagnosis.

substance abuse exist at their facility and/or genuinely believe that such abuse is of little consequence. To the extent their client population contains people who have engaged in MSA, the program can be said to be doing combined treatment, without even realizing it is doing so, albeit a less than effective variety of combined treatment.

To work with multiple substance-abusing clients, the vast majority of whom have most likely abused both alcohol and one or more other drugs, in effect is to be engaged in some form of combined treatment. Preferably, the service will be conscious and overt, since this variety of combined treatment offers the best possibilities for providing effective treatment. The only question then becomes one of deciding whether or not such a program will also admit people who insist that they have abused only one substance (e.g., alcohol).

A number of studies indicate that single substance abusers (SSAers) can be successfully mixed with MSAers for purposes of treatment.[33–35] For example, using Eagleville Hospital's experience as a guide and the percentage of SSA and MSA clients completing the inpatient program as a criteria for success (see Table II and Fig. 1), it can be seen that SSAers and MSAers achieve very nearly the same outcomes in treatment. Whether a particular program should choose to mix MSA and SSA clients together, however, is a matter to be decided by each program, depending on a variety of special considerations, including economic and political factors.

3.6. Specific Treatment Interventions

The generic goals of substance abuse rehabilitation were listed above. When and if an individual needs detoxification, this goal obviously must take priority over all other goals. The same can be said for goals 2 and 3, Restore Physical Health and Restore Emotional Stability. Serious problems in either area will necessitate immediate intervention until the client is stabilized. In this regard, a number of writers (e.g., Kaufman[36]) have addressed the need for psychiatric and psychological services for MSA clients.

Since the dominant form of MSA involves sequential and/or concurrent abuse of both alcohol and other drugs, MSA treatment programs would do well to provide both Alcoholics Anonymous (AA) and Narcotics Anonymous (NA) services. Although integrating AA and NA services will not be without some cost,[37] the overall gains will prove to be greater, especially with respect to goal 4, Motivate for Treatment, and the three Aftercare goals 5, 9, and 10.

AA and NA program components will have the effect of raising clients' consciousness of the real dangers of using "safe" substances (e.g., the use of alcohol by drug-dependent clients or the use of "minor tranquilizers" and/or "sleeping pills" by alcoholics). AA and NA will also provide access to valuable social networks that can help to overcome loneliness and the feeling of being different or stigmatized, as well as sustain commitment to sobriety.

MSA programs very definitely need to have an effective, reliable urine surveillance system, which will screen for a wide band of substances, especially marijuana. No treatment program can hope to be successful when clients are actively abusing substances. Abstinence is the recommended mode of treatment, although this does not rule out the use of antagonist, such as antabuse and naltrexone, or the judicious prescription of psychotropics.[38]

With respect to treatment goals 6, 7, and 8, Challenge Destructive Defenses, Facilitate Catharsis and Development of Insight, and Establishing a Chemically Free Sense of Identity, group-oriented therapeutic interventions are favored over individual sessions (although the latter certainly should not be prohibited). In this regard, judicious forms of confrontation and the provision of feedback from peers and staff are key elements for success.[39]

Therapeutic modalities that focus on putting the client in touch with feelings, sharing these feelings with others, and learning better strategies for coping with such feelings are preferable to cognitive and didactic interventions, although there is a place for the latter.[36,39,40] The reason for this recommendation is that when clients begin to share their deepest and most suppressed and repressed feelings, a very strong therapeutic bonding occurs among the clients. This bonding process cuts across all manner of differences in race, sex, age, and economic status.

A variety of feeling-oriented therapies can be employed (e.g., Gestalt therapy, psychodrama, etc.). The only caveat to this recommendation is that the emotional stability of the therapist becomes even more critical as the potency of the therapy increases, everything else being equal. Thus, this strong feeling-oriented approach calls for fairly well adjusted, insightful, sensitive, and tactful therapists.

In working with MSA clients, a wide range of ancillary services are needed. As previously noted, psychiatric and psychological services are most desirable.[38] Even if a program cannot afford full time services of this nature, they could be obtained on a case-by-case consultative basis.

Other ancillary services for MSA clients include: medical and nursing services, including dentistry; family therapy; remedial education; vocational counseling and job placement; occupational; recreational, and art therapy; legal and social services, and sex education and counseling. Also needed are services that address the spiritual needs of clients, an often ignored area.

Effective case management of the delivery of diverse services to the same client is a key component for success. Effective teamwork and good intrastaff communications and cooperation are also essential. Ideally, such teams should not be headed by any one particular profession (e.g., medicine); rather, experience and demonstrated competence should be the preferred basis for selection of team leaders.

4. Staffing Issues

In seeking to acquire a competent staff to treat MSA clients, program directors should consider the following guidelines. One, select those job applicants who appear to be the most flexible and adaptable with respect to the range of clients they would like to serve (e.g., blacks, whites, males, females, old, young). MSAers will prove to be a very heterogeneous group, although the majority will likely be below the age of 30. (As more attention becomes focused on the substance abuse problems of older adults [65 years or more], it is expected that considerable MSA will be observed, except that the drugs abused will more likely be prescriptive medications than illicit substances, such as marijuana or amphetamine).

Interest in working in a MSA program is important. To compel someone to work in a program whose philosophy and procedures s/he perceives to be repugnant or foolish is to invite failure. Anyone holding very firm views against mixing different types of substance dependence clients together will constitute a serious impediment to success; they should not be hired.

Program directors would do well to hire recovered men and women with varied histories of substance abuse, some who have abused alcohol principally and others who have abused drugs primarily. This will insure that the MSA clients in the program will have access to role models for recovery—a vital component in any successful substance abuse rehabilitative program.

4.1. Training

The quality of training provided the staff will be another key element affecting the success of the program. Special attention should be focused on how various subcategories of substance abusers are similar and how they are different, as well as how these similarities and differences are to be managed within the program.

Full and honest discussion of staff attitudes and beliefs (stereotypes) about particular subcategories of substance abusers (e.g., those whose primary substance of abuse is heroin or amphetamine or alcohol) should be encouraged. This requires creating an atmosphere of trust wherein respect for differing points of view must prevail.

In many respects, more emphasis must be given to preparing the staff to relate to and cope well with the diversity of human beings with MSA patterns they will encounter than to the pharmacologic reactions of particular substances used singularly or in combination with other substances. The ability of the treatment staff to work effectively with very heterogeneous clients, for example, in group therapy, is a major factor that will decide the success or failure of the program.

Program directors should consider inviting management, treatment staff, and even clients from other programs (both substance-specific and combined treatment programs) to provide some of this training. Such first-hand face-to-face encounters will do much to dissipate negative stereotypes and assumptions about particular subcategories of substance abusers.

A variation on this theme would be to send staff to other programs for brief periods of time to broaden their experience with different varieties of substance abuse patterns and how to treat such patterns.

Finally, encouraging the formation of formal and informal support groups within the program can also pay handsome dividends. Such groups can ease the pain of frustration associated with treatment failures and provide additional information and skills to staff who are relatively inexperienced in working with MSA patients, as well as provide a little relief from staff burnout.

4.2. Some Programmatic Considerations

As previously stated, MSA clients are a very heterogeneous lot. Residential treatment programs must, therefore, be prepared to accommodate a very wide range of client needs and interests. The medical, recreational, educational, vocational, and therapeutic needs of this population are extremely diverse. Program administrators, therefore, must insure that all elements of the treatment population have their unique complex of needs and interests addressed. This means that compromise must be the order of the day, and that every subcategory of client (e.g., women, blacks, young, old) must experience the process of effecting compromises (e.g., in choosing recreational activities, decorating rooms, and establishing visiting privileges) as fair and equitable.

5. Summary

The trend in substance abuse is definitely in the direction of MSA, especially MSA involving the sequential and/or concurrent abuse of alcohol and drugs. To continue to maintain the current segregation of alcohol dependence and drug dependence treatment prevents many MSAers from gaining admittance to treatment and/or leads to inadequate diagnosis of their substance abuse problems, incomplete treatment, inadequate understanding of the epidemiology of substance abuse in this country, and, worst of all, relapse to addiction subsequent to completing treatment.

Treatment staff must be alert to detect covert forms of MSA, and they must be properly trained to appreciate its significance. The generic perspective was described as one that would facilitate proper diagnosis and treatment of MSA. In this regard, the relationship between MSA and combined treatment approaches was discussed.

Except for detoxification, which necessitates specific medical interventions for specific combinations of substances abused, the treatment of the MSAers, as is the case for SSAers, follows a generic sequence.

Specific treatment interventions recommended include integrating AA and NA into the treatment program, providing psychiatric and psychological services, stressing feeling-oriented treatment modalities (e.g., Gestalt therapy and psychodrama), and providing a variety of ancillary services, such as family therapy, remedial education, and legal services. Offering such a wide range of services requires effective case management.

Staffing MSA treatment programs with interested, flexible people including recovered staff with mixed substance abuse histories will improve a program's chances for success. Training that prepares staff to deal effectively with the rich diversity of backgrounds to be found among MSAers is essential.

Finally, programmatic considerations designed to effect compromises that will accommodate the differences observed among MSAers, with respect to their therapeutic, recreational, social, and living-arrangement needs, was also stressed.

References

1. Carroll JFX, Malloy TE, Santo Y, et al: The meaning and evolution of the term multiple substance abuse. *Contemp Drug Probl* 6(2):101–134, 1977.
2. Marjot DH: Annotation: Alcohol, alcoholism and drugs. *Br J Alcohol Alcoholism* 14(2):69–73, 1979.
3. Carroll JFX (ed): National Drug/Alcohol Collaborative Project (NDACP) Final Report (NIDA Grant H81 DA 01113). Rockville, Maryland, National Institute on Drug Abuse, 1977.
4. Carroll JFX, Santo Y, Hannigan PC: Description of the total client sample: Analysis of substance use patterns, and individual program descriptions, in Gardner SE (ed): National Drug/Alcohol Collaborative Project: Issues in multiple substance abuse (Services Research Monograph Series, DHEW Publication No. [ADM] 89-957). Rockville, Maryland, National Institute on Drug Abuse, 1980, pp 25–62.
5. Kaufman E: The abuse of multiple drugs. I. Definition, classification and extent of problem. *Am J Drug Alcohol Abuse* 3(2):279–292, 1976.
6. Kaufman E: Polydrug abuse or multidrug misuse: It's here to stay. *Br J Addict* 72:339–347, 1977.
7. Carroll JFX, Malloy TE, Kendrick FM: Alcohol abuse by drug dependent persons: A literature review and evaluation, *Am J Drug Alcohol Abuse* 4(3):293–315, 1977.
8. Carroll JFX, Malloy TE, Dendrick FM: Drug abuse by alcoholics and problem drinkers: A literature review and evaluation. *Am J Drug Alcohol Abuse* 4(3):317–341, 1977.
9. General Service Office of Alcoholics Anonymous: Analysis of the 1980 Survey of the membership of AA. (Available from Alcoholics Anonymous World Services, Inc. 468 Park Ave South, New York, N.Y. 10016.)
10. Santo, Y, Friedman AS: Overview and selected findings from the National Youth Polydrug Study. *Contemp Drug Probl* 9(3):285–300, 1980.
11. Croughan JL, Miller JP, Whitman BY, et al: Alcoholism and alcohol dependence in narcotic addicts: A prospective study with a five year follow-up. *Am J Drug Alcohol Abuse* 8(1):85–94, 1981.
12. Morrissey EH: The measurement of multiple drug use and its relationship to the pattern of alcohol intake. *Am J Drug Alcohol Abuse* 8(3):311–328, 1981.
13. Lowman C: Facts for planning, No. 2: Alcohol use as an indicator of psychoactive drug use among the nation's senior high school students. *Alcohol Health Res World* 6(2):41–46, 1981/82.
14. Simpson DD, Lloyd MR: Alcohol use following treatment for drug addiction. *JAMA* 213:294–295, 1970.
15. Rounsaville BJ, Weissman MM, Kleber HD: The significance of alcoholism in treated opiate addicts. *J Nerv Ment Dis* 170(8):479–488, 1982.
16. Rounsaville BJ, Weissman MM, Wilber C, et al: Identifying alcoholism in treated opiate addicts. *Am J Psychiatry* 140(6):764–766, 1983.
17. Stimmel B, Cohen M, Hanbury R: Alcoholism and polydrug abuse in persons on methadone maintenance. *Ann NY Acad Sci* 311:99–109, 1978.

18. Stimmel B, Cohen M, Sturiano V, et al: Is treatment for alcoholism effective in persons on methadone maintenance? *Am J Psychiatry* 140(7):862–866, 1983.
19. Hoag J: Alcohol abstinence—Total drug freedom in the therapeutic community. *ALMACAN* 14(1):3–4, 1984.
20. Carroll JFX: Uncovering drug abuse by alcoholics and alcohol abuse by addicts. *Int J Addict* 15(4):591–595, 1980.
21. Schnoll SH: Alcohol and other substance abuse in adolescents, in Gottheil EH (ed): *Addiction Research and Treatment: Converging Trends*. New York, Pergamon Press, 1979, pp. 40–45.
22. Benzer D, Cushman P: Alcohol and benzodiazepines: Withdrawal syndromes. *Alcoholism Clin Exp Res* 4(3):243–247, 1980.
23. Schnoll SH: Guidelines for the care of the drug abusing patient. *Hosp Med* 12(10):85–97, 1976.
24. Smith DE, Wessor DR: A new method for treatment of barbiturate dependence. *JAMA* 213:294–295, 1970.
25. Carroll JFX, Schnoll SE: Mixed drug and alcohol populations, in Pattison EM, Kaufman E (eds): *Encyclopedia Handbook of Alcoholism*, New York, Gardner Press, 1982, pp 742–758.
26. Inaba D, Way EL, Blum K, et al: Pharmacological and toxicological perspectives of commonly abused drugs. *Med Monogr Ser* (No. 5) 1978.
27. Carroll JFX: Similarities and differences of personality and psychopathology between alcoholics and addicts. *Am J Drug Alcohol Abuse* 7:219–236, 1980.
28. Carroll JFX: Personality and psychopathology: A comparison of alcohol and drug-dependent persons, in Solomon J, Keeley KA (eds): *Perspectives in Alcohol and Drug Abuse: Similarities and Differences*. Boston, John Wright PSG Inc, 1982, pp 58–88.
29. Carroll JFX, Malloy TE, Roscioli DL, et al: Personality similarities and differences in four diagnostic groups of women alcoholics and drug addicts. *J Stud Alcohol* 42(5):431–440, 1981.
30. Carroll JFX, Malloy TE, Roscioli DL, et al: Similarities and differences in self-concepts of alcohol and drug addicted women. *J Stud Alcohol* 43(7):725–738, 1982.
31. Eagleville Hospital: *Eagleville Hospital Documentation Process Manual (proof edition)*. Unpublished manuscript, 1982 (Available from Public Relations Department, Eagleville Hospital, Eagleville, PA 19408.)
32. Carroll JFX, Malloy TE: Combined treatment of alcohol and drug dependent persons: A literature review and evaluation. *Am J Drug Alcohol Abuse* 4(3):317–341, 1977.
33. Ottenberg DJ, Carroll JFX: Combined treatment of alcoholism and drug addiction, in Solomon J, Keeley KA (eds): *Perspectives in Alcohol and Drug Aubse: Similarities and Differences*. Boston, John Wright PSG Inc, 1982, pp 117–144.
34. Greene BT: Treating drug and alcohol abusers in the same facilities: Process and implications. *J Drug Issues* 9(3):399–412, 1979.
35. Barr H, Antes D: Seven years after treatment: A follow-up study of drug addicts and alcoholics treated in Eagleville Hospital's Inpatient Program (excerpts and related findings). Unpublished manuscript, 1981 (Available from H. Barr, Director of Research, Eagleville Hospital, Eagleville, PA 19408.)
36. Kaufman E: The abuse of multiple drugs. II Psychological hypothesis, treatment. *Am J Drug Alcohol Abuse* 3(2):293–301, 1976.
37. Krupka LF, Blume ES: Alcoholics anonymous in a therapeutic community. *J Drug Education* 10(2):145–151, 1980.
38. Carroll JFX, Sobel BS: Integrating mental health personnel and practices into a therapeutic community, in De Leon G, Ziegenfuss J (eds): *Therapeutic Communities for Addiction*, Springfield, Illinois, Charles C Thomas (in press).
39. Carroll JFX: Do contemporary drug/alcohol treatment strategies create a basic conflict between ethical concerns and treatment effectiveness? *Contemp Drug Prob* 8(3):389–404, 1979.
40. MacDonough TS: Process research data on a potent, feeling-evoking residential treatment program for the simultaneous counseling of alcohol abusers and drug abusers. *Int J Addict* 16(6):973–1001, 1981.

II

Typologies of Alcoholics

Thomas F. Babor and Roger E. Meyer, Section Editors

Overview

Thomas F. Babor and Roger E. Meyer

Readers whose curiosity is likely to be aroused by the concept of alcoholic typologies will be richly rewarded by a careful reading of the chapters in this section. Its authors have been chosen to represent the best that contemporary alcohol studies have to offer with respect to typological research and theory. Yet, despite more than a century of research and speculation, the field is still struggling to carve out an identity for itself, develop a set of coherent concepts, and construct a scientific methodology that will bring order out of the complexity that is alcoholism.

One encouraging sign evident in these chapters, and the sole focus of the first, is the sense of historical perspective that typology theory must develop if research is to move beyond the cultural, disciplinary and methodological straightjacket it has so often been confined to. As Chapter 5 by Babor and Lauerman shows, those who fail to heed the lessons of history are doomed to repeat its failures. Typology theorists have tended to work in a time warp, independent of one another and independent of the work of their predecessors. Their failures are evident. With the notable exception of Jellinek's typological synthesis, very little of the past has been recognized by contemporary researchers, theorists, or clinicians as a significant contribution to the understanding or treatment of alcoholism. Although the verdict is not yet in, a similar indictment can be made about the recent past of typology research, which has been so heavily dominated by abnormal personality theory and the Minnesota Multiphasic Personality Test.

Fortunately, the chapters in this section not only recognize the limits of what has gone before them but also illustrate a broader and more sophisticated approach to the tasks of (1) finding whether or not distinct alcoholic typologies exist and, if they do (2) determining whether different approaches to identification, treatment, and prevention can do any more to relieve the personal and social costs of alcoholism than the present undifferentiated approach. These tasks should not be confused, because the second is relatively fruitless unless the first is accomplished successfully. It is therefore not surprising that contemporary typology research has focused on the problem of defining and

Thomas F. Babor and Roger E. Meyer • Alcohol Research Center, Department of Psychiatry, University of Connecticut Health Center, Farmington, Connecticut 06032.

validating distinctive and clinically meaningful subgroups of alcoholics rather than launching into treatment matching studies prematurely. In the process, the field has been advanced considerably by the development of conceptual ground rules, research methods, and validation procedures.

Conceptually, typology researchers are beginning to realize that the entire question of empirical validation and clinical relevance depends on the definition of typology. Before one can validate or use a typology of alcoholics, one must have a concept of types. Although the concept of type is rarely defined and loosely constructed in these chapters, there is some consensus concerning its nature. In part, this consensus has been forged by nomenclature, the rules for defining terms within a discipline. The long tradition of typological thinking within the social, behavioral, and medical sciences has clearly identified a "type" as an artificial construct. Types are idealized constructions of an observer, defined by numerous characteristics that only imperfectly describe the individuals fitted to them. As currently employed, the term is used to describe the integration of characteristic personality traits, habitual drinking behaviors, and alcohol-related consequences into meaningful *Gestalten* or clusters. Although types are impressionistic and synthetic, they do assemble into meaningful clusters numerous individuals who are similar in the majority of relevant respects. The beauty of a type is that, like any abstract concept, it summarizes a great deal of information about the individual case. To the extent that alcoholic types are readily identifiable, scientifically valid, and clinically meaningful, they can be extremely useful for the purpose of diagnosis and treatment.

Once there is agreement concerning the definition of a type, one can begin the search for the optimal typological classification system. The chapters in this section suggest that by past as well as current standards, a useful classification system should have the following characteristics:

1. *Homogeneity within categories.* Individuals within the purview of a given type should be similar with respect to the major distinguishing features of alcoholism. While there is still disagreement about the essential characteristics of alcoholism, a broad interpretation of the homogeneity criterion would suggest that, like other medical conditions, subtypes of alcoholism should be similar with respect to etiology or origins, natural history (progression of the biological disease process), the drinking career (the sequence of drinking experiences and role expectations resulting in the self-identification of the drinker as an alcoholic).

2. *Heterogeneity between categories.* A typological classification should differentiate among different homogeneous groups of alcoholics, not only with respect to etiology, natural history, and drinking career, but also in terms of treatment response and prognosis. The greater the differences between subtypes, the more easily they will permit reliable classification.

3. *Stability.* The chronicity of alcoholism results in a longitudinal sequence of age- and role-related consequences. Despite the variability and at times the

progressiveness of the disorder, the defining characteristics of many typologies (e.g., hereditary vulnerability, psychopathology) imply that there are common underlying type structures that remain fairly stable over time. One may therefore question the value of ephemeral typological defining characteristics, such as reactive depression, that may only be temporary states, or of characteristics that change as the disorder progresses, such as impaired memory function. In these cases the same individual may be classified as a different type at several different times in the drinking career.

4. *Comprehensiveness and specificity*. Typological classification systems should account for most, if not all, the cases in a representative sample of alcoholics, who are distinguished in relevant respects from a like sample of nonalcoholic controls. The more inclusive the typology, the more useful it will be for both theory and practice. It should be emphasized, however, that the defining characteristics should be closely related to alcoholism. While male and female alcoholics may differ from each other in many respects, this may tell us little about their varieties of alcoholism. If depression is a distinguishing characteristic of female alcoholics, it is important to determine if depressed female alcoholics differ from depressed male alcoholics before using gender to define a typology. Depression may do just as well. Thus it is important when searching for a typology to sample from the universe of characteristics that are specific to alcoholism. Antisocial alcoholics in treatment may be characterized by their youthfulness, but this is not necessarily germane to a typology of alcoholism unless sociopathic alcoholics require treatment at an earlier age. When comparing subtypes, care must be taken to control for confounding variables, such as age and socioeconomic status, that may distinguish certain subgroups regardless of their alcoholism.

5. *Multidimensionality*. In order to be comprehensive, a typological classification should be capable of differentiating alcoholics along a variety of alcohol-related dimensions. Alcoholism, after all, is a generic term that encompasses a variety of behaviors, symptoms, physical conditions, and social consequences. As the chapters in this section point out, typologies based on single dimensions such as personality functioning or family history may be of limited usefulness if they do not take into account other relevant aspects of the disorder.

6. *Utility*. Typological formulations are capable of serving a variety of useful purposes. As Kurt Lewin once said, nothing is as useful as a good theory. To the extent that typologies describe homogeneous varieties of alcoholism, they provide a theoretical basis for understanding how different individuals develop alcoholism and how different alcoholics progress through completely different drinking careers. In addition to their heuristic and predictive value, typological theories may be useful in suggesting more effective approaches to treatment and prevention. To be useful, typological classification systems should permit the efficient identification and assignment of patients to the most appropriate aspects of the treatment system. Because the health care system in which alcoholics are treated is complex and multifaceted,

the most useful typology would be one that suggests program assignment (e.g., inpatient vs. outpatient; psychiatric vs. medical care), treatment matching (e.g., psychotherapy vs. vocational counseling), treatment goals (e.g., abstinence vs. moderate drinking), intensity of treatment (short-term care vs. long-term care), and aftercare modality (Alcoholics Anonymous vs. behavioral programs).

Typologies may also have utility for prevention or prophylactic measures. Should the natural history of some types be especially virulent, secondary prevention measures could be initiated at an early stage of development. Should there be a type characterized by a history of familial alcoholism, this information could be used to educate the children of alcoholics. Not all typological classifications will have equal theoretical value, clinical relevance, and administrative feasibility. The search for an all-purpose, definitive typology may distract researchers from the practical value of developing different typologies for different purposes.

7. *Validity*. To be credible, a typological classification should permit external validation, and its robustness should be demonstrable across different samples of alcoholics. Ideally, a typology should have cross-cultural generalizability. This would constitute persuasive evidence that the typology is reflecting essential and universal elements of alcoholism. Validity can be established in a variety of ways, many of which are discussed in the chapters that follow.

In addition to these conceptual ground rules, a level of methodological sophistication heretofore unknown in typology research is displayed in the chapters that follow. The technology of differential assessment has improved dramatically in recent years. With the addition of biological tests, standardized medical and psychiatric ratings, personality and attitudinal inventories, neuropsychological assessments, family history interviews, and longitudinal research designs, it is possible for the first time to gain a comprehensive description of the variations among alcoholics. These data would be virtually impossible to summarize and interpret without the aid of high-speed computers and multivariate statistical techniques, which were not available until the last decade on a wide scale. These advances have added a new dimension to the armamentarium of typology research.

A final cause for optimism is the emergence of a cadre of researchers working independently on related aspects of typology. The scientific community can be a lonely place unless there is sufficient communication to provide stimulation, encouragement and a healthy climate for competitiveness. Considerable time, resources, and career investments are needed to produce the researchers represented herein. Without a basic infrastructure of like-minded research groups, progress in any field is unlikely.

Despite these encouraging developments, it would be false to conclude that typology research has come of age. The current resurgence of interest in alcoholic typologies has not resulted in any compelling systematic theories.

To a large extent the field is still characterized by disciplinary parochialism and methodological faddism. Typologies historically have been dictated more by the ideological biases of the typologists than by the rich clinical data available to the scientific observer. The dominating role personality typologies have assumed during the past two decades may have less to do with the importance of psychological disorder than with the popularity of the MMPI.

Perhaps the greatest shortcoming of contemporary typology theory is its failure thus far to exert any influence on differential diagnosis, clinical practice, or treatment policy. Few researchers have found the rationale or the resources to move beyond the pages of their journal manuscripts to the development of diagnostic criteria, therapeutic interventions, or specialized treatment programs. The so-called matching hypothesis, still heralded as the salvation of the treatment industry, is practically impossible to test without some credible theory suggesting the types of alcoholics who should be matched to the variety of available treatments. To date, matching research has focused on esoteric therapies while ignoring the major parameters of the treatment system through which most alcoholics are processed. Until typologies are developed having clinical relevance to the rational determination of such factors as length of treatment, compatibility with Alcoholics Anonymous, appropriateness of inpatient treatment, and the need for specialized therapies, typology research will continue to serve as not much more than an academic pastime. While it is indeed encouraging to see some evidence for the Jellinek typology in Chapter 6 (Morey and Skinner) it should be noted that, despite its nearly universal acceptance, the gamma-delta typology has inspired virtually no research in the 25 years of its popularity.

The central question is how effective will contemporary typology researchers be in fulfilling the promise that has sustained interest in this subject for so long.

ACKNOWLEDGMENT. The writing of this paper was supported in part by Grant No. 1 P50 AA 03510 from the National Institute on Alcohol Abuse and Alcoholism.

5

Classification and Forms of Inebriety

Historical Antecedents of Alcoholic Typologies

Thomas F. Babor and Richard J. Lauerman

Abstract. This chapter reviews 39 typological classifications of alcoholics published in the world alcohol literature between 1850 and 1941. After a brief discussion of the concept of typology within the Western intellectual tradition, the typologies are described in terms of classification criteria, cultural context, and historical trends. Four countries (France, Germany, England, and the United States) accounted for all but one of the typologies. Within countries, typological theories tended to be concentrated during specific historical periods, often reflecting prevailing trends in medicine, psychiatry, and clinical practice. Despite a number of common themes, there was little indication of the progressive development of typology theory in a predictable direction. Like their counterparts in contemporary times, these typologies failed to gain widespread acceptance as the basis for theoretical explanations or clinical practice. Rather, their function was more likely to serve as justifications for the disciplinary or policy orientations held by the typologists. It is concluded that unless typologies are formulated on the basis of careful research, sound theory, and clinical relevance, they are likely to be relegated to a similar status as historical artifacts.

1. Introduction

The infinite spectrum of human variability has been analyzed and classified in numerous ways. Descriptions of human types are as old as the inclination to reflect on human nature and have endured undoubtedly because they have proved useful as guides to understanding and to action.

In the naive psychology of everyday life, simple type systems are employed quite frequently, following the cognitive imperative to generalize and to classify. Stereotypes based on age (young, old), sex, intelligence (smart, dull), nationality (Irish, Italian), and psychological adjustment (normal, neurotic) pervade thinking about alcoholic as well as nonalcoholic individuals.

The pervasiveness of typological thinking about drinking is often reflected in the mythology, folklore, and language of a culture. Perhaps the most common popular typology of the alcoholic is that of the degenerate drinker

Thomas F. Babor and **Richard J. Lauerman** • Alcohol Research Center, Department of Psychiatry, University of Connecticut Health Center, Farmington, Connecticut 06032.

who has forsaken everything for the bottle. Vagabonds, alcoholics, and homeless men are known as Bowery bums in New York, Skid Row alcoholics in Seattle, and *clochards* in Paris. Related terms depicting this type of alcoholic are "rummy" and "lush." Other types of drinkers are described according to the setting where they drink, the pattern of their drinking, or the beverages they prefer. A "barfly" is a heavy drinker who spends a great deal of time in public drinking establishments. A "closet drinker" is a person (often a woman) who drinks excessively in the privacy of the home. A "bender" is an old Scottish name for a hard drinker, who was required to bend his elbow with great frequency during the long drinking bouts that also became identified with this term. Similar to the bender is the "carouser," who drinks intensively and episodically, but less for the alcohol than for the fun of engaging in revelry. The "tippler" takes his drams in measured doses, while the "wino" drinks the cheapest fortified wines because it is the most economical way to drink on a limited budget. A drunkard is one who habitually drinks to excess; a common drunkard is one who is arrested repeatedly for intoxication; and a "sot" is one who makes himself foolish and dull with intoxication.

Moving beyond the tendency to classify alcoholics according to popular stereotypes, the remainder of this chapter seeks to clarify the widely felt, but frequently ignored, distinction between anticipations and foundations in the history of typological theories of alcoholism. According to Sarup,[1] anticipations are "those antecedent ideas that have likeness to, but not developmental ties with, later modes of thought" (p. 478). In contrast, foundations are "the actual beginnings of later concepts and theories in the sense that the growth of thought is relatively continuous and the lines of influence are traceable" (p. 478). Anticipations are historically isolated instances of foreshadowing, while foundations have priority, similarity, and demonstrable continuity with respect to later developments. By way of introduction, the chapter begins with a brief discussion of the notion of typologies within the Western intellectual tradition. Building on the work of Thomas Crothers, Karl Bowman, and E.M. Jellinek, we next summarize the world literature on typological formulations dating from the late 19th century to 1940. This summary will serve as a basis for examining the extent to which antecedents and foundations constitute historical roots of current typological ideas. Special attention will be given to the ways in which typological concepts have emerged from particular ideological and cultural contexts and how they have been applied to the treatment of alcoholism as well as to the formulation of alcoholism treatment policy.

2. Types and Typologies in the Western Intellectual Tradition

Typology is the study of types. More specifically, it is a particular system for the classification of types. Before anything can be said about typologies, however, we must define what is meant by type. There are a number of ways to approach this concept, each one having different implications for the development, formulation, and usefulness of typologies.

Perhaps the most common meaning of the word type comes from the pre-Darwinian concept of ideal types. Ideal types are conceptions of fictitious or prototypical individuals who embody the characteristics of a category to its fullest measure. An ideal type is the central form about which all variations in the members of a class center. Derived from rational, not empirical methods, ideal types are not intended to cover real persons but rather exist in the eye of the observer. Prescientific theories of personality provide the most common examples of ideal types. The Greek physician, Galen, based his fourfold classification on the predominance of different "humors" in the body. His types were the sanguine, the choleric, the phlegmatic, and the melancholic. The German philosopher Eduard Spranger (1882–1963) proposed six types defined by the following value orientations: theoretical, economic, aesthetic, social, political, and religious. Other examples of ideal types are Carl Jung's classification of extroverted and introverted types; William James' division of tender-minded, tough-minded; and the psychoanalytic classification into hysterical, obsessive-compulsive, paranoid, masochistic, schizoid, dependent, and psychopathic character types.

Another approach to typology comes from the biological sciences. Here all members of a class or category are considered as somehow collectively embodying the defining qualities of the group. E.M. Jellinek,[2] a biometrist, may have had this approach in mind when he described alcoholism as a "genus" having various "species," of which two were described as disease processes (gamma and delta types).

Another underlying concept of type is statistical. A frequent meaning in typologies is that the individual has most of the defining qualities of the group. This is based on the concept of a type as a group average. Another statistical concept is the definition of types based on the extremes of a continuum or the peak instances of a bimodal distribution of a single variable. Perhaps the greatest advances in statistically based typology theory have come from the application of factor analysis and cluster analysis to the study of personality test data. Empirical investigation suggests that certain habits, traits, and attitudes are manifestations of personality types. These types represent a more embracing organization that stands conceptually between the level of traits and the level of the total personality.[3]

This brief introduction to different conceptual approaches suggests that typologies need to be understood in terms of their theoretical assumptions, classification rules, historical origins, and disciplinary context, since the basic approach implicit in a given typology will have an important influence on its purpose, content, and usefulness. The following sections will review clinically based classifications of the alcoholic before returning to these issues to organize a general critique of alcoholic typologies.

3. Overview: A Compendium of 19th and 20th Century Typologies

Table I provides summaries of 39 typological formulations identified from an historical review of the world literature on alcoholism. Twenty-four typologies were summarized by Bowman and Jellinek[4] in their 1941 paper on "Alcohol Addiction and Its Treatment." The remaining 15 typologies were found sources in the *International Bibliography of Studies on Alcohol*[5] or from various 19th century medical texts and journals. Although this compendium is not necessarily exhaustive, it is fairly comprehensive in that it includes and supplements the major bibliographic sources available.[4–7] Table I organizes the typological systems chronologically by country of origin. This provides a basis for examining historical developments within the context of such major cultural influences as the development of modern psychiatry. Included in the table are the results of a content analysis of the primary criteria used to define the subtypes. Four major criteria were sufficient to account for the content of almost all typologies. These were: (1) dependence or addiction, often described in terms of craving, tolerance, or withdrawal symptoms; (2) drinking pattern, usually labeled as either continuous or intermittent; (3) chronicity, i.e., whether the symptoms and consequences are acute, periodic or persistent; and (4) etiology. This last category includes hereditary causes, psychiatric disorder, and environmental influences.

Four countries account for all but one of the typologies identified: France, Germany, England, and the United States. Within countries, interest in typological formulations tended to be concentrated in relatively circumscribed periods. The French were active in the late 19th century, the Germans and British in the 1920s and 1930s. The Americans were active in two stages, one corresponding to the American Association for the Study and Cure of Inebriety (1870–1916) and the other between the repeal of Prohibition and the beginning of World War II (1933–1941).

The content analysis reveals that the French typologies were classified primarily according to differences in drinking pattern and etiology. Hereditary causes predominate. Classification criteria based on drinking pattern and etiology also dominate the early American typologies (1870–1916), but the Americans favored psychological causes over hereditary influences. Continuing in this tradition the later American typologies (1932–1938) were almost exclusively based on psychological criteria. The German typologies emphasized both psychological and hereditary causes and, to a lesser extent, drinking pattern and dependence criteria. The British classified their types most frequently according to dependence criteria. The content analysis shows that most typologies were based on multiple classification criteria. Psychological etiologies were cited most often (24 typologies), followed by hereditary causes (15 typologies). Drinking pattern and dependence criteria were used to classify 22 and 19 typologies, respectively. Chronicity was also used as a classification criterion in about one quarter of the typologies.

Table I. Typological Classification Systems Listed in Chronological Order of Publication by Country of Origin[a,b]

Author	Year	Classification	Major classification criteria: Dependence/addiction	Drinking pattern	Etiology	Chronicity
		French typologies				
Legrain[8]	1889	1. Moral degenerates: Excessive, psychopathic personalities 2. Escapists who enjoy mental effects 3. Dipsomaniacs		×	H,P	
Magnan[9]	1893	1. Periodic: infrequent, accidental intoxication 2. Chronic: characterized by three types of delirium a. Brief delirium b. Persistent delirium and somatic deterioration c. Delusional disorder following delirium		×	H	×
Lancereaux (cited in ref. 10)	1900	1. Oenilisme: consequences resulting from habitual use of wine 2. Alcoolisme: consequences resulting from habitual use of distilled spirits 3. Absinthisme: consequences resulting from habitual use of absinthe		×	S	×
Triboulet and Mathieu	1900	1. Dipsomaniacs 2. Hereditary regular drinkers 3. Habitual drinkers (*buveurs d'habitude*)	×	×	H,S	
Dromard[11]	1902	1. Classic chronic alcoholics 2. Latent alcoholics characterized by *alcoolomanie:* tolerance and craving 3. Dipsomaniacs	×	×		×
		American typologies				
Parker (cited in ref. 12)	1870	1. Hereditary alcoholics with irresistable craving 2. Nonhereditary alcoholics who begin as social drinkers 3. Young antisocial drinkers	×	×	H	
Parrish[12]	1883	1. Solitary, midnight inebriates 2. Violent inebriates 3. Traumatic inebriates 4. Hereditary inebriates		×	P,H	

(Continued)

Table I. (*Continued*)

Author	Year	Classification	Major classification criteria: Dependence/addiction	Drinking pattern	Etiology	Chronicity
Crothers[6]	1893	1. Inebriates	×	×	P,H,S	
		a. Habitual drunkards				
		b. Accidental				
		c. Emotional				
		d. Solitary				
		e. Pauper				
		2. Dipsomaniacs				
		a. Acute				
		b. Periodic				
		c. Chronic				
Palmer[13]	1898	1. Brutal criminal inebriate				
		2. Nervous animal type			P,H	
		3. Intellectual type				
		4. Domestic and religious type				
Ford[14]	1909	1. Accidental drunkards				
		2. Occasional drunkards				
		3. Habitual drunkards: Diseased alcoholics having craving, loss of self control	×	×		×
		a. Stress-induced habitual drunkards				
		b. Dipsomaniacs				
		c. Defectives and degenerates				
Parmelee[15]	1909	1. Occasional drunkards: First offenders not seriously dependent on alcohol	×	×	P	×
		2. Habitual drunkards: Physiological craving				
Crothers[7]	1911	1. Continuous drinkers				
		2. Periodic	×	×	P,H	×
		a. Irregular				
		b. Regular				

*Coriat[16]	1912	1. Steady tippler				
		2. Periodic drinker				
		a. Due to depression		×	P	
		b. Epileptic equivalent				
		c. Cyclothymic				
		d. As a psychasthenic impulsion				
Anderson[17]	1916	1. Habitual drinkers: Steady drinking leads to progressive deterioration		×	P	×
		2. Periodic drinkers: Neurotic individuals who exhibit drink paroxysms				
*Mangold[18]	1916	1. Degrading social customs and environmental factors cause normal drinker to become alcoholic			P,S	
		2. Persons who are weak, neurotic, feeble-minded, or defective in character				
*White[19]	1932	1. Drinking an expression of a psychosis but not its cause, especially early paresis and mild manic depressive				
		2. Drinking to drown troubles and escape; chiefly hysterics, psychoneurotics, dipsomaniacs			P	
		3. Highly susceptible groups, especially posttraumatic consititution				
		4. Alcoholism complicating other psychoses				
		5. Purely alcoholic psychosis				
*Fleming[20]	1937	1. Symptomatic drinking due to physical or mental pathologic condition for which alcohol provides relief	×		P	
		2. True addiction associated with habituation and characterized by specific craving				
*Allen[21]	1938	1. Psychopathic alcoholic having inadequate youth				
		2. Neurotic alcoholic			P	
*Knight[22]	1938	1. Essential: Maladjustment dating from childhood with first alcoholic episodes in teens				
		2. Reactive: Alcohol addiction occurs late in life as a response to stressful situation			P	
		3. Symptomatic alcoholics: Drink only incidentally				

(*Continued*)

Table I. (*Continued*)

Author	Year	Classification	Major classification criteria: Dependence/addiction	Drinking pattern	Etiology	Chronicity
*Menninger[23]	1938	1. Essential type (see Knight)				
		2. Reactive type (see Knight)				
		3. Neurotic characters: Excessive drinking evidence of maladjustment			P	
		4. Psychotic personalities: Alcohol a symptom of paranoid, schizoid, or psychotic system				
Bowman and Jellinek[4]	1941	1. True addicts				
		2. Symptomatic drinkers (endogenous)	×	×	P,H,S	
		3. Symptomatic drinkers (exogenous)				
		4. *Stammtisch* drinkers				
		<u>German typologies</u>				
*Bruhl-Cramer (cited in ref. 29)	1901	1. Constant alcoholism				
		2. Temporary alcoholism				
		a. *Nachlassende Trunksucht:* Daily craving for alcohol				
		b. *Intermittierende Trunksucht:* Binges several times a month	×	×	P	
		c. *Periodische Trunksucht* or *Quartalsuff:* Prodromal depressive state precedes drinking				
		3. Mixed alcoholism				
*Kretschmer[25]	1924	1. Pynic, cyclothymic type: Drinking develops from gregarious disposition			P,H	
		2. Schizoid types: Relief drinkers				
*Cimbal[26]	1926	1. Decadent drinkers				
		2. Impassioned drinkers			P,H,S	
		3. Self-aggrandizing drinkers				
		4. Stupid drinkers				
*Stockert[27]	1926	1. Convivial drinkers (*Stammtisch* alcoholics)				
		2. Alcohol addiction	×		P,S	
		a. Weaklings: Drink for pleasure				
		b. Psychopaths: Asocial repressed personalities				

*Grotjan (cited in ref. 28)	1928	1. Intemperate drinkers: Drink excessively, but can control amount	×	×		
		2. Addicts: Lack resistance to craving				
*Dittmer[29]	1932	1. Irregular drunkenness without pathological reaction				
		2. Frequent drunkenness with pathological reaction	×	×		
		3. Endogenous, addictive, continuous drinking				
*Gabriel[30]	1933	1. Genuine addicted drinker: Addiction is constitutional				
		2. Habitual drinkers	×	×	H	
*Pohlisch[31]	1933	1. Hyperthymic and depressive psychopaths				
		2. Schizoid drinkers				
		3. Excitable, irritable, explosive drinker; temporary drinkers with an accumulation of excesses but not true habituation	×	×	P,H	
*Mollenhof[32]	1935	1. Exuberant, reckless drinker				
		2. The *gemutlich* drinker			P,S	
		3. "Misery" drinker				
*Wuth[33]	1935	1. Exogenic etiology			P,H,S	
		2. Endogenic etiology				
*Gabriel and Kratzmann[34]	1936	1. Positivistic: Similar to Kretschmer's cyclothymic type				
		2. Negativistic: Similar to Kretschmer's schizothymic type			P,H	
Meggendorfer[35]	1940	1. Periodic alcoholism: Dipsomania from psychological predisposition				
		2. Chronic alcoholism	×	×	H,S	×
		a. Alcohol adiction: Constitutional alcoholics				
		b. Environmental alcoholics: Progressive, nonaddictive alcohol abuse				
		British typologies				
Carpenter[36]	1850	1. Acute oenomaniacs: Sudden desire to drink				
		2. Periodic: Binge drinkers	×	P,H,S		
		3. Chronic oenomanics: Continuous desire for stimulants				
*Wingfield[37]	1919	1. Pseudodipsomania: Craving and excessive drinking only after alcohol is taken				
		2. Chronic sober alcoholism: Regular and prolonged excessive drinking not due to intoxication	×	×		×
		3. Chronic inebriate alcoholism: Regular and prolonged excessive drinking to avoid becoming sober				
		4. True dipsomania: Spontaneous craving for alcohol				

(Continued)

Table I. *(Continued)*

Author	Year	Classification	Major classification criteria: Dependence/addiction	Drinking pattern	Etiology	Chronicity
Crichton-Miller[38]	1928	1. Steady drinkers				
		a. Hypopietic: Drink to relieve low blood pressure				
		b. Subthyroidic: Drink for general vasomotor stimulation				
		c. Sensorial type: Drink to modify sensory experience				
		d. Rebels: Sons of temperance reformers	×	×	P	
		2. Intermittent drinkers				
		a. Epileptic: Explosive craving for alcohol				
		b. Dual personality				
		c. Manic depressive				
*Dent[39]	1934	1. "Active": Drink to drown sorrow				
		2. "Habitual" drinker: Inability to give up alcohol	×		P	
*Carver *et al.*,[40]	1936	1. Intermittent				
		2. Regular				
		a. With intermittent exacerbation	×	×		
		b. Sober				
		3. Paroxysmal dipsomaniacs				
		Canadian typology				
*Stevenson[41]	1940	1. Well-built, sociable and indolent			H	
		2. Slight, moody, hard-working				

[a] Identified from refs. 4, 5, and other sources.
[b] (*)Reviewed in Bowman and Jellinek[4]; ×, criterion used to classify one or more types; H, hereditary causes cited; P, psychological causes cited; S, societal/environmental causes cited.

4. Nineteenth Century French Typologies

Toward the end of the 19th century, a number of typological theories were published in France by prominent alienists and physicians. Like Valetin-Jacques Magnan and Paul Maurice Legrain, many were associated with the fledgling French temperance movement. Following in the tradition of Pinel, Esquirol, and Morel, Magnan and his student Legrain were leading advocates for the institutional treatment of the insane and popularized a psychophysiological interpretation of Darwinian theory based on the concepts of inherited mental degeneracy (*dégénérescence*) and moral insanity. Mental degeneracy was thought to result from the cumulative influence of certain hereditary characteristics that predispose fragile individuals to psychoses and alcoholism. Moral insanity was considered to render the individual incapable of abiding by the rules of current morality.

In 1889, Legrain's typology was published in a book entitled *Hérédité et Alcoolisme*.[8] In it, he described three groups of "conscious alcoholics" based on certain clinical and psychological characteristics. The first group consists of morally insane alcoholics whose basic instincts take primacy over higher mental faculties. Because their moral sense is poorly developed, they do all things to excess. Often intoxicated and sometimes violent, these drinkers are particularly susceptible to accidents. The second group has an adequate moral development but lacks will power. These weak-willed alcoholics are either alcoholics by taste (*par goût*) or by habit (*par entraînement*). The latter drink by imitation, social necessity, or occupational pressures. The third group consists of the dipsomaniacs, impulsive individuals whose will power dissolves in alcohol.

Legrain's mentor, Magnan,[9] conceptualized alcoholism in terms of two extremes: (1) infrequent, accidental intoxication; and (2) chronic alcoholism. The latter was considered a permanent condition that could manifest itself differently as a function of three types or degrees of alcoholic delirium (*délire alcoolique*). In the first group, tremors, delirium, and digestive symptoms last several days following a drinking episode. In the second, the delirium persists for a longer time and hallucinosis often lasts for several months. These individuals usually have a long history of drinking, with previous episodes of delirium, and manifest greater impairment in physical and intellectual functioning. The third group is characterized by the development of a systematic delusional system that persists indefinitely. Hereditary antecedents account for the greater toxicity of alcohol among these individuals. The last group is relatively incurable, while the first two sometimes respond to a change in social milieu or occupation.

In addition to the identification of subtypes based on inherited tendencies, another theme in the 19th century French literature is the description and differentiation of chronic alcoholism. Modeling their concept after the *alcoholismus chronicus* of Magnus Huss, numerous writers described a disease condition attributable to alternations in the nervous system. Lancereaux (cited in ref. 10), as well as Triboulet and Mathieu,[10] described three types of chronic alcoholism according to the predominant beverage used. *Oenilisme* is a condition often observed among the 3-liter-a-day wine drinkers who first develop digestive and liver disorders and only later "nervous" problems such as delirium tremens. In contrast, *alcoolisme* results from the regular ingestion of distilled beverages. Drinkers with this condition first develop polyneuropathy and other neurological disorders, then digestive problems. A third condition, *absinthisme,* is developed by chronic users of absinthe, a popular mint-flavored liqueur made from toxic wormwood oil. The course of absinthism is rapid and the primary symptoms include convulsions, hallucinations, hyperreflexia, partial paralysis, cramps, hot flashes, nightmares, delusions, and delirium. According to Triboulet and Mathieu,[10] *absinthisme* and *alcoolisme* are more likely than *oenilisme* to be hereditary. Triboulet and Mathieu questioned the utility of the Lancereaux classification since the beverage preferences of many alcoholics are eclectic. They proposed a threefold classification: (1) dipsomaniacs; (2) hereditary regular alcoholics; and (3) nonhereditary *buveurs d'habitude* (habitual drinkers). Depending on the stage of development, three types of treatment are appropriate for the latter group. Simple moral treatment, consisting of simple advice, education, and support, is recommended for early *buveurs d'habitude.* At a more advanced stage, the authors recommend voluntary commitment to a special asylum where manual work, hydrotherapy, leisure activities, and moral treatment would be available. For recidivists and "moral degenerates," compulsory treatment in a regimented institution for at least a year is recommended.

Another theme implicit in late 19th century French literature is the differentiation of chronic alcoholism from a less pronounced form of latent alcohol dependence. In his book entitled *Les Alcoolisés Nonalcooliques,* Dromard[11] describes a widespread form of latent alcoholic intoxication that does not manifest itself with clearly defined symptoms. Termed *alcoolomanie* (alcohol mania), this condition is characterized by progressive habituation (*accoutumance*) to the toxic effects of alcohol, followed by an irresistible need (*besoin*) to drink. Mild tremulousness and other symptoms are relieved by morning drinking, and all subsequent activities are dictated by the need to drink in relatively small doses throughout the day. With the gradual deterioration of physical stamina, cognitive functioning, and personality adjustment, these *buveurs d'habitude* eventually require hospitalization. Unlike Tribolet and Mathieu, Dromard suggests that institutional treatment is useless, since the major solution for the alcohol problem in France lies in the improvement of living and working conditions for the lower classes.

Although these 19th century French alienists were read widely in the Anglo-Saxon countries, there is a distinct preference for subtypes reflecting culturally conditioned patterns of drinking. In particular, absinthism and latent alcoholism are varieties peculiar to France, which led the world in the *per capita* consumption of both absinthe and wine. Nevertheless, elements of the French typologies were influential in other countries, especially the neurobiological hereditary theories of Magnan and Legrain and the descriptions of chronic alcoholism by Lancereaux and others.

5. Early American Typologies

American typology theory before Prohibition was dominated by the American Association for the Study and Cure of Inebriety. The Association was organized in 1870 to bring together alienists and other medical practitioners interested in the scientific study of alcoholism. Their founding principles were based on the assumption that inebriety is a disease that is curable, especially when treated at specialized inebriate asylums. In the 1890s, the Association promoted what Jaffe[42] refers to as the psychological disease concept of alcoholism. The diagnosis of alcoholism and the classification of alcoholics were frequent topics in the pages of its scholarly review, the *Quarterly Journal of Inebriety*.

In his address before the Association in 1870, Dr. Willard Parker (quoted in Parrish,[12] pp. 124–125) observed that there are different classes of patients "whose condition varies, like their family history." Parker's groups, defined primarily on the basis of inherited characteristics, include: (1) inebriates who have healthy and temperate parents, but who nevertheless develop a disease after frequent social drinking manifested by a "depraved appetite" for alcohol; (2) descendants from "drinking stock," who have an inherited tendency or predisposition to develop "irresistible craving" that occurs in "paroxysms"; and (3) young drinkers who "are depraved in all their instincts." Although Parker's types are not well developed in terms of presenting symptoms and other characteristics, several treatment implications are discussed. The first group is thought to respond well to the care of specialized inebriate asylums. The second group is less curable, but these alcoholics are also candidates for the asylums. The third group is best dealt with through the legal system since they "do not desire either reformation or improvement."

A somewhat different typology was published in 1883 by Association member Joseph Parrish[12] in his book *Alcoholic Inebriety from a Medical Standpoint*. Parrish's typology is based on the belief that "there are certain peculiarities that are displayed with such remarkable uniformity in the career of some inebriates as to warrant their classification into separate groups" (pp. 51–52). Parrish's groups included: (1) the solitary, midnight inebriates, usually men of "learning, integrity and piety," whose secretive drinking leads to habitual craving and chronic alcoholism; (2) inebriates having a possible organic propensity to violence or other vices; (3) traumatic inebriates, whose exciting causes include injuries to the head and "psychical traumatism;" and (4) hereditary inebriates. Although Parrish argues that inebriate asylums are needed for "a more clear and satisfactory distinction in the varieties of its forms" (p. 125), there is little discussion of differential treatment or prognosis for these groups.

As founding editor of the Association's *Journal* and one of the leading treatment experts in the country, Thomas Crothers was familiar with the major trends and writings in the field. Thus, it is not surprising that when Crothers[6] published a volume in 1893 to summarize the first two decades of the Association's work, topics such as the classification and forms of inebriety would play a prominent part. Entitled *The Disease of Inebriety from Alcohol, Opium and Other Narcotic Drugs,* the volume largely consists of writings published in the *Journal of Inebriety* and provides a comprehensive synopsis of the major threads of typological thinking during the late 19th century.

The Association's typologies are loosely organized around two concepts, inebriety and dipsomania. Inebriety is a more general term referring to habitual drunkenness. It was especially popular in the nomenclature of the Association's medical establishment because it served to distinguish alcoholism (a disease) from drunkenness (a moral disorder). Inebriates, as a general class, are divided into four groups: (1) accidental inebriates, whose drinking is due to external environmental conditions or to organic functional disturbance; (2) emotional inebriates, "who are always on the borders of hysteria, with feeble and unstable will . . . all the time suffering from a constitutional unrest . . ." and for whom "spirits afford relief for this physical state . . ." (p. 28); (3) solitary inebriates, persons often occupying responsible positions, "who use spirits only at night or alone, and seem morbidly sensitive to conceal this fact" (p. 28); and (4) pauper inebriates, for whom inebriety is another symptom of their disadvantaged socioeconomic condition.

Dipsomania is used to describe a large and special class of inebriates "in which the drink impulse comes on suddenly and after a time dies out, and is succeeded by a free interval" (p. 29). In the 19th century, the term refers often to periodic alcoholism where the drinking bouts are precipitated by apparently spontaneous craving. Three principal forms are outlined with considerable attention given to etiology, natural history, prognosis, and treatment. The first, acute dipsomania, is considered to be uncommon. In this condition, the "drink craze" comes on suddenly from such influences as sunstroke, excessive stress, and exhaustion. Because it resembles mania in its violence and uncontrollability, it may constitute a manifestation of insanity. The second and more common type is periodic dipsomania. Large quantities of spirits are consumed during periodic attacks that occur without any apparent "premonitory" symptom. While drinking, periodic inebriates seem to lose conception of their moral obligations. In terms of etiology, "the periodic variety seems hardly ever to be induced by acquired habits of drinking alcohol, it being almost always the result of strong hereditary tendency to neurosis of some kind" (p. 32). Treatment consists of "elevating the moral nature by every possible means, improving the patient's general health, and getting him to employ his mind and body actively" (p. 34). Bromide of potassium is also recommended for treating periodic attacks of drinking, since it seems to work for epilepsy. In cases where the "moral nature is evidently low, weak or absent, no hope can be held out for cure" (p. 34). For these cases a "proper law" is required, presumably to sequester these individuals.

The third and most common form is chronic dipsomania. In these cases, drinking usually starts at an early age. Many die of alcohol-related causes before age 30. Hardly drunk, never sober, these continuous drinkers eventually develop constant craving and deteriorate physically and mentally. Delirium tremens is common. Where the disease is hereditary and begins early in life, a lack of "moral sensibility" dating from adolescence is found. In acquired dipsomania, moral degeneration is a direct result of drinking and develops later in life. The chronic form of inebriety is "very incurable." Although prolonged hot baths may be useful, this form of inebriety is best treated through the establishment of work-house hospitals "where the inebriate can be treated and restrained" (p. 200). Recurrent cases should be sentenced for as long as 10 years. These individuals "should be thoroughly organized into military habits of life and work, and kept in the best conditions of forced healthy living" (p. 200).

In addition to the global classes of inebriates, and the specific and clinically detailed types of dipsomaniacs, the Association's book also classifies inebriates as hereditary and acquired, borrowing heavily from the theories popularized by Magnan, Legrain, and others. According to Crothers,[6] 80% are hereditary (p. 156). In general, hereditary alcoholism is thought to begin earlier, and "shows itself by irritability, instability, and a vicious moral disposition, which seems to place the sufferer under some burden to find an excitement which will relieve him from his suffering" (p. 156).

In 1911, Crothers[7] published the crowning work of his 43-year career as an alcoholism specialist. Entitled *Inebriety: A Clinical Treatise,* it went far beyond his previous 1893 formulations in comprehensiveness and scope. Crothers' discussion of typologies begins with the admission that there are "innumerable classes of drinkers, and the effort to divide them is beset with difficulties, for the reason that the causes of the desire for spirits and the resistance of the body to spirits are at present largely unknown" (p. 40). Using case histories to illustrate the various types of inebriates, Crothers provides a general introduction to typologies formulated by himself and others. These include: (1) the "trained and cultivated inebriates" characterized by a long, gradual preliminary period of moderate drinking; (2) the erratic "explosive" drinker; (3) various types of periodic drinkers; (4) psychopathic drinkers; and (5) the senile inebriate whose drinking begins just before death. In addition, Crothers discusses a more general cultural typology based on the kinds of alcoholics found in Europe and America. The American inebriate, in particular, drinks to produce psychological effects, and exhibits a manialike alternation between heavy drinking and abstinence. Crothers attributes this pattern to rapid social change and to the intensity of life in America.

Crothers' most systematic treatment of typologies is contained in two chapters under the separate headings of "Continuous Drinkers" and "Periodic

Drinkers." The continuous drinker is similar to Crothers' "trained and cultivated" European variety of inebriate. These drinkers use spirits regularly and literally become paralyzed by the toxic effects of alcohol. They tend to be more diseased and degenerate than periodic drinkers. Several etiologies are described. The first is constitutional degenerations and defects due to heredity or to physical and psychical causes existing long before drinking began, such as dyspepsia, bad nutrition, or unhygienic living conditions. The second is physical and psychical exhaustion. In a large percentage of cases there is "a distinct neurotic and psychopathic condition, which is traceable to the ancestors, and is clearly transmitted to the next generation" (p. 109).

Crothers' second type of drinker, the periodic form, manifests itself in two basic patterns: (1) an irregular pattern in which the drinking period is variable in length and unpredictable in its timing; and (2) a regular pattern in which the "drink attack" is always the same with the nondrinking period constant. As the disease progresses, the nondrinking intervals become shorter and the patient eventually becomes a regular drinker. Periodic drinkers are always neurotic and psychasthenic, often secretive in their drinking, and sometimes exhibit emotional changes such as depression.

In a book entitled *Inebriety: Its Source, Prevention, and Cure,* Association member Charles F. Palmer[13] devoted a chapter to the "Moral Characteristics and Various Types of the Inebriate." The types he identified were: (1) the "brutal criminal inebriate of our cities," characterized as "the blackguard drunkard of our streets, big of limb, broad of chest, low of brow . . . thief and murderer by inherent qualities . . . always the concentrated living spawn of the accumulating growth of generations of depravity" (p. 98); (2) the nervous animal type, the "spoiled boy" of the *nouveau riche* whose "later education is of billiard halls, concert saloons, dance houses, gambling dens, and brothels" (p. 99); (3) the intellectual type who, when drinking "indulges in the intellectual form of pleasure rather than the animal . . ." (p. 100); and (4) the domestic and religious type, whose "periodical attacks of intoxicative mania seem to come as a resultant of his quiet, noncombative existence, his soft and yielding nature, the disturbing influences of uncongenial living, and as a corrective medicine for his mental and physical weakness" (p. 101). Palmer's last two types are "the product of hereditary disease" (p. 100), the latter "a congenital neurotic." Although little attention is given to treatment implications, he does suggest that by "turning our prisons and jails into schools of mental hygiene," the value of such a system would be incalculable with respect to the "brutal criminal inebriate."

About the same time as Crothers published his text on *Inebrity,* Isador Coriat[16] advanced a surprisingly comprehensive typological theory in a concise article in the *British Journal of Inebriety.* Borrowing liberally from various European writers such as Kraepelin and Janet, Coriat conceptualizes inebriety not as a disease but as "a species of an abnormal mental reaction." Like Crothers, Coriat distinguishes between the "steady tippler" and the periodic drinker. The steady tippler is the classic chronic alcoholic who initially uses alcohol for its stimulatory effect, either for social reasons or to relieve fatigue. Four types of periodic drinkers are also proposed, each having a distinctive etiology related to different psychological causes. The first type is due to mild depression and anxiety arising from business or social stressors. The second type, genuine or true dipsomania, is "a form of epilepsy in which the drinking is due to an uncontrollable impulse or obsession" (p. 141). The third variety is associated with cyclothymia, which is seen as a mild variant of manic depressive insanity. The last type of periodic drinker is characterized by "psychasthenic impulsion, so well described by Janet." As in the case of cyclothymia, constitutional factors may be involved. Since alcoholism is due to these kinds of "abnormal mental reactions" rather than physical causes, Coriat suggests that the most appropriate treatment is some form of psychotherapy. Indeed, "purely physical methods of treatment are not only unscientific, but are to be deprecated" (p. 146).

Psychotherapy is thought to work best for the steady tippler, least well for the true dipsomaniacs. Beginning with total abstinence, psychotherapy is intended to "increase the will power," to instill an indifference to alcohol and an intolerance for it, and to associate alcohol with nausea and disgust" (p. 147). Like many psychiatrists of the period, hypnosis was considered by Coriat as the best procedure to effect this change of mental attitude. While Coriat's typology is consistent with the Association's psychological disease concept of alcoholism, it goes beyond previous formulations in proposing psychological treatment for the types considered most amenable to psychotherapy.

A number of common themes are evident in the typology theories promoted by Crothers and other Association members. These include the description of ideal types, the use of case histories as the major form of illustration and validation, the introduction of psychological constructs such as neurosis, psychosis, mania and craving to explain etiology; the invocation of genetic constructs to account for individual differences in host susceptibility; careful description of natural history for different types; and specific discussion of differential therapeutic approaches.

6. Typologies of Public Inebriates

In the early part of the 20th century, several investigations of the Massachusetts penal system were devoted to differential treatment for different types of drunkenness offenders and to institutional alternatives to imprisonment. M.F. Parmelee's[15] study of *Inebriety in Boston* was published as a Ph.D. thesis in 1909. A total of 650 cases, randomly selected from eight courts, was studied by means of a 77-item interview schedule. The primary aim of the study was to describe the social and demographic characteristics of drunkenness offenders in relation to those of the general population.

In discussing the utility of imprisonment for these individuals, Parmelee adopted a twofold classification of "occasional and habitual drunkards." The criteria for the occasional drunkard are not clearly specified, but it is suggested that these individuals are likely to be first offenders who are not seriously dependent on alcohol. In contrast, the "rounder" or habitual drunkard has "a physiological craving for drink which results in an inebriety which is more or less constant or which returns at periodic intervals." Because it is assumed that "rounders" are in part a product of the existing penal system, it is strongly recommended that occasional drunkards be given probation and then be treated by social agencies. Habitual drunkards, on the other hand, "should be sent for an indefinite length of time to an institution, more like a hospital or asylum than a prison, where they will be subjected to examination and to treatment . . ." (p. 62). Parmelee recommends the establishment of a farm colony where therapeutic work is combined with medical treatment. Given the assumed hereditary nature of alcoholism, this approach amounts to substituting "artificial for natural selection. . . . By segregating these individuals from society, they are prevented from propagating themselves. Thus, in the course of time, this type of inebriate would be eliminated from society" (p. 64).

In a study similar in nature but less drastic in its recommendations, Anderson[17] provides a medical-psychiatric description of *The Alcoholic as Seen in Court*. Based on a random sample of 50 "habitual" and 50 "periodic" drinkers having long records of drunkenness arrests, Anderson notes these two types are "essentially different in makeup, and apparently requiring different methods of handling" (p. 5). The habitual drinker imbibes alcohol "more or less steadily, and perhaps in small quantities, for a prolonged period of years. He shows an insidious, progressive impairment of his nervous system and lowering of the functional activities of the entire organism" (p. 5). In contrast, the periodic drinker has "drink paroxysms which subside and are followed by periods of sanity and rational thought and conduct. . . . He is a neurotic individual with a nervous system that is unstable and poorly unbalanced" (p. 5). In perhaps the first statistical comparison of alcoholic subtypes, Anderson's data show that more of the habitual drinkers are found to be mentally defective and physically deteriorated, while greater numbers of the periodic drinkers are self-supporting and diagnosed as psychopaths.

Considering these physical and mental handicaps, Anderson concludes that the best interests of the individual would be served by medical rather than penal treatment. Prolonged hospital care and farm colony treatment are recommended for the habitual or chronic alcoholic, while the periodic alcoholic should be "incorporated back into society by means of well-directed medical and social service methods of treatment" (p. 11).

The last study devoted to the public inebriate problem was commissioned by the Massachusetts State legislature. In 1909, the Trustees of the Foxborough State Hospital were asked to "report upon the treatment of inebriates in

Massachusetts." James Ford, a Ph.D. and an instructor at Harvard University, was appointed by the Trustees to review court and institutional procedures for the treatment of drunkenness offenders. The report recommended a differential approach to the processing of drunkenness offenders based on certain medical and social assumptions about the underlying causes of drunken comportment: "Any plan for the disposition of drunkards must be sufficiently adaptable to conform to the needs of each specific case." Three types of drunkards were identified: accidental, occasional, and habitual. The latter condition was considered a disease characterized by craving and loss of self-control. Habitual inebriates were distinguished further into: (1) normally healthy individuals whose stressful or unhygienic environment lowered their resistance to alcohol; (2) periodic inebriates or dipsomaniacs; and (3) "defectives" and "degenerates." To satisfy the need for a differential treatment of the public inebriate, a graded approach was recommended. Occasional and accidental inebriates would first receive a combination of release, probation, and fines. Pathologic cases in their early stages were to be sent to Foxborough or to a similar treatment facility. Finally, incurable, chronic inebriates were to be given indeterminate sentences and sent to a proposed detention farm colony located in a rural setting "free of the temptations of alcohol."

Several important features distinguish these typologies from the medical and psychiatric approaches of the Association's contemporaries. First, statistical data rather than clinical case histories provide the empirical basis for the typologies. Second, the types are ordered along a continuum of severity and chronicity. Third, while the clinical characteristics and etiologies of the subtypes are not well developed, the policy implications of the typology are given special emphasis. Finally, the influence of the eugenics movement is translated into concrete policy recommendations.

7. Later American Typologies

As indicated in Table 1, no articles on typologies were published by American authors between 1916 and 1932. The climate of Prohibition, the demise of the American Association for the Study and Cure of Inebriety, and the ultimate dissolution of the alcoholism treatment system in the United States are possible reasons for this hiatus. With the notable exception of Fleming's[20] and White's[10] papers, the Post-Prohibition typologies have a distinct psychoanalytic flavor.

One of the more influential and enduring typologies in this group was proposed by psychoanalyst Robert Knight.[22] Knight's typology is based on the assumption that "alcoholism is only a symptom, not a clinical entity," and that "no excessive drinker is normal and well adjusted when sober" (p. 1444). Three types are proposed. Essential alcoholics are characterized by "oral fixation" and conflict between passive, feminine wishes and masculine strivings. These "psychopaths" drink excessively from adolescence and are unable to function well in school or occupational roles. Their prognosis is poor, especially in contrast to the second type, called "reactive" alcoholics. For these individuals a "discoverable precipitating event" initiates heavy drinking, which is often periodic. They tend to be better adjusted than the essential alcoholics and to have a better attitude toward treatment. In the third group, called symptomatic alcoholics, drinking is seen as only incidental to other prominent neurotic or psychotic symptoms. According to Knight, the treatment for those alcoholics who are intelligent and motivated is sanatorium care for a few months combined with psychoanalysis, which continues for several months after discharge.

Borrowing liberally from Knight's formulation, psychiatrist William Menninger[23] proposed a similar typology in a 1938 article. In addition to Knight's essential and reactive types, Menninger described "neurotic characters" and psychotic personalities. Both were elaborations of Knight's symptomatic alcoholics. Like Knight, Menninger recommends individualized psychoanalytic psychotherapy aimed at helping the patient "achieve a psychosexual maturity with an insight into the nature of his previous methods of attempted solution of conflicts" (p. 103).

A third psychoanalytic typology was outlined by psychiatrist E.B. Allen.[21] Similar to Knight's essential type, the psychopathic alcoholic is inadequate from youth, begins drinking at puberty and "never accomplishes anything worthwhile." Allen's second type is the neurotic alcoholic, who overcompensates in his career until failure leads to alcoholism. Rejecting hereditary etiology, Allen urges that "alcoholics are begotten of abstinent as well as convivial fathers" (p. 1500).

Not all psychiatrists of the period, however, based their typologies on psychoanalytic theory. In answer to Allen's contention that alcoholic drinking reflects fixation at the "oral liquid stage" of emotional development, Robert Fleming[20] notes that "only a superficial consideration of the other available orifices is necessary to make the scientist cautious in attaching much significance to the selection of the oral route" (p. 782). Fleming's typology divides alcoholics into two groups. The first is characterized by symptomatic drinking, where excessive alcohol use is a response to an underlying mental or physical pathologic condition. The second, true alcohol addiction, is characterized by habituation and specific craving. True addiction tends to develop later than symptomatic drinking, and at times is the cumulative result of symptomatic drinking. Treatment of symptomatic drinking consists of treating the underlying condition, while true addiction must be treated first by detoxification and then by substitution. The latter should take place in hospital over a period lasting from 6 to 12 months. By substitution is meant the exchange of drinking for some alternative type of satisfaction such as religion or abstinence clubs. Apomorphine counterconditioning is also suggested as a possible treatment of true addiction.

8. German Typologies

As indicated in Table I, almost all of the German typologies were published between 1924 and 1936. The 1920s in Germany were characterized by increased academic interest in cultural anthropology, laboratory science and the classification of mental disorders.[43] In the 1930s, all aspects of intellectual life in Germany were influenced by the rise of the Nazi state, which was particularly hostile to psychoanalytic theory. The typologies of alcoholics proposed in this period must be viewed as a culmination of interest in characterology beginning with Eduard Spranger and ending with Ernest Kretschmer (1888–1964). Kretschmer's[25] treatise on constitutional types was based on clinical observation of the physique and temperament of psychiatric patients. In 1924, he outlined two groups of chronic alcoholic: (1) a pyknic, cyclothymic type for whom alcoholism develops within a pliable, gregarious disposition; and (2) schizoid types who are nervous individuals using alcohol for relief of internal stress. Kretschmer's types were adopted with varying degrees of modification by Stockert,[27] Cimbal,[26] Pohlisch,[31] and Gabriel and Kratzmann.[34] All of these contrast the convivial or *Stammtisch* drinkers with more psychologically-based forms of alcoholism. For example, Stockert[27] proposes that alcoholism may develop in different constitutional types for different reasons. In addition to Kretschmer's cyclothymic type of convivial drinkers, Stockert identifies two varieties who use alcohol as a drug (*Trinksuchtigen*). The first group consists of "weaklings" who drink primarily to induce pleasant sensations. The second consists of psychopaths. These are asocial repressed personalities who use alcohol to adapt to their environment.

Cimbal's[26] formulations developed out of biographical studies of individual patients and their families. His types were labeled decadent, discordant, spineless, and self-aggrandizing. Decadent drinkers are thought to develop in families in which pampering and inbreeding have been going on for generations, extinguishing the "driving forces." The discordant or impassioned drinkers are persons lacking emotional maturity. Resembling Kretschmer's schizoid drinkers, they drink because they cannot deal with life's tension. Habituation and craving develop out of relief drinking. These individuals are considered good risks for therapy once the source of discordance can be identified and extinguished. The spineless or "stupid" drinkers include vagrants and criminals whose primitive drives are excited by drink. Drinking for them is a passive form of enjoyment, since liquor is the cheapest and lowest form of gregariousness available. The self-aggrandizing drinker is characterized by weak will power and high ambition. Tavern life provides a way of compensating for inferiority feelings, since the *Stammtisch* (table) is an ideal forum for their idle boasting.

The final typology identified in the German literature differs little from the previous constitutional theories in its general content. Nevertheless, Meggendorfer's[35] distinction between "constitutional" and "environmental" alcoholics epitomizes the Nazi conceptualization of alcohol-related deviant behavior and mental disorder. Constitutional alcoholics, estimated to comprise 70% of the alcoholic population, are characterized by a hereditary predisposition to alcoholism and other disorders. These individuals are further subdivided into "mental cases," psychopaths and "criminal antisocials". The smaller proportion of environmental alcoholics (30%), thought to be less addicted to alcohol and more responsive to rehabilitation, are the result of both environmental and genetic causes.

The main features of these German typologies are their reliance on hereditary constitutional theories for an explanation of endogenous etiology. The eclipse of typology theory in Germany in the 1930s was heralded by the nationalization of all alcohol and drug activities by the Nazis. This resulted in partial dissolution of the system of clinics developed for the management of alcoholics.[44] Other significant developments include the suppression of the freedom of inquiry in the universities and the enactment of "racial hygiene" laws, such as the 1933 statute for the "Prevention of Descendents Affected by Hereditary Disorders." That law made it possible to submit as many as 30,000 "hereditary" alcoholics to involuntary surgical sterilization on the basis of vague evidence that their drinking was chronic and therefore inherited.[44,45] Undisciplined, antisocial, constitutional alcoholics were deemed a menace to the Aryan race and therefore were prevented from procreating defective offspring. Since these individuals were considered incurable, they were refused admission to the established treatment system. Only the environmental alcoholics could be treated at the 25 existing inebriate sanitariums. Failure to respond to compulsory treatment could result in transfer to "secure custody", a euphamism for the concentration camp.[45]

9. British Typologies

One of the earliest and most enduring typologies was proposed by Dr. William Carpenter of England in his 1850 essay "On the Use and Abuse of Alcoholic Liquors, in Health and Disease."[36] In it, he described three types of "oenomania": (1) acute, in which the desire to drink occurred suddenly; (2) periodic, in which binges alternate with periods of abstinence; and (3) chronic, in which the drinker is continuously "under the most overwhelming desire for stimulants" (p. 47).

After Carpenter's essay there was little published material on typologies in the British Isles until the period between the two World Wars. Hugh Wingfield, a physician and former president of the British Psycho-Medical Society, published in 1919 a book devoted entirely to *The Forms of Alcoholism and Their Treatment*.[37] He proposed two types of chronic alcoholism and two types of dipsomania. In chronic sober alcoholism the patient regularly drinks to excess but is never intoxicated except by accident. Craving occurs in these patients only if alcohol is cut off. A second type, chronic inebriate alcoholism, resembles the first except the patient is never sober. The third type, pseudodipsomania, is similar to that described by Crothers and others. In these individuals craving appears only after alcohol is consumed. The final type, true dipsomania, is thought to be relatively uncommon. It differs from pseudodipsomania in that craving occurs spontaneously. In addition to these distinguishing characteristics Wingfield goes beyond previous formulations in describing specific differences among types in various dependence symptoms. The types differ primarily with respect to dysphoria (which is absent in the chronic sober alcoholic), tolerance (often diminished in the pseudo-dipsomaniacs), and paralysis of the will (very marked in the dipsomaniacs and absent in the chronic alcoholics). Treatment of the alcoholic is described in two stages: (1) withdrawal, which differs somewhat between the dipsomaniacs and the chronic alcoholics; and (2) measures to induce total abstinence. The latter stage is thought to be initiated with best results at a "voluntary retirement in a retreat for a limited period." To extinguish craving in the chronic alcoholics, a form of aversive conditioning is described in which the patient is forced to drink alcohol after injections of atropine and strychnine. Following institutional treatment, hypnosis is recommended, especially for dipsomaniacs.

Almost 10 years after Wingfield's typology, Crichton-Miller[38] proposed a quite different and original classification based on affective change. Subtypes of steady and intermittent drinkers were explained on the basis of affective states or psychological causes, consistent with the notion that alcohol is used primarily to modify "feeling tone" on either a somatic level (e.g., to relieve fatigue, thirst) or an emotional level (to relieve inferiority feelings). Steady drinkers were divided into four groups: (1) hypopietic drinkers who use alcohol to relieve low blood pressure; (2) subthyroidic drinkers for whom alcohol produces vasomotor stimulation; (3) sensorial types for whom sensation-seeking predominates; and (4) rebels who drink in psychological response to their fathers' complexes. Periodic or intermittent drinkers are also distinguished on the basis of psychological etiologies: (1) epileptic alcoholics, whose explosive craving is analogous to epilepsy, or for whom chronic drinking has produced seizures; (2) the dual personality type, characterized by profound personality dissociations; and (3) manic depressive alcoholics, where craving is a feature of either phase. According to Crichton-Miller, "no single aetiology will cover the pathogenesis of alcoholism" and the therapist who deals in a stereotyped treatment is "open to criticism." Nevertheless, aside from stating that the manic depressive group is resistant to virtually all types of treatment, no recommendations are made for the differential management of these types.

Another comprehensive typology was described by Carver *et al.* in their book on *Alcoholism in General Practice.*[40] In it, they first differentiate the "true alcoholist" from the symptomatic drinker. The former are predisposed to develop craving and use alcohol for its euphoric or tension-reducing effects. True alcoholics are classified into three types. The first are the intermittent cases having either regular or irregular periodicity. Tolerance is not pronounced in these individuals, but eventually the intervals between drinking bouts become shorter and the pattern merges into that of the regular or chronic alcoholist. The regular drinker acquires increased tolerance, which undermines his constitution and produces the classic signs of chronic alcoholism. Some of these individuals drink regularly but are always sober, while others demonstrate bouts of acute intoxication in addition to their regular drinking. The sober regular drinkers develop more physical impairments than the previous types. The third group, paroxysmal dipsomaniacs, are characterized by "paroxysmal attacks of depression associated with an intense craving for alcohol occurring in regular cycles" (p. 14). Like many other treatments of dipsomania, this type is thought to resemble epilepsy and to be precipitated by internal, metabolic factors. Despite some modifications in terminology and content, Carver *et al.*'s typology is similar to that proposed by Wingfield.[37] Although the authors give rather extensive description of the varieties of institutional treatment available, there is no mention of the usefulness or application of their typology to the clinical management of patients.

10. The Bowman–Jellinek Synthesis of 20th Century Typologies

In their classic 1941 review of the alcoholism treatment literature,[4] "Alcohol Addiction and Its Treatment," psychiatrist Karl Bowman (1888–1973) and biometrist E.M. Jellinek (1890–1963) devoted a major section to the description and integration of 24 of the typological formulations summarized in Table I. In their attempt to synthesize the meaning of these typologies, Bowman and Jellinek created a hierarchical classification system shown in Fig. 1. They argued that this would serve as an efficient way of identifying "ultimate" types, and would result in the greater predictive value of typologies. The typologies were differentiated first on the broadest, most general level of analysis: steady versus intermittent drinking. These groups were further subclassified on the basis of etiology (endogenous versus exogenous) and next into four "ultimate" subgroups: (1) steady, endogenous, primary addicts; (2) steady endogenous symptomatic drinkers; (3) intermittent (irregular) exogenous *Stammtisch* drinkers; and (4) intermittent (periodic) endogenous symptomatic drinkers.

Primary or "true" addicts are a group of types characterized by: (1) a definite need for alcohol; (2) definite functions for drinking; and (3) dependence and inability to abstain that are not determined by habit, mental disease, or physiological processes. Among true alcohol addicts, "the dependence upon alcohol is practically immediate and is psychologically motivated . . . his inability to give up alcohol is to all intents an initial phenomenon" (p. 108). In contrast, the secondary addict is initially not dependent on alcohol but develops habituation and physical dependence in the course

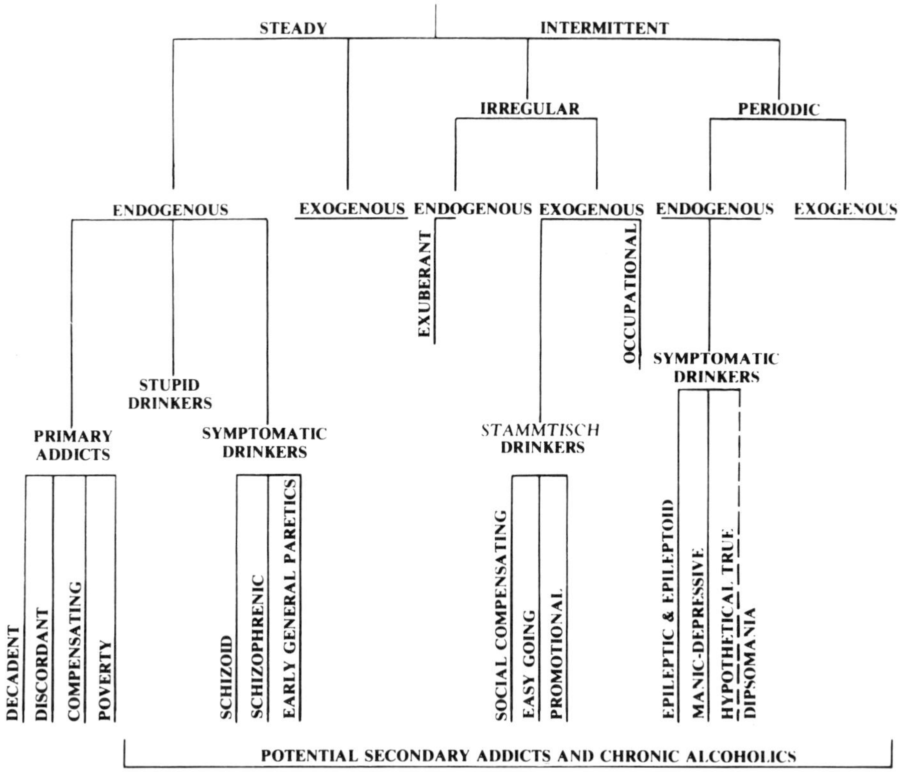

Figure 1. The Bowman–Jellinek[4] classification system of abnormal drinkers.

of prolonged drinking. With the exception of the primary addicts, all of the remaining major types are considered potential secondary addicts.

As indicated in Fig. 1, the subdivisions within the major classifications are defined by similar subtypes, all of which have been outlined in Table I. The "decadent" drinker is intended to be Cimbal's[26] subtype and is thought to be similar to Knight's[22] essential type and Legrain's[8] immoral individual. The discordant drinker is a schizoid personality for whom alcohol is the only means of temporary relief from conflict. While this type is identical to Cimbal's discordant or impassioned drinker, it also resembles Knight's reactive alcoholic. A third subtype is the compensating drinker who, like Cimbal's self-aggrandizing type, is motivated to drink primarily because of unconscious feelings of inferiority. The last group of primary addicts, the poverty drinkers, combine elements of endogenous readiness with an exogenous precipitating factor, such as unemployment, so that drinking is a basic solution to their problems. The classification of Cimbal's "stupid drinkers" is considered as a separate endogenous category because their excessive drinking is "determined by lack of resistance inherent in the feeble-minded constitution" (p. 135). For the "stupid drinker," neither a true addict nor a symptomatic drinker, "alcohol has no other function than to supply brute pleasure."

Another major group whose drinking is considered to be endogenously conditioned is termed the symptomatic drinkers. In this classification, drinking is only one of many symptoms of an underlying cause such as schizophrenia, manic depressive disorder, or epilepsy. Representative types include the symptomatic schizoid drinkers for whom drinking is incidental to personality difficulties; the schizophrenic drinker, characterized at times by violent drinking; and the early general paresis drinker whose wild, continuous drinking is the expression of grandiose personality disorder.

Another group of symptomatic drinkers is distinguished by virtue of its periodic drinking pattern. These include the epileptic and epileptoid drinkers who exhibit wild drinking bouts; manic-depressive drinkers whose drinking is just one of many symptoms; and hypothetical true dipsomaniacs whose periodic drinking is a symptom of an organic disease.

The so-called exuberant drinker is a hypomanic type who "avails himself of any special occasion to go into excess." These individuals, according to Bowman and Jellinek, seem to return to moderate drinking or abstinence with maturity.

The group designated as the *Stammtisch* drinkers are "socially conditioned excessive drinkers who use alcohol practically every day around the cafe or restaurant table in conformity with their cultural group" (p. 531). Their high degree of tolerance nevertheless contributes to the development of alcohol-related diseases. Other names for this type are the "good-fellow" and "gregarious" drinker. The subtypes included within this classification are: (1) social compensating drinkers who drink to overcome "fairly conscious" feelings of social inadequacy; (2) the easy-going drinker who tends to be an unsophisticated, good-natured, cyclothymic type; and (3) the promotional drinker who utilizes the camaraderie of drinking to promote his business.

Another group of exogenously determined, socially conditioned alcoholics is the occupational drinkers. This group includes brewery and distillery employees, waiters and barmen, and manual laborers who "through their constant exposure to alcoholic beverages, frequently become excessive drinkers" (p. 136).

According to Bowman and Jellinek, *Stammtisch* and occupational drinkers comprise a large part of the drinking population. True addicts are a comparatively small group, "perhaps exceeded even by symptomatic drinkers." In commenting on the eclectic nature of this typology, Floch[46] states that "the Bowman–Jellinek schedule is more significantly inclusive than any other schedule encountered thus far, providing for the largest number of concretely described categories meaningful with regard to prediction" (pp. 532–533).

In what is perhaps the first empirical evaluation of alcoholic typologies since the 1919 study of Anderson,[17] Floch[46,47] attempted to apply the Bowman–Jellinek system to a sample of 276 institutionalized prisoners having a history of abnormal drinking. Drawing on information obtained from case histories, psychiatric examinations, psychometric tests, clinic reports, official records, and interviews with relatives, the author attempted to classify the sample into the 17 subgroups outlined by Bowman and Jellinek.

Contrary to Bowman and Jellinek's contention that the *Stammtisch* and occupational drinkers would be most prevalent, Floch found the stupid drinker as most numerous (43.8%), followed by the discordant (15.6%), compensating (6.5%), and decadent (4.7%) drinkers. These latter groups are all from the category of primary addicts. Subgroups, such as the social compensating, the exuberant, and the promotional drinkers, were not identified in Floch's sample, and 6.8% were unclassifiable.

11. Conclusion: Retrospect and Prospect

This chapter has considered the roots of alcoholic typology theory, its growth and application in various countries and historical eras, and the major typological systems developed. Our interest throughout has not been to describe a museum of oddities or antiquities, although numerous efforts have seemingly led into blind alleys and absurdities, at least by contemporary standards. Rather, the review has shown that alcoholic typologies are embedded in a rich tradition of speculation, theory, and clinical observation, whose insights may serve as useful guideposts for contemporary efforts to understand and provide treatment for alcoholism. This concluding section of the chapter will, therefore, focus on historical trends in typology theory, similarities and differences among typologies, the apparent functions served by typological formulations, and the limitations of typology theories.

From the beginning of medical and scientific interest in alcoholism as a disease, there has been a concomitant interest in differential diagnosis, the identification of separate etiological paths into alcoholism, the description of distinctive symptom patterns, and the matching of different kinds of treatment to distinct types of patients. Although this interest has been consistent and continuous over almost a century, there have been clearly defined trends within certain countries and during various historical periods.

Like the growth of other areas of knowledge, typological theory resulted from the interaction of multiple factors: the theory of evolution, the development of modern medicine, the emergence of psychiatry as a separate branch of medicine, the acceptance of the psychological disease concept of alcoholism and the growth of a separate system for the institutional treatment of alcoholics. Seen in this light, typology theories are often a reflection of trends existing in other sciences and of the *Weltanschauung* of an era.

In France, typology theories were concentrated in the last quarter of the 19th century when alcoholism was becoming recognized as a major public health problem. As the birthplace of modern psychiatry and the exemplar of humane treatment of the insane, France was the logical country to stimulate the formulation of alcoholic typologies. Although the notions of moral insanity and hereditary degeneration have not stood the test of time, they were influential concepts that were incorporated into numerous German and American typologies. The French were also the first to identify a culturally patterned typology, *buveurs d'habitude,* that suggested social origins rather than biological or psychological etiologies.

Numerous American typologies in the late 19th century and the first two decades of the 20th assimilated many of the concepts of the Europeans. American typologies are characterized by their pragmatism and emphasis on psychological causes. In contrast to the French interest in organic explanations and neurological theories, the Americans were more interested in clinical typologies that could be studied and treated in institutional settings, preferably inebriate asylums. American typologies of the 1930s show little continuity with the theories formulated prior to Prohibition. With their tendency to focus almost exclusively on psychological etiology, these typologies seem considerably less ambitious and comprehensive than their predecessors.

In many respects, the British typologies of the 1920s and 1930s are the most sophisticated in terms of the attention given to etiology, manifestational symptoms, natural history, the concept of addiction, and treatment implications. With their emphasis on constitutional and hereditary typologies, the German formulations of this same period share much in common with earlier French theories. Yet, the German typologies are also very modern in their use of the emerging classification system that was to dominate Western psychiatry until the present.

Viewing the long history of typology theory, it is thus possible to discern a series of eras, each dominated to a certain extent by a theme. There is, however, little progressive movement in a predictable direction, if one defines progress as increasing knowledge and improving practice.

Despite the apparent differences in classification criteria and the relative emphasis given to theoretical or practical implications, there are a number of common themes running through these typologies. These germs of insight should not be overlooked, since they say a great deal about the similar functions and common content of typological theories. First, almost all typologies are multidimensional, deriving their classification criteria from various combinations of etiological, behavioral, or psychophysiological variables. Hereditary, psychopathological, and socially conditioned factors are often cited as separate and distinct paths into alcoholism. The presence, absence or scheduling of craving is frequently used to differentiate patterns of consumption and types of addiction. The pattern of consumption (continuous versus periodic) is explained on the basis of dependence and etiological variables. Finally, the notion of chronicity appears as a separate typological category and, at times, as the final common pathway of all typologies. These commonalities, first identified and synthesized by Bowman and Jellinek[4] have unfortunately not resulted in any consensus in the field as to the classification and forms of alcoholism. Although many aspects of these typologies bear striking resemblance to contemporary formulations (see, for example, refs. 48–50), there is little to suggest that current theorists have derived inspiration from them. One exception is the Bowman–Jellinek synthesis, which 20 years later appeared as the foundation for Jellinek's[2] five species of alcoholism.

The ultimate failure of typological theories to gain widespread acceptance, even within their own time, is perhaps a reflection of the limitations of these theories, especially when viewed by contemporary standards. Although current typology theory shows a similar lack of consistency and consensus, there have been significant attempts to establish scientifically based ground rules for an optimal approach to study alcoholic typologies.[48–50]

Implicit in the notions of typology reviewed in this chapter are a number of assumptions about the definition, derivation, and verification of alcoholic subtypes. These assumptions include the relative homogeneity of persons within typological groups, the presence of different etiological paths into alcoholism, dissimilar manifestations of alcohol problems and symptoms, differences in prognosis and natural history, and different approaches to selection and treatment. These assumptions for a theory of typology are not unlike those proposed by contemporary theorists,[48–50] and can serve as a basis for a brief critique of these typologies in terms of their scientific rigor and clinical relevance.

By these standards it seems that the 39 typologies suffer from a number of shortcomings. First, the classification rules and criteria required to make reliable assignments are often absent or ambiguous. Nowhere in the discussions of hereditary types is there mention of a procedure for determining the presence or absence of familial alcoholism. Similarly, there are no criteria provided in the typologies based on dependence to evaluate the quality or frequency of craving. The lack of an operational definition makes it unlikely that these typologies could lend themselves to reliable classification into homogeneous groups. It also reduces the possibility that they could be subjected to scientific validation, then or now.

Although the typologies are often rich in clinical description and are frequently based on case histories that serve as ideal types or exemplars, there is little effort to provide external validation for the theories. Indeed, with the exception of Anderson's[17] and Parmelee's[15] statistical studies and Floch's[46,47] evaluation of the Bowman–Jellinek classification, there are no empirical data available to support or refute these theories. It may be unfair to expect empirical validation of the early typologies, but the total lack of research interest in post-World War I typologies suggests that neither group was heuristic. The typologies can also be faulted for their lack of comprehensiveness. Many are unrealistically specific in their differentiation of types based on psychopathology,[19,21–23] excluding completely any types without psychiatric disorder. Many types lack comprehensiveness, owing to an exclusive reliance on just one classification criterion.[13,18,21–23,25,26,32,33,41] A number of the etiological types, for example, say nothing about the nature of dependence, the pattern of drinking, or the chronicity of the disorder. The most glaring limitation in terms of comprehensiveness is the total exclusion of any reference to female alcoholics in these typologies. Without exception, the typologies apply to male alcoholics, with only passing reference given to females, most often with respect to the connection between menstrual distress and acute dipsomania. Although a number of typologies mention treatment implications and propose the possibility of rational treatment matching, there is no organized theory of treatment types. The possible exception is the psychoanalytic theories.[21–23]

Given these ostensible limitations, it may be instructive to ask what functions have been served by typology theory in the past and what lessons may be learned for future work. One apparent function of most typologies is theoretical, either as explanations of alcoholism or as secondary theories of psychopathology and behavioral genetics. The first function is obvious in that most typologies begin as an attempt to comprehensively explain the behavior of alcoholics. A number of typologies, however, seem to represent attempts to impose genetic,[19] constitutional,[25] or personality[22] theories on alcoholics. To the extent that nonalcoholics differentiate into the same groups as alcoholics in these models, it is very questionable whether these theories are exclusively alcoholic typologies.

In addition to their theoretical or explanatory functions, typologies have been advanced for practical reasons: either to facilitate treatment planning or to suggest procedures for societal management of alcoholics. With the unfortunate exception of Meggendorfer's[35] ill-fated theory, there is little evidence that typologies have served this purpose. Rather, typology theories most often have served to reinforce and rationalize preexisting notions of therapeutic practice or social policy. For example, typological theories have been advanced to justify medical management of the alcoholic in specialized inebriate asylums,[6,7,10,12,37] reform of the judicial processing of public inebriates,[14,15,17] expansion of social services for alcoholics,[15,17] intensive and long-term psychoanalytic psychotherapy,[21–23] the involuntary sequestering of chronic inebriates,[14,15,17] and the forcible sterilization and genocide of presumed incurable alcoholics.[35]

If the conclusions of this review seem harsh, it is important to note that a similar judgment has been made with respect to contemporary typology theories. In his review of 29 studies designed to identify empirical subtypes, Skinner[49] concludes that these studies have not been well received, nor have they led to improvements in diagnosis or clinical practice. The lesson for the contemporary typology theorist is clear. Unless typologies are formulated on the basis of careful research, sound theory, and clinical relevance, they are likely to provide little more than historical artifacts for the next historian.

ACKNOWLEDGMENT. The writing of this paper was supported in part from grants awarded to the University of Connecticut Alcohol Research Center by the National Institute on Alcohol Abuse and Alcoholism (Nos. 5 T32 AA07290 and 1 P50 AA 03510).

References

1. Sarup G: Historical antecedents of psychology, The recurrent issue of old wine in new bottles. *Am Psychol* 33:478–485, 1978.
2. Jellinek EM: *The Disease Concept of Alcoholism.* New Haven, College and University Press, 1960.
3. Eysenck HJ: *Dimensions of Personality.* London, Routledge and Kegan Paul, 1947.
4. Bowman KM, Jellinek EM: Alcohol addiction and its treatment. *Q J Stud Alcohol* 2:98–176, 1941.
5. Jordy SS: *International Bibliography of Studies on Alcohol, References 1901–1950.* New Jersey, Rutgers Center of Alcohol Studies, vol 1, 1966.
6. Crothers T (ed): *The Disease of Inebriety from Alcohol, Opium and Other Narcotic Drugs.* New York, Arno Press, 1893.
7. Crothers TD: *Inebriety: A Clinical Treatise on the Etiology, Symptomatology, Neurosis, Psychosis and Treatment and the Medico-Legal Relations.* Cincinnati, Harvey Publishing Co., 1911.
8. LeGrain PM: *Hérédité et Alcoolisme.* Paris, Dion, 1889.
9. Magnan LV: *Recherches sur Les Centres Nerveux.* Paris, Masson, 1893.
10. Triboulet H, Mathieu F: *L'Alcool et L'Alcoolisme.* Carre et Naud, Paris, 1900.
11. Dromard DR: *Les Alcoolises non Alcooliques.* Steinheil, Paris, 1902.
12. Parrish J: *Alcoholic Inebriety: From a Medical Standpoint.* Philadelphia, P. Blakiston, Son & Co., 1883.
13. Palmer CF: *Inebriety, Its Source, Prevention, and Cure.* New York, Fleming H. Revell, 1898.
14. Ford J with Woods RA, Mulready E, Allen PR, Locke FL, Foley TJ, Peabody WR: Drunkenness in Massachusetts, conditions and remedies. Special report of the board of trustees of the Foxborough State Hospital. Boston, Wright & Potter, 1910.
15. Parmelee M: *Inebriety in Boston.* Ph.D. Thesis, New York, Columbia University, 1909.
16. Coriat IH: The psycho-pathology and treatment of alcoholism. *Br J Inebr* 9:138–147, 1912.
17. Anderson VV: The alcoholic as seen in court. *Boston Med Surg J* 74:492–495, 1916.
18. Mangold GB: Public treatment of drunkenness in St. Louis. *Wash Univ Stud Sc Tech* 3:271–309, 1916.
19. White WA: *Outlines of Psychiatry. The toxic psychoses.* Washington, Nervous Mental Disease Publishing Co., 1932.
20. Fleming R: Treatment of chronic alcoholism. *N Engl J Med* 217:779–783, 1937.
21. Allen EB: Alcoholism as a psychiatric medical problem. *NY State J Med* 38:1492–1505, 1938.
22. Knight RP: Psychoanalytic treatment in a sanatorium of chronic addiction to alcohol. *JAMA* 111:1443–1448, 1938.
23. Menninger WC: Treatment of chronic alcohol addiction. *Bull Menninger Clin* 2:101–112, 1938.
24. Gaupp R: *Die Dipsomanie. Eine Klinische Studie.* Jena, 1901.
25. Kretschmer E: Die veranlagung zu den endogenen seelenstorungen, in Kehrer F, Kretschmer E (ed): *Die Veranlagung zu Seeligchen Storungen.* Berl, pp. 164–165, 1924.
26. Cimbal W: Trinkerfursorge als Teil der Verwahrlostenfursorge. *Allg Z Psycht* 84:52–86, 1926.
27. Stockert FG: Zur Frage der Disposition zum Alkoholismus chronicus. *Z Ges Neur Psycht* 106:379–400, 1926.
28. Meggendorfer F: Intoxikations Psychosen, in Bumke O (ed): *Handbuch der Geisteskrankheiten,* 7 (spec pt. 3), Berl, 1928, pp 165–286.
29. Dittmer A: Versuch einer Klassifizierung der Alkoholkranken. *M Weit* 6:1256, 1932.
30. Gabriel E: Uber die "Ursachen" des Alkoholismus. *Psychiatr Neurol Wohenschr* 35:90–92, 108–111, 115–117, 1933.
31. Pohlisch K: Die Klinik des Alkoholismus. *Allg Z Psychiatr* 99:193–202, 1933.
32. Mollenhoff L: Liber den stand der Suchtenbehandlung. *Fortschr Ther* 11:275–284, 1935.
33. Wuth O: Zur Erbanlage der Suchtigen (Kombinierte Suchtigkeit). *Z Ges Neurol Psychiatr* 153:495–505, 1935.
34. Gabriel E, Kratzmann E: *Die Suchtigkeit. Eine Seelenkunde.* Berl, 1936, pp 47–98.

35. Meggendorfer F: Der schwere alkoholismus, in Gutt A (ed): *Handbuch der Erbkrankheiten.* Leipzig, 3:271–438, 1940.
36. Carpenter WB: *On the Use and Abuse of Alcoholic Liquors in Health and Disease.* Philadelphia, Lea & Blanchard, 1850.
37. Wingfield H: *The Forms of Alcoholism and Their Treatment.* New York, Oxford University Press, 1919.
38. Crichton-Miller H: Etiology of alcoholism. *Proc R Soc Med* 21:1356–1357, 1928.
39. Dent JY: Apomorphine in the treatment of anxiety states, with a special reference to alcoholism. *Br J Inebr* 32:65–88, 1934.
40. Carver AE, Hunt TH, Wilson W (eds): *Alcoholism in General Practice.* London, Constable & Co., 1936.
41. Stevenson GH: Psychological and medical aspects of the excessive use of alcohol. *Can Med Assoc J* 42:57–61, 1940.
42. Jaffe A: Reform in American medical science: The inebriety movement and the origins of the psychological disease theory of addiction, 1820–1920. *Br J Addict* 73:139–147, 1978.
43. Kraepelin E: *Psychiatrie: ein Lehrbuch,* ed 8, 4 vols. Leipzig, Germany, J.A. Barth, 1909–1915.
44. Fleming R: The management of chronic alcoholism in England, Scandinavia and Central Europe. *N Engl J Med* 216(7):279–289, 1937.
45. Fahrenkrug WH: Conceptualization and management of alcohol-related problems in Nazi Germany, 1933–45. Presented at Conference "Social History of Alcohol: Drinking in Modern Society," January, 1984.
46. Floch M: Imprisoned abnormal drinkers: Application of the Bowman–Jellinek Classification Schedule to an institutional sample, Part I. Review and analysis of data. *Q J Stud Alcohol* 7:518–566, 1947.
47. Floch M: Imprisoned abnormal drinkers: Application of the Bowman–Jellinek Classification Schedule to an institutional sample, Part II. Illustrative case histories and conclusions. *Q J Stud Alcohol* 8:61–120, 1947.
48. Meyer RE, Babor TF, Mirkin PM: Typologies in alcoholism: An overview. *Int J Addict* 18(2):235–249, 1983.
49. Skinner HA: Statistical approaches to the classification of alcohol and drug addiction. *Br J Addict* 77:259–273, 1982.
50. Morey LC, Blashfield RK: Empirical classifications of alcoholism. *J Stud Alcohol* 42(11):925–937, 1981.

6

Empirically Derived Classifications of Alcohol-Related Problems

Leslie C. Morey and Harvey A. Skinner

Abstract. In recent years a number of investigators have utilized empirical techniques to develop classification schemes for alcohol related problems. This chapter examines this literature, reviewing both dimensional and categorical models that have been proposed. Despite much consistency in the methodologies that have been used, relatively few consistent substantive findings have emerged from these studies. However, increasing sophistication in the use of these empirical techniques over the past decade has produced some interesting results. One such study which yielded a hybrid model for alcoholism incorporating advantages of both categorical and dimensional approaches, is discussed in some detail. Finally, promising directions for future research are outlined with references to the implications of such taxonomy for alcoholism treatment and course.

1. Introduction

In his book *Aspects of Scientific Explanation,* G. C. Hempel states, "The concept of type has played a significant role in various phases of the development of empirical science."[1] Hempel goes on to point out that the nature of the relationship between types can vary a great deal under different models of typology and classification. This observation is particularly accurate as applied to the typology literature in alcoholism. A reading of the present section of this volume will make it apparent that a number of diverse viewpoints exist concerning the classification of alcohol problems. A major division between many of the extant models of alcoholism concerns the nature of the relationship between types. In models for classification of alcoholism, a primary division exists between *dimensional* as opposed to *categorical* models.

A dimensional model of alcoholism orders individuals along an axis (or axes) in some dimensional space. This approach places an emphasis on quantitative differences between types, as opposed to all-or-none variations. An example of a dimensional model in the alcoholism literature can be found in the World Health Organization's description of the alcohol dependence syn-

Leslie C. Morey • Department of Psychology, Vanderbilt University, Nashville, Tennessee 37240. **Harvey A. Skinner** • Addiction Research Foundation, Toronto, Ontario M5S 2S1, Canada.

drome.[2] In this model, alcohol dependence is held to exist in degrees, and the severity of an individual's disorder represents the dimension of classification. A somewhat different example of a dimensional typological model would be Jellinek's stage model of alcoholism,[3] which views alcoholism as a developmental disorder characterized by qualitatively different stages.

A second commonly used approach to modeling types of alcoholics is *categorical*, which seeks to identify internally cohesive, nonoverlapping classes of problem drinkers. Categorical models place an emphasis on the qualitative differences between classes of disorder, in contrast to the quantitative emphasis of the dimensional approach. Categorical classification structures have enjoyed a long history of popularity in medicine and psychiatry,[4] and this approach is embedded in the American Psychiatric Association's nosology, the DSM-III. In addition to the stage model described above, Jellinek[5] also proposed a well-known categorical model of alcoholism in which he identified five discrete types of alcoholics, with hypothesized qualitative differences in etiology and drinking style.

Since most conceptual approaches to typology in alcoholism are representative of either a dimensional or a categorical model, it is not surprising to find that empirical approaches to this problem are similarly differentiated. There exist a number of different methods that represent a realization of both dimensional and categorical models. The empirical classification literature is further complicated by the number and complexity of different methods, even within a particular abstract model, available for creating typologies.[6] For example, *factor analysis* is a generic term for a number of methods that assume a dimensional model, such as principal components analysis, common factor analysis, or multidimensional scaling. The results of a factor analysis yield a simplified dimensional presentation of the data. In contrast, *cluster analysis* represents the implementation of a categorical model of classification. The family of methods subsumed under this label share the purpose of identifying discrete, homogeneous classes of entities. Degerman[7] has reviewed a number of different geometric representations of classification structure, many of which have been applied in empirical classification research.

The aim of this chapter is to provide an overview of the attempts to create empirically based classifications of alcoholics. For organizational purposes, the review of this literature will be divided into two sections: one examining categorical approaches and the second reviewing the the dimensional approaches used in this area. A final section of this chapter will describe a recent attempt to devise a hybrid model for classification in alcoholism that integrates the relative advantages of categorical and dimensional approaches.

2. Categorical Empirical Models

In the past 20 years, a number of researchers have attempted to create classifications using a variety of multivariate procedures. These procedures are referred to generically as cluster analysis techniques. These methods share the purpose of attempting to create homogeneous classes by placing "similar" individuals into the same class. A number of critical decisions are made by the experimenter in selecting a cluster analysis procedure. First, the definition of similarity must be articulated in some empirical fashion. Examples of commonly used similarity metrics include correlation (q-type) and Euclidean distance. Second, an algorithm, or rule, must be used to assign individuals into clusters. For instance, a simple algorithm might dictate that an individual is to be placed into the class containing that person most similar to the individual in question. This algorithm is called "single linkage," a simple hierarchical clustering technique.[8] Third, a decision must be made concerning the number of clusters which exist in a particular data set. A large number of possible combinations of these different parameters exist. For example, there are at least 150 different algorithms [9–14] and at least 50 different similarity measures [10,13] which have been proposed. These different techniques can generate decidedly different classifications from identical data sets.[15,16] To further complicate matters, it is generally accepted that no particular cluster analytic technique has gained clear ascendancy as the method of choice.[17] This technology is still at an early stage of development, and as such, it is crucial that any classification generated by these techniques be extensively validated before being adopted for general use. For a more complete description of these methods, the reader is referred to texts such as Sneath and Sokal,[10] Hartigan,[13] and Everitt.[14]

Because of the extensive and repetitive calculations involved in performing a cluster analysis, these techniques were not commonly used before the advent of high-speed computers, even though methods had been proposed much earlier.[18] Thus, the first application of statistical techniques to create a classification of alcoholics occurred in the mid-1950s.[19,20] However, the study which seemed to act as a catalyst for research in this area was a study performed by Goldstein and Linden.[21] These investigators utilized a sample of 513 alcoholics who were inpatients at a short term treatment unit from a state hospital. These patients had completed the MMPI at the beginning of their hospitalization. Goldstein and Linden used a cluster analysis method proposed by Lorr [22] to create a classification based upon this MMPI data. The following four clusters were obtained:

Type I. This type was characterized by elevations on scale 4. Goldstein and Linden describe this type as representative of an emotionally unstable personality, exhibiting poorly controlled anger and/or psychopathy.

Type II. This type, a 2-8-7-4 profile, was frequently diagnosed as reactive depression or anxiety reaction. Somatic complaints, significant dependency, and chronic severe alcoholism were common. This type was considered to be at particular risk for suicidal ideation and/or behavior.

Type III. With a 4-9-2 group profile, this type was seen as chronically alcoholic with sporadic attempts at abstention. Denial of difficulties, uncooperative attitudes toward treatment, and a generally poor prognosis were also features associated with this type.

Type IV. The 4-9 group profile of this type was identified as diagnostic of alcoholism with secondary characteristics of drug addition and paranoid features. This type may often mix alcohol consumption with other drugs or non-beverage alcohol (such as aftershave lotion). Relatively lengthy periods of abstinence were characteristic of this class of alcoholic.

In 1971, Whitelock *et al.* (23) published a study that was conceptually very similar to the one performed by Goldstein and Linden. Whitelock studied MMPIs gathered on 136 male alcoholics who were inpatients in a state hospital. These authors concluded that they had closely replicated the findings reported by Goldstein and Linden. They obtained four types of MMPI profile high points as follows: Type A, 4; Type B, 2-8-1-4-7; Type C, 4-2-7; and Type D, 2.

The studies described above seemed to serve as catalysts for similar studies in this area, as a number of papers similar to the Goldstein article were published after its appearance. In earlier reviews, [24,25] we examined 28 articles [26–53] that used cluster analysis to create classifications of alcohol abusers. Many of the studies were quite similar in methodology and the studies tended to share common shortcomings, which will be described later. Research interest in this area seems to have continued undiminished, as a number of alcoholic clustering studies have appeared since these reviews were published.[54–59]

Recently, there have been attempts to provide integrative reviews of this literature in the hope of outlining any potential consistencies in the results of the cluster analytic research. Reviews by Conley [60] and Nerviano and Gross [61] describe a fairly high level of agreement in the literature on cluster analytic approaches to alcoholism, although they reach somewhat different conclusions as to what these consistencies are.

In his review of the MMPI literature, Conley[60] noted a correspondence between the results of clustering studies of alcoholics and more general studies of MMPI subtypes. In particular, Conley felt that the molar MMPI subtypes identified by Skinner and Jackson, [62] which will be discussed in more detail in a following section, had also been consistently identified in the alcoholism investigations. To the Skinner and Jackson subtypes (neurotic, psychotic, and character disorder) Conley added a fourth group, which he termed *classic alcoholic*. He proposed the following decision rules for assignment to these four classes:

1. *Neurotic:* Scales Hs, D, Hy, and Pt must be above 60t, with three of these among the four highest scale scores. The two highest scales must involve some combination of Hs, D, Hy, and Pt.
2. *Psychotic:* Sc must be highest scale, with second highest either Pa, Pt, or Ma. Both high points are to be above 60t.
3. *Psychopathic* (*character disorder*): Scaled Pd and Ma must be the two high points, and both must be above 60t.
4. *Classic alcoholic:* Scales D, Pd, and Pt must be above 60t, with all three among the four highest scales. The two high points must include some combination of D, Pd, and Pt.

Conley[60] assigned individuals referred for treatment of alcohol problems and found that roughly 48% could be classified into one of the four types described above. He then compared these four types on a number of measures, including biodemographic and follow-up variables. A number of interesting results were reported. For example, the psychopathic group were found to have an early age of onset of problem drinking, and also were found to report the largest improvement following treatment, even though no differences were found in pre- and post-treatment MMPI comparisons. The remaining three types demonstrated notable reductions in scale elevations following treatment, with depression in particular significantly reduced in the classic alcoholic group. Conley concluded that this partitioning of alcoholics held promise for future research in the area.

In a different review of the alcoholism clustering literature, Nerviano and Gross[61] described some consistencies that they observed across studies utilizing the MMPI. These authors felt that the following seven subtypes had been generally replicated across several cluster analytic studies:

1. *Chronic severe distress* (MMPI code type 2-7-8). This type is characterized by a general and severe psychosocial impairment, marked depression, and obsessionality and anxiety. Personality adjustment in the borderline of schizotypal range would be expected.
2. *Passive-aggressive and sociopathic* (MMPI code type 4-2). This group is seen as resentful, rebellious, and egocentric, but are noted to have relatively low levels of alcohol consumption, fewer complications associated with drinking, and less serious psychopathology than other groups described.
3. *Antisocial sociopathic* (MMPI code type 4-9). This group is described as impulsive, immature, and hyperactive. Extraversion and superficial sociability without emotional attachment may be expected, as is heavy drinking
4. *Reactive-acute depression* (MMPI code type 2-4). In this type, impulsivity and antisocial conduct might be expected but is typically followed by distress and guilt over the consequences. Long-term prognosis for this group is seen as poor.
5. *Severe neurotic-psychophysiological* (MMPI code type 1-2-3-4). This group is seen as manifesting a psychophysiological reaction with anxiety and depression. Personality characteristics in this type are described as dependent and demanding.
6. *Mixed character-dysphoria* (MMPI code type 2-4-7). Individuals in this group may present with diagnoses of dysthymic disorder, passive-aggressive personality, or atypical psychosis. Anxiety and obsessionality are seen as hallmarks of this type. Acting-out behavior in this type tends to be inhibited by compulsive defenses.
7. *Paranoid-alienated* (MMPI code type 8-2-4 or 8-6). This group is characterized by immaturity, hostility, and suspiciousness or frank delusional symptomatology. This group may be aggressive while intoxicated. Other features associated with this group had high levels of drinking, poor social histories, polydrug abuse, and possibly lower verbal IQs.

In sum, both Conley[60] and Nerviano and Gross[61] describe what seems to be an impressive amount of consistency in the results of cluster analytic studies of alcoholism. However, a closer inspection of the specific findings of these studies suggests that this consistency may be illusory. Although many of the prose descriptions of obtained subtypes are fairly similar, there has been little attempt at providing empirical evidence of such similarity. Therefore, we made an attempt to examine the average group profiles obtained in alcoholism clustering studies in order to determine if any generality was present.

This analysis included the centroids, or "average individuals," from each study that utilized the MMPI and reported these mean values, a total of 12 studies.[21,23,29,32,34,36,38,40,41,47,55,56] These group profiles were entered into a computer and examined for intercorrelation. There were a total of 66 cluster profiles, plus an additional 9 profiles that were replicates. Table I represents an attempt to place the results of this analysis into the conceptual framework provided by Nerviano and Gross. The first three of Nerviano and Gross's types are examined, as these three types had been frequently identified according to their review. As an anchor point for each of these three types, the group profiles obtained in the Goldstein and Linden study that correspond to the Nerviano types are used as reference points. Thus, Goldstein and Linden's Type II alcoholic served as the modal profile for Nerviano's chronic severe distress group; the Goldstein Type I profile represents Nerviano's passive aggressive and sociopathic alcoholic; and the Goldstein and Linden Type III profile is the reference point for Nerviano's antisocial-sociopathic alcoholic. This table is patterned after Nerviano and Gross's Table 1, in which they identify the different studies that had yielded subtypes similar to their proposed typology. The columns in our Table I contain the highest Q-type correlation between *any* group profile from the listed studies and the three Goldstein and Linden profiles described above. Also included is a column

Table I. Generality of Three MMPI Alcoholic Types

	Chronic severe distress[a] (Goldstein Type II)	Passive aggressive sociopath[a] (Goldstein Type I)	Antisocial sociopath[a] (Goldstein Type III)	Highest within-study[b] correlation
Bean and Karasievich[34]	.942	—	.640	.937
Donovan *et al.*[40]	.947	.546	—	.897
Eshbaugh *et al.*[41]	.959	.460	.580	.820
Glen *et al.*[32]	.826	.259	.419	.809
Hetler[36]	.929	.745	.803	.736
Loberg[56]	.925	.583	—	.839
Nerviano *et al.*[47]	.900	.530	.339	.876
Warner[38]	.741	—	—	.997
Whitelock *et al.*[23]	.525	.678	—	.963
Median	.925	.546	.580	.876

[a] Highest Q-Type correlation between Goldstein Type and any type obtained in listed studies.
[b] Highest Q-Type correlation between any two types obtained in listed studies.

that contains the highest correlation of types *within the same study*. Thus, in the Bean and Karasievitch[34] study, two of their obtained types correlated .937 with each other.

An examination of Table I reveals a number of interesting trends. First, the replication of Goldstein and Linden's Type II alcoholic (Nerviano's chronic severe distress group) is quite impressive. Most of the studies listed found a type that was quite similar to this modal profile (median correlation = .925). This correspondence suggests that the Type II alcoholic proposed by Goldstein and Linden represents a viable construct worthy of further investigation. However, the results for their Type I and Type III alcoholics (Nerviano's passive-aggressive/sociopathic and antisocial/sociopathic alcoholics) are not as impressive. Despite the finding that most studies found types with moderate similarity to these modal profiles (median correlations = .546 and .580, respectively), the similarity of clusters within studies was, on the whole, much greater. This conclusion is supported by the high correlations obtained when examining clusters from the same study. As an example, Whitelock *et al.*[23] suggested that their results successfully replicated the findings of Goldstein and Linden.[21] However, when the actual obtained group profiles are examined, it is apparent that the Whitelock types are actually much more similar to each other than they are to the Goldstein types. This point is illustrated in Table II, which presents the intercorrelation among the Goldstein[21] and Whitelock[23] types. In our correlation analysis, the *smallest* correlation of the nine possible correlations among the Whitelock types was .853. This suggests that their clusters were not adequately distinct from one another, let alone successful replicates of the Goldstein typology. The Whitelock *et al.* study was not alone in this regard; there was a general trend for a relatively high degree of similarity of clusters within studies in this literature, as compared to similarity across studies. This finding indicates that the consistencies in the literature noted by Conley[60] and Nerviano and Gross[61] may be somewhat misleading, as the prose descriptions are often more similar than the empirical configurations.

Table II. Intercorrelations among Goldstein and Whitelock Alcoholic Types

	Goldstein and Linden[21] types				Whitelock *et al.*[23] types			
	I	II	III	IV	1	2	3	4
Goldstein Types								
I	—	.166	.090	.420	.678	.390	.388	.384
II		—	.379	.277	.214	.525	.416	.347
III			—	.413	−.012	.013	.061	−.060
IV				—	.525	.548	.580	.436
Whitelock Types								
1					—	.857	.899	.894
2						—	.951	.963
3							—	.954
4								—

A number of other methodologic problems affect the generality and interpretability of the findings of the cluster analytic research.[24,25,63] Some of these difficulties center about the selection of subjects and variables in these studies, while others involve concerns with the implementation of the clustering procedures

2.1. Samples

An inspection of the studies in this area reveals a remarkable consistency among these studies in terms of the characteristics of their samples. Most studies utilized inpatient males from state hospital or Veterans' hospital facilities. The age range of these samples tended to be quite constricted, with an average of about 45 years. Very few women alcoholics had been included in these samples. In addition, samples were universally composed solely of alcoholics in treatment, another source of potential bias.[64] Given the rising concern about alcoholism in youth,[65] the aged,[66,67] and women,[68] the applicability of clusters derived from lower socioeconomic status, middle-aged male veteran inpatients appears limited. It is important to note that more recent studies,[46,48,55,59] have made the attempt to include more women in their samples.

2.2. Variable Selection

Another striking consistency across the studies in this literature concerns the choice of the variables used to form the basis of classification. Most of these studies used an objective personality inventory (generally the MMPI) to collect data. Given that most conceptual classifications of alcoholics (for example, Jellinek's models) have been based upon alcohol use behavior, it is unfortunate that the focus of these studies has been nearly exclusively upon personality configuration. More recent efforts[40,43,69] have focused upon identifying stylistic differences in alcohol abuse between types, and hopefully this trend will continue in subsequent studies. However, even this alcohol use data have been largely self-reported in nature. Despite evidence suggesting that such data are generally valid,[70,71] studies using alternative sources of information, such as observational techniques or laboratory data, have yet to be performed. In sum, the variable domains which have served as basis for classification, as well as for the validation of the classification, have been disappointingly narrow in scope.

2.3. Clustering Methodology

As might be expected given the current state of the art in clustering methodology, the studies in this literature were quite diverse in terms of specific techniques utilized. Morey and Blashfield[24] in interviewing the parameters of many of the studies in this area, identified Lorr's method[22] and

Ward's method[72] of cluster analysis as the most frequently used clustering techniques. With regard to similarity metrics, the studies were about evenly divided between use or correlational and distance measures.

Given the diversity of these methods and the relative lack of knowledge about their characteristics, it is exceedingly important that this methodology be used with caution. Blashfield[63] has proposed five criteria that may be used as guidelines in performing a cluster analytic study. The first four criteria concern the clear description of the specific technique utilized. If, according to Blashfield, the algorithm is not clearly specified, if the similarity measure is not adequately described, if the computer software used to perform the analysis is not referenced, and if the procedure used to select number of clusters is not delineated, then the study cannot be replicated due to insufficient information. Very few of the studies in the alcoholism literature meet these criteria for adequacy of description. Although editorial constraints often preclude the inclusion of such information, it is essential if an informed reader is to evaluate the meaningfulness of any obtained results, since different methods can (and do) generate different results from the same data set.

The fifth criterion for clustering studies suggested by Blashfield[63] is use of a validating procedure. Given the differences between methods, it is important to test the results of any cluster analysis for validity. Most of the studies in this area did attempt to provide some evidence of validity. In many cases this validation effort was limited to the subjects and variables upon which the classification had been derived. This procedure provides little evidence of the validity of a classification.[13,14] However, as the difficulties with clustering methodology are becoming better understood, some recent studies[42,59,69] have been particularly impressive in terms of validation efforts. Also procedures for establishing the validity of a clustering solution are becoming increasingly sophisticated.[73,74] It is hoped that such recent trends will continue and that future researchers will make every effort to establish the validity of their proposed classification.

In sum, there are a number of limitations in the literature on the cluster analysis of alcoholics, both in the studies themselves and in the conclusions that can be drawn from them. There do seem to be some limited conclusions which can be drawn from these studies. First, as is evident from Table I, a group of alcoholics described as chronic severe distress drinkers by Nerviano and Gross[61] has been impressively replicated in nearly every study that has utilized the MMPI. However, even though a number of other types have seemingly been replicated across studies, most types obtained in this literature appear to be sample specific.

Another consistency notable in this literature is the importance of variables related to the problem drinker's interpersonal style. This variable domain has been identified in studies using instruments such as the 16PF, and PRF, as opposed to the MMPI, as the basis for classification.[27,29,30,35,39,42,69] For example, Nerviano and Gross[30] noted that their clusters were differentiated most effectively by "a single dimension best described as one of social inadequacy, introversion, and anxiety" (p. 373). The dimension noted by Nerviano has been found to be bipolar in some studies (e.g., ref. 27) with group dependency and conformity at one extreme and an asocial withdrawal at the other. It is not surprising that the studies that have utilized the MMPI have not found this variable to be particularly salient, since the standard clinical scales of the MMPI are not sensitive measures of this construct.

3. Dimensional Models

Another approach to classification in alcoholism has involved the construction of dimensional models. Multivariate statistical methods such as factor analysis[75] have been used in an attempt to identify dimensions that might successfully discriminate differences among alcohol abusers. The aim of this approach to empirical classification has been to identify important dimensions upon which alcoholics vary. Although not as numerous as studies utilizing a categorical model, a number of investigators have begun constructing dimensional models of individuals' differences among alcoholics. Such models have varied in scope, but examples include models of alcoholic personality characteristics,[76] vocational adjustment,[77] self-report measures of alcohol use,[71] and treatment outcome.[78] This section will focus on two influential dimensional models: one model based upon psychopathology, originally proposed by Skinner and Jackson,[62] and another suggested by Horn, Wanberg and their associates,[79,80,81] which is primarily based upon stylistic features of alcohol use.

3.1. Model Based on Psychopathology

Skinner[62,82,83] has proposed a model of psychopathology based on the MMPI that characterizes individuals in terms of three clinical syndromes: *neurotic, psychotic,* and *sociopathic.* The three syndromes are hypothesized to reflect fundamental ways in which individuals differ, with each syndrome having certain biological and environmental determinants. Each syndrome is defined empirically by a configuration of scores on the MMPI clinical scales. The neurotic syndrome has high points on 1, 2, and 3, and is characterized by somatic complaints, depression symptoms, and an immature or egocentric orientation. The psychotic syndrome is defined by elevations on 8, 7, and 6. This syndrome is evidenced by unusual thought content, inappropriate affect, emotional agitation, fearfulness, and to a lesser extent by a suspiciousness of others. The sociopathic type, with high points on 4 and 9, and a low point on 0, represents a character disorder with a tendency toward sociopathic extraversion.

Each MMPI syndrome defines an orthogonal axis (Fig. 1). Given the MMPI clinical scales in T-score format, one may readily compute the coordinants for individual profiles in this three-dimensional space. For example,

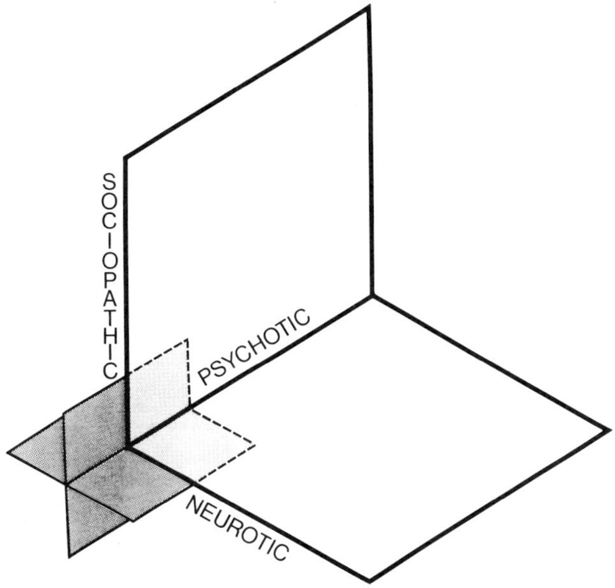

Figure 1. Three-dimensional representation of the MMPI dimensional model.

if a person has elevations on 1, 2, and 3, his vector in Fig. 1 is determined by the MMPI profile *shape*, that is, the actual pattern of "ups and downs" across the 13 clinical scales. Three shape parameters are generated one describing the resemblance of an individual to each of the three clinical syndromes. It is hypothesized that the shape represents the clinical pattern or type of disorder and that this parameter should be relatively constant over time.

Another important parameter of the model is profile *elevation*, which is the mean score of an individual across all 13 MMPI clinical scales. It is postulated that elevation provides a more situationally determined index of symptom severity. Thus, by distinguishing shape and elevation parameters, one may integrate aspects of the trait (shape) and situational (elevation) approaches to the study of psychopathology.[83]

The MMPI model of psychopathology provides a useful framework for integrating various studies of alcohol abuse patients. For example, Table III illustrates how the model may be used with the four types identified by Goldstein and Linden.[21] Type I has a moderate weighting on both the neurotic and sociopathic axes. Individuals with this profile have been described as having poorly controlled anger and emotional instability. The second type has a substantial weighting on the psychotic axis, with a secondary correlation on the neurotic axis. Since these individuals have been described as manifesting the most severe, chronic evidence of alcoholism, it is consistent to observe that the Goldstein and Linden[21] Type II has the highest elevation

Table III. Alcohol Abuse Subtypes Classified According to the MMPI Model

Types	Maladjustment (elevation)	Clinical syndrome		
		Neurotic	Psychotic	Sociopathic
Alcoholic[a]				
Type I	57	.44	−.11	.51
Type II	68	.59	.73	.00
Type III	52	−.27	.45	.27
Type IV	59	−.05	.26	.92
DUI offenders[b]				
Type 1	55	.22	−.44	.53
Type 2	55	−.55	.45	.57
Type 3	57	.57	.32	.19
Type 4	57	−.13	−.04	.65

[a] Goldstein and Linden[21]
[b] Sutker *et al.*[49]

parameter of the four types. Also, the resemblance to the psychotic syndrome denotes fairly severe symptoms (e.g., thought disorder, generalized anxiety). Type III is characterized by a moderate weighting on the psychotic syndrome. The fourth type has a marked similarity to the sociopathic syndrome. These individuals tend to exhibit a concomitant drug addiction.

In comparison, Sutker *et al.*[49] identified four MMPI types among 500 males arrested for driving under the influence (DUI) of alcohol. Since the DUI sample was an earlier stage of problem drinking, one might expect their MMPI profiles to reflect lower of psychopathology. This difference between the two studies may be seen in Table III, where the profile elevation parameters are all around a T-score of 55-57 for the DUI types versus 60+ for the alcoholic types. Also, there are some interesting similarities among the types with respect to the three clinical syndromes. The fourth type in each study has a salient weighting on the sociopathic axis, whereas the DUI Type II and alcoholic Type III have a similar pattern of absence of neurotic symptoms (negative weight) combined with elevations on the psychotic and sociopathic dimensions. The DUI Type III reported the highest level of drinking, and this type has certain resemblances to the alcoholic Type II, which reported the most severe drinking histories in the state hospital sample.

In Table IV, the MMPI model parameters have been computed for two longitudinal studies of alcoholic patients. Kammeier *et al.*[84] compared the MMPI profiles of men when they enter college and when they first entered an alcoholism treatment facility an average of 13 years later. There is a clear increase in profile elevation (55 versus 62) on the second testing, which indicates a rise in the degree of pathology. Also, there is an interesting shift in profile shape. While college freshmen, the men resembled the sociopathic syndrome, which signified a tendency toward rebellious attitudes and high energy levels, although the level of symptoms was generally within the normal range. However, at the time these men entered treatment there was a substantial weighting on the psychotic axis as well. This weighting very likely represents consequences of alcohol use, such as impaired concentration and withdrawal symptoms.

Finally, Bean and Karasievitch[34] tested alcoholic clients at three stages of treatment: 5 days, 30 days, and 60 days. As treatment progressed, a decrease in the elevation parameter is evident which corresponds to a lower level of symptom severity. However, the shape parameters are relatively stable.

3.2. Wanberg and Horn's Differential Assessment Model

Perhaps the most extensive research program utilizing a dimensional model for alcoholism is that of Horn and Wanberg and their associates.[79,80,81,85] Their research program, operating under the assumption that problems associated with alcohol are very diverse, sought to identify the major dimensions along which these problems vary. Beginning with a compilation of presenting concerns and complaints typically expressed by new admissions to alcohol treatment, these authors[79,80] eventually developed a hierarchical model of factors within the domain of alcohol use using factor analytic techniques. The three tiers of this hierarchy are presented in Table V and include 16 primary factors tapping specific stylistic features of alcohol use, six second-order scales, and a general factor representing a broad measure of involvement with alcohol use.

Wanberg, Horn, and associates have extended this model into an examination of background and psychosocial functioning. Specifically, these researchers have looked at factors related to life situations, both past and present[81]; personality dimensions[86]; and immediate response to treatment.[81] Again, multilevel dimensional models were constructed, outlining factors central to these domains. The higher order factors from each of these three domains are presented in Table VI.

Wanberg and Horn[81] have recently begun to examine the interrelationships of these factors across domains. For example, both introversion and extraversion are related to the use of alcohol for social benefit, with shy individuals seeming to use alcohol as a disinhibitor and outgoing individuals enhancing their preferred interpersonal style. Also, loss of behavioral control when drinking seems related to childhood rebelliousness and aggressiveness, while social role difficulties as a result of drinking are associated with unstable living conditions in childhood. Finally, treatment response differences also emerge, with individual drinking in an obsessive style least likely to remain abstinent after 1 year follow up.

The work of these researchers stimulated the development of instruments designed to assess the dimensions which they had identified as crucial. Perhaps the most important instrument to come out of their work has been the *Alcohol Use Inventory* (AUI).[85] The AUI was derived from the model of drinking patterns described in Table V. It was designed to encompass differences in style of alcohol use, unfavorable consequences from drinking, and perceived

Table IV. Longitudinal Studies of Alcoholics

Types	Maladjustment (elevation)	Clinical syndrome		
		Neurotic	Psychotic	Sociopathic
Kammeier *et al.*[84]				
Tested when college freshman	55	.01	.34	.62
Tested when entered treatment (13 years later)	62	.18	.60	.53
Bean and Karasievich,[34] stages of treatment				
At 5 days	65	.52	.72	.34
At 30 days	62	.54	.69	.40
At 60 days	60	.47	.61	.54

benefits from drinking.[80] The 23 scales of the AUI are arranged in the hierarchical structure presented in Table V. Subsequent psychometric evaluation of the AUI has determined that this measure is internally consistent, relatively free from response style biases, and concurrently valid with respect to other important variables related to alcohol use.[87]

The AUI itself has served as the basis for further factor-analytic investigations into significant dimensions of alcoholism. For example, Skinner[88] identified four major syndromes of alcohol abuse within the domain tapped

Table V. Alcohol Use Domain Factors Derived by Horn, Wanberg, and Associates

Primary	Second order	General
1. Social benefit	A. Enhanced functioning	G. Involvement with alcohol use
2. Mental benefits	B. Obsessive-sustained drinking	
3. Changes mood	C. Awareness of problem	
4. Manages loss	D. Anxiety and concern	
5. Cope with marital problems	E. Severe alcoholism: direct	
6. Gregarious vs. solo use	F. Severe alcoholism: indirect	
7. Obsessive-compulsive drinking		
8. Sustained vs. periodic use		
9. Quantity of daily use		
10. Loss of behavioral control		
11. Social role maladaptation		
12. D.T.'s		
13. Physical withdrawal		
14. Causing marital problems		
15. Guilt, worry, and fear		
16. Help-seeking behavior		

Table VI. Psychosocial Domain Factors Derived by Horn, Wanberg, and Associates

Life situation dimensions
1. General childhood instability
2. General living instability
3. Social withdrawal/restricted activities
4. Health problems
5. Antisocial/legal problems
6. Employment instability
7. Marital problems
8. General treatment needs
Personality dimensions
1. Expedient, deviant vs. conscientious morality
2. Introversion vs. extraversion
3. Anxiety/depression vs. self-confidence
4. Suspicious/distrustful vs. accepting/trustful
Treatment outcome dimensions
1. Employed/productive vs. unemployed/unproductive
2. Social involvement vs. withdrawal/uninvolved
3. Abstinence vs. nonabstinence
4. Lack of symptoms/disruptions vs. many symptoms/disruptions
5. Good health vs. health problems
6. Lack of emotional stress vs. high stress
7. Involvement in treatment vs. low level of involvement
8. Perceived treatment benefit vs. little or no benefit
9. Good marital relations vs. marital problems

by the AUI and correlated these dimensions with variables assessing personality, intellectual, and demographic characteristics. The first factor, alcohol dependence, was represented by loss of control when drinking, a compulsive drinking style, symptoms of physiological dependence on alcohol, and repeated attempts to stop drinking. This factor was associated with chronic social debilitation and psychopathology. The second factor, perceived benefits from drinking, involved the belief that alcohol use facilitates social and mental functioning. This factor was associated with a sustained drinking style and anxiety, particularly in social situations. A third factor, marital discord, involved drinking problems that may have either resulted from or instigated marital problems. The final factor, polydrug abuse, was marked by the use of illicit drugs as well as by a gregarious drinking style. High scorers on this factor tended to be younger and have marked antisocial attitudes.

Subsequent investigation into these major factors related to alcohol use have demonstrated their utility.[88] In particular, the alcohol dependence measure has been found to be a powerful discriminator among alcoholics. Skinner and Allen,[89] in following up on their factor analytic work with the AUI, proposed a brief subscale that could be calculated from the AUI to place individuals along this dimension. Scores on their proposed scale seemed to be distributed normally along the hypothesized continuum, supporting a dimensional or quantitative approach. In addition, this scale was meaningfully associated with a number of important variables. For example, higher levels of alcohol dependence were related to greater quantity of alcohol consumed, increased social consequences of drinking, and noncompliance with treatment. The degree of alcohol dependence was also associated with thought disorder, depression, anxiety, and hypochondriasis, as well as with a complicated medical condition. Skinner and Allen,[89] in interpreting their scale, point out that this construct is quite similar to the *alcohol dependence syndrome* concept utilized by the World Health Organizations.[2]

4. A Hybrid Model for Classification of Alcohol Disorders

From the preceding sections it is apparent that dimensional and categorical models of alcoholism represent very different conceptual approaches to classification in this area. Proponents of each type of model have offered plausible evidence in support of their proposed structure, and yet each model also suffers inherent weaknesses. It is unlikely that empirical analysis alone will help resolve which type of model is "best" for alcoholism, since even empirical criteria for "best" can vary as a function of assumptions underlying a particular model. A plausible resolution to this problem may lie in the consideration of hybrid models which integrate key elements of these different conceptual structures.[90] Other sciences, faced with a similar dilemma, have constructed such models.[7] For example, the theory of quantum mechanics in physics evolved from an integration of the seemingly disparate wave theory and particle theory of light.

In a recent project, an effort was made to construct a hybrid classificatory model of alcoholism which combined features of both dimensional and categorical approaches.[69,73] This project will be examined in some detail as an example of how hybrid models may be used to understand the concordant validity of seemingly disparate approaches to the problem of classification in alcoholism. These studies involved a series of cluster analyses which formed classifications based upon the multidimensional framework provided by Wanberg *et al.*[80] A multilevel, sequential validation method was used to compare classifications generated by over 20 different strategies of cluster analysis.[73] Many of the most commonly used clustering methods were included in this project, and it represented one of the most ambitious applied studies of cluster analysis to date. The different classifications were derived from the dimensions of the Alcohol Use Inventory,[85] the instrument devised to place individuals within the multidimensional space described in the previous section. These classifications were then validated in psychosocial domains such as personality, psychopathology, intellectual and neuropsychological variables, sociodemographic status, and other variables tapping features of alcohol abuse. The classification generated by Ward's method[72] of cluster analysis was determined to be well validated, both in an absolute sense and by comparison to the other models examined.[73] This model included the following three types of alcoholics:

Early-stage problem drinkers. This class was a relatively heterogenous group that tended to have the least severe drinking problems of the three types. These individuals tended to begin drinking later in life than the other types, demonstrated a relatively low average daily alcohol intake, and were undifferentiated with respect to beverage preference. In this group, denial of drinking problems may have been prominent; they were less likely to see alcohol as a problem (66%) or to consider themselves alcoholic (53%) than the other two types, even though all had been referred for treatment of alcohol abuse.

This class of drinkers also tended to have fewer complications of the type generally associated with alcoholism. For example, it was family difficulties, as opposed to legal or occupational problems, that most often led to referral for treatment. This group had the most stable living conditions of the three types, with higher incomes, higher employment rates, and fewer instances of lost jobs. The largest part of this group was presently married and living with spouse (and children, if any). This group made fewer reports of psychiatric symptoms, and there was no evidence of neuropsychological compromise as a result of drinking.

Personality configuration in this study was assessed using the Personality Research Form.[91] The early-stage problem drinker had a mean profile which was quite similar to the normative sample for the PRF. In other words, no particular personality patterns distinguished this type of drinker from the general population. However, this group could be differentiated from the other two groups with respect to personality. This group was more achievement oriented and had higher needs for mastery and for accomplishment. Also, this type had a relatively low need for aggression, making them less likely to see force as necessary as a means to overcoming their obstacles. Likewise, this group was less impulsive than their counterparts in the other two types. The early-stage problem drinker also manifested a greater need to understand their world, to analyze and ask questions. Finally, this type of person maintained an internal locus of control, seeing the outcomes of an event as contingent upon their behavior.

Affiliative alcoholic. Individuals within this second group of alcohol abusers were experiencing more severe problems related to alcoholism than were the early-stage problem drinkers, although these difficulties were not as severe as those noted in the third type obtained. With respect to alcohol use, a striking feature of this type was the relatively high preference for beer as the beverage of choice. This group also tended to drink in a more or less continuous fashion, with relatively brief periods of abstinence noted. Also noted was the tendency for this group to seek company in drinking; hence the name affiliative alcoholic.

Individuals within the affiliative alcoholic group demonstrated an intermediate level of severity of consequences of drinking as compared to the other types. For example, this type rated lower than the early-stage problem drinker in social stability and social class and had lost more jobs as a function of alcoholism. The affiliative alcoholic also reported more symptoms of depression, anxiety, and thought disorder than the early-stage type and also described more interpersonal problems. This type also had experienced significantly more stressful life events in the previous year than had the type described above.

The personality characteristics of the affiliative alcoholic were somewhat more pronounced than those described for the early stage drinker. As mentioned above, this type tended to be affiliative and less socially introverted, particularly as compared to the type to be described below. In addition, the affiliative drinker demonstrated higher needs for aggression and impulsivity and a lower need for understanding than the early-stage alcoholic. Finally, the locus of control for this type was predominantly external, in contrast to the internal locus of control noted for the early-stage problem drinker.

Schizoid alcoholic. The dominant feature of schizoid alcoholics was a chronic and severe problem with alcohol. These individuals reported being obsessed with alcohol, drinking with a great sense of guilt, fear, and worry. An overwhelming majority (92%) considered themselves alcoholic and most had experienced physiological and psychological effects of withdrawal from alcohol at some point in their drinking "careers." In contrast to the affiliative alcoholic, these individuals consumed primarily wine or liquor as the beverage of choice. Furthermore, the schizoid alcoholic tended to drink in a solitary fashion, primarily for the purpose of getting away from others as opposed to being with them. Another difference between the schizoid group and the affiliative group involved the pattern of alcohol consumption; schizoid drinkers were more likely to drink in binges, with relatively lengthy periods of abstinence in between.

As might be expected, this type had the most severe consequences of drinking of the three types. The schizoid alcoholics tended to score lowest in social class and social stability, had lost the most jobs as a consequence of their drinking problem, and scored lowest on measures of cognitive functioning as compared to the other types. Individuals in this type tended to endorse antisocial attitudes and were prone to risky and reckless action. Of the three types, the schizoid alcoholic reported the most anxiety (both trait and state), depression, low self-esteem, and tended to endorse more items characteristic of thought disorder. While these individuals had been subjected to more stressful life events in the past year than the early-stage problem drinker, there was little difference between the affiliative and schizoid alcoholics in this regard.

The personality organization of the schizoid alcoholic was fairly stereotyped and was characterized by extreme aggressiveness, social withdrawal, and impulsivity. Needs for achievement, autonomy, and understanding were quite low as compared to the other three types. The schizoid alcoholic dem-

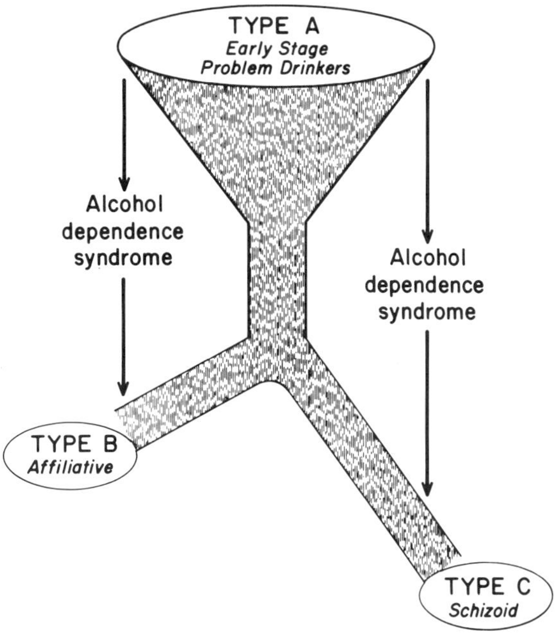

Figure 2. A hybrid model for classification of alcohol-related problems.

onstrated a predominantly external locus of control, as did the affiliative drinker, although the schizoid group tended to be more extreme in this regard.

Morey *et al.*[69] proposed a hybrid categorical/dimensional model relating these three types. A representation of this model is portrayed in Fig. 2. In this model, the early-stage problem drinker represents a fairly heterogeneous group of individuals who demonstrated significant signs of alcohol abuse, but who had not accrued severe symptoms of physical dependence on alcohol. In contrast, the affiliative and schizoid alcoholic types were both at a more advanced level of alcohol dependence, suggesting a developmental model similar to Jellinek's[3] phase model of alcoholism. However, the model in Fig. 2 also suggests a bifurcation into one of two categorical types, differentiated by both interpersonal style as well as features of alcohol use. Thus, there may be two "outcomes" of the developmental process described by Jellinek: one, a schizoid adaptation characterized by binge drinking and extremely severe symptoms of alcohol dependence; the other, an affiliative adaptation manifesting a preference for beer and drinking in a continuous fashion. It is interesting to note that many of the features characteristic of these latter two types may be found in Jellinek's species model of alcoholism; thus, a moderate correspondence is noted between the affiliative alcoholic and Jellinek's delta alcoholic, as well as between the schizoid alcoholic and Jellinek's description of the gamma alcoholic.

This hybrid model suggests a number of hypotheses regarding differential treatment planning for the different types. The early-stage problem drinker generally believed that it was possible to cut down successfully on their drinking, and that a controlled drinking strategy[92] was a desirable goal for treatment. In contrast, the majority of individuals in the affiliative and schizoid types expressed the belief that the only potentially successful approach to treatment would involve abstinence.[69] Hence, one would expect that a controlled drinking strategy, given no contraindications,[93] would be most effective with the early-stage drinkers, whereas affiliative and schizoid alcoholics would tend to require abstinence-based methods. This aspect of the model is consistent with the dimensional model of Skinner and Allen,[89] who similarly note differences in beliefs about treatment as a function of degree of alcohol dependence. In addition, this finding adds to the growing body of evidence pointing to the differential effectiveness of abstinence versus controlled drinking with different types of problem drinkers.[54,94–96]

The nature of the differences between affiliative and schizoid alcoholics also suggest different treatment approaches within an abstinence framework. Given the gregarious, affiliative nature of the affiliative alcoholic, the approach of Alcoholics Anonymous (AA), which stressed abstinence as well as interpersonal support,[97] might be particularly well suited to their needs. On the other hand, the generally withdrawn schizoid group would likely have difficulty, particularly at first, complying with the interpersonal demands of the AA approach. Given their more introspective nature, as well as their generally more troubled psychological condition, an intensive, broad-based individualized treatment aimed at producing internal controls might be optimal for the schizoid alcoholic.

These hypotheses are representative of what Glaser[98] has called the "matching hypothesis"; namely, that suitable matching between different patients and different treatment strategies might lead to better outcome. This assumption underlies nearly all work in typological strategies for alcohol problems; whether such typologies are empirically derived or based upon some other partitioning strategy.[99] However, despite the promise which has been recently shown in this literature, the empirical classification of alcoholism is still at a largely preliminary stage. It is encouraging to see official recognition of many of the important findings in this field; for example, the continuing evolution of the alcohol dependence syndrome concept by the World Health Organization. However, as Skinner and Blashfield[100] have demonstrated, a number of factors work against the introduction and widespread use of typologies based upon empirical methods. Nonetheless, the increasing degree of sophistication in the use of these methods, combined with better assessment instrumentation, have resulted in encouraging findings from recent studies. It is hoped that the results of such studies will yield an increased understanding of the disorders currently organized under the rubric of "alcoholism."

In conclusion, this chapter has underscored the increased recognition of multiple syndromes of alcohol abuse and has suggested a hybrid model for integrating the relative advantages of categorical and dimensional classification systems. The various syndromes of alcohol abuse that have been identified in previous studies suggest some clear avenues for the differential treatment of patients. The present challenge is to conduct rigorous evaluations of these models for differential diagnosis and treatment. As refinements are made in the tailoring of treatment services to specific syndromes, real gains should be achieved in alcoholism treatment effectiveness.

References

1. Hempel CG: Aspects of scientific explanation. New York: Free Press, 1965.
2. Edwards G, Gross MM: Alcohol dependence: Provisional description of a clinical syndrome. *Br Med J* 1:1058–1061, 1976.
3. Jellinek EM: Phases of alcohol addiction. *Q J Stud Alcohol* 13:673–684, 1952.
4. Menninger K: *The Vital Balance*, New York, Viking Press, 1963.
5. Jellinek EM: *The Disease Concept of Alcoholism*. New Haven, College and University Press, 1960.
6. Blashfield RK, Aldendertfer MS: The literature on cluster analysis. *Multivariate Behav Res* 13:271–295, 1978.
7. Degerman RL: The geometric representation of some simple structures, in Shepard RN, Romeny, AK, Nerlove SB (eds): *Multidimensional Scaling*. New York, Seminar Press, Vol. 1, 1971.
8. Sokal RR, Sneath PHE: *Principles of Numerical Taxonomy*. San Francisco, Freeman, 1963.
9. Anderberg MR: *Cluster Analysis for Applications*. New York, Academic Press, 1973.
10. Sneath PHE, Sokal TR: *Numerical Taxonomy*. San Francisco, Freeman, 1973.
11. Bailey KD: Cluster analysis, in Heise D (ed): *Sociological Methodology*. San Francisco, Jossey-Bass, 1974.
12. Clifford JH, Stephenson W: *An Introduction to Numerical Classification*. New York, Academic Press, 1975.
13. Hartigan, J: *Clustering Algorithms*. New York, Wiley, 1975.
14. Everitt BS: *Cluster Analysis*, (ed 2). London, Halstead Press, 1980.
15. Bartko JJ, Strauss JS, Carpenter WJ: An evaluation of taxometric techniques for psychiatric data. *Classif Soc Bull* 2:2–28, 1971.
16. Blashfield RK, Morey LC: A comparison of four clustering methods using MMPI Monte Carlo data. *Appl Psycholo Measurement* 4:57–64, 1980.
17. Milligan GW: A review of Monte Carlo tests of cluster analysis. *Multivariate Behav Res* 16:37–407, 1981.
18. Tryon RC, Bailey DE: *Cluster Analysis*. New York, McGraw-Hill, 1970.
19. Button AD: A study of alcoholics with the Minnesota Multiphasic Personality Inventory. *Q J Stud Alcohol* 16:263–281, 1955.
20. Swenson CH, Davis HC: Types of workhouse inmate alcoholics. *Q J Stud Alcohol* 20:757–766, 1959.
21. Goldstein SG, Linden JD: Multivariate classification of alcoholics by MMPI. *J Abnorm Psychol* 74:661–669, 1969.
22. Lorr, M: *Explorations in Typing Psychotics*. New York, Pergamon Press, 1966.
23. Whitelock PR, Overall JE, Patrick JH: Personality patterns and alcohol abuse in a state hospital population. *J Abnorm Psychol* 78:9–16, 1981.
24. Morey LC, Blashfield RK: The empirical classification of alcoholism: A review. *J Stud Alcohol* 42:925–937, 1981.
25. Skinner HA: Statistical approaches to the classification of alcohol and drug addiction. *Br J Addict* 77:259–273, 1982.

26. Partington JT, Johnson FG: Personality types among alcoholics. *Q J Stud Alcohol* 30:21–34, 1969.
27. Lawlis GF, Rubin SE: 16-PF study of personality patterns in alcoholics. *Q J Stud Alcohol* 32:318–327, 1971.
28. Whitelock PR, Overall JE, Patrick JH: Personality patterns and alcohol abuse in a state hospital population. *J Abnorm Psychol* 78:9–16, 1971.
29. Stein KB, Rozynko V, Pugh LA: The heterogeneity of personality among alcoholics. *Br J Soc Clin Psychol* 10:253–259, 1971.
30. Nerviano VJ, Gross WF: A multivariate delineation of two alcoholic profile types on the 16 PF. *J Clin Psychol* 29:371–374, 1973.
31. Evenson RC, Altman H, Sletten IW, et al. Factors in the description and grouping of alcoholics. *Am J Psychiatry* 130:49–54, 1973.
32. Glen A, Royer FL, Custer R: A study of MMPI-profile types of hospitalized alcoholic veterans. *Newslett Res Mental Health Behav Sci* 15:53–56, 1973.
33. Skinner HA, Jackson DN, Hoffman H: Alcoholic personality types: Identification and correlates. *J Abnorm Psychol* 83:658–666, 1974.
34. Bean KL, Karasievitch GO: Psychological test results at three stages of inpatient alcoholism treatment. *J Stud Alcohol* 36:838–852, 1974.
35. Nerviano VJ: Common personality patterns among alcoholic males: a multivariate study. *J Consult Clin Psychol* 44:104–110, 1976.
36. Hetler JH: A critical examination of the adequacy of typological analyses provided by several clustering techniques. Ph.D. dissertation, University of Minnesota, 1976.
37. Replogle WH, Hair JF, Jr: A multivariate approach to profiling alcoholic typologies. *Multivariate Exp Clin Res* 3:157–164, 1977.
38. Warner JS: Personality clusters in MMPI protocols of alcoholics. Ph.D. dissertation, Columbia University, 1977.
39. Costello RM, Lawlis GF, Manders KR, et al: Empirical derivation of a partial personality typology of alcoholics. *J Stud Alcohol* 39:1258–1966, 1978.
40. Donovan DM, Chaney EF, O'Leary MR: Alcohol MMPI subtypes: Relationship to drinking styles, benefits, and consequences. *J Nerv Mental Dis* 166:553–561, 1978.
41. Eshbaugh DM, Tosi DJ, Hoyt C: Some personality patterns and dimensions of male alcoholics: a multivariate description. *J Personality Assess* 42:409–417.
42. Finney JW, Moos RH: Treatment and outcome for empirical subtypes of alcoholic patients. *J Consult Clin Psychol* 47:25–38, 1979.
43. Steer RA, Fine EW, Scoles PE: Classification of men arrested for driving while intoxicated, and treatment implications: a cluster-analytic study. *J Stud Alcohol* 40:222–229, 1979.
44. Hart LS, Stueland D: Relationship of sociodemographic and drinking variables to differentiated subgroups of alcoholics. *Community Ment Health J* 15:47–57, 1979.
45. Hart LS, Stueland D: An application of the multidimensional model of alcoholism to program effectiveness: Rehabilitation status and outcome. *J Stud Alcohol* 40:645–655, 1979.
46. Hart LS, Stueland D: Classifying women alcoholics by Cattell's 16 PF: A preliminary investigation of an alcoholic typology. *J Stud Alcohol* 41:911–921, 1980.
47. Nerviano VJ, McCarty D, McCarty SM: MMPI profile patterns of men alcoholics in two contrasting settings. *J Stud Alcohol* 41:1143–1152, 1980.
48. Eshbaugh DM, Tosi DJ, Hoyt CN: Women alcoholics: A typological description using the MMPI. *J Stud Alcohol* 41:310–317, 1980.
49. Sutker PB, Brantley PJ, Allain AN: MMPI response patterns and alcohol consumption of DUI offenders. *J Consult Clin Psychol* 48:350–355, 1980.
50. Zivich JM: Alcoholic subtypes and treatment effectiveness. *J Consult Clin Psychol* 49:72–80, 1981.
51. Nerviano VJ: Personality patterns of alcoholics revisited: Delineation against the MMPI and clinical implications. *Int J Addict* 16:723–730, 1981.
52. O'Leary MR, Donovan DM, Chaney EF, et al: Relationship of alcoholic personality subtypes of treatment follow-up measures. *J Nerv Ment Dis* 168:475–480, 1980.

53. Gibbs LE: A classification of alcoholics relevant to type-specific treatment. *Int J Addict* 15:461–488, 1980.
54. Polich JM, Armor, DJ Braiker HB: Patterns of alcoholism over four years. *J Stud Alcohol* 41:397–416, 1980.
55. Svanum S, Dallas CL: Alcoholic MMPI types and their relationship to patient characteristics, polydrug abuse, and abstinence following treatment. *J Pers Assess* 45:278–287, 1981.
56. Loberg T: MMPI-based personality subtypes of alcoholics. *J Stud Alcohol* 42:766–782, 1981.
57. Donovan DM, Marlatt GA: Personality subtypes among driving-while-intoxicated offenders: Relationship to drinking behavior and driving risk. *J Consult Clin Psychol* 50:241–249, 1982.
58. Conley JJ, Prioleau LA: Personality typology of men and women alcoholics in relation to etiology and prognosis. *J Stud Alcohol* 44:996–1010, 1983.
59. Filstead WJ, Drachman DA, Rossi JJ, et al: The relationship of MMPI subtype membership to demographic variables and treatment outcome among substance misusers. *J Stud Alcohol* 44: 917–921, 1983.
60. Conley J: An MMPI typology of male alcoholics: Admission, discharge, and outcome comparisons. *J Pers Assess* 45:33–39, 1981.
61. Nerviano V, Gross W: Personality types of alcoholics in objective inventories. *J Stud Alcohol* 44:837–851, 1983.
62. Skinner HA, Jackson DN: A model of psychopathology based on the interrelation of MMPI actuarial systems. *J Consult Clin Psychol* 46:231–238, 1978.
63. Blashfield RK: Propositions regarding the use of cluster analysis in clinical research. *J Consult Clin Psychol* 48:456–458, 1980.
64. Rubington E: The hidden alcoholic. *Q J Stud Alcohol* 33: 667–683, 1972.
65. Sackin C: Youthful and aged alcohol abusers: Some policy implications. *J Alcohol Drug Educ* 26:6–75, 1980.
66. Zimberg S: The elderly alcoholic. *Gerontologist* 55:221–224, 1974.
67. Schuckit MA, Miller PL: Alcoholism in elderly men: A survey of a general medical ward. *Ann NY Acad Sci* 273:558–571, 1975.
68. Lender ME: Women alcoholics: Prevalence estimates and their problems as referenced in turn of the century institutional data. *Int J Addict* 16:443–448, 1981.
69. Morey LC, Skinner HA, Blashfield RK: A typology of alcohol abusers: correlates and implications. *J Abnorm Psychol* 93:408–417, 1984.
70. Maisto SA, Sobell LC, Sobell MG: Comparison of alcoholics self-report of drinking behavior with reports of collateral informants. *J Consult Clin Psychol* 47:106–112, 1979.
71. Hesselbrock M, Babor TF, Hesselbrock V, et al: Never believe an alcoholic? On the validity of self-report measures of alcohol dependence and related constructs. *Int J Addict* 18:593–609, 1983.
72. Ward JH: Hierarchical grouping to optimize an objective function. *J Am Stat Assoc* 58:236–244, 1963.
73. Morey LC, Blashfield RK, Skinner HA: A comparison of cluster analysis techniques within a sequential validation framework. *Multivariate Behav Res* 18:309–329, 1983.
74. Blashfield RK, Aldenderfer MA, Morey LC: Validating a cluster analytic solution, in Hudson H (ed): *Classifying Social Data*. San Francisco, Jossey-Bass, 1982.
75. Gorsuch RL: *Factor Analysis*. Philadelphia, Saunders, 1974.
76. Nerviano VJ: Common personality patterns among alcoholic males: a multivariate study. *J Consult Clin Psychol* 44:104–110, 1976.
77. Hart L: Rehabilitation need patterns of men alcoholics. *J Stud Alcohol* 38:504–511, 1977.
78. Foster FM, Horn JL, Wanberg KW: Dimensions of treatment outcome. *Q J Stud Alcohol* 33: 1079–1098, 1972.
79. Horn JL, Wanberg KW: Symptom patterns related to excessive use of alcohol. *Q J Stud Alcohol* 30:35–58, 1969.
80. Wanberg KW, Horn JL, Foster FM: A differential assessment model for alcoholism: The scales of the alcohol use inventory. *J Stud Alcohol* 38:512–543, 1977.

81. Wanberg KW, Horn JL: Assessment of alcohol use with multidimensional concepts and measures. *Am Psychol* 38:1055–1069, 1983.
82. Skinner HA: A model of psychopathology based on the MMPI, in Newmark CS (ed): *MMPI: Current Clinical and Research Trends*. New York, Praeger Publishing, 1979.
83. Skinner HA: Models for the description of abnormal behavior, in Adams H, Sutker P (eds): *Comprehensive Handbook of Psychopathology*. New York, Plenum, 1984.
84. Kammeier ML, Hoffman H, Lopez RG: Personality characteristics of alcoholism as college freshmen and at time of treatment. *Q J Stud Alcohol* 34:390–399, 1973.
85. Horn JL, Wanberg KW, Foster FM: The alcohol use inventory—AUI. Denver, Center for Alcohol Abuse Research and Evaluation, 1977.
86. Horn JL, Wanberg KW, Appel M: On the internal structure of the MMPI. *Multivariate Behav Res* 8:131–171, 1973.
87. Skinner HA, Allen BA: Differential assessment of alcoholism: Evaluation of the alcohol use inventory. *J Stud Alcohol* 44:852–862, 1983.
88. Skinner HA: Primary syndromes of alcohol abuse: Their measurement and correlates. *Br J Addict* 76:63–76, 1981.
89. Skinner HA, Allen BA: Alcohol dependence syndrome: Measurement and validation. *J Abnorm Psychol* 91:199–209, 1982.
90. Skinner HA: Dimensions and clusters: A hybrid approach to classification. *Appl Psychol Measurements* 3:327–341, 1979.
91. Jackson DN: *Personality Research Form Manual*. Goshen, New York, Research Psychologists Press, 1974.
92. Sobell MB, Sobell LC: Controlled drinking: A concept coming of age, in Blumstein KR, Polivy J (eds): *Self-Control and Self-Modification of Emotional Behavior*. New York, Plenum, 1982.
93. Miller WR, Caddy GR: Abstinence and controlled drinking in the treatment of problem drinkers. *J Stud Alcohol* 38:986–1003, 1977.
94. Mulford HA: Stages in the alcoholism process: Toward a cumulative, nonsequential index. *J Stud Alcohol* 38:563–583, 1977.
95. Oxford J, Oppenheimer E, Edwards G: Abstinence or control: The outcome for excessive drinkers two years after consultation. *Behav Res Ther* 14:409–418, 1976.
96. Sanchez-Craig M: Random assignment to abstinence and controlled drinking in a cognitive behavioral program. *Addict Behav* 5:35–39, 1980.
97. Osborne AC, Glaser FB: Characteristics of affiliates of Alcoholics Anonymous. *J Stud Alcohol* 42:661–675, 1981.
98. Glaser FB: Anybody got a match? Treatment and the matching hypothesis, in Edwards G, Grant M (eds): *Alcoholism Treatment in Transition*. London, Crown Helm, 1980.
99. Meyer RE, Babor TF, Mirkin PM: Typologies in alcoholism: An overview. *Int J Addict* 18:235–249, 1983.
100. Skinner HA, Blashfield RK: Increasing the impact of cluster analysis research: The case of psychiatric classification. *J Consult Clin Psychol* 50:727–735, 1982.

7

An Examination of Selected Typologies

Hyperactivity, Familial, and Antisocial Alcoholism

Arthur I. Alterman and Ralph E. Tarter

Abstract. In exploring potential alcoholism typologies, this chapter critically examines findings of adoption, high-risk, and familial alcoholism studies and studies of psychiatric syndromes in alcoholic individuals and their families. The adoption studies revealed that familial alcoholism and childhood conduct disorder and hyperactivity are associated with subsequent alcoholism. However, the relationship between childhood hyperactivity and alcoholism is probably coincidental to the conjoint presence of aggressive and antisocial behaviors in the same individuals. Psychiatric diagnosis and family psychiatric history studies suggest a synergistic relationship between alcoholism and sociopathy. Clinical studies of familial and antisocial alcoholism indicate that both are associated with early onset, more severe alcoholism, and poorer treatment outcome. Both meet clinical criteria for an alcoholism typology, although the evidence is more compelling for antisocial alcoholism.

The findings of metabolic, electrophysiological, and neuropsychological differences between high- and low-risk subjects are of potential import, although their present significance is uncertain. Further clinical evaluation of antisocial and familial alcoholism and their relationship to each other is necessary. High risk and familial alcoholism findings may be confounded by the subject's antisocial characteristics.

1. Introduction

The last two decades of research have produced an increased recognition of the heterogeneity of the alcoholic population.[1–3] One implication of this conclusion is that alcoholic individuals with different problems may respond differentially and be more susceptible to different treatments. Assuming that appropriate treatment strategies could be developed and implemented, the

Arthur I. Alterman • Veterans Administration Medical Center, Philadelphia, Pennsylvania 19104; and University of Pennsylvania School of Medicine, Philadelphia, Pennsylvania 19104. **Ralph E. Tarter** • Department of Psychology, University of Pittsburgh School of Medicine, Pittsburgh, Pennsylvania 15213.

ultimate outcome of such a set of circumstances would be an improvement in the treatment outcomes of alcohol-dependent persons. The most cited inquiry into such a question was conducted by Kissin *et al.*,[4] who randomly assigned alcoholic patients to an outpatient drug therapy program, outpatient group psychotherapy, inpatient rehabilitation, or a nontreatment control condition. Socially stable individuals were more likely to prefer an outpatient treatment, while the socially unstable tended to opt for inpatient treatment. Socially stable and intellectually sophisticated outpatients fared best with psychotherapy, while those less psychologically oriented did best in drug treatment. Intellectually intact, but unstable, individuals seemed to do best in inpatient treatment. This study therefore demonstrated that alcoholic patients differed in their susceptibility to different treatments and that such differences could conceivably be employed in optimizing treatment effectiveness.

Since the above study was conducted, a considerable amount of information has been produced concerning the characteristics of the alcoholic population. New ways of subgrouping and classifying alcoholics have emerged that could conceivably have considerable impact on our understanding of the etiology of alcoholism and for increasing treatment effectiveness. This chapter will be concerned with several potential subgrouping and typological variables and the related issues associated with two, partially converging lines of inquiry; that is, the investigations concerned with genetic influences in alcoholism and studies of the coexistent psychiatric diagnoses of individuals with diagnoses of alcoholism. Findings from the first body of work have shown that some alcoholics may have inherited a predisposition for childhood hyperactivity/MBD and conduct disorder.[5] Related work has sought to investigate potential electrophysiological, physiological, and biochemical differences between subjects who are at high risk (HR+) and are not at high risk (HR−) for the development of alcoholism.[6] The latter line of inquiry noted above, concentrating on additional psychopathology in alcoholics, was also concerned with the possible genetic etiologies of various diagnostic constellations in alcoholics and accordingly investigated the family psychiatric histories of these individuals.[7,8] Within this context, we will focus in this chapter on the relationship between adult sociopathy and childhood hyperactivity and conduct disorder and also examine the relationship between adult sociopathy, familial alcoholism, and the findings for individuals at risk for alcoholism. Our review of the above variables and conditions will incorporate an examination of their relationship to the severity of alcoholism, to psychosocial and neuropsychological functioning, and to treatment outcome. It should be emphasized at the outset that the typologies discussed only apply to males, since research has mainly been conducted with this population and many of the issues and variables concerned, i.e. sociopathy and hyperactivity, appear to be more common in male alcoholics and to have a clearer genetic association in males.

2. Genetic Research

2.1. Adoptee Studies

As most of us are currently aware, adoption studies conducted by Goodwin *et al.*[9] and Cadoret and Gath[10] in the 1970s provided some support for the notion that there may be genetic influences in male alcoholism. Specifically, adopted biological sons of alcoholics were found to be more likely than biological sons of nonalcoholics to develop alcoholism in their early adulthood. Both of these investigations suffer from relatively small numbers in the experimental group. The Goodwin *et al.* research reported, but did not comment, on the presence of higher proportions of heavy and problem drinkers among the control group subjects. As Murray *et al.*[11] have commented, "if the cut off for abnormality is widened to include not just alcoholism, but also problem drinking, then evidence for any genetic predisposition vanishes." The subjects in the Goodwin *et al.* study were about 30 years of age. It may be early-onset alcoholism is inherited, as contrasted with later-onset alcoholism, i.e., the control subjects who at age 30 were problem and heavy drinkers and who may yet become alcoholic. Indeed, there appears to be considerable evidence supporting the notion that early-onset alcoholism is inherited. This evidence will be discussed later in the paper.

The Cadoret *et al.* research suffered from an extremely large subject attrition rate and a rather broad definition of alcoholism. Additionally, when secondary alcoholism is also included, the experimental and control groups do not differ.[11] Since the distinction between secondary and primary alcoholism is somewhat questionable, and the information collection procedures employed in this study were relatively weak, this distinction is even more suspect.

More recently, Cloninger *et al.*[12] have provided evidence for two forms of inherited alcohol abuse in males. One form, consisting of moderate alcohol abuse, was found to be highly heritable and independent of environmental influences. The fathers were likely to have a history of criminality and severe alcohol abuse. The second form consisted of either mild or severe alcohol abuse. The fathers were not criminals, but were mild to moderate alcohol abusers, and the mothers were also often alcohol abusers. Both genetic and environmental factors are considered to be important for its development, with genetic factors presumably contributing the alcohol abuse and environmental factors apparently affecting the severity of the alcohol abuse. It should be noted that the definition of environment employed in this investigation was rather restrictive.

One problem with the Cloninger *et al.* investigation was that information on alcohol abuse was obtained from Temperance Board registrations. The relationship of these vis a vis alcoholism is certainly imperfect and except for the severe abusers, the investigation appears to be concerned with alcohol abuse rather than alcoholism. The Temperance Board registrations also point to a significant consideration that probably applies to all of the adoptee studies. That is, registrations are likely to be higher in antisocial individuals. Similarly, individuals who adopt out their children are also more likely to have antisocial characteristics. Thus, the subject population in the adoptee studies of alcoholism are probably biased toward sociopathy. The relationship between alcoholism and sociopathy will be considered later in this chapter.

2.2. High-Risk and Familial Alcoholism Studies

The findings for genetic influences in alcoholism described above have led to a number of studies directed toward specifically determining what characteristics are genetically transmitted. Inasmuch as the adoption study is very costly, two other research strategies have been employed. One approach, called the "high-risk" paradigm, involves comparing the characteristics of nonalcoholic, usually male, preadult relatives of alcoholics (HR+ subjects) with nonalcoholic relatives of nonalcoholics (HR− subjects). In other words, nonalcoholic subjects with and without familial alcoholism are compared. Presumably, the HR+ subjects are more likely than HR− subjects to have inherited a predisposition for alcoholism, so that any differences between these two groups may reflect genetic differences. The second strategy compares the characteristics of already affected alcoholics who either do (FH+ alcoholics) or do not (FH− alcoholics) have relatives who suffer from alcoholism. This strategy also assumes that alcoholics positive for a family history of alcoholism are more likely to have a genetic loading for alcoholism than alcoholics without alcoholism in their family. The greater accessibility of eligible research subjects provided by these approaches makes them very useful for preliminary investigations of genetic hypotheses, although they are much less able than adoption or twin studies to separate out possible environmental influences.[5] The HR strategy presumably has an advantage over the FH strategy vis a vis etiological considerations in avoiding possible contaminating consequential effects of alcohol abuse.[13] At the same time, it is not clear what proportion of the HR+ population carry the genetic vulnerability, so that when HR+ and HR− subjects are compared, actual genetic-based differences may be diluted. For example, Schuckit[6] found that HR+ subjects had higher blood acetaldehyde levels following alcohol consumption than HR− subjects. However, he noted that one third of the HR+ subjects showed marked effects, one third moderate effects, and the remaining one third responded like HR− subjects. Could these differences have reflected differences in genetic vulnerability within the HR+ group? By contrast, the familial alcoholism approach probably includes a higher proportion of "genetic alcoholics" in the FH+ group. One possible approach to resolving the problem with the HR design would be to compare HR+ subjects in their late teens or early twenties who are and are not problem drinkers. Since "genetic" alcoholism is believed to have an early onset, those individuals more likely to have inherited alcoholism would already be manifesting such problems, and those without this inherited vulnerability would be free of the problem. To our knowledge, only one high-risk investigation has included a comparison of HR+ problem drinkers and HR+ nonproblem drinkers.[14]

Several other problems of both the HR and FH research strategies should be mentioned. These procedures become much more costly when the family history information provided by the subjects has to be corroborated with informants. Unfortunately, subjects are often unaware of alcoholism in their relatives, and this therefore results in individuals being inappropriately assigned to either the positive or negative groups. One might speculate that HR subjects are more susceptible to this problem than alcoholic subjects, because the latter are more familiar with alcoholism problems. In a study in which adopted sons of alcoholics were compared with their siblings who were raised at home by the alcoholic parent, Goodwin *et al.*[15] found that only 60% of the subjects in the latter group were aware of the alcoholism of their parent. Another difficulty with the FH and HR paradigms is that subjects frequently are not aware that the fathers with whom they were raised are not their biological fathers.[11] As a result, subjects can be classified improperly. The need to corroborate subjects' reports on family psychiatric histories is therefore stressed.

3. Evaluation of Potential Typologies

3.1. Coexistent Psychiatric Diagnoses

Penick *et al.*[16] describe a number of criteria that should be met to demonstrate the clinical validity of any method of subtyping. That is, the method of subtyping should be both reliable and stable over time; developmental course, prognosis, and treatment outcome should vary as a function of the subtype; and the subtypes should be distinguished in terms of their histories of psychiatric disorders. Noting that a number of investigations have shown that individuals who carry an alcoholism diagnosis also suffer from symptoms common to other psychiatric syndromes, they present evidence lending preliminary support for a typology of alcoholism based on the coexisting psychiatric syndromes of the alcoholic. The history and development of such a concept is described in the immediately following sections of this paper.

The work of Winokur and his colleagues[7,8] was perhaps the first to draw attention to coexisting psychiatric syndromes in persons diagnosed as alcoholic. Winokur *et al.*[7] proposed a classification of alcoholics based on their secondary psychiatric diagnoses. Three groups were enumerated: primary alcoholics, i.e., those with no secondary diagnoses, and depressed and sociopathic alcoholics. Although alcoholism was found to be the most common psychiatric diagnosis in the relatives of all three groups of male alcoholics, sociopathic and depressed alcoholics were more likely to have a greater proportion of relatives with these psychiatric diagnoses in their families than the primary alcoholics. Evidence such as this,[2,17] and the finding that relatives of persons with a diagnosis of antisocial personality (ASP) are much more likely to have an ASP diagnosis[17] than alcoholism, has led to the conclusion that alcoholism and ASP are etiologically, and perhaps genetically, distinct entities. Vaillant,[18] employing multiple regression statistical procedures, concluded that alcoholism and ASP were attributable to different antecedent variables—the former to a family history of alcoholism and certain sociocultural variables, the latter to a disruptive family environment during childhood. At the same time, we mentioned previously that Cloninger *et al.*[12] described a form of inherited alcoholism that was dependent upon the conjoint existence of severe alcohol abuse and criminality in the father. Additionally, Reich *et al.*[2] found that male relatives of alcoholic + ASP probands are more likely than relatives of pure alcoholics to be alcoholics themselves and that ASP male relatives of alcoholics are much more likely to be alcoholic (81%) than relatives without an ASP diagnosis (44%). As these investigators point out, the presence of ASP in a family elevates the familial risk of alcoholism. It seems clear that there is some synergistic interaction between ASP and alcoholism.

One condition that ASP appears to foster is heavy drinking and this is believed to be a necessary minimum requirement for the development of alcoholism.[2,12,17,19] An amazing 98% of the male relatives of alcoholic probands, who themselves qualified for an ASP diagnosis, were likely to be heavy drinkers, and 77% of the male relatives of alcoholic probands were heavy drinkers even when they did not qualify for an ASP diagnosis.

Although Winokur *et al.*[7] included primary depressed (prior onset of depression) alcoholics as one of three subgroups in his classification system, this category was not meaningful for the male patients, since almost all of the primary depressed alcoholics were women. Thus, a breakdown of male alcoholics into primary and sociopathic alcoholics would have more directly reflected the diagnostic distribution for men. Fowler *et al.*[20] also found little evidence for depression in male alcoholics. It is of interest that both of these investigations employed the Feighner (or Feighner-like) diagnostic criteria,[21] which requires symptom duration of at least 1 month for the determination of a diagnosis of depression, while other studies which have found higher proportions of depressed alcoholics have instead employed either the RDC[22] (see refs. 23, 24, 25), which requires only one week duration of symptoms, or the DSM-III criteria[26] (see refs, 16, 27), which requires 2 weeks of symptom duration. Thus, it appears that depression is more commonly diagnosed in alcoholics when no more than 2 weeks of depressive symptomatology are required for a positive diagnosis, whereas it is less commonly diagnosed in men when the depressive symptomatology must last for a month or more. Hewett and Martin[28] concluded that nearly three fourths of the alcoholics they studied would have qualified for an ASP diagnosis and that sociopathy in the preadult years is a pervasive characteristic of alcoholics and drug addicts. The research of Reich *et al.*[2] and Lewis *et al.*[17] described previously found that a majority of their alcoholics qualified also for an ASP diagnosis, and Goodwin *et al.*[29] found that a majority of the convicts they interviewed were alcoholic and sociopathic. Thus, the evidence we have reviewed indicates that a combination of alcoholism and sociopathy is relatively common. On the other hand, the status of coexistent depression in male alcoholics is not as clear. Hewett and Martin[28] have argued that alcoholics do not really suffer from depression but from low mood states that come and go over relatively short periods of time and are commonly found in addicts. Cadoret *et al.*[27] have obtained some evidence in support of this contention.

Recognizedly, the relative distribution of various psychiatric diagnoses may vary depending upon the population of alcoholics encountered,[30] the instrument and diagnostic criteria employed, and possibly even with the point in time in which the diagnostic interview takes place.[31] At present, the relative importance of depression in male alcoholics is somewhat in question, but the evidence for ASP as a coexisting psychiatric disorder in a large number of alcoholics is substantial. We would suggest that a sociopathic vs. primary alcoholic distinction may provide a useful foundation for an alcoholism typology.

3.2. Childhood Hyperactivity and Conduct Disorder

Other investigators[32–34] have proposed a typological distinction between inherited and noninherited alcoholism, represented empirically by familial and nonfamilial alcoholism. The comparison of high-risk and non-high-risk subjects would seem to reflect a similar distinction to some degree. We review below the evidence from studies of familial alcoholism and high risk studies, which attempt to differentiate commonalities that could serve as the basis for an inherited vs. noninherited alcoholism typology. In keeping with the criteria set forward by Penick *et al.*[16] we examine the data with respect to the onset, developmental course, prognosis, and treatment outcome of these subgroups, attempting thereby to determine whether the evidence is sufficient to support a typological distinction. Finally, as we suggested previously, the findings from the studies investigating the genetic basis for alcoholism and those from the study of coexisting psychiatric diagnoses of alcoholics converge to some extent. We suggest that the childhood hyperactivity and conduct disorder found in adopted biological children of alcoholics, rather than being evidence of genetically transmitted behavioral vulnerability, are probably instead the precursors and correlates of adult sociopathy. A similar hypothesis for the findings of familial alcoholism and high-risk research will also be explored to the extent that this is presently possible given the limited available data. First, we discuss childhood hyperactivity and conduct disorder and their relation to adult sociopathy, and we then review the experimental and clinical evidence obtained in high-risk and familial alcoholism studies.

3.2.1. Childhood Hyperactivity and Alcoholism. In a subsequent analysis of their adoption study data, Goodwin *et al.*[35] examined the childhood characteristics of the 14 adoptees (ten had alcoholic biological fathers and four had nonalcoholic fathers) who ultimately became alcoholic. The paper emphasized the presence of childhood hyperactivity, in particular, in a large proportion (50%) of their alcoholic sample. It is important to note, however, that although childhood antisocial behavior was not found in a large proportion of subjects, aggressiveness was found in 50%. Cadoret *et al.*[10,36] also pointed out in their research that the only significant predictor of adult alcoholism, beside familial alcoholism, was childhood conduct disorder. Until relatively recently, however, the role of childhood hyperactivity in relation to alcoholism has received the bulk of attention, and the role of childhood conduct disorder has received relatively little attention. The evidence concerning the relation between both of these conditions and alcoholism will be examined in the following sections, beginning with hyperactivity.

In addition to the Goodwin *et al.*[35] study described above, a number of studies have pointed to a relationship between childhood hyperactivity and alcoholism. Three longitudinal studies of children[37–39] have described the subjects who ultimately became alcoholic as having been restless and impulsive as children, i.e., hyperactive. Cantwell,[40] Goodwin *et al.*,[9,35] and Morrison and Stewart[41] found that adopted hyperactive children were more likely than nonhyperactive children to have a biological father who was alcoholic. Longitudinal research has shown that hyperactive adolescents have more problematic encounters with alcohol.[42,43] Wood, Wender, and their colleagues[44–46] found that many adults in treatment for alcoholism are likely to have suffered from hyperactivity and MBD as children. Tarter *et al.*[47] and DeObaldia *et al.*[48] have also contributed findings linking childhood hyperactivity to alcoholism. Tarter *et al.* found that a subgroup of early-onset, severe "primary" alcoholics retrospectively reported significantly more symptoms of childhood hyperactivity/MBD than "secondary," late-onset alcoholics. Primary alcoholism was found to be significantly related to familial alcoholism,[47] suggesting a genetic link for the childhood hyperactivity. In other research, Alterman *et al.*[49] found that familial alcoholics reported significantly more symptoms of childhood hyperactivity than FH alcoholics. In a latter study, however, Alterman *et al.*[50] failed to find a significant relationship between childhood hyperactivity and familial alcoholism. Hesselbrock *et al.*[14] also failed to find more childhood hyperactivity in a high-risk sample. Nevertheless, sufficient evidence has been cumulated for a relationship between alcoholism and childhood hyperactivity that the question may arise whether hyperactive alcoholics should be considered to be a separate subgroup from nonhyperactive alcoholics.

3.2.2. Childhood Conduct Disorder, Alcoholism, and Sociopathy. One problem with the diagnosis of the syndrome of hyperactivity has been the broadness and looseness of the symptoms included. As August and Stewart[51] have noted, "although overreactivity, inattentiveness, and impulsivity comprise the core of the syndrome, some investigators also include aggression, noncompliance, antisocial behavior and learning problems." Thus, essentially all of the studies described above as supporting a relationship between childhood hyperactivity and alcoholism also yielded evidence for a relationship between childhood aggressiveness/conduct disorder and alcoholism. As mentioned previously, Cadoret *et al.*[36] found that the only variable significantly predicting alcoholism in their adoptee population, besides familial alcoholism, was childhood conduct disorder. Similarly, childhood aggressiveness was found in as many of Goodwin's alcoholic adoptees as hyperactivity.[35] The three longitudinal studies[37–39] of boys who ultimately became alcoholic, mentioned above, all reported aggression or antisocial behaviors in their subjects, in addition to hyperactivity; the two longitudinal studies[42,43] that described problematic drinking in adolescents who were hyperactive as children, as well as the three studies by Wood *et al.*[44–46] all employed definitions of hyperactivity that included aggressiveness and antisocial behaviors. A similar description applies to the work by Tarter *et al.*[47] and DeObaldia *et al.*[48] who primarily used items suggested by Wender in their checklists. Finally, the fathers of adopted hyperactive children in the studies mentioned were just as likely to be sociopathic as alcoholic.

Guze[52] has hypothesized that childhood hyperactivity leads to a greater risk of sociopathy. Given the distinctions just made and some that will soon be presented, it is probably more accurate to conclude that childhood aggressiveness and antisocial behavior are more directly associated with adult sociopathy than is childhood hyperactivity. In this connection, research by Stewart *et al.*[53] has revealed that childhood aggressiveness and resistance to discipline are associated to a greater degree with an antisocial disposition in the parent, rather than hyperactivity. The results of several investigations by the present authors should therefore come as no surprise. Alterman *et al.*[50] compared alcoholics high and low in childhood "hyperactivity" and found a personality pattern reflective of an underlying character disorder in the high "hyperactivity" alcoholics. Tarter *et al.*[54] compared delinquent sons of alcoholics with delinquent sons of nonalcoholics for hyperactivity and found no differences between the groups. Thus, the risk for alcoholism was not found to be associated with hyperactivity when conduct disorder was held constant in the subjects. These findings suggest that studies that have been interpreted as indicating a relationship between childhood hyperactivity and alcoholism may have been confounded by the presence of antisocial behavior in their subjects.

The findings of several other recent studies need to be emphasized. Gomez *et al.*[55] evaluated adult psychiatric inpatient veterans for self-report of symptoms of childhood and adulthood hyperactivity, attentional deficit, and impulsivity. In both childhood and adulthood, character disorder patients reported a higher incidence of target symptoms than either patients diagnosed as alcoholic, psychotic, having an affective disorder, or control subjects. Although alcoholics reported more symptoms of hyperactivity than control subjects, they did not differ significantly from the other patient groups. Character/personality disorder patients were far more likely than any of the other groups to have retained their hyperactivity into adulthood. The results of this study therefore suggest that the linkage between hyperactivity and character disorder is much stronger than that for hyperactivity and alcoholism and that the presence of hyperactivity in alcoholics may often be attributable to the concurrent existence of a character disorder, rather than to the alcoholism per se. Further support for this conclusion can be found in two studies with drug addicts. In a study with substance abusers, Loney[56] found that childhood hyperactivity alone did not predict subsequent substance abuse, but hyperactivity coupled with aggression, or the aggression alone, did. Thus, aggression appeared to be the critical predictor of subsequent substance abuse. Eyre *et al.*[57] also found that over 20% of their opiate addict subjects reported childhood histories of hyperactivity. This subgroup of addicts was described by the investigators as appearing highly antisocial even within an addict population.

August and Stewart[51] compared hyperactive children having a parent with a disorder in the antisocial personality spectrum (ASP, alcoholism, drug abuse, or hysteria for women) with hyperactive children whose parents were free of these disorders. They found that the behavior of the first group of hyperactive children was deviant for aggressiveness, noncompliance, inattention, egocentricity, and reactivity, while the latter group was deviant only on inattention and reactivity. The siblings of the FH+ subjects were also found to suffer from similar problems. Interestingly also, the FH− group suffered from significantly more academic problems and tended to have lower IQs. Thus, the group with parents with disorders in the antisocial spectrum had the symptoms of hyperactivity plus conduct disorder, while the hyperactive group whose parents did not suffer from disorders in the antisocial spectrum were pure hyperactives. As indicated by August and Stewart, these findings form a mirror image of their recent findings that boys with conduct disorder have parents with personality disorders and alcoholism, while the parents of hyperactive boys do not have these disorders.[53] August and Stewart concluded that pure hyperactivity and conduct disorder have independent etiologies. These findings provide additional reinforcement for these conclusions: (1) Conduct disorder, rather than hyperactivity, is etiologically linked to alcoholism; (2) the apparent association between alcoholism and hyperactivity is actually attributable to the co-occurrence of hyperactivity with conduct disorder in many individuals.

3.3. High-Risk Studies and Familial and Antisocial Alcoholism

We suggested earlier that the distinction between "inherited" and "noninherited" alcoholism may provide the basis for an alcoholism typology. Numerous familial history (FH) and high-risk (HR) studies have been conducted toward establishing the validity of such a distinction. The preceding discussion, indeed, examined hyperactivity, a behavioral characteristic considered to be such an inherited vulnerability, and concluded that what was previously believed to be the result of hyperactivity was more likely attributable to antisocial characteristics and that although ASP is frequently co-occurrent and synergistic with alcoholism, it is nevertheless etiologically independent of it. We consequently suggested that the distinction between antisocial and primary alcoholism might represent a useful alcoholism typology. The remaining sections of this chapter review the findings of studies concerned with HR subjects FH, and sociopathic alcoholics in relation to some of the criteria suggested by Penick *et al.* for establishing the validity of a clinical typology, i.e., developmental course, current functioning, and treatment outcome.

3.3.1. Electrophysiological, Physiological, and Metabolic Studies. Schuckit has conducted a number of investigations with college-aged male populations, comparing subjects with alcoholic first-degree relatives (HR+) with subjects having no first-degree relatives who were alcoholic. In most of these studies, the metabolic reactions and behavioral responses of the subjects were evaluated after they had consumed a small dose of alcohol. The family alcoholism information provided by the subjects in these studies was not corroborated by informants.

In one such study,[58] blood acetaldehyde levels of HR+ subjects were found to be significantly higher than that of HR− subjects. In another investigation by Schuckit and Duby,[59] more alcohol-related flushing was demonstrated in HR+ subjects. The flushing response was found to be correlated +0.83 with blood acetaldehyde levels and at least +0.60 with heart rate and skin temperature. These findings appear paradoxically to be consistent with the hypothesis that persons "not at risk" for alcoholism are protected by a low tolerance for alcohol.[6,33] A low tolerance for alcohol would be reflected in flushing and other adverse effects, e.g., nausea, that presumably occur with acetaldehyde accumulation. However, such effects are inconsistent with the findings of several other studies by Schuckit *et al.* that have revealed lower prolactin levels,[60] lower levels of subjective intoxication,[61] less behavioral and cognitive impairment,[60] and less upper body sway[62] following alcohol consumption in HR+ subjects. In addition, they conflict with the high-risk status of the subjects and the associated assumption that high-risk individuals have high levels of tolerance for alcohol.[2,17,33]

An alternative explanation for the acetaldehyde findings has been offered by Schuckit and Rayses.[58] They suggested that individuals predisposed to alcoholism are more vulnerable to organ damage from acetaldehyde. This hypothesis, then, conflicts somewhat, but may not be totally incompatible, with the notion that one necessary characteristic of alcoholics is their ability to tolerate large amounts of alcohol.[2,17,33] Instead, alcoholics may be seen as individuals who may be able to consume large amounts of alcohol but also, in the process, suffer organ damage—the end product of which results in their being labeled alcoholics. Seen in these terms, individuals who can tolerate long-term consumption of large amounts of alcohol and not suffer organ damage would presumably not be labeled alcoholics.

In the acetaldehyde investigation, the authors described, as noted, three subgroups of HR+ responders. It would have been informative to know whether the flushing/acetaldehyde responders could have been differentiated on some other basis. For example, inasmuch as we have described the common co-occurrence of alcoholism and sociopathy, it would have been of interest to know if the acetaldehyde responders were more likely to have been sociopathic. The findings could then have been attributed to the sociopathy, rather than to inherited vulnerabilities associated with alcoholism. Although antisocial behavior of the subjects was not examined in this investigation, Schuckit[63] reported that HR+ subjects had more alcohol and drug problems and psychopathology but unfortunately reported no specific data on other forms of antisocial behavior. It is evident that this syndrome should be taken into account in future HR and FH studies.

A number of other studies of high-risk populations have revealed electrophysiological differences between HR+ and HR− subject groups. Several investigators[64,65] have found evoked potential differences. Gabrielli *et al.*[66] reported an excess of high-frequency EEG activity in HR subjects. They argued that although many of the parents of HR subjects were also sociopathic, the results were specific to parental alcoholism, because sociopathy is associated with an excess of low-speed EEG. Propping *et al.*[67] found deficient alpha activity, and Pollock *et al.*[68] found that HR men exhibited greater increases of slow-alpha energy and greater decreases of fast-alpha energy after alcohol consumption than control subjects. The authors concluded that HR+ subjects are differentially sensitive to alcohol and theorized that this may be related to differential acetaldehyde levels, though they recognized other possible explanations for the results.

Several other studies of upper body sway (static ataxia) have been reported in addition to that by Schuckit mentioned earlier. Lipscomb *et al.*[69] found greater body sway in HR+ college-aged subjects after alcohol consumption, but a subsequent study by the same investigators failed to replicate the original finding.[70] On the other hand, Hegedus *et al.*[71] found more static ataxia in 9- to 17-year-old sons of alcoholics than in sons of social drinkers or depressed persons. Alcohol was not consumed in this study. Thus, metabolic/electrophysiological studies thus far conducted on high-risk populations have been conflicting, and their ultimate significance is unclear. It is certainly not evident at this point whether high-risk populations carry genetically transmitted characteristics that could be employed to predict, prevent, or treat such individuals.

Before proceeding to an examination of neuropsychological studies of HR and FH populations, a study by Sher and Levenson[72] will be described briefly, basically for its heuristic merits. These investigators selected a high-risk group of college-aged males based on their scores on the MacAndrew Alcoholism Scale and found a greater amount of stress response dampening of alcohol on the physiological and affective responses of HR+ subjects. The MacAndrew Alcoholism scale is of particular interest, because high scores on it, which are found in both alcoholics and drug addicts, are thought to reflect a boisterous, gregarious, uninhibited personality style akin to sociopathy.[73] In line with the conceptual framework we have described, individuals at risk for alcoholism would be expected to score high on this scale.[74]

3.3.2. Neuropsychological Studies of HR Populations. An evaluation of neuropsychological functioning is important not only because it provides information on current functioning but also because neuropsychological functioning has been found to be predictive of treatment outcome in alcoholics.[75] An early finding by Kaij[76] indicated that children of alcoholics may suffer from cognitive deficits that antedate alcoholism. Taken in conjunction with the findings of EEG and evoked-potential differences between HR+ and HR− subjects, it is reasonable to anticipate that these groups may differ neuropsychologically. Group differences, if obtained, would be difficult to interpret solely in genetic terms, however, since numerous investigations have described early environmental disruption and familial disorganization in alcoholic families, including family psychiatric disorder, poor nutrition, and child abuse, that could adversely affect neuropsychological functioning.[13,29,77,78]

Tarter *et al.*[79,80] found poorer language-related neuropsychological functioning and academic achievement in delinquent sons of alcoholics and Gabrielli and Mednick[81] found lower verbal, but not performance, IQs in HR+ subjects. Tarter *et al.*[82] conjecture that such language impairment may result in insufficient ability to verbally mediate impulse control. Ervin *et al.*[83] also found inferior IQ and achievement scores in children of both sexes raised by alcoholic fathers. The majority of the fathers were not the biological fathers, however, and the authors did not provide separate data for the biological and nonbiological fathers. Hesselbrock *et al.*[14] compared sons of alcoholic parents with HR− sons and found no differences in performance on an extensive neuropsychological test battery. There was suggestive, but not significant, evidence that the heavier-drinking HR+ subjects did more poorly than the lighter drinkers. These investigators also compared familial alcoholics having either one or two alcoholic parents with FH− alcoholics on the same test battery and found no group differences. A study conducted by Schaeffer *et al.*[84] constitutes both a familial history and high-risk study. This study compared middle-aged alcoholic men who were positive or negative for familial alcoholism and also nonalcoholic middle-aged men who were FH+ and FH−. Overall, a positive family history for alcoholism was associated with poorer neuropsychological functioning. However, the group differences were statistically significant for the nonalcoholic subjects, but not for the alcoholic subjects. These findings are difficult to explain on a genetic basis. The genetic loadings for the FH+ alcoholics and nonalcoholics are not equivalent, since the FH+ alcoholics have a high probability of carrying a genetically transmitted vulnerability, while the FH+ nonalcoholics are much less likely to be carrying that vulnerability. This is particularly the case, since they have passed the age of maximum risk for alcoholism. The most parsimonious explanation for the findings are in terms of antecedent environmental effects. Overall, therefore, the findings of studies of neuropsychological functioning of HR+ and FH+ populations for alcoholism are mixed. It is noteworthy that the studies with positive outcomes appear to be those that have indirectly controlled sociopathy in the comparison groups, by comparing either two groups of delinquents[79,80] or adopted subjects.[81]

3.3.3. Course, Prognosis, and Treatment Outcome of FH and ASP Alcoholics. As we have indicated, familial and antisocial alcoholism are highly interrelated. A number of studies have revealed that familial alcoholism has an earlier onset and tends to be more severe, but there is also evidence that alcoholism is earlier and more severe for sociopathic alcoholics; only one study has attempted to distinguish between the effects of the two conditions.[19]

3.3.3a. Familial Alcoholism Studies. Penick *et al.*[85] found an earlier onset of excessive drinking in FH+ alcoholics and greater likelihood of prior treatment. Although FH+ alcoholics did not have more medical complications associated with their alcohol abuse, they reported more alcohol-related social and personal problems. No major differences were found in the mood and personality status of the groups.

Ohayon[23] and Alterman *et al.*[49] also failed to find personality differences associated with familial alcoholism, although FH+ subjects in Ohayon's study reported a greater tendency to get sick after intoxication. Frances and his colleagues[34] reported more severe alcoholism symptomatology in FH+ alcoholics (hangovers, hallucinations, number of times receiving treatment), *more antisocial behavior*, poorer academic and social performance in school, less stable employment histories, and a background of large families with lower SES and more psychopathology. In a recent 2-year follow-up of this population, Frances *et al.*[86] discovered that FH+ alcoholics had poorer treatment outcomes, although it should be appreciated that the group differences obtained were quite small.

Fitzgerald and Mulford[87] also reported somewhat more severe alcoholism, as measured by a self-report inventory, but the authors emphasized that their results may have been the spurious product of an alcoholic labeling process that may be more evident in alcoholics with relatives in their family. FH+ alcoholics were also found to be somewhat more recidivistic. McKenna and Pickens[88] found FH+ alcoholics to be significantly younger when first intoxicated and first admitted to treatment. They had been drinking for fewer years, *had significantly more alcohol related arrests and days spent in jail, and more of them had been suspended from school.* On the other hand, the severity of drinking and treatment outcome did not differ as a function of familial alcoholism.

Volicer *et al.*[89] have reported more physical dependence, binge drinking and morning drinking, and an accelerated rate of development for alcoholism in FH+ alcoholics. Some of the negative effects appeared to be greater for alcoholics with mothers who were alcoholic. Finally, Stabenau[19] found more impairment of control over drinking, more psychosocial problems, and more pathologic problems (physical symptoms) in bilineal familial alcoholics than in either unilineal familial or nonfamilial alcoholics.

3.3.3b. Antisocial Alcoholics. A number of investigators have found an earlier onset of alcoholism in antisocial alcoholics.[16,27,90] Stabenau[19] failed to find more symptoms of impaired control, physical problems, or symptoms associated with chronic alcohol use in ASP alcoholics; but Rimmer *et al.*[91] reported that ASP alcoholics were more likely to experience blackouts, arrests and driving difficulty, but that they were not more likely to suffer from withdrawal symptoms or liver cirrhosis. Virkkunen[92] found that ASP alcoholics had fewer symptoms of alcohol dependence and medical complications than non-ASP alcoholics. Lewis *et al.*[17] also found that ASP alcoholics had fewer years of heavy drinking, but had a higher prevalence of loss of control over their drinking and of trying to limit intake. Goodwin *et al.*[29] reported more recidivism in sociopathic alcoholics.

The two most extensive studies of ASP alcoholics thus far conducted have been completed by Cadoret *et al.*[27] and Penick *et al.*[16] The first group of investigators compared ASP alcoholics with primary alcoholics and found that many of their childhood and adult behavioral differences were naturally reflective of the ASP diagnosis of the first group. ASP alcoholics were also more likely to be binge drinkers, to have suffered blackouts and other alcohol-related symptoms such as fighting, job problems, arrests for public intoxication, and more physical symptoms (vomiting, blurred vision). ASP alcoholics also had more problems with anxiety and depression, a greater likelihood of a drug problem, and more prior treatments for alcoholism. The latter two symptoms suggest a poorer prognosis and treatment outcome for ASP alcoholics.

Penick *et al.*[16] compared ASP alcoholics with subgroups of depressed, manic, and primary alcoholics. ASP alcoholics, in addition to having the earliest onset, had the worst psychosocial status (job, education, marital status), had more alcohol-related hospitalizations, arrests, alcohol abuse symptoms, medical complaints, and familial psychopathology. In a preliminary 1-year follow-up study, Penick *et al.* compared primary alcoholics and a combination of the three groups with additional psychiatric diagnoses. Although the primary alcoholics did not manifest relatively more improvement than the other alcoholics, they were doing better than the others because they were generally less impaired initially. Unfortunately, the treatment outcome findings for ASP alcoholics were not presented separately from those for the depressed or manic alcoholics. Since ASP alcoholics were the worst group in terms of almost all of the characteristics reviewed above, it is quite likely that they were functioning more poorly than the other alcoholics following treatment. We anticipate that studies will soon be completed which will answer this questions.

3.3.4. Summary. A number of studies have found metabolic/electrophysiological differences between HR+ and HR− groups, usually after controlled alcohol consumption. The significance of these findings is uncertain at this point in time. Neuropsychological studies of high-risk and familial alcoholism populations have provided some indication that the "at risk" alcoholic population exhibits cognitive deficits compared to individuals not at risk for alcoholism. However, there is some reason to suspect that the findings are confounded with "antisocial dispositions" of the subjects. Additionally, it is very difficult to attribute any differences obtained to genetic vulnerabilities, as contrasted with antecedent environmental influences.

There is considerable evidence that both FH+ and ASP alcoholics experience an earlier onset of alcoholism. Studies also reveal that the alcoholism is more severe and, by inference, the prognosis worse for both of these subgroups. However, the evidence for greater severity of alcoholism seems thus far to be stronger for ASP than for familial alcoholics. There is more evidence, by contrast, for poorer treatment outcome in FH+ than in ASP alcoholics, but this appears to be largely due to a dearth of research studies of treatment outcome in ASP alcoholics. More treatment outcome research is needed for both groups. Wood and Wender's research,[45,46] which reported some success in treating with stimulant medication alcoholics suffering from attentional deficit disorder, residual type, is a further illustration of the potential value of specialized treatment for specific alcoholic subgroups. Whether the positive effects of the medication were specific to the attention deficit characteristics of the patients, or to the antisocial characteristics also encompassed within that diagnosis, is not presently known.

Undoubtedly, there is considerable overlap between ASP and FH+ alcoholics. Only one clinical study has attempted to distinguish between the effects of these two categorizations.[19] Interestingly, ASP appeared to contribute more directly to early onset of alcohol abuse, while FH+ seemed to be associated more with loss of control over drinking and physical problems. It should be pointed out that the FH+ and ASP subjects in many of the studies conducted had been drinking for fewer years, and the effects of this variable were not controlled. The evidence for greater severity in FH+ and ASP alcoholics might therefore have been even more marked, if this variable had been controlled or taken into account. Finally, some of the findings of FH and HR studies might have been inconclusive or conflicting, because the definition of alcoholism in the subject's family has varied from study to study and has often been so loose as to include subjects with only second-degree alcoholic relatives, along with those with first-degree relatives, in the positive familial category. Fortunately, more recent research appears to be requiring the presence of at least one first-degree relative for inclusion in the positive familial category.

4. Conclusions

This chapter has reviewed and evaluated the evidence for at least three potential alcoholism typologies: hyperactive vs. nonhyperactive, antisocial vs. nonantisocial, and familial vs. nonfamilial alcoholism. High-risk studies have also been evaluated as a corollary to the familial alcoholism distinction. The following conclusions can be suggested with respect to the validity of these typologies:

1. *Hyperactivity,* although once believed to be a strong candidate for a genetically transmitted characteristic of alcoholism, appears now to be a correlate of elements or variants of conduct disorder in children and sociopathy in adults. These latter syndromes seem to be more intimately associated with the development of alcoholism.

2. As suggested, *childhood aggressive and antisocial behavior and adult sociopathy* appear to be characteristics of many alcoholics, and an alcoholism typology based on the distinction between sociopathic and nonsociopathic alcoholics appears to have merit. Such a typology can only be tentative, given the limited available evidence. Nevertheless, the existing information indicates that an ASP/non-ASP alcoholism typology satisfies a number of requirements needed to support a valid clinical typology. The diagnosis of antisocial alcoholism can be made fairly reliably and is more or less stable. There is evidence that the course and treatment outcome of such individuals differ and that the psychiatric family histories of their relatives is distinctive. Obviously, more research needs to be conducted on the functional characteristics and clinical course of this syndrome and its relation to other variables such as familial alcoholism.

3. *Familial alcoholism* also appears to have some merit as an alcoholism typology, although the results do not appear to be as compelling as for sociopathic alcoholism. Some questions remain and need to be resolved concerning inclusion criteria and the most effective procedural means of ensuring the reliability and validity of this classification. Some evidence is available that the clinical course and treatment outcome of familial alcoholics is poorer than that of nonfamilial alcoholics. More research is needed, however, in order to more fully evaluate the adequacy and clinical utility of this distinction. The extent to which familial alcoholism effects can be explained by the conjoint existence of sociopathy or other concurrent or antecedent variables most definitely needs to be investigated. For as Stabenau[19] has noted, "it is possible that . . . alcoholism in family history positive probands is principally related to undiagnosed or uncontrolled effects of antisocial personality."

4. The findings of the *high-risk studies* are interesting, but their significance is unclear. Just as for familial alcoholism, issues concerning the most appropriate inclusion criteria and the most effective procedural means for ensuring classificatory reliability and validity need to be resolved. Within the above context, high-risk investigations are conceivably of potential import for understanding the etiology of alcoholism and preventing, inhibiting, or minimizing its occurrence.

ACKNOWLEDGMENT. The authors wish to express their appreciation to the Veterans Administration for its support of this work.

References

1. Pattison EM: The selection of treatment modalities for the alcoholic patient, in Mendelson JH, Mello NK (eds): *The Diagnosis and Treatment of Alcoholism*. New York, McGraw-Hill, 1979, pp. 125–228.
2. Reich T, Cloninger C, Collins L, et al: Some recent findings in the study of genotype-environment interaction in alcoholism, in Meyer R, Glueck R, O'Brien J, et al (eds): *Evaluation of the Alcoholic: Implications for Research Theory and Treatment*. Rockville, Maryland, USDHSS, 1981, pp. 145–165.
3. Tarter R: Minimal brain dysfunction as an etiological predisposition to alcoholism, in Meyer R, Glueck R, O'Brien J, et al (eds): *Evaluation of the Alcoholic: Implications for Research Theory and Treatment*. Rockville, Maryland, 1981, USDHHS, pp. 167–191.
4. Kissin B, Platz A, Su WH: Social and psychological factors in the treatment of chronic alcoholism. *J Psychiatr Res*, 8:13–27, 1979.
5. Alterman AI, Tarter RE: The transmission of psychological vulnerability: Implications for alcoholism etiology. *J Nerv Ment Dis* 171:147–154, 1983.
6. Schuckit M: Biological markers: Metabolism and acute reactions to alcohol in sons of alcoholics. *Pharm Biochem Behav* 13:9–16, 1980.
7. Winokur G, Reich T, Rimmer J, et al: Alcoholism. III. Diagnosis and familial psychiatric illness in 259 alcoholic probands. *Arch Gen Psychiatry* 23:104–111, 1970.
8. Winokur G, Rimmer J, Reich T: Alcoholism. IV: Is there more than one type of alcoholism. *Br J Psychiatry* 118:525–531, 1971.
9. Goodwin DW, Schulsinger F, Hermansen L, et al: Alcohol problems in adoptees raised apart from alcoholic biological parents. *Arch Gen Psychiatry* 28:238–243, 1973.
10. Cadoret R, Gath A: Inheritance of alcoholism in adoptees raised apart from alcoholic biologic relatives. *Br J Psychiatry* 132:252–258, 1978.
11. Murray RM, Clifford CA, Gurling HMD: Twin and adoption studies: How good is the evidence for a genetic role? in Galanter M (ed): *Recent Developments in Alcoholism. Genetics, Behavioral Treatment, Social Mediators and Prevention, and Current Concepts in Diagnosis.* New York, Plenum, vol 1, 1983, pp. 25–47.
12. Cloninger R, Bohman M, Sigvardsson S: Inheritance of alcohol abuse: Cross-fostering analysis of adopted men. *Arch Gen Psychiatry* 38:861–867, 1981.
13. Tarter RE, Alterman AI: Neuropsychological deficits in alcoholics: Etiological considerations. *J Stud Alcohol* 45:1–9, 1984.
14. Hesselbrock VM, Stabenau JR, Hesselbrock MN: Minimal brain dysfunction and neuropsychological test performance in offspring of alcoholics, in Galanter M, Goodwin DW (eds): *Recent Developments in Alcoholism* New York, Grune & Stratton, vol 3, 1984.
15. Goodwin D, Schulsinger F, Moller W, et al: Drinking problems in adopted and non-adopted sons of alcoholics. *Arch Gen Psychiatry* 31:164–169, 1974.
16. Penick EC, Powell BJ, Othmer E, et al: Subtyping alcoholics by co-existing psychiatric syndromes: Course, family history, outcome, in Goodwin DW, Van Dusen RT, Mednick SA (eds): *Longitudinal Research in Alcoholism*. Kluwer-Nijhoff Publishing Co., Hingham, Mass., 1984, pp 167–196.
17. Lewis CE, Rice J, Helzer JE: Diagnostic interactions: Alcoholism and antisocial personality. *J Nerv Ment Dis* 171:105–113, 1983.
18. Vaillant GE: Natural history of male alcoholism. V: Is alcoholism the cart of the horse to sociopathy? *Br J Addict* 78:317–326, 1983.
19. Stabenau JR: Implications of family history of alcoholism, antisocial personality, and sex differences in alcohol dependence. *Am J Psychiatry* 141:1178–1182, 1984.
20. Fowler R, Liskow B, Tanna V, et al: Psychiatric illnesses and alcoholism. *Alcoholism* 1:125–128, 1977.
21. Feighner JP, Robins E, Guze SB, et al: Diagnostic criteria for use in psychiatric research. *Arch Gen Psychiatry* 26:57–63, 1972.

22. Spitzer R, Endicott J, Robins E: Research diagnostic criteria: rationale and reliability. *Arch Gen Psychiatry* 35:773–782, 1978.
23. Ohayon J: Familial and nonfamilial alcoholics. Master's thesis. University of Pittsburgh, 1981.
24. Stabenau J, Hesselbrock V: Assortative mating, family pedigree and alcoholism. *Subst Alcohol Actions Misuse* 1:375–382, 1980.
25. Weissman MM, Meyers JK, Harding PS: Prevelance and psychiatric heterogeneity of alcoholism in a United States urban community. *J Stud Alcohol* 41:672–681, 1980.
26. American Psychiatric Association, Diagnostic and Statistical Manual of Mental Disorders, ed 3. Washington, D.C., The Association, 1980.
27. Cadoret R, Troughton E, Widmer R: Clinical differences between antisocial and primary alcoholics. *Compr Psychiatry* 25:1–8, 1984.
28. Hewett B, Martin W: Psychometric comparisons of sociopathic and psychophysiological behavior and alcoholics and drug abusers versus a low drug control population. *Int J Addict* 15:77–105, 1980.
29. Goodwin DW, Crane JB, Guze SB: Felons who drink; and eight-year follow-up. *Q. J Stud Alcohol* 32:136–147, 1971.
30. Robins L: The diagnosis of alcoholism after DSM III, in Meyer R, Glueck R, O'Brien J, et al. (eds): *Evaluation of the Alcoholic: Implications for research, theory, and treatment.* USDHSS, Rockville, Maryland, 1981.
31. Rounsaville BJ, Cacciola JS, Weissman MM, et al: Diagnostic concordance in a follow-up study of opiate addicts. *J Psychiatr Res* 16:191–201, 1981.
32. Goodwin DW: Genetic and experimental antecedents of alcoholism: a prospective study. *Alcoholism* 1:259–265, 1977.
33. Goodwin D: Alcoholism and heredity: A review and hypothesis. *Arch Gen Psychiatry* 36:57–61, 1979.
34. Frances R, Timm S, Bucky S: Studies of familial and nonfamilial alcoholism. I. Demographic studies. *Arch Gen Psychiatry* 37:564–566, 1980.
35. Goodwin D, Schulsinger F, Hermansen L, et al: Alcoholism and the hyperactive child syndrome. *J Nerv Ment Dis* 160:349–353, 1975.
36. Cadoret R, Cain C, Grove W: Development of alcoholism in adoptees raised apart from alcoholic biologic relatives. *Arch Gen Psychiatry* 37:651–563, 1980.
37. Jones H, MacFarlane J, Eichorn D: A progress report on growth studies at the University of California. *Vita Humana* 3:17–31, 1960.
38. McCord W, McCord J, Gudeman J: *Origins of Alcoholism.* Stanford, California, Stanford University Press, 1960.
39. Robins L: *Deviant Children Grow Up: A Sociological and Psychiatric Study of Sociopathic Personality.* Baltimore, Williams and Wilkins, 1966.
40. Cantwell D: Psychiatric illness in the families of hyperactive children. *Arch Gen Psychiatry* 27:414–417, 1972.
41. Morrison J, Stewart M: A family study of the hyperactive child syndrome. *Biol Psychiatry* 3:189–195, 1971.
42. Blouin A, Bornstein R, Trites R: Teenage alcohol use among hyperactive children: A five year follow-up study. *J Pediatr Psychol* 3:188–194, 1978.
43. Mendelson W, Johnson N, Stewart M: Hyperactive children as teenagers: A follow-up study. *J Nerv Ment Dis* 153:273–279, 1971.
44. Wood DR, Reimherr FW, Wender PH, et al: Diagnosis and treatment of minimal brain dysfunction in adults. *Arch Gen Psychiatry* 33:1453–1460, 1976.
45. Wender PH, Reimherr FW, Wood DR: Attention deficit disorder (Minimal brain dysfunction) in adults. *Arch Gen Psychiatry* 38:449–456, 1981.
46. Wood D, Wender PH, Reimherr FW. The prevalence of attention deficit disorder, residual type, or minimal brain dysfunction, in a population of male alcoholic patients. *Am J Psychiatry* 140:95–98, 1983.
47. Tarter RE, McBride H, Buonpane N, et al: Differentiation of alcoholics: Childhood history

of minimal brain dysfunction, family history, and drinking pattern. *Arch Gen Psychiatry* 34:761–768, 1977.
48. DeObaldia R, Parsons O, Yohman R: Minimal brain dysfunction symptoms claimed by primary and secondary alcoholics: Relation to cognitive functioning. *Int J Neurosci* 20:173–182, 1983.
49. Alterman AI, Petrarudo E, Tarter RE, et al: Hyperactivity and alcoholism: Familial and behavioral correlates. *Addict Behav* 7:413–421, 1982.
50. Alterman AI, Tarter RE, Baughman TG, Bober BA, Fabian SA: Differentiation of alcoholics high and low in childhood hyperactivity. *Drug Alcohol Depend* 15:111–121, 1985.
51. August GJ, Stewart MA: Familial subtypes of childhood hyperactivity. *J Nerv Ment Dis* 171:362–368, 1983.
52. Guze SB: The validity and significance of the clinical diagnosis of hysteria (Briquet's syndrome). *Am J Psychiatry* 32:138–141, 1975.
53. Stewart MA, DeBois CS, Cummings S: Psychiatric disorder in the parents of hyperactive boys and those with conduct disorder. *J Child Psychol Psychiatry* 21:283–292, 1980.
54. Tarter RE, Hegedus AM, Gavaler JS: Hyperactivity in sons of alcoholics. *J Stud Alcohol* 46:259–261, 1985.
55. Gomez RL, Janowsky MD, Zetin M, et al: Adult psychiatric diagnosis and symptoms compatible with the hyperactive child syndrome: A retrospective study. *J Clin Psychiatry* 42:389–394, 1981.
56. Loney J: The Iowa theory of substance abuse among hyperactive adolescents, in Lettieri DJ, Sayers M, Pearson HW (eds): *Theories on Drug Abuse.* National Institute of Drug Abuse Research Monograph 30. Washington, D.C., U.S. Department of Health and Human Services, 1980, pp. 132–132–136.
57. Eyre SL, Rounsaville BJ, Kleber HB: History of childhood hyperactivity in a clinical population of opiate addicts. *J Nerv Ment Dis* 170:522–529, 1982.
58. Schuckit M, Reyses V: Ethanol ingestion: Differences in acetaldehyde concentrations in relatives of alcoholics and controls. *Science* 203:54–55, 1979.
59. Schuckit MA, Duby J: Alcohol-related flushing and the risk for alcoholism in sons of alcoholics. *J Clin Psychiatry* 43:415–418, 1982.
60. Schuckit MA, Parker DC, Rossman LR: Ethanol-related prolactin responses and risk for alcoholism. *Biol Psychiatry* 18:1153–1159, 1983.
61. Schuckit MA: Subjective responses to alcohol in sons of alcoholics and control subjects. *Arch Gen Psychiatry* 41:879, 1984.
62. Schuckit MA: Personal Communication.
63. Schuckit MA: A study of young men with alcoholic close relatives. *Am J Psychiatry* 13:791–794, 1982.
64. Begleiter H, Porjesz B, Kissin B: Event related brain potentials in children at risk for alcoholism. *Science* 225:1493–1496, 1984.
65. Elmasian R, Neville H, Woods D, et al: Event-related brain potentials are different in individuals at high and low risk for developing alcoholism. *Proc Natl Acad Sci USA* 79:7099–7903, 1982.
66. Gabrielli WF, Mednick SA, Volavka J, et al: Electroencephalograms in children of alcoholic fathers. *Psychophysiology* 19:404–407, 1982.
67. Propping P, Kruger J, Mark N: Genetic disposition to alcoholism: An EEG study in alcoholics and their relatives. *Hum Genet* 59:51–59, 1981.
68. Pollock VE, Volavka J, Goodwin DW, et al: The EEG after alcohol administration in men at risk for alcoholism. *Arch Gen Psychiatry* 40:857–861, 1983.
69. Lipscomb T, Carpenter J, Nathan P: Static ataxia: A predictor of alcoholism. *Br J Addict* 74:289–294, 1979.
70. Lipscomb TR, Nathan PE: Blood alcohol level discrimination: The effects of family history of alcoholism drinking pattern, and tolerance. *Arch Gen Psychiatry* 37:571–576, 1980.
71. Hegedus A, Tarter R, Hill SYU, et al: Static ataxia: A possible marker for alcoholism. *Alcoholism* 8:580–582, 1984.

72. Sher KJ, Levenson RW: Risk for alcoholism and individual differences in the stress-response-dampening effect of alcohol. *J Abnorm Psychol* 91:350–367, 1982.
73. MacAndrew C: On the possibility of the psychometric detection of persons who are prone to the abuse of alcohol and other substances. *Addict Behav* 4:11–20, 1979.
74. Saunders GR, Schuckit MA: MMPI scores in young men with alcoholic relatives and controls. *J Nerv Ment Dis* 169:456–457, 1981.
75. Parsons OA, Farr SP: The neuropsychology of alcohol and drug abuse, in: Filskov S, Boll T (eds): *Handbook of Clinical Neuropsychology*. New York, John Wiley and Sons, 1981.
76. Kaij L: Studies on the Etiology and Sequels of Abuse of Alcohol, Lund, Department of Psychiatry, University of Lund, 1960.
77. El Guebaly N, Offord DR: On being the offspring of an alcoholic: An update. *Alcoholism* 3:148–157, 1979.
78. Haberman PW: *Marriage Family* 28:152–154, 1966.
79. Tarter RE, Hegedus AM, Goldstein G, et al: Adolescent sons of alcoholics: Neuropsychological and personality characteristics. *Alcoholism* 8:216–222, 1984.
80. Hegedus AM, Alterman AI, Tarter RE: Learning achievement in sons of alcoholics. *Alcoholism* 8:330–333, 1984.
81. Gabrielli W, Mednick S: Intellectual performance in children of alcoholics. *J Nerv Ment Dis* 171:444–447, 1983.
82. Tarter RE, Alterman AI, Edwards KL: The vulnerability to alcoholism in men: A behavior-genetic perspective. *J Stud Alcohol* (in press).
83. Ervin CS, Little RE, Streissguth A, et al: Alcoholic fathering and its relation to child's intellectual development: A pilot investigation. *Alcoholism* 8:362–365, 1984.
84. Schaeffer KW, Parsons OA, Yohman JR: Neuropsychological differences between male familial and nonfamilial alcoholics and nonalcoholics. *Alcoholism* 8:347–351, 1984.
85. Penick E, Read R, Crowley P, et al: Differentiation of alcoholics by family history. *J Stud Alcohol* 39:1944–1948, 1978.
86. Frances RJ, Bucky ST, Alexopoulos GA: Outcome study of familial and nonfamilial alcoholism. *Am J Psychiatry* 141:1469–1471, 1984.
87. Fitzgerald J, Mulford H: Alcoholics in the family? *Int J Addict* 16:349–357, 1981.
88. McKenna T, Pickens R: Alcoholic children of alcoholics. *J Stud Alcohol* 42:1021–1029, 1981.
89. Volicer L, Volicer B, D'Angelo N: Relationship of family history of alcoholism to patterns of drinking and physical dependence in male alcoholics. *Drug Alcohol Depend* 13:215–223, 1984.
90. Hesselbrock M, Hesselbrock V, Babor T, et al: Antisocial behavior psychopathology and problem drinking in the natural history of alcoholism, in Goodwin D, Van Dusen K, Mednick S (eds): *Longitudinal Research in Alcoholism*. Boston, Nijhoff, 1984.
91. Rimmer J, Reich T, Winokur G: Alcoholism. V Diagnosis and clinical variation among alcoholics. *Q J Stud Alcohol* 33:658–666, 1972.
92. Virkkunen M: Alcoholism and antisocial personality. *Acta Psychiatr Scand* 59:493–501, 1979.

8

Alcoholic Typologies

A Review of Empirical Evaluations of Common Classification Schemes

Michie N. Hesselbrock

Abstract. This chapter reviews literature examining two typological classifications of alcoholism: typologies derived empirically by employing multivariate statistical techniques and typological classification schemes formulated from theoretical frameworks. Most of the empirical classifications were based on personality measures such as the MMPI, 16PF, and others. Examinations of theoretically based typologies included gender, psychopathology, and family history. The usefulness and limitations of these typological approaches are discussed.

1. Introduction

Efforts to subclassify alcoholics go all the way back to the turn of the century. When Bowman and Jellinek reviewed various classifications of alcoholics in 1942, they identified 24 main classifications by various writers.[1] While most classifications were descriptions of patterns of drinking (i.e., steady and intermittent drinkers), some studies described three or more etiological types (e.g., reactive and symptomatic types, psychopathic and neurotic alcoholics, and others). More recent attempts to examine alcoholism by subclassifying alcoholics into several homogeneous groups have been influenced by Jellinek's formulation of the "disease concept of alcoholism" and public interpretation of his concepts.[2] The thrust of Jellinek's formulation is that alcoholism is a progressive disease that follows an inexorable development through a distinct series of phases. Pattison and colleagues[3] have identified several basic concepts in Jellinek's formulation: (1) alcoholism can be identified and described despite its variations; (2) alcoholics may experience cravings for alcohol and/or a compulsion to drink; (3) "loss of control" over drinking will develop and may progress to an inability to stop drinking; (4) once permanent alcohol-induced biological changes occur, alcoholism becomes a permanent and irreversible condition. Jellinek warned that his theory was only

Michie N. Hesselbrock • Department of Psychiatry, University of Connecticut Health Center, Farmington, Connecticut 06032.

a working hypothesis and not based on empirical evidence. However, the alcohol studies field has adopted his ideas as virtual gospel, and, over the years, even dissenting voices have generaly acknowledged the wide appeal of Jellinek's formulation. "The work of this extraordinary individual has framed most aspects of the current debate on the nature of alcoholism and its treatment."[4] Despite the popular interpretation of his hypothesis depicting alcoholism as a unitary entity, Jellinek considered alcoholism a generic, rather than a specific, term. He was aware of the variability among alcoholics with regard to the etiological elements, alcoholic process, and types of damage resulting from drinking, and attempted to present a schematic form incorporating all of these aspects.[5] Jellinek classified alcoholics into five types: alpha, beta, gamma, delta, and epsilon. Alpha alcoholics are characterized by a psychological dependence on alcohol. The main addictive feature of this group is deliberate undisciplined drinking rather than an actual loss of control over drinking behavior. Very slight progression of the disorder is observed, with no major psychological or social behavior changes occurring. Beta alcoholics may exhibit a number of medical problems without physical or psychological dependence. This type of alcoholic can be found in certain social groups whose customs include heavy drinking. Gamma alcoholics show marked progression of the disorder in terms of changes in social and psychological behavior. Changes may be due to the addictive process and the emergence of chronic alcoholic disease. In this phase of alcoholism psychological dependence progresses to physical dependence. "Loss of control" may be witnessed, but gamma alcoholics still retain the ability to abstain from alcohol without withdrawal symptoms. Delta alcoholics show the same characteristics as gamma alcoholics except for their physical inability to abstain from alcohol. Delta alcoholics can control the amount of their intake, but rapid onset of withdrawal symptoms after cessation of drinking prevents them from abstaining. The disease concept of alcoholism applies only to gamma and delta alcoholics, as they represent addiction in the strict pharmacological sense. Alpha and beta alcoholics, on the other hand, are neither physically addicted nor are they considered to have disease symptomatology. Thus, the criteria for alpha and beta alcoholics are similar to the DSM-III criteria[6] of alcohol abuse, while the descriptions of gamma and delta alcoholics conform to the DSM-III criteria of alcohol dependence.

Since Jellinek first formulated his classification of alcoholics, his hypothesis regarding the progressive nature of alcoholism has come under increasing criticism for its failure to account for the individual variability of those alcoholics who do not follow the prescribed sequence of stages. The most frequently voiced criticism holds that Jellinek's approach to alcoholism does not adequately deal with the diversity and multidimensional nature of alcoholism.

A growing number of clinical and research efforts have attempted to provide more accurate descriptions of the varied and complex factors involved in alcoholism. Many studies have employed multivariate statistical approaches (e.g. cluster analysis and factor analysis) to identify homogeneous groupings of alcoholics based on various observations and measures. Other studies have utilized classification systems often based on dichotomous theories. In this chapter, both empirical and theory-oriented approaches to the classification of alcoholics will be reviewed.

2. Empirical Approaches to Classification

A frequent empirical approach to the categorization of alcoholics has employed the application of factor analysis to a large data base. Findings from this approach indicate that alcoholics differ on a variety of dimensions and each dimension may vary in degree of severity.[7,8] In a strict sense, the factor analytic, multidimensional approaches are not always typological studies. Rather, these approaches are a means of identifiying individual similarities and differences among alcoholics in terms of their unique profiles on the various dimensions.[9] Clustering techniques have also been used to subclassify alcoholics into types. Most efforts to categorize alcoholics, whether by factor analysis or cluster analysis, have been made according to personality type.[10,11]

2.1. Classification Based on Personality Inventories

Typically alcoholics are classified into personality subtypes based on their responses to the Minnesota Multiphasic Personality Inventory (MMPI).[12,13–23] Several comprehensive review articles have summarized the major findings of personality subtypes of alcoholics.[24–26] Morey and Blashfield[24] discuss Goldstein and Linden's findings, which have been replicated by other studies. Goldstein and Linden[14] derived three major clusters of alcoholic subtypes: psychopathic personality with emotional instability characterized by an elevated MMPI Pd scale, depressive-anxiety neurosis with elevated Sc, D/and Pt scales, and secondary psychopathic personality style with a 4-2-9 profile (elevated Pd, D, and Ma scales). Based on these clusters, Goldstein and Linden then divided alcoholics into neurotic and personality disorder categories. Subsequent studies reviewed by Morey and Blashfield seem to establish Goldstein and Linden's classification with only a few exceptions.[24] Morey and Blashfield[24] also described a similar typological classification in Whitelock *et al.*,[16] whose four types were comprised of three clusters characterized by anxiety neurosis and one by personality disorder.

Nerviano and Gross[26] describe several MMPI prototypes in their review: (1) chronic and severe distress characterized by a high degree of general psychosocial incapacity; (2) passive-aggressive and sociopathic with an elevated Pd scale characterized by irritability, frustration, and dependence; (3) sociopathic with elevated 4 and 9 scales characterized by antisocial personality and emotionally unstable personality; (4) reactive acute depression reflected by dysphoric characteristics and an elevation on the D scale; (5)severely neurotic-psychophysiological prototype preoccupied with a psychophysiological reaction; (6) mixed character-dysphoria that includes a mixture of depressive neurosis, passive-aggressive personality, and anxiety reaction, and (7) paranoid-alienated type with a tendency toward poor social histories and the greatest severity of consequences from excessive drinking.

Nerviano and Gross[26] also reviewed studies utilizing the 16PF questionnaire.[27] They found a comparison of these studies more difficult than those using the MMPI because of variations in test forms, sample size and subject composition.[28–32] Nerviano and Gross nonetheless were able to derive some common subtypes that can be characterized as follows:

1. Conforming (compulsive-high impulse control and high social poise).
2. Impulsive (histrionic-low impulse control and moderate social poise).
3. Aggressive (impulsive and defensive).
4. Submissive (low defendency and dependent).
5. Avoidant (schizoid-low social poise & high autonomy).
6. Asocial (schizoid-independent but inhibited).
7. Narcissistic (low emotional attachment and low self blame).
8. Hostile (withdrawn-low social poise and high defensiveness)(26).

In sharp contrast to the MMPI subtypes who are sociopathic or estranged individuals, these subtypes show that excessive drinking seems to "occur in the context of obsessive perfectionalism, characterological dependency or odd self-perception."[26] Reviews of subclassification based on personality measure, therefore, can probably be divided into two major domains: psychopathological and nonpathological personality types. The extent to which these domains interact needs further investigation.

Despite the progress made in systematic approaches to subtyping alcoholics using personality inventory profiles, efforts to subclassify alcoholics according to personality sub-types have several limitations. First, most studies have used older males in Veteran Administration Hospitals, thereby excluding younger alcoholics and women.[25] With the development of new treatment programs to attract greater numbers of youths and women, studies based on VA patients may no longer be as generalizable to the broader population of alcoholics. A second limiting factor is that of sample size. While most studies had an adequate sample size (up to 1500), some studies included samples of less than 100 alcoholics. The most important limiting factor, however, was discussed by Skinner[25] in his review of the literature on clustering studies in alcoholism. His concern was based on the degree to which these derived subtypes are unique to individuals who abuse alcohol. Reviewing some of his own work, Skinner *et al.*,[15] found that, "aside from maladaptive drinking behavior, alcoholic patients may be little different from the clinical syndrome of other types of psychiatric patients." They were able to generalize personality subtypes found in alcoholics to prison inmates, psychiatric patients and college students.[33] Lack of a standard or normal profile to which alcoholic profiles can be compared may contribute to the failure to find a typical profile for alcoholism.[34] Another limitation of typological studies based on personality variables is the instability of personality measures over time. The MMPI D Scale has been criticized for being state dependent and very sensitive to the respondent's mood at the time of assessment. In addition, it should be noted that elevated scales do not necessarily mean the presence of a psychiatric diagnosis. For example, Hesselbrock *et al.*[35] compared a diagnosis of major depression (DSM-III), DSM-III criteria for depressive symptoms, and the MMPI D-scale in a sample of alcoholics. They found both very low diagnostic concordance and low correlation between the DSM-III symptoms and the MMPI D scale. One contributing factor to this discordance was the MMPI's focus on individual symptoms over time as contrasted with the DSM-III requirement of a clustering of symptoms persisting for at least one week. Changes in the MMPI configuration at the time of hospital admission and discharge have been examined by Conley,[36] who classified 337 male alcoholics treated at the Hazelden Foundation into four groups (neurotic, classic, psychotic, and psychopathic alcholics) based on the admission MMPI. The "neurotic" profile showed a general decline in elevation at discharge but maintained the basic admission configuration. The "classic" alcoholic also showed a forshortening with some alteration of shape from admission to discharge. The D scale, which had the highest elevation at admission, declined sharply. The "psychotic" profile maintained its basic shape with greatly reduced elevation across scales, while "psychopathic" alcoholics remained the same in terms of elevation and configuration from admission to discharge. Considering the sharp decline on some MMPI scale scores during hospitalization, one needs to be cautious about drawing conclusions based on the admission MMPI Profile.

Despite the methodological limitations discussed thus far, examination of alcoholic typologies based on personality assessment remains popular. At the same time, others have attempted to focus their efforts on integrating subtypes derived from personality assessment with different aspects of alcoholism, i.e., treatment outcome.[21,37] However, such studies are relatively few in number.

2.2. Classification of Alcoholics According to Alcohol Use Patterns and Related Variables

Studies attempting to classify alcoholics according to alcohol use patterns and related variables are based on the assumption that alcoholism has several dimensions along which individual alcoholics can be identified. Using factor analysis, Horn and Wanburg[7] derived several factors from a questionnaire completed on 2300 subjects admitted to a state mental health center for alcoholism treatment. The factors included drinking patterns (styles and types), perceived social and psychological benefits of drinking, antisocial problems, family adjustment, willingness to accept treatment, and gender. Using a second-order factor analysis of the same data, Wanburg and Knap[8] derived four broad dimensions: general severity, tension relief, self-enhancement, and periodic drinking patterns. Their findings indicate that these dimensions are statistically independent rather than being related on a continuum or to subjects' chronological age.

Horn, Wanberg and associates developed the Alcohol Use Inventory (AUI), a comprehensive assessment of alcoholics.[38] An empirical evaluation of the AUI was reported by Skinner and Allen.[39] The AUI contains several dimensions, including style of alcohol use, negative consequences of alcohol use, and perceived benefits of alcohol use. Skinner and Allen found the validity and reliability of the AUI to be respectable. Factor analysis of the 16-item AUI identified four factors,[40] with the first factor describing the alcohol dependence syndrome as postulated by Edward and Gross.[41] Edward and Gross described the clinical syndrome of alcohol dependence, which included several elements: a narrowing of the drinking repertoire, salience of drink-seeking behavior, increased tolerance to alcohol, repeated withdrawal symptoms and attempts to avoid withdrawal by further drinking, compulsion to drink, and reinstatement of the syndrome after abstinence.[41] Additional factors included perceived benefits of drinking, polydrug abuse, and marital discord. Higher levels of alcohol dependence were associated with social consequences and higher levels of alcohol consumption. In addition, the degree of alcohol dependence was also related to psychopathology and physical symptoms.[42] While Skinner and associates indentified severity of alcohol dependence as one dimension, other investigators have found the alcohol dependence factor to be more complex. Chick[43] found two dimensions within the alcohol dependence factor. The main dimension included subjective need, withdrawal, and salience of drinking behavior, while narrowing of the drinking repertoire and impaired control over drinking behavior formed a separate dimension. Hesselbrock *et al.*[44] have also produced an "alcohol dependence syndrome" factor using a questionnaire based primarily on the NCA criteria.[45] It is not clear, however, how these dimensions are related to each other or to other formulations of alcohol dependence. The alcohol dependence syndrome described by Edward and Gross is a general term describing alcoholism with different characteristics. It does not necessarily differentiate sub-types of alcoholism.

2.3. Subclassification Based on Treatment Needs

While typologies focusing on alcohol dependence can describe alcoholics with regard to behavior patterns and related experiences, few studies have attempted to examine typologies based on treatment needs. Hart and Stueland examined 563 alcoholics on the basis of rehabilitation needs.[46] They used the Human Service Scale (HSS),[47] an 80-item instrument designed to assess rehabilitation needs in terms of physiological status, emotional severity, economic, family and social status, self-esteem, and vocational needs. A cluster analysis was utilized and five homogeneous subgroups were identified. The subgroups ranged from those subjects experiencing no severe disabling effects due to heavy drinking to groups of severely affected individuals on all the above-mentioned dimensions of rehabilitation needs. Sociodemographic variables, including age, living arrangements, number of dependents, drinking variables, and subjects' own perceptions of drinking type, were most strongly related to the different subgroups.[46] Similarly Gibbs developed 50 prognostic indicators, personal characteristics of alcoholics, which were shown empirically to be related to various treatment outcomes. He derived two clusters and classified alcoholics into mutually exclusive types on the basis of social stability and intellectual functioning.[48]

The empirical typologies discussed thus far have been derived from only one domain of data, i.e., psychopathology based on the MMPI or drinking behavior). Thus, it is difficult to compare various classifications since no common mechanism exists to examine various typologies across samples and domains of data. It is essential, however, to derive typologies using a variety of data, i.e., alcohol use patterns, psychopathology, and family history, in order to develop prognostically and therapeutically meaningful assessment programs.[9] Kivlahan *et al.*[49] attempted to derive subtypes from several assessment areas, including age, social position, average hours worked per week, years of problem drinking, alcohol dependence scales, neuropsychological functioning, WAIS subtests (vocabulary and arithmetic scales), and psychopathology. Their findings indicate that complicated relationships exist among demography, drinking behavior, level of neuropsychological functioning, and psychopathology. The six clusters of derived patients had different responses to aftercare participation and outcome 9 months after discharge from the hospital.

Kivlahan *et al.*'s study demonstrates that many empirically derived typologies have limited application to treatment programs because they are based on only one aspect of the person. Failure to consider other types of data probably makes any subsequent description of the population of alcoholics incomplete. Studies examining subtypes across domains should be encouraged. Empirical multi-dimensional approaches that classify alcoholics may, however, lack a clear description of severity or chronicity of the disorder. Severity, when considered, is often measured by scales developed using the factor analytic method. However, the relationship between these scales measuring dependence and the chronicity of alcoholism is unknown. A recent study evaluating the DSM-III criteria for alcohol abuse/dependence and an empirically derived alcohol dependence scale found a positive but low correlation between the sum of alcohol dependence symptoms that alcoholic patients experienced during the six months prior to admission and DSM-III lifetime symptoms of alcohol abuse.[44]

3. Theoretical Classification Approaches

The lack of clinical applicability of empirically derived typologies has forced alcohol researchers to reconsider the utility of theoretically based classification schemes of alcoholism. Several such classification approaches have been attempted, including gender, psychopathology, and family history. Each will be reviewed here separately.

3.1. Gender Differences

Studies of alcoholism have only recently included female alcoholics in their samples, despite efforts to identify characteristics of alcoholic women as long as 25 years ago.[50] This lack of interest was due in part to the difficulty of identifying women alcoholics and in recruiting adequate sized samples of females.[51] However, with an increase in the number of women seeking treatment for alcoholism, the need for knowledge about women alcoholics has become crucial.

Reasearch findings on male and female alcoholics show that gender differences ranging from childhood antecedent behaviors to the adult alcoholic careers exist. Several studies have found that more female alcoholics report parental drinking problems (especially fathers).[50,52,53] As children, male alcoholics tend to be more antisocial and encounter more school problems than female alcoholics.[54,55] Generally, the prevalence of conduct-related psychopathology is higher among men than women alcoholics, while the rates of affective disorder, phobia, and panic disorders are higher among women than men.[56;-58] Hesselbrock *et al*, investigated DSM-III[59] psychopathologies in a sample of 321 hospitalized alcoholics that included 231 men and 90 women. Antisocial personality (ASP) was by far the most prevalent psychopathology among men (49%), while only 20% of the women were diagnosed as having antisocial personality disorder. The rate of substance abuse was also higher among men than women (44% and 39%, respectively). However, major depressive disorder among women was twice as prevalent for women (55%) as for men (32%). A higher prevalence of phobia and panic disorder was also found in women alcoholics. It should be noted that when behavior disorders (e.g., ASP or substance abuse) were considered, the proportion of men and women alcoholics who were free of other types of psychopathologies was similar (26% and 21%, respectively). The relationship of the age of onset of alcohol abuse to other psychopathologies also distinguished men and women alcoholics. The onset of most additional psychopathologies (i.e., depression, substance abuse, obsessive-compulsive disorder, phobia, and panic disorder) preceded the abuse of alcohol among women while alcohol abuse preceeded substance abuse, depression, and obsessive compulsive disorder among alcoholic men. The results support previous findings describing women as drinking for reasons of relief, i.e., to relieve stress, or to self-medicate dysphoric mood.[60–62]

The natural history of alcoholism also seems to differ between men and women. Women usually begin drinking at a later age than men.[51,52,63–65] However, the progression from the first drink to regular drinking, regular intoxication, realization of problem drinking, and entering treatment is more rapid for women than for men.[51] The natural history of alcoholism among women may be greatly influenced by differential cultural influences on men and women in our society. American culture is generally more permissive toward men drinking heavily and becoming intoxicated, while women are often stigmatized for such behavior. Cultural factors may also influence women entering treatment at a much earlier age than men. Women generally seek help for illness, whether physical or psychiatric, more frequently than men. This may help explain why women alcoholics enter treatment much sooner than men. Thus, subtypes of alcoholism based on gender do distinguish alcoholics in terms of the natural history of the disorder and in terms of their clinical picture (i.e. associated psychopathology) on admission. Whether the male–female distinction is an important prognostic factor for treatment outcome is not clear.

3.2. Psychopathology

The presence of additional psychiatric disorders among persons with alcoholism has been well documented.[66–68] In this section, the classification of alcoholics based on the DSM-III criteria of antisocial personality and major depression will be reviewed.

ASP is often associated with alcoholism, especially among young males. Criteria for the diagnosis of ASP according to the DSM-III includes conduct problems before age 15 and the continuation of antisocial behavior into adulthood. Thus, the age of onset of ASP generally precedes that of alcoholism. Even though ASP is often described as an etiological factor for alcoholism, it is difficult to establish a causal relationship between the two disorders since antisocial behaviors are often the consequence of heavy drinking. Distinguishing between the two disorders is sometimes difficult. Nevertheless, the prevalence of ASP among alcoholics remains high.[69–71] Alcoholics with the additional diagnosis of ASP tend to begin abusing alcohol at an earlier age,[60] consume more alcohol,[72] and abuse other drugs.[73] Hesselbrock *et al.*[73] examined hospitalized alcoholics by subclassifying them into two groups: those alcoholics with the diagnosis of ASP and those without. ASP and non-ASP alcoholics varied greatly along a number of dimensions. Demographic differences were noted in terms of age, education and occupational achievement. The ASP alcoholics were much younger at admission, less educated, and had fewer occupational skills. The drinking style of the relatives of ASP and non-ASP alcoholics were also different. The frequency of alcoholism was generally higher among both first- and second -degree relatives of probands with ASP compared to the relatives of probands without ASP. The frequency of alcoholism among the fathers of ASP probands was particularly high. While similar rates of alcoholism were found for both the first- and second-degree relatives of ASP probands, the rate of alcoholism among first-degree relatives of the non-ASP probands was twice as high as that for the second-degree relatives.

ASP alcoholics could also be distinguished in terms of the natural history of alcoholism. ASP alcoholics reported significantly more childhood conduct problems and hyperactivity prior to age 12 than non-ASP alcoholics. Alcoholics with ASP reported having their first drink at a much younger age than non-ASP alcoholics. Once they began drinking to regular intoxication, they progressed to alcoholism much faster than non-ASP alcoholics. Further, ASP alcoholics were much younger than their non-ASP counterparts, but had a drinking problem as long as the older subjects without ASP. Although a high prevalence of alcoholism is found among the first- and second-degree relatives of ASP probands and early childhood behavior problems are associated with an early onset of abusive drinking, the nature of the etiological relationship is not clear. In adolescents, heavy drinking may interact with the antisocial life style and accelerate the progression to chronic alcohol abuse.

Major depressive disorder is another important psychopathology often associated with alcoholism. Several studies have found a high prevalence of major depression among alcoholics.[67,68] However, it can be difficult to distinguish major depression from the effects of chronic alcohol abuse. Dysphoric mood is often associated with heavy alcohol consumption, while acute intoxication and withdrawal from alcohol can also produce dysphoric mood among heavy drinkers. Depressed alcoholics tend to have more binges and are more likely to make suicide attempts than alcoholics without depression, particularly as they get older.[72]

Recently, the effect of major depression on the course and consequences of alcoholism was investigated among hospitalized alcoholics.[59,74] Major depression, whether primary or secondary to alcohol abuse/dependence, did not significantly affect the course of alcoholism. However, alcoholics with the additional diagnosis of major depression reported higher levels of affective disturbances and experienced more psychological problems than alcoholics without major depression.[59] In addition, alcoholics with a history of major depression could be distinguished on the basis of motivational factors for drinking. Alcoholic men with a diagnosis of major depression reported drinking alcohol to relax, to forget problems, to cheer up, to relieve tension, and to facilitate social interaction. Alcoholic women with depression also reported drinking to forget their worries, but the women in general tended to drink for the same reasons as the men.[74] However, alcoholics may have experienced some difficulty in remembering their exact affective state while intoxicated and used the "escape hypothesis" as an excuse for heavy drinking. It is not clear whether alcohol does relieve dysphoria.[75]

Although depression is a frequent concurring condition with alcoholism, the usefulness of subtyping alcoholism by major depression seems to be limited. There is little evidence to suggest depression's importance as an etiological factor and a recent study by O'Sullivan *et al.*[76] has cast doubt on the importance of alleviating depression for improving abstinence after alcoholism treatment. O'Sullivan *et al.* found that alcoholics with affective disorder were more frequently treated for both their alcoholism and their mood disorder, but could not be distinguished from nondepressed alcoholics on the basis of alcoholic symptoms, previous drinking history, or periods of abstinence after treatment.

3.3. Family History

Alcoholism runs in families and is considered to be a familial disorder. Whether the nature of the familial association is genetic, environmental or a combination of both remains an empirical question. Goodwin[65] has suggested subclassifying alcoholics into familial versus nonfamilial groupings. According to this classification familial alcoholics should have a positive family history of alcoholism, an early onset of alcoholism, and severe symptoms requiring early treatment intervention. Francis *et al.*[77] and Schuckit[78] have shown that familial alcoholics had more antisocial behavior, poor academic performance, and severe alcoholism symptoms. Penick *et al.*[79] found that alcoholics with alcohol abusing parents or grandparents began drinking at an early age, and had severe social and personal problems. While the association between familial alcoholism and the course and consequences of alcoholism seems to have solidified in recent years, the effect of additional contributory factors (e.g., the diagnosis of ASP) has seldom been considered. A recent study suggested that the presence of ASP in alcoholics might exert a stronger influence on the course of alcoholism than the type of family history for alcoholism. Hesselbrock *et al.*[80] found that the course of alchoholism in male alcoholoic probands with different types of family history for alcoholism was similar after the effects of ASP were removed. However, alcoholics with a positive family history of alcoholism reported experiencing higher levels of impaired control over drinking and physical and psychosocial problems than probands with a negative family history. While the presence of ASP in alcoholics might have contributed to the consequences of alcoholism, the effects due to ASP are separate and additive to the effects attributable to a positive family history for alcoholism.[80]

The usefulness of a subtype of alcoholism based on family history is equivocal at this point but does show some promise. Several studies have indicated that there are important etiological differences between family history positive and family history negative alcoholics. If these differences are substantiated by other studies, the findings would have important implications for primary prevention and early intervention programs. Although it is clear that having a family history of alcoholism is a risk factor for the development of alcoholism, it is possible that other variables exert a more powerful effect on the course and consequences of alcoholism once the individual becomes affected. There is some evidence to indicate that ASP is one such potentially potent contribution variable.[80]

3.4. Interrelationship among Different Subclassifications

The overlap among different subclassification schemes, including gender, antisocial personality, depression, and parental alcoholism, is summarized in Fig. 1. This data came from a study of 321 hospitalized alcoholic men and women in greater Hartford-area alcoholism treatment centers. A detailed de-

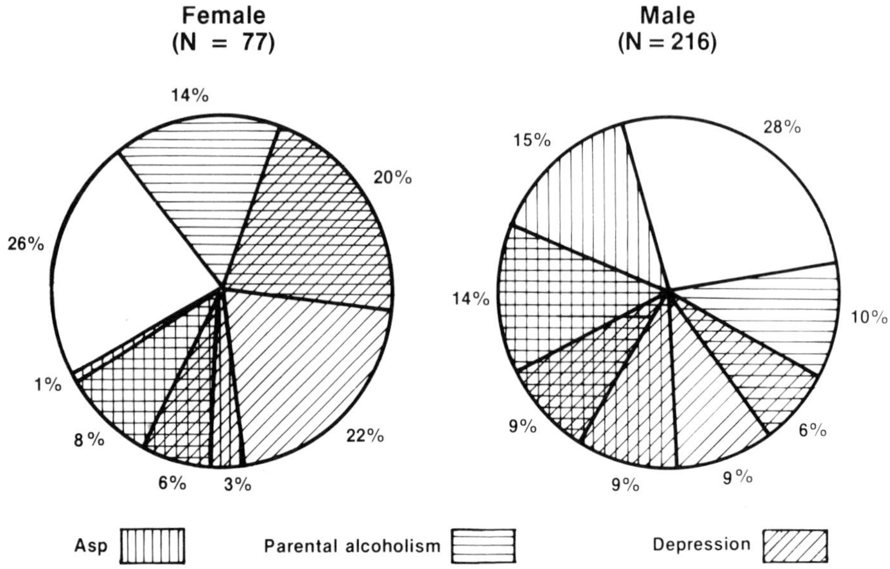

Figure 1. Interrelationship among different subclassifications.

scription of the sample is presented elsewhere.[59] Striking differences are seen in terms of the prevalence of depression and ASP between male and female alcoholics. In general, a higher proportion of women than men have an additional diagnosis of psychopathology and parental alcoholism. Persons with the diagnosis of ASP, regardless of sex, tend to be less problem free. Depression is more common among women than men, but the rates of major depression are similar for ASP and non-ASP alcoholics. While parental alcoholism is more common among ASP than the non-ASP alcoholics, the amount of overlap between depression and parental alcoholism is similar for ASP and non-ASP alcoholics. This figure does not provide data concerning possible etiological factors of alcoholism or associated variables, but it does indicate the complexity of different classification schemes. Although different classifications are discussed and compared as if they are independent, this is not the case. There is considerable overlap among the classification schemes considered in this report, suggesting the need for future investigation to clarify the extent of overlap and the theoretical efficacy of each type.

4. Conclusion

This chapter has reviewed two (empirical and theoretical) typological approaches to alcoholism and a variety of classification schemes based on personality, treatment needs, gender, psychopathology, family history, and other characteristics. An examination of the different subclassifications indicates that complicated interrelationships and overlap between the various subtypes exist. An important point to consider, but not discussed by the investigators reviewed, is the purpose for which any classification scheme of alcoholics will be used. As indicated by this review, it seems that different classification systems of alcoholism have different uses and that no single typology is able to efficiently explain etiology, is useful for the treatment planning purposes, and is a powerful predictor of treatment outcome. This may be due to the fact that only limited domains of data have been used in the construction of the typologies reviewed here. If a broader range of data are considered, a more comprehensive typology may be derived. It is also possible, however, that due to the multidimensional nature of the disorder, a single typology will not suffice to serve the many and varied purposes of those interested in the prevention, epidemiology, nosology, and treatment of alcoholism.

References

1. Bowman KM, Jellinek EM: Alcohol addiction and its treatment.*QJ Stud Alcohol* 2(1):98–176, 1941.
2. Jellinek EM: *The Disease Concept of Alcoholism*. New Haven, Hillhouse Press, 1960.
3. Pattison EM, Sobell MB, Sobel LC: *Emerging Concepts of Alcohol Dependence*. New York, Springer Publishing Company, 1977.
4. Lender ME: Jellinek's typology of alcoholism—some historical antecedents. *J Stud Alcohol* 40(5): 361–375, 1979.
5. Jellinek EM: Alcoholism: a genus and some of its species. *The Can Med Assoc J* 83(26): 1341–1345, 1960.
6. American Psychiatric Association Diagnostic and Statistical Manual of Mental Disorders (DSM-III), Washington, D.C., American Psychiatric Association Press, 1980.
7. Horn JL, Wanberg KW: Symptom patterns related to excessive use of alcohol. *Q J Stud Alcohol* 30:35–58, 1969.
8. Wanberg KW, Knap J: A multidimensional model for research and treatment of alcoholism. *Int J Addict* 5:69–98, 1970.
9. Meyer RE, Babor TF, Mirkin PM: Typologies in alcoholism, an overview. *Int J Addict* 18:235–249, 1983.
10. Replogle WH, Hair JF: A multivariate approach to profiling alcoholics typologies. *Multivariate Exp Clin Res* 3:157–164, 1977.
11. Nerviano V: Common personality patterns among alcoholic males, a multivariate study. *J Consult Clin Psychol* 44:104–110, 1976.
12. Dahlstrom WG, Welsh GS, Dahlstrom LE:*An MMPI Handbook*. Minneapolis, University of Minnesota Press, 1972.
13. Burton AD: A study of alcoholics with the Minnesota Multiphasic Personality Inventory. *Q J Stud Alcohol* 17:263–281, 1956.
14. Goldstein SG, Linden JD: Multivariate classification of alcoholics by means of the MMPI. *J Abnorm Psychol* 74:661–669, 1969.
15. Skinner HA, Jackson DN, Hoffman H. Alcoholic personality types: Identification and correlates. *J Abnorm Psychol* 83:658–666, 1974.
16. Whitelock PR, Overall J. Patrick JA: Personality patterns and alcohol abuse in a state hospital population. *J Abnorm Psychol* 78:9–16, 1971.
17. Bean KL, Karasievich GO: Psychological test results at three stages of inpatient alcoholism treatment. *J Stud Alcohol* 36:838–852, 1975.

18. Donovan DM, Chaney EF, O'Leary MR: Alcohol MMPI subtypes: Relationship to drinking styles, benefits and consequences. *J Nerv Ment. Dis* 166:553–561, 1978.
19. Esbaugh DM, Tosi DJ, Hoyt C: Some personality patterns and dimensions of male alcoholics, a multivariate description. *J Pers Assess* 42:409–417, 1978.
20. Sutker PB, Brantley PJ, Allain AM: MMPI response pattern and alcohol consumption in DWI offenders. *J Consult Clin Psychol* 48:350–355, 1980.
21. O'Leary MR, Donovan DM, Chaney EF, et al: Relationship of alcoholic personality subtypes to treatment follow-up measurement. *J Nerv Ment Dis* 168:475–480, 1980.
22. Nerviano VJ, McCarty D, McCarty SM: MMPI profile patterns of men alcoholics in two contrasting settings. *J Stud Alcohol* 41:911–921, 1980.
23. Loberg T: MMPI based personality subtypes of alcoholics. J N Stud Alcohol 42:766–782, 1981.
24. Morey LC, Blashfield RK: Empirical classifications of alcoholic. *J Stud Alcohol* 42:925–937.
25. Skinner HA: Statistical approaches to the classification of alcohol and drug addiction. *Br J Addict* 77:259–273, 1982.
26. Nerviano VJ, Gross HW: Personality types of alcoholics on objective inventories. *J Stud Alcohol* 44:837–851, 1983.
27. Cattell RB, Ebner WH, Tatsuoka MM: *Handbook for the Sixteen Personality Questionnaires (16PF).* Champaign, Illinois, Institute for Personality and Ability Testing, 1970.
28. Lawlis GF, Rubin SE: 16 PF Study of personality patterns in alcoholics. *Q J Stud Alcohol* 30:21–34, 1971.
29. Nerviano VJ, Gross WF: A multivariate delineation of two alcoholic profile types on the 16 PF. *J Clin Psychol* 29:371–374, 1973.
30. Nerviano VJ: Common personality patterns among alcoholic males: A multivariate study. *J Consult Clin Psychol* 44:104–110, 1976.
31. Costello RM, Lawlis GF, Manders KR, et al: Empirical derivation of partial personality typology of alcoholics. *J Stud Alcohol* 39:1258–1266, 1978.
32. Hart LS, Stueland D: Clasifying women alcoholics by Cattell's 16 PF: A preliminary investigation of an alcoholic typology. *J Stud Alcohol* 41:911–921, 1980.
33. Skinner HA, Reed PL, Jackson DN: Toward the objective diagnosis of psychopathology: Generalizability of model personality profiles. *J Consult Clin Psychol* 44:111–117, 1976.
34. Miller WR: Alcoholism scales and objective assessment methods: A review psychological bulletin. 83:649–674, 1976.
35. Hesselbrock MN, Hesselbrock VM, Tennen H, et al: Methodological considerations in the assessment of depression of alcoholics. *J Consult Clin Psychol* 51:399–405, 1983.
36. Conley JJ: An MMPI typology of male alcoholics: Admission, discharge and outcome comparison. *J Pers Assess* 45:33–39, 1981.
37. Zivich JM: Alcoholic subtypes and treatment effectiveness. *J Consult Clin Psychol* 49:72–80, 1981.
38. Horn JL, Wanberg KW, Foster FM: The Alcohol Use Inventory. Denver, Center for Alcohol Abuse Research and Evaluation, 1974.
39. Skinner HA, Allen BA: Differential assessment of alcoholism evaluation of the Alcohol Use Inventory. *J Stud Alcohol* 44:852–862, 1983.
40. Skinner HA: Primary Syndromes of alcohol abuse: Their measurement and correlates. *Br J Addict* 76:63–76, 1981.
41. Edward G., Gross MM: Alcohol dependence: Provisional description of a clinical syndrome. *Br Med J* 1:1058–1061, 1976.
42. Skinner HA, Allen BA; Alcohol dependence syndrome: Measurement and validation. *J Abnorm Psychol* 91:199–209, 1982.
43. Chick J: Is there a unidimensional alcohol dependence syndrome? *Br J Addict* 75:265–280, 1980.
44. Hesselbrock MN, Choquette KA, Margoles SM, et al: *Comparison of the DSM-III Alcohol Abuse/Dependence Criteria with Empirically Derived Scales of Alcohol Related Symptomatology.* Farmington, University of Connecticut Health Center, 1984.
45. National Council on Alcoholism Criteria Committee: Criteria for diagnosis of alcoholism. *Am J Psychiatry* 129:127–135, 1972.

46. Hart LS, Stueland D: An application of the multidimensional model of alcoholism, differentiation of alcohlics by mode analysis. *J Stud Alcohol* 40:283–289, 1979.
47. Reagles KW, Butler AS: The Human Service Scale; a new measure for rehabilitation. *J Rehab* 42:34–38, 1976.
48. Gibbs LE: A classification of alcoholics relevant to type specific treatment. *Int J Addict* 15:461–488, 1980.
49. Kivlahan DR, Donovan DM, Walker RD: Alcoholic subtypes; validity of clusters based on multiple assessment domains. Presented at the Annual Meeting of the American Psychological Association, Anaheim, California, 1983.
50. Lisansky ES: Alcoholism in women; social and psychological concomitants. 1, social history data. *Q J Stud Alcohol* 18:588–623, 1957.
51. Hesselbrock MN: Women alcoholics: A comparison of the natural history of alcoholism between men and women, in: Meyer RE, Babor TF, Glueck BC, et al,(eds): *Evaluation of the Alcoholic: Implications for Research, Theory and Treatment.* National Institute on Alcohol Abuse and Alcoholism Research Monograph #5, Rockville, Maryland, National Institute on Alcohol Abuse and Alcoholism, 1981 pp.129–144.
52. Bromet E, Moos R: Sex and marital status in relation to the characteristics of alcoholics. *J Stud Alcohol* 37:1302–1312, 1976.
53. Hesselbrock VM, Stabenau JR, Hesselbrock MN, et al: The nature of alcoholism in patients with different family histories for alcoholism. *Progr Neurol Psychopharmacol Psychiatry* 6:607–614, 1982.
54. Rimmer J, Pitts F, Reich T, et al: Alcoholism. II. Sex, socioeconomic status and race in two hospitalized samples. *Q J Stud Alcohol* 32:942–952, 1971.
55. Schuckit MA, Morrissey ER; Alcoholism in women, some clinical and social perspective with an emphasis on possible subtypes, in: Greenblatt M, Schuckit MA (eds): *Alcoholism Problems in Women and Children.* New York, Grune and Stratton, 1976.
56. Woodruff RA, Guze SB, Clayton PJ, et al: Alcoholism and Depression. *Arch Gen Psychiatry* 28:97–100, 1973.
57. Schuckit MA, Morrissey ER: Psychiatric problems in women admitted to an alcoholic detoxification center. *Am J Psychiatry* 136:611–616, 1979.
58. Cloninger CR, Reich T, Wetzel R: Alcoholism and affective disorders, in: Goodwin DW, Erickson CK (eds): *Alcoholism and Affective Disorders.* Jamaica, New York, Spectrum Publications, 1979.
59. Hesselbrock MN, Meyer RE, Keener JJ: Psychopathology in hospitalized alcoholics. *Arch Gen Psychiatry* (in press).
60. Schuckit MA: Alcoholism and sociopathy–diagnostic confusion. *Q J Stud Alcohol* 34:157–164, 1973.
61. Beckman LJ: Alcoholism problems and women: An overview, in: Greenblatt M, Schuckit MA (eds): *Alcoholism Problems in Women and Children.* New York, Grune and Stratton, 1976.
62. Gomberg EL: Alcoholism in women, in: Kissin B, Begleiter H (eds): *The Biology of Alcoholism* vol. 4, *Social Aspects of Alcoholism.* New York, Plenum Press, 1976.
63. Elder TC: Alcoholism and its onset in a population of admitted alcoholics: An AA study. *Br J Addict* 68:291–294, 1973.
64. Beckman LJ: Women alcoholics, a review of social and psychological studies. *J Stud Alcohol* 36:797–824, 1975.
65. Goodwin DW: *Is Alcoholism Hereditary?* New York, Oxford University Press, 1976.
66. Fleeson W, Gildea EF: A study of the personality of 289 abnormal drinkers. *Q J Stud Alcohol* 3:409–432, 1942.
67. Weissman MM, Myers JK, Harding PS: Prevalence and psychiatric heterogeneity of alcoholism in a United States urban community. *J Stud Alcohol* 41:672–681, 1980.
68. Woodruff RA, Guze SB, Clayton PJ: Alcoholism and depression, in: Goodwin DW, Erickson CK (eds): *Alcoholism and Affective Disorders.* Jamaica, New York, Spectrum Publications, 1979.
69. Robins LN: The diagnosis of alcoholism after DSM-III, in: Meyer RE, Babor TF, Glueck BC, et al (eds): *Evaluation of the Alcoholic: Implications for Treatment.* National Institute on Alcohol

Abuse and Alcoholism Research Monograph #5, Rockville, Maryland, National Institute on Alcohol Abuse and Alcoholism, 1981 pp. 85–105.

70. Fowler RC, Liskow BI, Tanna VL: Alcoholism, depression and life events. *J Affect Dis* 2:127–135, 1980.
71. Lewis CE, Helzer J, Cloninger CR, et al: Psychiatric diagnostic predisposition to alcoholism. *Comp Psychiatry* 23:451–461, 1982.
72. Goodwin DW, Guze SB: *Psychiatric Diagnosis* ed 2. New York, Oxford University Press, 1979.
73. Hesselbrock MN, Hesselbrock VM, Babor TF, et al: Antisocial behavior, psychopathology and problems drinking in the natural hisotyr of alcoholism, in: Goodwin DW, VanDusen KT, Mednick SA (eds): *Longitudinal Research in Alcoholism.* Boston, Kluwer-Nijhoff Publishing Co., 1983.
74. Hesselbrock VN, Hesselbrock MN, Workman-Daniels, KL: The effect of major depression and antisocial personality on alcoholism: Course and motivational patterns. *J Stud Alcohol* (in press).
75. Avery DH, Overall JE, Calil HM, et al: Alcohol-induced euphoria alcoholics compared to nonalcoholics. *Int J Addict* 17:823–845, 1982.
76. O'Sullivan K, Whillans P, Daly M, et al: A comparison of alcoholics with and without coexisting affective disorder. *Br J Psychiatry* 143:133–138, 1983.
77. Francis RJ, Timm S, Bucky S: Studies of familial and nonfamilial alcoholism. *Arch Gen Psychiatry* 37:564–566, 1980.
78. Schuckit MA: Relationship between the course of primary alcoholism and family history. *J Stud Alcohol* 45:334–338, 1984.
79. Penick EC, Powell BJ, Othmer E, et al: Subtyping alcoholics by coexisting psychiatric syndromes; course, family history outcome, in: Goodwin DW, VanDusen KT, Mednick SA (eds): *Longitudinal Research in Alcoholism.* Boston, Kluwer-Nijhoff Publishing Co. 1984.
80. Hesselbrock VM, Hesselbrock MN, Stabenau JR: Subtyping of alcoholism in male patients by family history and antisocial personality. *J Stud Alcohol 49:89–98, 1985.*

9

Alcoholic Subtypes Based on Multiple Assessment Domains

Validation against Treatment Outcome

Dennis M. Donovan, Daniel R. Kivlahan, and R. Dale Walker

Abstract. Research in the area of subtype development within alcoholic populations has undergone a number of changes over the recent years. First, there has been a shift from subtype derivation based on *a priori* comparative approaches toward a more recent use of *a posteriori* correlational approaches such as cluster analysis. Second, there has been an increased multivariate focus in which multiple measures from a number of practically and/or theoretically relevant assessment domains are entered into the classificatory process. Third, there has been an increased emphasis on the external validation of derived clusters. The present chapter briefly reviews these issues, using examples of research from the Seattle Veterans Administration Medical Center to illustrate each of these shifts across a series of studies focusing on the development of alcoholic subtypes. Finally, the results of a recent subtype identification and validation study will be presented to illustrate the difficulties in and advantages of a multidomain cluster analytic strategy.

1. Introduction

Much of the initial work attempting to understand factors associated with the etiology, maintenance, and prognosis of alcoholism involved comparing individuals defined as alcoholic with nonalcoholic individuals on a variety of theoretically relevant variables. These early studies, often focusing on personality characteristics and dynamics, provided both interesting and useful information about aspects of alcoholism. However, such a methodological approach had a number of practical limitations. First, it was a theory-bound

Dennis M. Donovan, Daniel R. Kivlahan and R. Dale Walker • Department of Psychiatry and Behavioral Sciences, University of Washington, Seattle, Washington 98195; and Alcohol Dependence Treatment Program, Veterans Administration Medical Center, Seattle, Washington 98108.

approach that often limited the scope of the variables and hypotheses to be explored.[1–3] As Jackson[1] noted, many authors paid lip service to the sociocultural, psychological, and physiological processes involved in alcoholism, but their actual research would focus on only one facet of a single area. Second, such group comparisons typically revealed significant differences. However, subsequent research[3,4] has suggested that alcoholics share many features in common with a number of other patient and nonpatient groups; such findings have helped to dispel the myth of a unique "alcoholic personality." Third, viewing alcoholics as a "generic" group in such comparison studies accentuated the homogeneity among such individuals; however, in so doing, the contribution of individual differences across alcoholic individuals was minimized. The fourth limitation involves the clinical utility of the results derived from such a comparative approach. Treatment personnel would not be surprised that alcohlics differed from nonalcoholics but would be interested in knowning that certain alcoholics differed from other alcoholics. From this clinical standpoint, greater appreciation of the distinctiveness of certain subgroups of alcoholics could be used to tailor more appropriate and effective interventions.[5]

These factors, among others, have helped to shift the focus of more recent research onto salient distinctions within groups of alcoholics or on the empirical derivation of alcoholic subtypes.[1–8] The process of subtype development has evolved considerably as both methodological sophistication and conceptual understanding of alcoholism have increased. The present chapter is intended to describe briefly a number of the major developments in subtype identification. Examples from research conducted at the Alcohol Dependence Treatment Program of the Seattle Veterans Administration Medical Center (VAMC) will be utilized to illustrate these developmental shifts. Table I presents an overview of the nature of these changes in methodological strategies from earlier studies of subtype derivation and validation to more recent investigations. Each of these methodological strategies will be described more thoroughly in the next two sections. Finally, a more detailed description of

Table I. Characteristics of Earlier and More Recent Approaches to the Derivation and Validation of Subtypes among Alcoholics

Phase of subtype development	Stage of subtype research	
	Earlier research	Recent research
Derivation phase	Univariate criterion	Multivariate criteria
	Single assessment domain	Multiple assessment domains
	A priori comparative approach	*A posteriori* correlation approach
Validation phase	Single assessment domain	Multiple assessment domains
	Within-domain criteria	Across-domain criteria
	Concurrent validation	Predictive validation

our recent research, embodying many of the previously described developments, will be presented.

2. Issues in Subtype Identification

Meyer *et al.*[2] have presented an overview of empirical studies attempting to classify alcoholics into meaningful typologies. Early subtype development relied heavily on an *a priori comparative approach*. In this strategy two or more groups of alcoholics are classified according to differences on an *a priori* criterion, often dichotomous in nature. These subgroups are then compared on a number of variables thought to have particular relevance to a given theoretical view of alcoholism.

Much of our early work at the Seattle VAMC followed the *a priori* comparative approach and was directed by social-learning theory, focusing on alcoholics' perceptions of control.[9,10] After initial research comparing alcoholics and nonalcoholics on this construct, the focus shifted to looking for alcoholic subtypes based upon their scores on Rotter's[11] locus-of-control scale. Significant differences were found between alcoholics having internal versus external perceptions of control. The former reflects the belief that the outcome of significant life events is within one's own personal control; an external locus of control suggests that the individual attributes the responsibility for the outcome of such events to factors beyond one's control, such as fate, chance, or powerful others. External subjects were found to perceive less control over interpersonal and intrapersonal sources of stress; higher levels of anxiety, depression, and psychopathology; a different pattern of defensive style; and a tendency to drink as a means of enhancing their ability to relate socially.[10]

This early line of research on perceived control also reflects another point raised by Meyer and colleagues,[2] namely, the classification of alcoholics into subtypes was based on a single variable. Such reliance on a *univariate approach* was relatively common in early studies of alcoholic typologies. As our research evolved, the breadth of assessment was increased to a *multivariate level*. At first, there was the expansion from looking at two groups based upon locus of control to four subtypes based on differing levels of both perceived and experienced control. This initial step toward a multivariate classification strategy also helped clarify many of our previous findings. For example, it was found[12] that while both locus of control and the experience of control were related to depression among alcoholics, a significant interaction effect was obtained. The subgroup that had an external locus of control and experienced minimal control over sources of stress had the highest level of depression; no differences were found among the remaining three groups.

These findings reflect a number of potential advantages of a mulitvariate classification system. First, it allows an increased breadth of coverage of theoretical variables in the derivation process. Second, the addition of variables allows further refinement and differentiation of the subgroups that are formed. Third, it allows the exploration of possible interactions between or among the variables of interest. However, this approach continued to be relatively limited, in that only two variables from a *single theoretical domain* (control orientation) were investigated. Other aspects of our work have included a broader range of variables within a given domain, such as psychopathology[6] or neuropsychological status[13]; however, there is again the exclusion of other variable domains that may be of relevance. The relatively limited utilization of data from different domains has characterized many of the earlier subtype classification systems.[1–3]

More recent multivariate studies on subtype derivation among alcoholics demonstrate an increased level of methodological and statistical sophistication.[2,3,8] There has been an increased emphasis upon the use of multivariate measures from a number of practically and/or theoretically relevant *multiple assessment domains.* On a statistical level, there has been an increased reliance on *a posteriori correlational approaches,*[2] employing techniques such as cluster analysis. Subtypes are defined empirically based upon the similarity among their members on a wide array of measures; these derived subtypes are characterized by a higher degree of intragroup homogeneity and intergroup differentiation. While there are limitiations in the use of techniques such as cluster analysis,[2,8,14,15] the *a posteriori* correlational strategy appears to be less dictated by theoretical considerations as well as being able to accommodate data from multiple assessement domains.

While certain of our previous investigations involved the use of *a posteriori* cluster analytic techiques on multivariate data from either a single assessment domain[6,13] or multiple domains,[16] our work in the area of neuropsychological function is most illustrative of the gradual departure from an *a priori* univariate perspective. We originally were interested in the perceptual style of alcoholics along the dimension of field dependence–independence.[17] Individuals who are classified as field dependent have considerable difficulty, being more bound to the background in a perceptual task; field-independent individuals, on the other hand, are able to make accurate perceptual judgements regardless of distractions in the context. In our original study,[18] alcoholic subjects were classified into three groups (field dependent, intermediate, field independent) based on their scores on the Group Embedded Figures Test. In this and a subsequent study, field dependence, within both alcoholic and nonalcoholic samples, was related to deficits in a wide array of cognitive and neuropsychological measures, particularly those related to nonverbal problem-solving ability.[18,19]

In a more recent study,[13] the Group Embedded Figures Test was again used. However, rather than being the only variable involved in defining alcoholic subtypes, it was one of 13 cognitive and neuropsychological variables. These scores were entered into a cluster analystic procedure that resulted in three subtypes that were large enough to be subjected to validation procedures. These groups were found to differ on a number of cognitive variables not included in the derivation process, as well as on certain demographic, drinking history, and treatment outcome measures. This represented a major advance over our earlier, cruder method of defining the three groups based on a trichotomization of the distribution of Group Embedded Figures Test scores.[18,19]

3. Issues in Subtype Validation

The previous example reflects the movement in our research toward a *multivariate, single domain* (e.g., neuropsychological funtion) assessment model with the use of *a posteriori* correlational clustering methodology. Our attempts to identify neuropsychological subtypes also illustrate two important points relevant to external cluster validation. Blashfield[14] has noted that it is possible to derive empirical subtypes regardless of the nature of the variables involved. Therefore, it is necessary to provide evidence of the meaningfulness of derived clusters by relating them to variables other than those used in the composition of the subtypes. A central issue noted in the previously described research on neuropsychological subtypes involved the selection of the criterion variables against which clusters were validated. These may be either within the neuropsychological domain or from other domains. In our original studies of perceptural style,[18,19] the subtypes were validated against a variety of cognitive and neuropsychological variables. This represented a form of *within-domain validation,* since variables involved in both subtype derivation and validation represented aspects of neuropsychological functioning. The more recent study of neuropsychological clusters[13] involved both *within-domain* (other measures of cognitive function) and *cross-domain* strategies. The latter is exemplified by comparing these subtypes on pretreatment drinking-related measures and treatment outcome. While knowing how the clusters differed on other aspects of cognitive function helped clarify the success of the derivation process, the differences among the clusters within other variable classes such as demographics, personality functioning, and drinking history documented their clinical meaningfulness. It should also be noted that this study employed validating criterion variables from multiple domains.

A second point has to do with the time frame involved in the collection of data used in both the cluster derivation and validation process. These data may be collected concurrently or longitudinally. If the former case, the *concurrent validity* of the clusters can be determined. In the latter situation, the *predictive validity* can be examined. Morey and Blashfield[3] have noted that studies to date have failed to provide convincing evidence for either type of external validity of empirically derived alcoholic subtypes. This appears to be especially true of predictive validity. Skinner[8] indicated that although a number of studies have evaluated the descriptive, concurrent validity of alcoholic subtypes by exploring variables either within or across domains, only three of 29 studies reviewed had attempted to address the predictive validity of a typology with respect to treatment outcome. While there are difficulties involved in conducting adequate follow-up studies on alcoholic subtypes,[7] the issue of prognostic utility is critical to the validation of any typological process.[2] This would appear particularly important given the stated goal of most researchers in this area to find an optimal match between alcoholic subtypes and type of treatment.[3]

4. An Empirical Investigation of Subtype Identification and Validation

Based upon the present review, as well as previous ones,[1–4,8] we have adopted several principles in our subsequent studies. First, these studies should be multivariate and multidomain. This proposition is consistent with the growing belief that alcoholism is a multifaceted disorder. The examination of variables from mulitple domains allows the exploration of complex interactions among sociocultural, psychological, and physiological processes thought to be important to the development and maintenance of alcoholism. Potential variables to be included in the derivation process might reflect premorbid demographic characteristics of the individual, the pattern of alcohol use, the degree of alcohol dependence, and the pattern of both psychological and physical alcohol-related consequences.[2] It is of interest to note that the majority of previous studies on alcoholism subtypes have not included measures of drinking patterns or alcohol dependence.[3,8] Second, studies should utilize appropriate *a posteriori* correlational methods, such as cluster analysis. As Skinner[8] noted, clustering methodology is yet in its relative infancy. It is important for investigators to maintain an awareness of issues related to the appropriate use and potential misuse of such techniques.[14,15] Finally, studies should focus attention on the process of validation. Ideally, attempts at external validation would utilize a multiple, cross domain approach and address the prognostic value of the derived subtypes.

The most recent of our attempts to develop an alcoholic typology[20] incorporated this more formalized set of recommendations. The subtype investigation represented a component of a larger research program investigating the relationship between neuropsychological deficits, length of inpatient hospitalization, and treatment outcome among alcoholics.[21] Our initial findings suggesed that neuropsychological status was significantly related, although at low levels, to treatment outcome. Overall, the length of inpatient stay to which individuals were randomly assigned (either 2 weeks or 7 weeks) was not related to outcome. In thinking about these findings, we speculated that our focus on neuropsychological deficits (a multivariate, single domain) had failed to reflect the complexity of the patient population. The movement to a multidomain approach and the use of cluster analytic techniques were chosen to allow the identification of more refined and homogeneous subtypes. Further, based upon our follow-up data collection strategies, it was possible to determine both the descriptive and the predictive validity of the subtypes. The remainder of the present section examines this study in more detail.

4.1. Method

4.1.1. Subjects. The subjects were 245 male veterans participating in a prospective treatment outcome study described in detail elsewhere.[21] A total of 245 subjects meeting the inclusion criteria were randomly assigned to 2 or 7 week length of stay (LOS), and all patients contracted for 9 months of weekly outpatient aftercare following the completion of their respective hospital stay.

The overall sample had a mean age of 45.7 years (S.D. = 11.9) and a mean of 12.4 years of education (S.D. = 2.8). The sample was predominantly Caucasian (90.3%). Most patients were from the lower middle or lower social classes (42.9% and 43.3%, respectively). A total of 52.3% of the subjects reported cohabiting in a maritallike relationship within the 6 months prior to admission. Based upon self-reported employment status during the 90 days prior to admission, only 20.8% of the subjects were employed full-time. Drinking was reported to have been a problem for at least 10 years by 61.6% of the patients. On average, subjects reported drinking approximately 9–10 drink equivalents per day. Subjects evidenced a number of symptoms indicative of alcohol dependence such as blackouts (81.4%) and withdrawal shakes (77.3%). The majority (62.0%) had been in prior treatment for alcohol-related problems.

4.1.2. Assessment. Patients were typically assessed within the first week of hospitalization (mean = 6.3 days after admission; S.D. = 3.2). Patients reported an average of 23.7 days (S.D. = 23.1) between their last drink and the first day of testing. Patient's drinking behavior, aftercare attendance and employment status were assessed at follow-up interviews 3, 6, and 9 months after hospital discharge. Aftercare completion rates and relapse status were determined for all 245 subjects over the 9-month follow-up, while employment status was determined for 78% of the subjects.

4.1.3. Variable Selection Considerations. As noted by Morris, *et al.*[22] decisions about variable selection have a crucial impact on the results of a cluster analysis. They identified three considerations in variable selection: characteristics of the frequency distribution (with multimodal and/or skewed distributions more likely to reflect subtypes than normally distributed variables), psychometric properties of the variables, and theoretical relevance. Additionally, it is important to restrict the number of variables in order to reduce redundancy and random error variance and increase subtype interpretability.

Our selection process occurred at two stages: domains of assessment and particular measures within domains. As mentioned above, we have previously identified subtypes based on neuropsychological functioning[13] and MMPI profiles.[6] From within the neuropsychological domain we selected the brain age quotient (BAQ)[23] and an estimated verbal IQ[24] as the least redundant and best established summary measures of cognitive functioning in our previous studies. In addition, both measures are age adjusted, an important consideration since we were also including age among the demographic measures.

The BAQ is an index of problem solving ability comprised of subtests from the Halstead–Reitan Neuropsychological Battery and the performance scale of the WAIS. Verbal IQ was prorated from the vocabulary and arithmetic subscales of the WAIS. From the MMPI-168[25] we selected four clinical scales most frequently included in previously identified alcoholic subtype codes (depression, psychopathic deviate, psychasthenia, and schizophrenia). In addition, we used the MMPI-168 version of the Edwards Social Desirability Scale. Skinner[8] and Morey *et al.*[15] have noted the importance of incorporating indices of response style when using self-report data.

The two other assessment domains included were those that receive primary emphasis in clinical assessment but have been notably absent in previous attempts at empirical identification of alcoholic subtypes. The curious omission of data on alcohol use patterns in favor of personality variables has been noted by other reviewers.[3,8] We selected three measures from this domain based on theoretical relevance and a desire to be able to describe subtypes in terms that would be familiar to clinicians. Chronicity was reflected by the number of years of self-reported problem drinking. Second, an index reflecting alcohol use patterns was based on the number of days during the three months prior to admission on which five or more drink equivalents were consumed. Third, we used the Alcohol Dependence Scale[26] to address the important theoretical and diagnostic issue of the extent of alcohol dependence symptoms.

Demographic characteristics represented the final assessment domain from which we selected clustering variables. Despite evidence documenting age-related differences in alcoholics,[27,28] age has not previously been included as a clustering variable, but rather as a descriptive validity criterion. Based on reviews of predictors of treatment outcome,[29,30] two other demographic indices were included: the Hollingshead Index of Social Position,[31] based on a weighted combination of occupational status and educational background, and an index of recent employment status based on average number of hours worked per week during the three months prior to admission.

Taken together, we wanted to test whether these 13 variables from four assessment domains could generate, via cluster analysis, profiles of alcoholic subtypes that would be both clinically recognizable and predictively valid.

4.1.4. Cluster Derivation. The 13 variables were initially standardized and entered into the CLUSTAN program,[32] using the single linkage method[33] with squared Euclidean distance as the similarity measure. This procedure was used as an initial screening process to identify outliers. Edelbrock[34] has previously shown that the accuracy of hierarchical clustering algorithms is a function of the degree of coverage. In his tests, accuracy values increased when outliers were excluded. Results of the single linkage method identified 11 cases that each had extreme values on one or more of the 13 measures.

With these outliers excluded, three procedural decisions were necessary in order to identify the subtypes to be validated: selection of a similarity measure, selection of a clustering algorithm, and determination of the optimal number of clusters. A recent comparative validation study of 23 different clustering methods on alcohol use data[15] demonstrated Ward's minimum variance clustering algorithm[35] using squared Euclidean distance as the similarity measure, to be particularly powerful. We had originally used this method on split halves of our larger sample in order to determine the optimal number of clusters. Inspection of the dendrograms, clustering coefficients, and profile means suggested a six-cluster solution within each half of the sample.

When results of the same clustering algorithm (Ward's method) were compared for the full sample and the smaller sample of 234 that excluded outliers, there was a reliable association between them ($\chi^2[25] = 359.2$, $p < .0001$). However, nearly half of the cases (47.9%) did not remain in the same cluster in both solutions. This lack of consistency demonstrates the potent order effect that occurs in hierarchical clustering procedures. Ward's method, along with other hierarchical techniques, does not guarantee an optimal cluster solution because objects merged at one step in the clustering algorithm are never unmerged at subsequent steps. Thus, the presence of a small proportion of outliers (less than 5%) in the original sample appears to have produced a cluster solution that, while not entirely independent of the solution on the reduced sample, is substantially different.

In light of these findings, we sought to improve upon the stability and homogeneity of clusters by using one of CLUSTAN's nonhierarchical clustering algorithms, the *k*-means relocation procedure with error sum of squares as the similarity measure. This approach began by randomly assigning cases to ten clusters and then iteratively removing and reassigning cases to other clusters according to the error sum of squares similarity criterion. Once the solutions to these ten clusters had stabilized, the two most similar clusters were combined and the iterative relocation procedure continued. Morey *et al.*[15] found this technique to be the most replicable of the 23 methods they tested. In addition it showed the closest correspondence to the solution based on Ward's method. Similarly in our data, these two different methods used on the refined sample of 234 resulted in greater consistency (67.5% overlap) than the results from Ward's method on the original and refined samples.

Results of the *k*-means solution showed a discontinuity in the clustering coefficient between the five- and six-cluster solutions indicating increased heterogeneity of the five-cluster solution. Consistent with our previous analyses, we pursued the validation phase of the analysis with six clusters.

4.2. Results

4.2.1. Characteristics of Clusters. Means of all 13 clustering variables within each of the six *k*-means clusters are presented in Table II. For convenience the subtypes are ordered along a continuum of age from youngest (cluster 1) to oldest (cluster 6). It should be noted that age is not the only

Table II. Means of the 13 Clustering Variables for the Six Empirically Derived k-Means Clusters

Clustering variable	Clusters 1 (n = 27)	2 (n = 37)	3 (n = 48)	4 (n = 51)	5 (n = 33)	6 (n = 38)
Age	31.3	39.1	42.2	49.9	53.2	54.7
Social position index[a]	58.5	59.7	58.1	50.8	46.0	61.3
Average hours worked per week[b]	29.2	12.5	9.9	20.2	12.9	14.2
Days of five or more drinks[b]	29.0	43.7	57.9	50.5	74.0	28.9
Chronicity (in years)	8.5	7.0	13.1	17.2	10.7	25.9
Alcohol Dependence Scale[c]	19.2	11.4	20.9	13.5	15.3	20.1
Brain age quotient	88.1	82.7	86.9	99.7	93.5	82.8
WAIS verbal IQ (prorated)	102.1	97.8	107.8	116.7	119.2	104.7
MMPI-168 depression	66.0	60.6	87.2	58.2	79.2	69.9
MMPI-168 psychopathic deviate	76.4	58.6	80.5	59.3	68.6	64.1
MMPI-168 psychasthenia	72.9	53.5	84.8	54.4	72.3	60.5
MMPI-168 schizophrenia	73.7	51.6	85.6	54.4	66.0	57.3
MMPI-168 social desirability	9.2	11.3	7.5	11.4	8.9	9.6

[a] Hollingshead[31]; lower values indicate higher social position.
[b] Based on the 90 days prior to admission.
[c] Skinner and Allen.[26]

discriminating variable. Even among clusters 4, 5, and 6, which are comparable with respect to age, the profiles reflect considerable differences on the remaining demographic, alcohol-related, neuropsychological, and personality measures.

4.2.2. Discriminant Validity of Clusters. External validity of the clusters was assessed by examining differences on pretreatment measures other than those from which the clusters were derived (see Table III). Chi-square analyses revealed differential rates between clusters for marital status with the two oldest clusters (5 and 6) having significantly higher proportions of married members ($\chi^2[10] = 20.3$, $p < .05$). There were marginally significant associations with previous alcohol treatment ($\chi^2[5] = 10.2$, $p < .10$) and previous psychiatric treatment ($\chi^2[5] = 10.9$, $p < .10$). There was no relationship between cluster membership and assignment to length of inpatient stay, a relevant finding since subsequent analyses explore the interaction of length of stay and cluster membership on treatment outcome.

Scores on several assessment instruments not included in the cluster analysis also differed significantly among the cluster groups. The AUI Drug Use Scale,[36] a summary score of somatic symptoms derived from the Cornell Medical Index Health Questionnaire,[37] Drinking-Related Internal/External Control Scale,[38] and Beck Depression Inventory[39] all reflected highly reliable differences among clusters. These results contribute corroborative evidence of the distinctiveness of the cluster patterns on demographic, drinking-re-

Table III. Discriminant Validity of Clusters

Variable	Cluster 1	2	3	4	5	6	F/χ^2
Married (%)	22.2	21.6	29.2	31.4	45.5	42.1	20.3**
Prior alcohol treatment	63.0	56.8	52.1	64.7	51.5	81.6	10.2*
Prior psychiatric treatment	33.3	24.3	33.3	9.8	21.2	15.8	10.9*
Drinking-Related Internal External Control Scale	5.1[a]	5.4[a]	7.1[b]	4.6[a]	8.3[b]	4.8[a]	5.9***
AUI Drug Use Scale	3.1[c]	1.4[b]	1.7[b]	.5[a]	.4[a]	.6[a]	13.9***
Beck Depression Inventory	10.4[bc]	8.0[ab]	17.5[d]	6.7[a]	13.5[c]	11.6[c]	16.5***
Cornell Medical Index somatic symptoms	19.3[a]	15.2[a]	27.8[b]	17.6[a]	26.0[b]	29.3[b]	9.7***

Note: Means with different superscripts differ significantly at $p < .05$ by Duncan's multiple range test.
* $p < .10$; ** $p < .05$; *** $p < .01$

lated, affective, and health measures. It should also be noted that these concurrent measures are not monotonically related to age.

4.2.3. Predictive Validity of Clusters. The crucial test of cluster validity for our purposes was the extent to which subtypes could be identified that had differential outcome from a given treatment program. Even more importantly, we hoped to reveal a significant interaction between length of treatment and outcome. Table IV presents data on the predictive validity of the clusters relative to three outcome parameters at 9-month followup: drinking status, completion of the 9-month posthospitalization aftercare program, and employment status. Among the six clusters, chi-square analyses showed a differential pattern of aftercare completion (range = 18.5–57.6% completers; ($\chi^2[5] = 13$, $p < .05$) and follow-up employment status (range = 27.8–56.1% employed full-time; $\chi^2[10] = 24.2$, $p < .01$). A categorization of drinking outcome as successful (i.e., no more than 1 heavy drinking day over the 9-month follow-up; 40.2% of the sample) versus relapsed (48.9%) or lost to follow-up (10.7%) did not show any overall difference among clusters, although the range of success rates was large (29.2–51.5%).

4.2.4. Differential Outcome Related to Length of Stay (LOS). Among patients randomly assigned to the briefer 2-week LOS, cluster membership was significantly associated with aftercare completion (range = 5.9–69.2% completion rate; $\chi^2[5] = 14.9$, $p < .01$) and final employment state (range = 10–70.8% full-time employment; $\chi^2[10] = 31.2$, $p < .001$), and showed a marginally significant relationship to drinking outcome (range = 20–57.1% success rate; $\chi^2[5] = 9.5$, $p < .10$). Conversely, there were no significant associations within the sample assigned to 7-week LOS.

Table IV. Predictive Validity of Clusters by Length of Stay

	Length of stay		
Treatment outcome	2-week (%)	7-week (%)	Total (%)
Aftercare completion			
Cluster 1 (n = 27)	5.9	40.0	18.5
Cluster 2 (n = 37)	29.4	30.0	29.7
Cluster 3 (n = 48)	30.0	32.1	31.3
Cluster 4 (n = 51)	46.4	26.1	37.3
Cluster 5 (n = 33)	69.2	50.0	57.6
Cluster 6 (n = 38)	40.0	39.1	39.5
Total (n = 234)	36.4	35.5	35.9
χ^2	14.9[a]	3.6[b]	11.6[b]
Treatment success			
Cluster 1 (n = 27)	29.4	50.0	37.0
Cluster 2 (n = 37)	52.9	25.0	37.8
Cluster 3 (n = 48)	20.0	35.7	29.2
Cluster 4 (n = 51)	57.1	34.8	47.1
Cluster 5 (n = 33)	53.8	50.0	51.5
Cluster 6 (n = 38)	35.7	43.5	40.5
Total (n = 234)	42.2	38.7	40.3
χ^2	9.5[c]	3.7	5.4
Employment status (working full-time)			
Cluster 1 (n = 27)	55.6	42.9	50.0
Cluster 2 (n = 37)	35.7	50.0	43.3
Cluster 3 (n = 48)	13.3	38.1	27.8
Cluster 4 (n = 51)	70.8	35.3	56.1
Cluster 5 (n = 33)	38.5	37.5	37.9
Cluster 6 (n = 38)	10.0	38.1	29.0
Total (n = 234)	41.2	39.8	40.4
χ^2	31.2[a]	9.39	24.2[a]

[a] $p < .01$.
[b] $p < .05$.
[c] $p < .10$.

5. Discussion

The present study reports results on empirically derived alcoholic subtypes and addresses a number of more general issues relevant to subtype development. The present findings indicated that it was possible to define six distinctive subtypes within our current sample of alcoholic inpatients. An inspection of the scores on the 13 clustering variables found in Table II reveals that the groups evidence different patterns both within and across the demographic, drinking-related, neuropsychological, and personality/psychopathology domains assessed. Each of the subtypes also appears to correspond to types of individuals often seen within our clinical setting. These include individuals such as those in cluster 1 who are relatively young, socially unstable men of average intelligence but with subtle deficits in problem-solving skills. Patients in this group evidence considerable psychological distress coupled with a high level of alcohol dependence despite a relatively short period of reported problem drinking. There are also individuals seen within our clincial setting who could seem to fit each of the remaining five derived subtypes. This match between empirically derived clusters and clinically observed constellations of characteristics among our alcoholic patients may represent a form of "face validity" that helps corroborate the clinical meaningfulness of the derived groups.

As is the case in other areas of psychological assessment, the presence of such face validity is insufficient to insure the practical and prognostic utility of a classificatory scheme. The actual meaningfulness of derived subtypes must be judged on the basis of documented external validation. While this validation stage has been stressed as a crucial element in subtype development, it often has received minimal attention.[1,3,8] The present results address both concurrent and predictive validity.

As an example of concurrent validity, cluster 3, which was composed of middle-aged men with a high degree of psychopathology, was found to have had the highest rate of past psychiatric treatment and the highest level of depression as assessed by the Beck Depression Inventory. Cluster 6, characterized by older patients with the longest self-reported period of problem drinking and a high level of symptoms defining an alcohol dependence syndrome, was found to have the highest rate of prior alcoholism treatment and the most somatic symptomatology. Cluster 1, composed primarily of young men with considerable psychological distress, was found to have the highest level of drug use. These findings provide a form of convergent validation, in that salient characteristics of the clusters were related in a predictable way to variables outside those used in the derivation process.

Predictive validity was also examined. As a number of authors have pointed out,[1–3,8] a primary goal of classifying alcoholics into subtypes is to explore the feasibility of patient–treatment matching based upon evidence of differential treatment outcomes. The present findings represent an initial step toward this goal. In previous analyses of data from this project[71] we found no overall differences in outcome as a function of length of hospitalization. It appears that looking at the alcoholic sample as a whole obscured significant differences that emerged once more homogeneous subtypes were derived. As an example, it appears that there was no differential treatment success for cluster 5 as a function of either a 2-week or 7-week hospitalization. This was not the case for clusters 1 and 4, however. For cluster 1 patients the longer hospitalization was associated with better outcome while the shorter length of stay appeared more beneficial for members of cluster 4. These findings, in conjunction with those focusing on concurrent validity, indicate that the derived subtypes reflect clinically meaningful typologies that may be useful in predicting outcome.

As noted earlier, our results also have a bearing on several unresolved general issues related to cluster analytic methodology. Morey and Blashfield[3] indicated a need for careful selection of subjects, clustering techiques, and variables in this process. Our patient population of male veterans represents a select group from which generalization may be limited. The choice of an appropriate clustering strategy involved a number of subjective decisions since there are no firm and fast rules in this regard. It is instructive to note the shifts in cluster composition both before and after outliers were removed. It is also of interest to note that the subtypes ultimately identified through our sequential clustering process, while relatively homogeneous, still evidenced a considerable degree of intragroup variability. With respect to decisions concerning variables to include in the clusters, we attempted to follow a set of explicit[22] and implicit guidelines. We wanted to utilize measures that might be readily available to clinicians and could be understood by them. However, we chose a disproportionate number of measures from the MMPI-168, which may have inadvertantly weighted the resultant subtypes more heavily with respect to the level of psychopathology. This may be appropriate given recent findings,[5] but such results remain to be corroborated by methods giving equal weighting to each domain. Also, in retrospect, it might have been equally feasible to derive subtypes from those variables we used as concurrent criterion measures or other variables not assessed such as family history of alcoholism. Although the *a posteriori* correlational techniques have been recognized as not being theory bound,[2] the decisions concerning the means of collecting data, the variables to be included, and the method of cluster analysis to be employed will continue to be influenced by the researcher's theoretical perspective.[3]

The present review and empirical study reflect the movement and evolution that has occurred in our research specifically as well as in the area of alcoholic subtype development more generally. We feel that the use of multidomain assessments in conjunction with sequential cluster analytic strategies provides a viable direction for future research. However, as we look at the many unresolved and misunderstood aspects of this approach, it is clear that there is yet considerable room for growth.

References

1. Jackson DN: Differential personality inventory types among alcoholics, in Cox WM (ed): *Identifying and Measuring Alcoholic Personality Characteristics.* San Francisco, Josey-Bass, 1983, p 87–99.
2. Meyer RE, Babor TF, Mirkin PM: Typologies in alcoholism: An overview. *Int J Addict* 18:235–249, 1983.
3. Morey LC, Blashfield RK: Empirical classifications of alcoholism: A review. *J Stud Alcohol* 42:925–937, 1981.
4. Nerviano VJ, Gross HW: Personality types of alcoholics on objective inventories: A review. *J Stud Alcohol* 44:837–851, 1983.
5. McLellan AT, Woody GE, Luborsky L, et al: Increased effectiveness of substance abuse treatment: A prospective study of patient–treatment "matching." *J Nerv Ment Dis* 171:597–605, 1983.

6. Donovan DM, Chaney EF, O'Leary MR: Alcoholic MMPI subtypes: Relationship to drinking styles, benefits, and consequences. *J Nerv Ment Dis* 166:553–561, 1978.
7. Shelly CH, Goldstein G: An empirically derived typology of hospitalized alcoholics, in Goldstein G, Neuringer C (eds): *Empirical Studies of Alcoholism.* Cambridge, Ballinger, 1976, pp 195–229.
8. Skinner HA: Statistical approaches to the classification of alcohol and drug addiction. *Br J Addict* 77:259–273, 1982.
9. Donovan DM, O'Leary MR: Control orientation among alcoholics: A cognitive social learning perspective . *Am J Drug Alcohol Abuse* 6:487–499, 1979.
10. Donovan DM, O'Leary MR: Control orientation, drinking behavior, and alcoholism, in Lefcourt HM (ed): *Research with the locus of control construct,* vol 2. *Developments and Social Problems.* New York, Academic Press, 1983, pp 107–153.
11. Rotter JB: Generalized expectancies for internal versus external control of reinforcement. *Psychol Monogr* 80 (1, Whole No. 609), 1966.
12. O'Leary MR, Donovan DM, Cysewski B, et al: Perceived locus of control, experienced control, and depression: A trait description of the learned helplessness model of depression. *J Clin Psychol* 33:164–168, 1977.
13. Donovan DM, Kivlahan DR, Walker RD, et al: Derivation and validation of neuropsychological clusters among alcoholics. *J Stud Alcohol* 45:205–211, 1985.
14. Blashfield RK: Propositions regarding the use of cluster analysis in clinical research. *J Consult Clin Psychol* 48:456–459, 1980.
15. Morey LC, Blashfield RK, Skinner HA: A comparison of cluster analysis techniques within a sequential validation framework. *Multivar Behav Res* 18:309–329, 1983.
16. Donovan DM, Marlatt GA: Personality subtypes among driving-while-intoxicated offenders: Relationships to drinking behavior and driving risk. *J Consult Clin Psychol* 50:241–249, 1982.
17. Karp SA: Field dependence and overcoming embeddedness. *J Consult Psychol* 27:294–302, 1963.
18. Donovan DM, Queisser HR, O'Leary MR: Group Embedded Figures Test performance as a predictor of cognitive impairment among alcoholics. *Int J Addict* 11:725–739, 1976.
19. O'Leary MR, Donovan DM, Chaney EF: The relationship of perceptual field orientation to measures of cognitive functioning and current adaptive abilities in alcoholics and nonalcoholics. *J Nerv Ment Dis* 165:275–282, 1979.
20. Kivlahan DR, Donovan DM, Walker RD: Alcoholic subtypes: Validity of clusters based on multiple assessment domains. Presented at the American Psychological Association, Anaheim, California, August, 1983.
21. Walker RD, Donovan DM, Kivlahan DR, et al: Length of stay, neuropsychological performance, and aftercare: Influences on alcohol treatment outcome. *J Consult Clin Psychol* 51:900–911, 1983.
22. Morris R, Blashfield R, Satz P: Neuropsychology and cluster analysis: Potentials and problems. *J Clin Neuropsychology* 3:79–99, 1981.
23. Reitan R: Behavioral manifestations of impaired brain function in aging. Presented at the American Psychological Association, Montreal, Canada, August, 1973.
24. Wechsler D: *Wechsler Adult Intelligence Scale: Manual.* New York, Psychological Association, 1955.
25. Overall J, Hunter S, Butcher J: Factor structure of the MMPI-168 in a psychiatric population. *J Consult Clin Psychol* 41:284–286,1973.
26. Skinner HA, Allen BA: Alcohol dependence syndrome: Measurement and validation. *J Abnorm Psychol* 92:199–209, 1982.
27. Smart RG: Young alcoholics in treatment: Their characteristics and recovery rates at followup. *Alcohol Clin Exp Res* 3:19–23, 1979.
28. Fillmore KM, Midanik L: Chronicity of drinking problems among men: A longitudinal study. *J Stud Alcohol* 45:228–236, 1984.
29. Gibbs L, Flanagan J: Prognostic indicators of alcoholism treatment outcome. *Int J Addict* 12:1097–1141, 1977.

30. Ogborne AC: Patient characteristics as predictors of treatment outcome for alcohol and drug abuse, in Israel Y (ed): *Research Advances in Alcohol and Drug Problems.* New York, Plenum Press, 1978, p 177–223.
31. Hollingshead A: Two-factor index of social position. Unpublished manuscript, Department of Sociology, Yale University, 1957.
32. Wishart D: CLUSTAN 1c user manual (computer program and manual). London, Computer Center, University College, 1975.
33. Sneath PH: The application of computers to taxonomy. *J Gen Microbiol* 17:201–226, 1957.
34. Edelbrock C: Mixture model tests of hierarchical clustering algorithms: The problem of classifying everybody. *Multivar Behav Res 14:367–384, 1979.*
35. Ward J: Hierarchical grouping to optimize an objective function. *J Am Statistical Assoc* 58:236–244, 1963.
36. Wanberg K, Horn J, Foster F: A differential assessment model of alcoholism: The scales of the Alcohol Use Inventory. *J Stud Alcohol* 38:512–543, 1977.
37. Brodman K, Erdmann Jr. A, Wolff H: *Manual: Cornell Medical Index Health Questionnaire.* New York, Cornell University Medical College, 1949.
38. Donovan D, O'Leary M: The Drinking Related Locus of Control Scale: Reliability, factor structure and validity. *J Stud Alcohol* 39:759–784, 1978.
39. Beck A, Ward C, Mendelson M, Mock J, Erbaugh J: An inventory for measuring depression. *Arch Gen Psychiatry* 4:53–63, 1963.

III

The Alcohol Withdrawal Syndrome

Alfonso Paredes, Section Editor

Overview

Alfonso Paredes

The physiological and behavioral events that follow the cessation of drinking in an alcohol-dependent person deserve careful examination. Justifiably much interest has been focused on those clinical manifestations that appear within the first 7–10 days after drinking has ceased and in particular on the symptoms that constitute the acute withdrawal syndrome. Three categories of symptoms have attracted the interest of clinicians: Clouding of sensorium, tremor, and diaphoresis; hallucinations; and, in general, hyperexcitability of the central nervous system. It must be pointed out that most alcoholics experience only mild symptoms such as slight tremor and malaise and irritability following the cessation of drinking. Many do not report serious discomfort and only 1–15% exhibit severe symptoms such as delirium tremens.[1,2] Considering the fact that alcohol has marked effects on most organ systems we must postulate the existence of significant changes with long-lasting consequences. Changes may be expected at the molecular, neuroendocrine, and neuropharmacological levels. Several other physiological systems are also involved. Furthermore, there is the possibility that a protracted withdrawal period exists, characterized by physiological and behavioral disturbances that may last weeks and even months. The alterations during this period may have an impact on the clinical course of alcohol dependence. The chapters included in this section were designed with this perspective in mind. It is possible that a better understanding of the mechanisms affected during the period indicated, as well as improved methods of management, may impact favorably on aspects such as risk or relapse. A good knowledge of the mechanisms should be of importance even in the management of those alcohol-dependent individuals who do not give signs of serious discomfort or who appear relatively asymptomatic.

The chapters that constitute this section address the several levels affected during withdrawal. In Chapter 10, Goldstein reviews the withdrawal phenomena at the molecular level and examines some of the animal models. She indicates that after the development of tolerance and dependence, CNS hy-

Alfonso Paredes • Department of Psychiatry, The Neuropsychiatric Institute, Alcohol Research Center, University of California, Los Angeles, California 90024.

perexcitability follow the withdrawal from alcohol. This state of increased responsiveness may be conditioned by cell membrane changes. Spectrometric techniques such as electron spin resonance and fluorescence polarization reveal that cell membranes of ethanol-withdrawn animals are often abnormally rigid and resistant to ethanol-induced disorder. Chemical changes may also account for the altered physical properties of membranes. Perhaps there is an increase in cholesterol or changes in the ratio of saturated to unsaturated fatty acids in the phospholipid components of the membrane. Some of the alterations in neurotransmitter metabolism and release and in the characteristics of neuronal receptors during the alcohol withdrawal period may be related to the physical properties of the neuronal membranes.

Wilkins and Gorelick examine in Chapter 11 the neuropharmacologic and neuroendocrine mechanisms underlying the process of withdrawal. Among the neuropharmacologic aspects, a most interesting GABA–benzodiazepine–barbiturate complex interaction with alcohol is discussed.

The ubiquity of systems affected by alcohol is illustrated by the studies of endocrine systems reviewed by Wilkins and Gorelick. The two most important systems implicated are the hypothalamic-pituitary-adrenal (HPA) axis and the endogenous opiates (endorphines). These systems are affected by the acute and chronic exposure to alcohol and significant alterations following the discontinuance of the drug. Along these lines, increases have been observed in plasma cortisol and ACTH levels. Alcoholics during acute withdrawal show a blunted rise in plasma cortisol following insulin-induced hypoglycemia. Interestingly, this response may remain abnormal for 3 to 6 weeks after cessation of alcohol intake. Persistent dysfunction of the HPA axis has been further demonstrated in cases of alcohol induced pseudo-Cushing's syndrome.

The levels in the brain of the endogenous opiates β-endorphin and met-enkephalin are lowered during withdrawal from alcohol. The broad neuroendocrine changes taking place in alcoholics are illustrated by a recent study showing blunted TSH response to TRA stimulation in a group of alcoholics without depression or hepatic disease. Serum prolactin is initially decreased and then returns to normal in patients undergoing alcohol withdrawal. High vasopressin levels have been found in alcoholics with clinical symptoms of withdrawal. During alcohol ingestion vasopressin release is inhibited and a rebound effect is observed during withdrawal.

Dose–response relationships between CNS amine metabolism and the severity of alcohol withdrawal has been reported in experimental animals. This phenomenon explains the CNS hyperirritability. In humans there is a close relationship between the signs and symptoms of autonomic nervous system disturbance and increased central norepinephrine turnover. It is possible that changes in biogenic amines and their metabolites during acute withdrawal and the recovery phase may be related to the severity of the withdrawal syndrome. Other interesting effects reviewed by Wilkins and Gorelick are a decrease in β receptor binding activity during withdrawal. Also, a probable relationship has been found to exist between alcohol withdrawal syndrome delirium and decreased CNS dopaminergic activity. Finally it has been demonstrated that decreases in brain cyclic AMP levels occur during withdrawal.

In Chapter 12, Naranjo and Sellers review recent developments in the clinical assessment and nonpharmacologic and pharmacologic treatment of the alcohol withdrawal syndrome. This progress makes possible a more effective treatment of the syndrome. The objectives of therapy, the authors contend, should be the relief of subjective symptoms, prevention and treatment of the more severe complications, such as seizures, hallucinations, and delirium, and preparation of the patient for long-term rehabilitation. Within this scheme it is important to minimize the hazards of creating a new drug dependence or exposing the patient to direct drug-induced toxicity.

Treatment of alcohol withdrawal syndrome should be standardized, humane and as economical as possible. It should be based in a sound pharmacokinetic and pharmacodynamic rationale and meet good standards of safety and efficacy. This needs to be established by studies conducted with sound methodology.

The authors indicate that in the management of over two thirds of the uncomplicated cases of alcohol withdrawal, monitoring of signs and symptoms, personal attention, and general nursing care suffice. The treatment recommended includes the administration of vitamins particularly thiamine. The use of benzodiazepines is favored since these drugs have a cross-tolerance with alcohol and do not cause enzyme induction. A novel procedure is recommended for the detoxification process: the authors suggest loading doses of diazepam 20 mg administered hourly until the patient shows clinical improvements or becomes mildly sedated.

In Chapter 13, Gorelick and Wilkins have addressed issues of considerable clinical importance seldom considered in the literature. Among these included are the management of withdrawal in patients who have concurrent psychiatric illness or mixed substance dependence. Concurrent illness may precipitate withdrawal in most patients. Certain complications are of particular importance. In many patients, elevated blood pressure during acute withdrawal is a manifestation triggered by the cessation of drinking rather than a direct result of primary hypertension. Thus the diagnosis of primary hypertension and the initiation of antihypertensive medication may be unwarranted in many of these cases. If medication is used, it might be more appropriate to use an adrenergic agent such as clonidine or propanolol rather than a thiazide diuretic. Drug pharmacokinetics may be altered during withdrawal; changes in drug plasma protein binding have been found in patients who experience acute withdrawal. For example warfarin and propanolol binding are decreased while diazepam binding is increased.

Psychiatric symptoms complicate the clinical picture observed during withdrawal. Significant depression has been observed in as many of 98% of the alcoholic patients who appear for treatment. Depression may be misdiagnosed for primary disorder; however, the depressive pictures in alcoholics resolve spontaneously in most cases.

Important aspects of management have to be considered in patients who show dependence on alcohol and another (cross-tolerant) hypnotic drug and in cases of dependence on alcohol plus another (non-cross-tolerant) drug such as an opiate or a stimulant. In the first situation, the course of the withdrawal symptoms may be prolonged and resemble the course of alcohol withdrawal alone. A bimodal course may also be observed. In the case of combined alcohol–nonsedative withdrawal the clinical picture may be a mixture of alcohol and opiate or stimulant withdrawal syndromes. Valuable suggestions for the management of these syndromes are included.

An important possibility discussed is the existence of the protracted withdrawal mentioned earlier and its likely clinical implications. Lastly, the need for more studies on the influence of withdrawal and its management on the outcome of alcohol dependence is presented. There is already some evidence that suggests that patients who receive medically oriented treatment during withdrawal are more likely to remain in treatment for their addiction.

A final comment on an area not fully covered in the chapters following deserves mention. Cessation of drinking in an alcohol-dependent individual may have been precipitated by the discomfort caused by symptoms associated with drinking, by the threat to health, or by the social consequences of drinking excessively. Whatever the reasons might be, this is a period of crisis during which the patient becomes aware of his or her psychological vulnerability and of the social consequences of drinking. It is a time when the person with a relatively clear mind has an opportunity to decide to accept help and more importantly assess the decision to discontinue or change their drinking behavior. Several options may be considered at this time. A decision to discontinue drinking has many implications for the patient's pattern of social relationships. The need to accept many responsibilities that in the past may have been neglected may also become apparent. Appreciation of serious interpersonal problems are evident and major changes in life style will have to be considered. It is therefore not surprising that patients experience considerable stress and anxiety during this phase. There may be feelings of guilt, bewilderment, and fear. Patients may describe feelings such as "feeling torn apart inside," "want badly to scream," or manifest psychological and conflict through somatizations. For these patients alcohol has been a steady and reliable companion that will not be given up without a sense of loss or grief. The period of withdrawal therefore provides an opportunity to encourage the patient to accept help with the behavioral aspects of the dependence on alcohol and to structure a long-term rehabilitative plan. The concern, therefore, with the demands created by the physiological disturbances should not overlook the fact that the withdrawal phase is a critical point in the psychological treatment of alcohol dependence.

References

1. Gross MM, Lewis E, Hastey J: Acute alcohol withdrawal syndrome, in Kissin and Begleiter (eds): *Biology of Alcoholism*, vol 3, *Clinical Pathology*. New York, Plenum Press, 1978, p 195–256.
2. Gross MM, Lewis E, Best S, et al: Quantitative changes of signs and symptoms associated with alcohol withdrawal: Incidence severity and circadian effects in experimental studies in alcoholics. *Adv Exp Biol Med* 59:615–631, 1975.

10

The Alcohol Withdrawal Syndrome

A View from the Laboratory

Dora B. Goldstein

Abstract. Animal models of the alcohol-dependent state, now readily available in many species, show that a withdrawal reaction can be produced whenever intoxication has been continuously maintained, even for short periods of time. The development of the tolerant/dependent state resembles a physiological adaptation in two ways: (1) the animal is no longer much affected by the drug, and (2) withdrawal reveals a condition of CNS hyperexcitability that is the opposite of the primary drug effect. This adaptation is believed to arise in response to ethanol's disordering effect in cell membranes (increased membrane fluidity). Spectrometric techniques such as electron spin resonance and fluorescence polarization reveal that cell membranes of ethanol-withdrawn animals are often abnormally rigid and resistant to ethanol-induced disorder, and it is thought that these changes may correspond to physical dependence and tolerance, respectively. Alterations in the chemical composition of the membranes can often (but not always) explain the abnormal physical properties. The relation between membrane order and ethanol-induced behavioral states is not known in detail, but these observations form a basis for a rational picture of the biochemical changes responsible for the withdrawal syndrome.

1. Introduction

Even as late as the first half of this century, clinicians and researchers were puzzled by the observation that a serious illness often followed the termination of a period of alcohol intake. It was only after Himmelsbach[1] suggested an analogy to physiological adaptations that the process began to be understood. The withdrawal reaction displays a state that has been produced during a period of drug administration, a state that is masked by the actions of the drug and is eventually revealed because it outlasts the presence of the drug in the body. The production of this dependent state is a predictable effect of the drug under appropriate conditions. Therefore, a withdrawal reaction can be studied by any of the pharmacological techniques used for the investigation of the direct effects of drugs, even though the events under observation occur after removal of the drug rather than during its period of action. Time courses, dose relations, and mechanisms of action are suitable topics for investigation.

Dora B. Goldstein • Department of Pharmacology, Stanford University School of Medicine, Stanford, California 94305.

The withdrawal reaction is more difficult to study than are acute effects of drugs only because the doses are more difficult to define. The effective dose that determines the severity of the ensuing withdrawal syndrome is the product of the drug concentration at its target site and the duration of its presence there. In addition it is important to consider the timing of the exposure to the drug, whether continuous or intermittent, because some degree of recovery may occur during periods when the drug is absent.

Animal models of a great variety are now readily available for study of this syndrome. The methodological aspects of these models have been reviewed.[2–4] Many biochemical, neurochemical, and endocrinological changes have been noted in such models. These must be important for the health of the subject, but we do not yet understand how they fit together or in what manner they have been evoked by ethanol.[5] By contrast, the alterations in the physical properties of membranes are the subject of a relatively coherent body of information that is agreed upon by most workers. Physical chemical methods unequivocally show that ethanol disorders the structure of biomembranes *in vitro*, and a compensatory change in the physical condition of membrane lipids can often be demonstrated after withdrawal of chronically administered ethanol. Whereas the physical change is reproducible in different models, it seems to be accompanied by different kinds of chemical alterations in the composition of membrane lipids. It is reasonable to ascribe these diverse adjustments to the same telic process, an attempt to retain a normal degree of membrane fluidity despite the presence of ethanol. This concept can be dealt with under the rubric of the homeostat hypothesis, the notion that cells adapt to any persistent, drug-induced disruption by the same physiological mechanisms they have available for offsetting a change in the external environment. On this basis, we can predict that adaptation to ethanol takes place in cell membranes.

2. Animal Models

The experimental production of an authentic alcohol withdrawal reaction in human subjects by Isbell *el al.*[6] in 1955 and the detailed analysis of its clinical manifestations by Victor and Adams at about the same time[7] opened the way for rational study of the syndrome. Isbell's experimental design assured that the subjects were kept in a state of continuous intoxication throughout the period of drug administration. This principle turned out to be the key to the long-sought animal models of physical dependence. When, in 1968, Essig and Lam[8] kept dogs intoxicated day and night for a few weeks, an alcohol withdrawal reaction was recognized in animals for the first time. Since then, many such models have been developed in a wide variety of species. Physical dependence can be produced when ethanol is administered in a liquid diet, by intubation, intraperitoneally, or by inhalation, but it is difficult to produce this state when the alcohol intake is limited to the amounts that animals will voluntarily consume in their drinking water.

The possibility of confounding alcohol effects with those of malnutrition is a frequent concern in this research. The two conditions often occur together, both in the lab and on the ward. Among the animal models, the liquid diet method of alcohol administration provides the best available control of nutrition. Here the controls are pair-fed a diet that is isocaloric with the ethanol diet but contains another carbohydrate (such as sucrose) replacing the ethanol. Thus, the controls eat little if the ethanol-treated animals are off their feed. Perfect nutritional controls do not exist because ethanol can interfere with the absorption (not just the ingestion) of nutrients.

Timing is important. Physical dependence apparently develops progressively during the periods when the drug is present in the body and it subsides quickly during interludes of sobriety. At least in mice, the dependent state arises extremely rapidly, in a matter of hours, and decays again with a similar time course when ethanol is withdrawn.[9] A mild but definite withdrawal reaction can be seen after a single dose of ethanol[9–10] (an observation that suggests that withdrawal hyperexcitability may contribute to hangover and to disruption of sleep after an evening's drinking). But a single daily injection of ethanol, even when continued over a long time, does not suffice to evoke a severe dependent state. What does suffice is to maintain elevated blood ethanol concentrations continuously over a period of days. The alcohol must be given in many small doses each day to avoid exceeding lethal levels. Success depends upon arranging some method of feedback control so that the individual animals that are already strongly intoxicated do not receive maximum doses at the next time point. This is often done by grading the doses according to the degree of intoxication of each animal.[11] In experiments where ethanol is administered in a liquid diet,[12] the animals are simply unable to continue drinking when they are severely intoxicated. In some inhalation models pyrazole is used to control the blood ethanol levels by inhibiting alcohol dehydrogenase competitively with ethanol.[13] The necessity for maintaining continuous intoxication in these models is evidence that the dependent state subsides rapidly after elimination of the ethanol. The rate of decay of this state has also been measured directly, but the generalizability of the results is in doubt. In our experiments with mice,[9] there is no cumulation of the intensity of withdrawal reactions in successive cycles of intoxication and withdrawal if the interval between cycles is more than a day, indicating that recovery was complete in about 24 hr. But other investigators have evidence for "carryover" of dependence during intervals as long as 2 or 3 weeks between periods of intoxication.[14] This important point has not been resolved by the animal models. Poldrugo and Snead[15] suggest that carryover may be a manifestation of kindling, i.e., a progressive, long-term increase in CNS excitability following repeated episodes of convulsions. Clinicians often observe that the abstinence syndrome becomes progressively more severe in individual patients after repeated binges and they ascribe this change to carryover,[16] but other explanations are possible, including a tendency to drink ever larger amounts of alcohol during successive binges.

The withdrawal reaction in animals is complex but several of its components can be scored at least semiquantitatively. The signs most easily identified are those of CNS hyperactivity such as tremor and convulsions. Scoring systems have been developed, including detailed, reliable schemes worked out by Majchrowicz for rats[11] and by Okamoto for studies of barbiturate and ethanol dependence in cats.[17,18] Mice often have spontaneous convulsions in the alcohol withdrawal state but rats are much less likely to do so; audiogenic seizures are commonly elicited and scored in rat models.[19] Mice (and sometimes rats) convulse when picked up by the tail in this and other states of hyperexcitability; this provides the basis for a commonly used rating system for ethanol withdrawal in these species.[20] Gross and his co-workers developed a quantitative scheme for scoring the alcohol withdrawal reaction in humans.[21]

The severity of the graded withdrawal syndrome in animals is dose-related, according to the alcohol exposure (blood levels × time).[20] Thus, a blood level of 300 mg% for one day produces a withdrawal reaction of about the same severity as a blood level of 100 mg% maintained for 3 days. After a week or two of intoxication the severity of the withdrawal reaction reaches a plateau.[9] The most useful models are those in which the alcohol exposure can be varied so that biochemical correlates of different degrees of dependence can be studied. Few models are sufficiently versatile, however.

An animal's genetic makeup strongly influences the severity of its withdrawal convulsions after a standard alcohol exposure. For example, when mice were subjected to two successive (well-separated) cycles of intoxication and withdrawal, individual animals with consistently high withdrawal scores and others with consistently low scores could be identified. Breeding the high-scoring males with high-scoring females and the lows with lows produced offspring whose sensitivity to withdrawal convulsions matched that of their parents.[22] By this method, Crabbe and co-workers have been breeding lines of withdrawal syndrome-prone and withdrawal syndrome-resistant mice for use in biochemical studies.[23] The long-sleep and short-sleep lines of mice that were selectively bred for differences in sensitivity to the hypnotic effect of ethanol also differ greatly in intensity of withdrawal reactions; the short-sleep mice have much higher withdrawal scores than the long-sleep mice.[24] Thus it is reasonable to expect that the intensity of the withdrawal reaction in patients will be affected not only by the alcohol dose but also by the individual's genetic background.

The nature of the withdrawal reaction in animals resembles only a part of the more complex human abstinence syndrome. None of the animal models can reproduce the characteristic time course of the human withdrawal reaction, which begins to develop as soon as the blood alcohol falls below the level maintained during the binge and gets worse progressively for a length of time that seems to be dependent on the alcohol dose. If the dose has been high and the binge prolonged, the syndrome progresses to delirium tremens, which is a subjective state of disorientation that cannot be recognized in animal models. Although there is some evidence of hallucinatory behavior in animals,[8] an animal version of an entire withdrawal syndrome has never been produced.

3. Ethanol Dependence as an Adaptation

When the continuous presence of a drug in the tissues disrupts their function, the body is likely to adjust itself in a compensatory manner. Just as in a physiological adaptation, the organism may use different responses simultaneously or in succession. Some changes are presumably suitable primarily for dealing with an emergency whereas other mechanisms are more efficient for use over the long haul. What they have in common is the ability to offset the original disruption.

Applying this notion to ethanol, we begin with the observation that ethanol increases the fluidity of cell membranes. This concentration-related effect can be seen with EPR,[25] fluorescence polarization,[26] differential scanning calorimetry,[27] and optical methods.[28] Other aliphatic alcohols also disorder membranes; their potencies in this respect increase with chain length, presumably reflecting their increasing lipid solubility. Furthermore, the disruption of membrane structure *in vitro* seems closely related to the ability of alcohols to cause intoxication. Longer chain alcohols are more potent as hypnotics for mice in proportion to their increased ability to disorder membranes.[29] Mice of different degrees of sensitivity to intoxication, obtained by genetic selection or by prior treatment with ethanol, are found to have synaptosomal plasma membranes with corresponding differences. The more sensitive mice have the more sensitive membranes, relatively easily disordered by ethanol *in vitro* compared to membranes taken from alcohol-resistant animals.[30] Thus, it appears possible that membrane disorder affects membrane function in such a way as to cause intoxication. This disorder might be the abnormality to which an animal adapts. Membranes may be the site of the compensatory changes. One would expect membranes to become more rigid during the period of ethanol administration, offsetting the alcohol-induced disorder, and perhaps to retain the rigidity into the withdrawal period after the ethanol has been eliminated. A similar adaptation in poikilotherms allows them to stiffen their membranes to offset increased ambient temperature, a process called homeoviscous adaptation.[31] Could this stiffness counteract the alcohol-induced disorder and thus account for tolerance? Could it cause neuronal hyperexcitability and thus explain the withdrawal reaction?

4. Chemical and Physical Changes in the Withdrawal Period

Focussing on the cell membrane, several investigators have observed changes that are similar to those predicted by the concept of homeoviscous adaptation, although more complex. Just as the disordering effect of ethanol occurs in any membrane, the changes seen after withdrawal can be found in many tissues.

The physical changes consist of increased rigidity of membranes and resistance to ethanol-induced disordering *in vitro*. Synaptosomal plasma membranes from alcohol-treated mice or rats are more rigid than controls. In our laboratory this effect has been seen with the spin probe 12-doxylstearic acid[32] and the fluorescent probe diphenylhexatriene,[33] both of which send signals from sites deep in the bilayer, but not with 5-doxylstearic acid, a label that resides nearer the surface.[32] Other investigators report that the increased rigidity of synaptosomal membranes from alcohol-treated mice can be observed with surface probes as well as deep ones. Harris *et al.*[34] have seen this effect in fluorescence polarization experiments with several probes, including one (TMS-DPH) that labels the surface polar groups of the membrane. Similarly, liver microsomes[35] and (less convincingly) liver mitochondrial membranes[36,37] from chronically ethanol-treated rats show increased order parameters with 5-doxylstearic acid. Thus, abnormal rigidity of membranes in animals treated chronically with ethanol is a common finding.

Spectroscopic techniques such as electron spin resonance or fluorescence polarization sometimes reveal a form of ethanol tolerance in membranes. Addition of alcohol to membranes from animals that have been chronically treated with ethanol produces less than the usual amount of disordering. This membrane tolerance has been seen with synaptosomal plasma membranes,[32,34,36,38] and some intracellular membranes.[35,37] Two reports disagree as to whether the membrane tolerance can[39] or cannot[34] be seen in lipid extracts of membranes from treated animals, so it is not yet clear whether tolerance is mediated by lipids or by proteins. In some reports, an associated tolerance to the disruption of membrane function by ethanol *in vitro* has been described, e.g., calcium transport in microsomes.[35] The reduction in the response to ethanol can perhaps be explained by decreased solubility of ethanol in these membranes; Rottenberg *et al.*[36] have directly measured a reduction in the partition coefficient of ethanol and halothane in membranes from alcohol-treated rats. It is thought that ethanol may be excluded from the membranes as a result of their increased order.

Chemical changes must be present to account for the altered physical properties of the membranes, but it has been difficult to define them consistently. The most obvious possibilities are an increase in cholesterol or in the ratio of saturated to unsaturated fatty acids in the phospholipids. Cholesterol is known to increase the order of biomembranes under most conditions, and it has also been shown to decrease the response of membranes to ethanol.[40] Thus, an increase in membrane cholesterol would be an appropriate adaptation. Under some conditions, ethanol administration does cause an increase in the cholesterol content of plasma membranes in the brain[39,41,42] or liver.[43] No such change was seen in liver mitochondria, which contain very little cholesterol.[37] Furthermore, tolerant and dependent mice can be produced whose synaptosomal plasma membranes are rigid and resistant to ethanol but do not contain excess cholesterol.[32,34] Besides cholesterol, the other likely possibility is increased saturation of fatty acid acyl chains, which makes membranes more ordered. This is the mechanism by which microorganisms and fish achieve homeoviscous adaptation. This change has also been observed in mouse brain[44] and rat liver[37] after chronic alcohol treatment but less reproducibly than the sterol changes. In contrast, other workers reported that acyl chains become more unsaturated after chronic alcohol administration,[45] and in one laboratory the changes in fatty acid composition of erythrocytes were in opposite directions in two replications of the same experiment.[46,47] Such data do not rule out the concept of homeoviscous adaptation, which is a mechanism for maintaining a constant degree of membrane order in the face of disordering influences such as ethanol or warming. This adaptation may be accomplished by means of various chemical changes, some of which have probably not yet been examined. To test this hypothesis we measure membrane order first—if we find a change then we may be able to explain it by examining the chemical composition of the membranes.

Changes in phospholipid head groups do not seem to be relevant in this connection. Gangliosides may be important, though. Harris and co-workers have recently reported that addition of rat brain gangliosides to model membranes dramatically increased their sensitivity to ethanol.[48] This suggests that the ganglioside fraction, which has received little attention and is usually discarded in the "upper phase" when lipid extracts are prepared, may be an important determinant of membrane order, especially in the presence of drugs. However, Harris *et al.*[34] did not detect any change in the brain membrane ganglioside fractions in rats that had been chronically treated with ethanol.

The concept that the alcohol withdrawal syndrome inheres in membranes is attractive, especially under conditions where cholesterol increases, because the observations fit together well and make sense. However, it is not universally accepted and much more evidence is needed. A relationship between membrane disorder and intoxication (or anesthesia) is plausible but not proven. The probes measure very small drug-induced changes in the motion of membrane lipids, whereas larger effects on hydrophobic portions of proteins would perhaps better explain the gross behavioral changes of ethanol intoxication and withdrawal. Any theory of the mechanism of action of ethanol must be quite general, since physical effects, not chemically specific ones, are invoked. But this generality makes it difficult to test. One does not know which proteins to examine because most membrane-bound proteins are likely to be affected by any substance that reduces membrane order. Although we can show excellent correlations between membrane disordering and intoxication, and we can demonstrate a "withdrawal state" in membranes that is opposite to the disordered condition that prevails during intoxication, we ignore hundreds or thousands of steps in a causative chain of disrupted function in membranes, synapses, neurons, and pathways. We have not yet even defined the second step, the direct result of membrane disorder on membrane function.

Neurochemists describe a great variety of alterations in neurotransmitter metabolism and release and in the characteristics of neuronal receptors during the ethanol withdrawal period.[5,49] All the known transmitters are affected. It is not clear which of these changes are directly related to the physical properties of neuronal membranes although it is reasonable to suppose that increased membrane order in the dependent state would influence the processing of transmitters in many ways. Some of the neurochemical abnormalities are doubtless the result rather than the cause of the withdrawal hyperexcitability but at present it is not possible to say which is which.

The alcohol withdrawal reaction in humans includes many aspects not directly related to adaptation to ethanol, such as the effects of impaired liver function, trauma, infection, and malnutrition. It will be difficult to analyze in detail. But understanding of the central pathology may come from animal studies and may lead to prevention or more rational treatment of the abstinence syndrome.

References

1. Himmelsbach CK: Can the euphoric, analgetic and physical dependence effects of drugs be separated? IV. With reference to physical dependence. *Fed Proc* 2:201–203, 1943.
2. Goldstein DB: Animal studies of alcohol withdrawal reactions, in Israel Y, Glaser FB, Kalant H, et al (eds): *Research Advances in Alcohol and Drug Problems,* vol 4. New York, Plenum Publishing Co, 1978, pp 77–109.
3. Cicero TJ: Alcohol self-administration, tolerance and withdrawal in humans and animals: theoretical and methodological issues, in Rigter H, Crabbe JC, Jr (eds): *Alcohol Tolerance and Dependence.* Amsterdam, Elsevier/North Holland, 1980, pp 1–51.
4. Friedman HJ: Assessment of physical dependence on and withdrawal from ethanol in animals, in Rigter H, Crabbe JC, Jr (eds): *Alcohol Tolerance and Dependence.* Amsterdam, Elsevier/North Holland, 1980, pp 93–121.
5. Goldstein DB: *Pharmacology of Alcohol.* New York, Oxford University Press, 1983.
6. Isbell H, Fraser HF, Wikler A, et al: An experimental study of the etiology of 'rum fits' and delirium tremens. *Q J Stud Alcohol* 16:1–33, 1955.
7. Victor M, Adams RD: The effect of alcohol on the nervous system. *Res Publ Assoc Res Nerv Ment Dis* 32:526–573, 1953.
8. Essig CF, Lam RC: Convulsions and hallucinatory behavior following alcohol withdrawal in the dog. *Arch Neurol* 18:626–632, 1968.
9. Goldstein DB: Rates of onset and decay of alcohol physical dependence in mice. *J Pharmacol Exp Ther* 190:377–383, 1974.
10. McQuarrie DG, Fingle E: Effects of single doses and chronic administration of ethanol on experimental seizures in mice. *J Pharmacol Exp Ther* 124:264–271, 1958.
11. Majchrowicz E: Induction of physical dependence upon ethanol and the associated behavioral changes in rats. *Psychopharmacologia* 43:245–254, 1975.
12. Ritzmann RF, Tabakoff B: Body temperature in mice: A quantitative measure of alcohol tolerance and physical dependence. *J Pharmacol Exp Ther* 199:158–170, 1976.
13. Goldstein DB: Inhalation of ethanol vapor, in Rigter H, Crabbe JC, Jr (eds): *Alcohol Tolerance and Dependence.* Amsterdam, Elsevier/North Holland, 1980, pp 81–92.
14. Branchey M, Rauscher G, Kissin B: Modifications in the response to alcohol following the establishment of physical dependence. *Psychopharmacologia* 22:314–322, 1971.
15. Poldrugo F, Sneal OC III: Electroencephalographic and behavioral correlates in rats during repeated ethanol withdrawal syndromes. *Psychopharmacology* 83:140–146, 1984.
16. Gross MM, Hastey JM, Lewis E, et al: Slow wave sleep and carry-over of functional tolerance and physical dependence in alcoholics. *Adv Exp Med Biol* 59:477–493, 1975.
17. Okamoto M, Rosenberg HC, Boisse NR: Withdrawal characteristics following chronic pentobarbital dosing in cat. *Eur J Pharmacol* 40:107–119, 1976.
18. Okamoto M, Hinman DJ, Aaronson LM: Comparison of ethanol and barbiturate physical dependence. *J Pharmacol Exp Ther* 218:701–708, 1981.

19. Falk JL, Samson HH, Winger G: Behavioral maintenance of high concentrations of blood ethanol and physical dependence in the rat. *Science* 177:811–813, 1972.
20. Goldstein DB: Relationship of alcohol dose to intensity of withdrawal signs in mice. *J Pharmacol Exp Ther* 180:203–215, 1972.
21. Gross MM, Lewis E, Nagarajan M: An improved quantitative system for assessing the acute alcoholic psychoses and related states (TSA and SSA). *Adv Exp Med Biol* 35:365–376, 1973.
22. Goldstein DB: Inherited differences in intensity of alcohol withdrawal reactions in mice. *Nature* 245:154–156, 1973.
23. Crabbe JC, Kosobud A, Young ER: Genetic selection for ethanol withdrawal severity: Differences in replicate mouse lines. *Life Sci* 33:955–962, 1983.
24. Goldstein DB, Kakihana R: Alcohol withdrawal reactions in mouse strains selectively bred for long or short sleep time. *Life Sci* 17:981–986, 1975.
25. Chin JH, Goldstein DB: Effects of low concentrations of ethanol on the fluidity of spin-labeled erythrocyte and brain membranes. *Mol Pharmacol* 13:435–441, 1977.
26. Harris, RA, Schroeder F: Ethanol and the physical properties of brain membranes. Fluorescence studies. *Mol Pharmacol* 20:128–137, 1981.
27. Jain MK, Gleeson J, Upreti A, et al: Intrinsic perturbing ability of alkanols in lipid bilayers. *Biochim Biophys Acta* 509:1–8, 1978.
28. Rowe ES: The effects of ethanol on the thermotropic properties of dipalmitoylphosphatidylcholine. *Mol Pharmacol* 22:133–139, 1982.
29. Lyon RC, McComb JA, Schreurs J, et al: A relationship between alcohol intoxication and the disordering of brain membranes by a series of short-chain alcohols. *J Pharmacol Exp Ther* 218:669–675, 1981.
30. Goldstein DB, Chin JH, Lyon RC: Ethanol disordering of spin-labeled mouse brain membranes: Correlation with genetically determined ethanol sensitivity of mice. *Proc Natl Acad Sci USA* 79:4231–4233, 1982.
31. Sinensky M: Homeoviscous adaptation—a homeostatic process that regulates the viscosity of membrane lipids in *Escherichia coli*. *Proc Natl Acad Sci USA* 71:522–525, 1974.
32. Lyon RC, Goldstein DB: Changes in synaptic membrane order associated with chronic ethanol treatment in mice. *Mol Pharmacol* 23:86–91, 1983.
33. Perlman BJ, Goldstein DB: Ethanol and sodium valproate disordering of membranes from chronic ethanol treated mice. *Fed Proc* 42:2123, 1983.
34. Harris RA, Baxter DM, Mitchell MA, et al: Physical properties and lipid composition of brain membranes from ethanol tolerant-dependent mice. *Mol Pharmacol* 25:401–409, 1984.
35. Ponnappa BC, Waring AJ, Hoek JB, et al: Chronic ethanol ingestion increases calcium uptake and resistance to molecular disordering by ethanol in liver microsomes. *J Biol Chem* 257:10141–10146, 1982.
36. Rottenberg H, Waring A, Rubin E: Tolerance and cross-tolerance in chronic alcoholics: Reduced membrane binding of ethanol and other drugs. *Science* 213:583–585, 1981.
37. Waring AJ, Rottenberg H, Ohnishi T, et al: Membranes and phospholipids of liver mitochondria from chronic alcoholic rats are resistant to membrane disordering by alcohol. *Proc Natl Acad Sci USA* 78:2582–2586, 1981.
38. Chin JH, Goldstein DB: Drug tolerance in biomembranes: A spin label study of the effects of ethanol. *Science* 196:684–685, 1977.
39. Johnson DA, Lee NM, Cooke R, et al: Ethanol-induced fluidization of brain lipid bilayers: Required presence of cholesterol in membranes for the expression of tolerance. *Mol Pharmacol* 15:739–746, 1979.
40. Chin JH, Goldstein DB: Membrane-disordering action of ethanol: Variation with membrane cholesterol content and depth of the spin label probe. *Mol Pharmacol* 19:425–431, 1981.
41. Chin JH, Parsons LM, Goldstein DB: Increased cholesterol content of erythrocyte and brain membranes in ethanol-tolerant mice. *Biochim Biophys Acta* 513:358–363, 1978.
42. Smith TL, Gerhart MJ: Alterations in brain lipid composition of mice made physically dependent to ethanol. *Life Sci* 31:1419–1425, 1982.

43. Smith TL, Vickers AE, Brendel K, et al: Effects of ethanol diets on cholesterol content and phospholipid acyl composition of rat hepatocytes. *Lipids* 17:124–128, 1982.
44. Littleton JM, John G: Synaptosomal membrane lipids of mice during continuous exposure to ethanol. *J Pharm Pharmacol* 29:579–580, 1977.
45. Sun GY, Sun AY: Effect of chronic ethanol administration on phospholipid acyl groups of synaptic plasma membrane fraction isolated from guinea pig brain. *Res Commun Chem Path Pharmacol* 24:405–408, 1979.
46. Wing DR, Harvey DJ, Hughes J, et al: Effects of chronic ethanol administration on the composition of membrane lipids in the mouse. *Biochem Pharmacol* 31:3431–3439, 1982.
47. Wing DR, Harvey DJ, Belcher, SJ, et al: Changes in membrane lipid content after chronic ethanol administration with respect to fatty acyl composition and phospholipid type. *Biochem Pharmacol* 33:1625–1632, 1984.
48. Harris RA, Groh GI, Baxter DM, et al: Gangliosides enhance the membrane actions of ethanol and pentobarbital. *Mol Pharmacol* 25:410–417, 1984.
49. Tabakoff B, Hoffman PL: Alcohol and neurotransmitters, in Rigter H, Crabbe JC Jr (eds): *Alcohol Tolerance and Dependence.* Amsterdam, Elsevier/North Holland, 1980, pp 201–226.

11

Clinical Neuroendocrinology and Neuropharmacology of Alcohol Withdrawal

Jeffery N. Wilkins and David A. Gorelick

Abstract. A number of alcohol research groups have measured anterior and posterior pituitary hormones, the endogenous opiates, CNS peptides, and putative neurotransmitters during alcohol withdrawal. The data are often complex and contradictory, though a number of themes have emerged. Activity of the hypothalamic–pituitary–adrenal axis (HPA) is increased during chronic alcohol exposure and appears to remain altered for at least 2 to 4 weeks after cessation of drinking. There is increased turnover of norepinephrine and enhanced binding of CNS adrenergic receptors. By contrast, there are decreases in CNS activity of select endogenous opiates and GABA. Other CNS compounds that may play a role in alcohol withdrawal are prolactin, thyrotropin-releasing hormone (TRH), vasopressin, cyclic 3′5′-adenosine monophophate (cAMP), Delta-sleep-inducing peptide (DSIP), and iron. Despite many studies in humans and animals, the roles of CNS dopamine and serotonin in withdrawal remain unclear. A number of peptides, including cholecystokinin (CCK), neurotensin, and bombesin, have been shown to interact with the CNS actions of alcohol and may play a role in alcohol withdrawal. Inadequate work has been performed on acetylcholine (ACh), human growth hormone (HGH) and luteinizing hormone (LH).

Studies of the recently identified GABA-benzodiazepine-barbituate receptor complex indicate that this system is likely to be involved in the pathophysiology of alcohol withdrawal. Perturbation studies with corticotropin-releasing factor (CRF) and TRH (with measures of ACTH and cortisol and TSH and prolactin, respectively), may identify patients with withdrawal-related autonomic dysfunction.

1. Introduction

Advances in measurements of CNS-regulated hormones (neuroendocrinology) and neurotransmitters (neuropharmacology) now allow for more highly refined studies to be conducted of alcohol withdrawal. Improvements in study

Jeffery N. Wilkins • Crisis Oriented Psychiatric Evaluation Service, Clinical Psychopharmacology Unit, Brentwood Division, West Los Angeles Veterans Administration Medical Center, Los Angeles, California 90073; and Department of Psychiatry, School of Medicine, University of Los Angeles, Los Angeles, California 90024. **David A. Gorelick** • Alcohol and Drug Treatment Program, Behavioral Pharmacology Laboratory, West Los Angeles Veterans Administration Medical Center, Los Angeles, California 90073; and Department of Psychiatry, School of Medicine, University of Los Angeles, Los Angeles, California 90024.

design and methodology have paralleled the advances in biotechnology. The goal of the following review of human and animal studies is to determine whether the results of current studies (1) assist the clinician in treatment decisions (including choice of and duration of treatment and prediction of complications, e.g. seizures and delirium tremens) and (2) provide insight into the complex reaction of the CNS to the abrupt removal of a chronic exogenous substance (e.g., alcohol).

In this review we (1) outline a number of proposed biological models of withdrawal, (2) relate the results from hormone and neurotransmitter studies of withdrawal to these models, (3) present a model involving the recently discovered GABA–benzodiazepine–barbituate receptor complex, and (4) offer suggestions for related future research, including the potential use of perturbation techniques in testing the function of hormone and neurotransmitter systems in patients who have recently stopped drinking. The review includes source material from the Medline Data Base (1966–1984) of the National Library of Medicine.

1.1. Background

Several investigators[1–5] have theoretically linked the pathophysiology of withdrawal with that of alcohol tolerance and dependence. Cicero[4] has postulated that acute and chronic alcohol administration are on a "biological continuum" and that alcohol produces its immediate pharmacological effect by altering the activity of biological systems. Beginning with the first administration and continuing through chronic exposure, the systems gradually adapt to alcohol. Thus, more alcohol is required to produce an equivalent effect (tolerance), and the continued presence of alcohol is required to maintain the status quo of the biological system (physical dependence). If the alcohol is removed, a disruption of this balance occurs (withdrawal). The models discussed below are differentiated by the presumed location of alcohol-induced pathophysiology. The reader is referred to Chapter 10 by Goldstein for a more in-depth review of models of alcohol withdrawal.

For the purposes of this chapter we assume the following: (1) the development of withdrawal behavior in an organism, after cessation of exposure to alcohol, indicates the presence of physical dependence; (2) the CNS mechanisms of tolerance, dependence, and withdrawal overlap; (3) altered neurotransmitter activity and hormone levels seen during alcohol withdrawal are the result of adaptations performed by the CNS during chronic alcohol exposure; and (4) the time required for hormone and neurotransmitter systems to return to prealcohol baseline reflects the time required for the brain to "heal" from the insult of alcohol.

1.2. CNS Models of Alcohol Withdrawal

1.2.1. Neurotransmitter Synthesis. Goldstein and Goldstein[2] have postulated that alcohol may inhibit a rate-limiting enzyme necessary in the biosynthesis of a neurotransmitter. They believe that depressed production of the affected neurotransmitter results in the acute effects of alcohol. Alteration of feedback inhibition would therefore occur over time, and this would result in an increase in synthesis and release of the neurotransmitter. More alcohol would then be required to suppress this neurotransmitter synthetic machinery (tolerance). Abrupt cessation of alcohol exposure would allow this increased activity to proceed unchecked for a certain period time (withdrawal).

1.2.2. Postsynaptic Receptor. Collier[1] proposes that alcohol exerts its effects through a postsynaptic receptor site. Disruption in feedback regulation results in an increase in the number of postsynaptic receptors (formed via protein synthesis). Tolerance results when the number of receptors produced has achieved a homeostatic receptor–neurotransmitter balance, leading to a maintained level of function. Withdrawal ensues when the antagonist (alcohol) is removed, and an increased number of receptors are available to interact with the normal secretion of transmitter. This model of increased receptor quantity assumes that the postsynaptic cell requires a minimum number of receptors to be bound before an action potential can be initiated.

1.2.3. Potentiation of Neural Activity. Post and Ballenger[6] suggest that each episode of alcohol withdrawal, with its concomitant hyperexcitability in the CNS, contributes to the development of kindling and subsequently to the symptomatology of alcohol withdrawal, including seizures. Kindling is a CNS process whereby repeated electrical or chemical stimulation of a brain region leads to a decreased seizure threshold in that region.[7–9] It is possible, however that kindling may also occur as a consequence of repeated exposures to alcohol per se. Pinel and Van Oot[10] and Pinel and Cheung[11] have reported that amygdala-kindled animals had corresponding increases in severity of alcohol withdrawal behaviors (see Chapter 13 by Gorelick and Wilkins).

1.2.4. Neuronal Membrane. Hill and Bangham[3] propose that alcohol may increase the fluidity of neuronal membranes by its effects on phospholipids, causing a "disordering" of membrane function. A compensatory mechanism would "stiffen" the membrane via the addition of more structural proteins, thus restoring proper function (tolerance). Cessation of alcohol exposure would result in over-rigidity of the membrane, leading to CNS dysfunction (withdrawal).

1.2.5. Discussion. The models of alcohol withdrawal outlined above assume that during withdrawal there is either altered neurotransmitter synthesis and/or neurotransmitter receptor binding (models 1 and 2), facilitation of neurophysiological activity of specific neural pathways (model 3), or altered cellular function of the neurons through changes at the membrane level (model 4). Studies reviewed in Section 3 present data consistent with the neurotransmitter receptor binding and synthesis models, but do not support the membrane model. There is no direct evidence supporting the kindling hypothesis, although some anecdotal clinical findings are consistent with it (see Chapter 13 by Gorelick and Wilkins).

Since these models were proposed, exciting work has been conducted in the neurophysiology and neuropharmacology of the recently described

GABA–benzodiazepine–barbituate receptor complex (GBB). Studies of the interactions of alcohol with this receptor complex are constistent with the assumptions of the two neurotransmitter models and the kindling model. Involvement of the GBB could also account for the well-established clinical usefulness of sedative/hypnotics in the treatment of alcohol withdrawal (see Chapter 12 by Naranjo and Sellers).

2. Neuroendocrine Aspects of Alcohol Withdrawal

Acute and chronic administration of alcohol has been shown to significantly alter circulating levels of most hormones studied in humans and animals.[12,13] The discussion below covers most hormone systems, with special focus on the HPA axis, the endorphins, and newly identified peptides (see Tables I, II, and III). The material is organized into two divisions: (1) what occurs in the hormonal or neuropharmacological system during withdrawal, and (2) what effect manipulation of the hormonal or neuropharmacological system has on withdrawal.

2.1. Hypothalamic-Pituitary Adrenal Axis

During acute alcohol withdrawal, significant increases are seen in plasma levels of adrenal cortex hormones in the blood of animals[14–21] and humans[22–24] (Table I). Adrenal-corticotropic hormone (ACTH) is increased in humans[25];

Table I. Substances That Increase or Decrease during Alcohol Withdrawal

Increase	Decrease
Hormones	
ACTH (rat brain)	CSF β-endorphin (human)
ACTH (human blood)	Met-enkephalin (rat brain)
Cortisol (human blood)	MSH (rat pituitary)
Corticosterone (rat blood)	ACTH (rat pituitary)
Vasopressin (human blood)	Prolactin (human blood)
	TSH response to TRH (humans)
Neurotransmitters	
CSF NOR (human)	GABA (mouse brain)
Urinary NOR (human)	
CSF MHPG (human)	
CNS β-receptor activity	
Platelet MAO (human)	
Other	
cGMP	cAMP
Adenylate cyclase	
Iron (human blood)	
Ferritin	

Table II. Percent DST Nonsuppression at 4 and 11 PM in Alcoholics during Periods of Abstinence

No. of Subjects	Ref.	Week 1	Week 3	Week 4	Week 6
52	32	21%	0%	—	
43	35	33%	—	—	
14	38	64%	—	—	
83	39	19%	—	2 of 6 patients[a]	
72	40	28%	—	—	—
8	40	—		62% at 3–6 weeks	
72	41	—		28% at 3–6 weeks[b]	
75	42	23%	—	—	0%
30	43	63%	—	10%	—
32	44	20%	—	0%	—

[a] Six of initial 16 DST nonsuppressed patients retested at 4 weeks

[b] 4 PM only

this finding is consistent with depletions found in ACTH in mouse[26] and rat[27] pituitary. If alcohol is administered during withdrawal, plasma cortisol values return to normal.[24] In rare cases, chronic alcohol intake can induce a pseudo-Cushing's syndrome.[28–30]

Convergent lines of evidence indicate persistance of HPA dysfunction in the human after cessation of alcohol intake. For example, during acute withdrawal alcoholics manifested a blunted rise in plasma cortisol following insulin-induced hypoglycemia.[31] This response remained abnormal for 3–6 weeks

Table III. Neuropharmacologic Substances That Alleviate or Worsen Symptoms and Signs of Alcohol Withdrawal

Alleviate Withdrawal	Worsen Withdrawal
Neurotransmitters	
Dopamine (rat brain)	6 Hydroxydopamine (rat brain)
GABA (rat brain)	NOR (rat brain)
L-DOPA (mice)	5-HT (rat brain)
Drugs	
Amphetamine (mice)	Phentolamine (rat)
Bromocriptine (humans and rats)	Picrotoxin (rats)
Clonidine (humans)	
Delta sleep-inducing peptide (humans)	
GABA agonists (rats, mice)	GABA antagonists (rats, mice)
Iron chelators (mice)	
Morphine (mice)	
Naloxone (rats)	
Metoclopramide (rats)	
Pimozide (rats)	
Propranalol (humans)	

after the last alcohol intake in some patients, but returned to normal when the subjects were retested after 6 months.[31] In addition, basal circulating plasma cortisol levels remained elevated for as long as 3 weeks after the last alcohol intake.[32] Though the data is less robust, some evidence for prolongation of altered HPA function during abstinence, comes from studies of the dexamethasone suppression test (DST) in chronic alcoholics who have stopped drinking.

The DST is best known as a state-dependent marker for the identification of major depressive disorder.[33] Though the symptoms and signs of major depression have been reported to be common in alcoholics undergoing withdrawal, the large majority of these patients do not subsequently manifest a major depressive disorder (see Chapter 13 by Gorelick and Wilkins). The frequent nonsuppression response to the DST in alcoholics in the first few hours of abstinence (see discussion below) is not surprising, since recent alcohol intake can produce a false positive response to the DST.[33] Other common factors found in alcoholic patients that can produce false positive results with the DST include recent weight loss,[34] liver disease,[35] diabetes,[36] and cigarette smoking.[37]

To date, at least nine studies have been published that performed the DST in over 450 subjects undergoing alcohol withdrawal or in various stages of abstinence[38–44] (Table II); most of the studies controlled for the presence of major depressive disorder. Key methodological problems with these studies often include the lack of control for liver disease or other concurrent illness in subjects, for the duration and intensity of drinking prior to abstinence, and marked variance in the duration of abstinence across subjects at the time of DST tests.

Twenty-eight percent of chronic alcoholics manifested non-suppression responses (plasma cortisol >5 μg/ml) to dexamethasone during the first week of alcohol withdrawal. At 3 weeks after withdrawal, subjects in one study returned to normal, while in four other studies, 30% of subjects still manifested nonsuppression from 21 to 40 days after withdrawal onset. In one of these studies,[39] six patients who manifested nonsuppression of the DST were retested at 28 days and also followed clinically for a few months. Four of the 6 normalized by 28 days, but two did not. One of the two patients who had failed to normalize the DST at 28 days eventually relapsed to drinking, while the other 5 in the same period did not. One study[42] reported a positive correlation between the tendency to DST nonsuppression and having a primary relative with history of alcohol abuse.

2.2. Endogenous Opiates

Although acute alcohol administration (intoxication) has been found to cause increased peripheral endorphin levels, acute alcohol withdrawal is associated with decreased CNS endorphin levels. Two studies using a total of 67 alcoholic inpatients found decreased lumbar CSF levels of (undifferentiated) endorphin fractions[45] or of β-endorphin[46] 24 hr and 11–14 days, respectively, after the last drink. There was no change in plasma β-endorphin levels (and thus a decrease in CSF-to-plasma ratio), indicating that peripheral endorphin levels may not well reflect CNS activity. Levels of CSF ACTH were increased fourfold during withdrawal, while plasma ACTH levels remained normal,[46] again suggesting the dichotomy between central and peripheral hormone levels. This pattern of findings is consistent with the hypothesis that acute alcohol intoxication releases endorphin stores, resulting in increased levels, while chronic administration eventually depletes endorphin stores, resulting in decreased levels during acute withdrawal. As withdrawal resolves, stores are replenished, consistent with the finding that CSF endorphin levels are back to normal by 1 week after the last drink.[45]

In mice made alcohol dependent, concurrent administration of naloxone and ethanol suppressed ethanol-induced sleep time[47]; when both drugs were stopped, the common occurence of withdrawal seizures in the mice were also inhibited. Naloxone may inhibit the development of ethanol dependence, as evidenced by prevention of the withdrawal reaction occuring after sudden termination of chronic, intense ethanol intoxication in mice.[48,49] However, in another study, naloxone had no effect on either intoxication or the ethanol withdrawal syndrome in the rat.[50]

Conversely, administration of alcohol to opiate-dependent animals can alter opiate withdrawal. For example, naloxone-induced morphine withdrawal is suppressed by chronic alcohol.[51] In a study with intriguing findings,[52] five male alcoholics given intravenous nalorphine given after two weeks of daily alcohol administration (equivalent of 240 ml/day of 95 percent ethanol) manifested lacrimation in one patient, and weakness, anorexia, insomnia, disorientation and tremor in, one or more of the other patients. The mechanism for the development of these opliate withdrawal-like symptoms in this small number of patients is unclear.

2.3. Thyroid

In a review of previous studies, the majority of alcoholics (if free of liver disease) were found to be clinically euthyroid and have normal serum total and free thyroxine (T_4) and triiodothyronine (T_3) levels.[13] A more recent study[25] found mild diminutions of 5–21% in thyroid indices.

The subsequent response of thyroid-stimulating hormone (TSH) to intravenously administered thyrotropin-releasing hormone (TRH) has been used as a laboratory aid in psychiatry.[53,54] At the beginning of withdrawal, nine of 32 subjects, in the withdrawal study mentioned above,[25] manifested abnormal blunting of the TSH response to TRH. All subjects returned to normal in the TSH response after 1 week of abstinence, except for one male. However, in two other studies,[43,55] eight of 32 patients were found to have significant blunting of TSH by TRH after 3 weeks of abstinence, and three of 15 subjects had blunting of the response at 2 years, respectively.

2.4. Prolactin and Growth Hormone

In patients undergoing alcohol withdrawal, serum prolactin (Prl) is initially decreased, but returns to normal levels in 4 weeks.[56] In this study, the more severe the withdrawal from alcohol, the more the tendency for lower serum Prl levels. The Prl levels normalized with improvement or disappearance of symptoms and signs of withdrawal.

During acute exposure to alcohol, the slow wave sleep release of human growth hormone (HGH) is altered.[57] In the only published study of HGH during alcohol withdrawal, plasma HGH levels were decreased 70–75% during 9 days of evening chronic alcohol intake (0.8 per night),[58] but were immediately normalized on the first night when alcohol was discontinued.

2.5. Gonadotropins

Alcohol is well known to cause testicular atrophy in male chronic alcoholics.[59] In a recent study,[25] 7 of 32 men entering alcohol withdrawal manifested atrophy of the testes. Four of these subjects also had low circulating levels of testosterone. However, the effects of chronic alcohol on regulation of luteinizing hormone (LH), the anterior pituitary peptide that regulates the function of the testes, is unclear. Increases, decreases, and no change in circulating LH levels in the human have been found after exposure to chronic alcohol.[60] Despite the intense effort in determining the effects of alcohol on sexual functioning, no work appears to have been performed on the role of luteinizing hormone (LH), testosterone, or estrogens in alcohol withdrawal.

2.6. Vasopressin and Other Peptides

Administration of the posterior pituitary hormone, arginine vasopressin (AVP) did not alter the withdrawal syndrome in mice,[61] when administered after withdrawal had begun. When a vasopressin analogue, des-Gly^{9}-AVP dicitrate (DGAVP) was administered to mice in conjunction with alcohol or at the beginning of the withdrawal phase, withdrawal severity scores were increased and the time to return to baseline was lengthened.[62] In a human study, alcoholics showing symptoms of withdrawal had higher plasma vasopressin concentrations than alcoholics not showing withdrawal symptoms, or controls.[63]

In a study of 49 patients manifesting either alcohol or opiate withdrawal,[64] delta sleep-inducing peptide (DSIP) reportedly produced beneficial effect in 48 of the patients. No major side effects were observed by the investigators. Other peptides including neurotensin, β-endorphin, and bombesin,[65] melanocyte-stimulating hormone (MSH), and ACTH$^{D4\text{-}10}$,[66] a fragment of ACTH, have all been shown to interfere with ethanol-induced behaviors in animals. Cholecystokinin (CCK) is altered by administration of alcohol to rats.[67] These substances, along with prostaglandings, the synthesis of which is altered by alcohol,[68] remain to be studied during alcohol withdrawal.

2.7. Discussion

The DST has low specificity (i.e., close to one-third "false positive" nonsuppression rate) during the first few weeks of abstinence from alcohol and thus is not a valid marker for major depression during this period. Results of one of the DST studies[32] suggest that the DST may not be the most sensitive test of HPA axis dysfunction. In that study, about half the patients with elevated mean basal (i.e., predexamethasone) serum cortisol levels (>30 μg/dl) had normal DST responses at the beginning of withdrawal. Furthermore, even in those patients with abnormalities, the DST result normalized much faster than the elevated serum cortisol level (8 days vs. 3 weeks). Though even fewer patients in the above study might have been DST nonsuppressors with a dexamethasone dose of 2 mg, rather than the 1 mg dosage given, the use of the larger dose has been recently recommended.[69] The recommendation stems from the finding, in a study of depressed patients, that only the 2-mg dose of dexamethasone, when compared with the 1-mg dose, correlated with abnormally high urinary cortisol values.

Therefore, the response to 1 mg dexamethasone can be normal in the face of abnormal circulating levels of cortisol[62] and abnormal in the face of normal urinary cortisol.[69] Meanwhile, circulating levels of ACTH can be normal in the face of high CSF values[46] and circulating levels of cortisol can be normal in the face of elevated levels of plasma ACTH.[25] A more specific and sensitive HPA axis perturbation test might be a challenge with corticotropin-releasing factor (CRF). In animals, increases in ACTH covary with decreases in hypothalamic concentrations of CRF, while administration of anti-CRF serum blocks the alcohol-induced rise in serum ACTH and corticosterone levels.[27]

In addition to the decreases seen in CSF levels of the 31 amino acid β-endorphin, there are decreases in rat cerebral cortex of the pentapeptide endogenous opiate, methionine-enkephalin.[70] The processes of alcohol withdrawal seem closely connected with the endogenous opiates. Supplementing the opiate and naloxone data cited earlier is an additional animal study. In rats made alcohol-dependent and then withdrawn acutely, levels of circulating corticosterone and adrenal catecholamines norepinephrine and epinephrine) are found to increase significantly.[71] When naloxone is co-administered with the alcohol, the levels of adrenal catecholamines measured during subsequent withdrawal are unchanged from baseline.

3. Neuropharmacological Aspects of Alcohol Withdrawal

3.1. Neurotransmitters

During withdrawal, significant changes have been found in levels of CNS norepinephrine (NOR) and γ-aminobutyric acid (GABA). Parallel changes are found in β-adrenergic receptor activity. Some inconsistencies across research groups exist, but by in large the data are congruent. However, significant inconsistencies exist in withdrawal studies of dopamine (DA) and serotonin (5-HT). The role of acetylcholine (ACh) in alcohol withdrawal has not been adequately studied.

Special caution is required when interpreting studies of neurotransmitter systems. Specifically, brains levels of a given neurotransmitter (as opposed to its metabolites) and respective rates of synthesis of the neurotransmitter are difficult to interpret. For example, after electric foot-shock, in a nonalcohol research paradigm, a number of studies have found either an increase, decrease or no change in rat brain DA levels.[72–79] However consistent measures of elevated levels of brain DA metabolites were found in these same studies, suggesting a stress-induced enhancement of DA activity. This shows that brain levels of a neurotransmitter alone may be poor indicators of activity in that neurotransmitter system since levels can be altered in any direction in association with enhanced neurotransmitter turnover. Similar inconsistencies exist with the measurement of the rates of synthesis of neurotransmitters. For example, the synthesis of DA increases both in response to an increase in impulse flow as well as to a complete cessation of impulse flow in CNS DA neurons.[80] Neuropharmacological strategies that do not appear to have these problems include: measurement of CNS and body fluid neurotransmitter metabolites in animals, measurement of neurotransmitter metabolites in human body fluids, and electrophysiological measures in animal brain.

3.2. Effects of Withdrawal on Norepinephrine and β-Adrenergic Receptor

Urinary excretion of NOR,[81] CSF NOR,[82] and CSF 3-methoxy,4-hydroxyphenylglycol (MHPG),[83,84] a key metabolite of CNS NOR, in humans, and CSF or brain turnover of NOR[85,86] in rats all significantly increase during alcohol withdrawal. In the human studies[82–84] and one animal study,[86] the respective CSF or brain measures correlated with the clinical conditions of the subjects.

High correlations between CSF MHPG and clinical state were achieved in one study[8] when 32 alcoholic patients were divided into three groups (major withdrawal associated with delirium; minor withdrawal with tachycardia, sweating, tremor, but without hallucinations; and asymptomatic withdrawal). Correlations of $r > .6$ with $p < 10.02$ with the first classification and $r > 0.086$ with $p < .001$ for the second classification were reported. In this study, the CSF, MHPG values returned to control levels upon clinical recovery.

There are sequential changes in brain β-adrenergic receptor sensitivity in animals during long-term ethanol treatment and withdrawal. First, during chronic exposure to alcohol, there is decreased sensitivity to NOR,[87] then during early withdrawal, there is increased sensitivity to NOR.[88,89,90] The development of subsensitivity of the receptor during chronic ethanol treatment follows classical lines of ligand–receptor interactions (down-regulation of receptor by increased levels of ligand). What is unclear, is how the receptors increase in sensitivity during acute withdrawal, at a time when NOR turnover remains high.[85]

3.3. Effects of Norepinephrine on Withdrawal

Norepinephrine administered into the ventricles of the brain has been shown to lessen the severity of head twitching in mice during alcohol withdrawal.[91,92]

Presumed blockage of NOR interactions with the α-adrenergic receptor (with clonidine) and the β-adrenergic receptor (with propranalol) has been tested in humans. Clinical studies demonstrate therapeutic responses to clonidine in patients with tremor, aditation, insomnia, and "pre-delirium."[93–95] These findings are consistent with finding of improved clinical state in withdrawing animals seen after lesioning of the locus coeruleus, where approximately half of all brain CNS NOR originates.[93]

Therapeutic responses to propranalol in humans during withdrawal from alcohol have been reported,[96,97] but the responses are limited. For example, propranalol has no effect on tremor[98] and is apparently confined to stabilization of tachycardia, hypertension, and subjective anxiety. In fact, in one study,[99] both α receptor blockade with phentolamine and β receptor blockade with propranolol produced a transient increase in withdrawal severity in mice. Yet in a previous double-blind study in humans,[100] where alcoholic subjects received an average of 30 mg propanalol per day, 40% less diazepam was required for treatment of anxiety and related withdrawal symptoms during acute withdrawal.

3.4. Effects of Withdrawal on Dopamine

Despite the difficulties in interpreting the actions of DA during withdrawal (see below), one study showed an interesting correlation[84] between the presence of delirium and diminished homovanillic acid (HVA) levels in CSF. The reduction of CSF–HVA may be a specific result of alcohol withdrawal delirium since HVA did not change significantly in patients with minor or asymptomatic withdrawal syndrome.

Turnover of brain DA (measurement of HVA, the main metabolite) during alcohol withdrawal has been reported as decreased[86] or unchanged.[101] Similar confusion exists with measures of brain DA levels during withdrawal. During acute withdrawal in rodents, DA in the striatum is increased.[102] The levels then returned to baseline values in twelve hours after the acute withdrawal. Another group,[103,105] however, reported reductions in DA levels during alcohol withdrawal in the caudate nucleus.

3.5. Effects of Dopamine on Withdrawal

Dopamine and L-DOPA[92,105] and amphetamine and apomorphine[91] have been shown to lessen convulsions and head twitches in mice and rats. In another study,[106] bromocriptine, a DA agonist, and pimozide and metoclopramide, DA antagonists, were given to rats after bilateral lesion of the A10 nucleus was induced by 6-hydroxydopamine. Following the administration of 6-hydroxydopamine, the forebrain content of dopamine was 58% less than that of control animals. The rats receiving bromocriptine manifested diminished locomotor activity and diminished incidence of audiogenic seizures (seizures induced in rats by sound and used as a model during withdrawal).[107,108] Treatment with pimozide also diminished intensity of withdrawal seizures, but at higher doses enhanced motor activity. Metoclopramide, a more specific DA receptor antagonist, reduced motor and seizure activity.

In a treatment study of 60 alcoholic subjects, 2.5 mg p.o. t.i.d. of bromocriptine was found to be superior to placebo in the treatment of anxiety, restlessness, tremor, diaphoresis and nausea.[109] In order for bromocriptine to alleviate withdrawal in the same manner as pimozide and metoclopramide, the drug must inhibit DA transmission through actions on the DA presynaptic receptor.

3.6. Effects of Withdrawal on Serotonin and Serotonin on Withdrawal: Effects of Withdrawal on Acetyl Choline

No consistent trends have been found with regard to the effects of withdrawal from alcohol on serotonin (5-HT) concentrations. Studies have shown increases,[110] decreases,[111] and no effects at all.[112–114] Similarly, when compared with controls, no change was found in CSF of the serotonin metabolite 5-hydroxy-indoleacetic acid (5-HIAA) of patients with any type of alcohol withdrawal syndrome.[84] This is in agreement with earlier animal experiments that showed no direct relationship between alcohol withdrawal and central serotonin metabolism.[115] In sum, due to conflicting results obtained with 5-HT, its precursors, and its inhibitors, the role of 5-HT in alcohol withdrawal has not been clearly defined.

Administration of 5-HT usually appears to worsen rating scores of withdrawal in rodents.[92,116] In humans, positive therapeutic results have been reported with trazadone, presumably through uptake inhibition of 5-HT, in the treatment of 17 patients undergoing alcohol withdrawal.[117]

Two groups have reported decreases in the brain ACh levels during withdrawal.[118,119] In the first study mouse brain levels were still diminished 48 hr after beginning withdrawal, while in the second study, which found ACh changes in select areas of the brain, ACh levels had returned to normal 12 hr after initiation of withdrawal.

3.7. MAO; Cyclic Nucleotides

Following cessation of drinking and during the first week of abstinence, systematic, sequential increases in human platelet MAO activity have been reported.[120] The phenomenon is transient and is not accompanied by a corresponding increase in platelet count.

Levels of human CSF cyclic 3′5′-adenosine monophosphate (cAMP) have been reported to be significantly decreased during delirium, while increased levels of cyclic 3′5′-guanosine monophosphate (cGMP) were found during delirium.[121] The decrease in cAMP did not correlate with the ratings of withdrawal signs and returned to normal when clinical signs of withdrawal had abated.

Mice treated chronically with alcohol have been found to have decreased cerebellar brain levels of cAMP in cerebellum, cerebral cortex, and pons-medulla.[122] Consistent with this finding, another group reported that 7 days of exposure (intragastric) of rats to alcohol resulted in decreases of cAMP in the subcortex of rats.[123] Eight hours after cessation of alcohol, the cAMP levels had increased towards normal in three of the four brain areas studied. However, this is in conflict with the study demonstrating a 70% increase in cAMP levels in mice who received alcohol throughout the day for 8 days.[124] Adenylate cyclase activity was also found to increase in this latter study.

The findings of increases and decreases of cAMP during withdrawal may be related to changes in sensitivity of the cAMP system to NOR. For example, French and his colleagues[88,125,126] have demonstrated that chronic ethanol shifted the dose–response curve to the right, resulting in subsensitivity by 4.3-fold. Three days after cessation of alcohol, the curve had shifted to the left resulting in supersensitivity by 2.4-fold. This down-regulation of the cAMP system is consistent with the previously mentioned increases in NOR turnover during chronic alcohol and withdrawal.[85,86,110] What is unclear is how, in the face of persistent increases in NOR turnover during withdrawal, the cAMP response can shift from subsensitive to supersensitive.

3.8. Effects of Withdrawal on GABA; Effects of GABA on Withdrawal

The majority of studies in animals have found GABA to increase during acute and chronic exposure to alcohol and then to decrease during withdrawal. One study[127] found the decrease in levels of GABA in mouse brain to be maximal at 8 hr after the beginning of withdrawal, when withdrawal symptoms were at their peak. In a second study of mice[118] brain GABA levels were detected during chronic alcohol and 48 hr after the beginning of withdrawal. At the 48 hr time period GABA levels were within the normal range, since they had decreased from the previous stimulated values. Complicating the picture is data demonstrating decreases in brain GABA during chronic administration of ethanol.[128,129] However, as noted by Tabakoff,[80] these studies may be difficult to interpret without the knowledge of when the samples were taken relative to the time of the last dose of alcohol.

Goldstein[99] has demonstrated that a number of drugs with GABA-ergic activity influence alcohol withdrawal seizures induced by handling mice. Picrotoxin, a GABA inhibitor, enhanced the development of the seizures, while injections of the GABA agonist aminooxyacetic acid reduced the rate of convulsions. GABA and GABA-ergic agents have also been tested using the model of susceptibility to audiogenic seizures during alcohol withdrawal in the rat.[130] Audiogenic seizures were antagonized by ethanol and intracisternal injections of GABA and GABA agonists muscimol, β-guanidinoacetic acid, and β-guanidinopropionic acid. The response to muscinol and GABA followed a dose-response paradigm. Seizures were also antagonized by ethanolamine-*O*-sulfate, a selective irreversible GABA-transaminase (GABA-T) inhibitor, and by *N*-dipropylacetate (DPA), a compound which elevates levels of GABA. In another study, DPA prevented ethanol withdrawal symptoms induced by either a monotonic or a heterotonic stimulus.[131] In a study that confirmed the earlier findings of Goldstein, intranigral administration of muscimol produced a dose-related suppression of audiogenic motor convulsions.[132]

3.9. Iron

Rats made dependent through exposure to persistent alcohol vapors demonstrate significant prevention of withdrawal if given iron chelating agents during the period of alcohol withdrawal.[133] Administration of iron (250 mg/kg) once prior to ethanol treatment and once during ethanol exposure resulted in a significant increase in the withdrawal ratings. In a study of 12 males, undergoing alcohol withdrawal, blood levels of iron and its carrier protein ferritin were significantly increased during withdrawal and returned to baseline levels from 1 to 2 weeks after initiation of abstinence.[134]

3.10. Cerebral Blood Flow

In a study of 12 male alcoholics undergoing withdrawal, using the xenon-133 inhalation method of measuring cerebral blood flow (rCBF),[135] the rCBF was found to be substantially reduced in all patients. The largest decreases were found in patients with a clouded sensorium and extended preceding drinking period. Aggravated withdrawal symptoms were coupled with high temporal and low parietal flows. Parenthetically, elevated rCBF values were found in the temporal, sylvian, and occipital regions of the two patients who reported withdrawal related auditory and visual hallucinations. Further studies are needed to confirm these findings.

3.11. Discussion

The data strongly suggest that enhanced activity of NOR is involved in a central position in the pathophysiology of alcohol withdrawal. To a lesser extent the data also support a central role for diminished activity of GABA. Increases in β-adrenergic activity and diminished cAMP likely reflect a downstream relationship to NOR. Although the data is now very inconsistent, the activities of DA, 5-HT, and ACh will become clear with future studies. Some relationship with these neurotransmitter systems and NOR and GABA is likely, since there are regulatory interrelationships between DA, 5-HT, and ACh, and NOR and GABA.[80] Specifically, NOR is interdependent with DA,[137]

5-HT,[137,138] ACh,[139] and cAMP.[80] GABA is known to interact with DA and Ach,[140] especially in the striatum.

The neurotransmitter and receptor models of Goldstein and Goldstein[2] and Collier[1] are supported by the NOR and β-adrenergic data. The membrane fluidization theory of alcohol dependence[3] could help explain the adrenergic receptor changes; however, the membrane theory is argued against by the finding of similar brain membrane fluidity in rats genetically sensitive or insensitive to alcohol withdrawal phenomena.[141]

3.12. Unified Model

The authors speculate that some of the symptoms of ethanol withdrawal might be explained by the interaction of ethanol with GABA receptors. It is possible to construct a model of sedative/hypnotic drug dependence and withdrawal (including alcohol) by focusing on ethanol interactions with the GBB, the data of respective activities of GABA and NOR during withdrawal, and the aforementioned models of dependence and withdrawal. Ticku *et al.*[142] have demonstrated that ethanol partially inhibits binding of the benzodiazepine-GABA receptor-ionophore complex (GABA-benzodiazepine-barbituate receptor complex, or GBB).

Clinical and animal evidence indicates that benzodiazepines, barbituates, GABA agonists, clonidine, and propranalol alleviate withdrawal symptomatology, whereas GABA antagonists worsen alcohol withdrawal. Clonidine inhibits NOR release and NOR cell firing by stimulating α_2-adrenergic autoreceptors.[143] Diazepam inhibits [^{3}H]-NOR release from rat brain by interacting with the GBB receptor complex.[144] Enhancement of GABA function also appears capable of inhibiting NOR release since GABA agonist lowered rat brain MHPG.[145] A number of alcohol and barbituates interact with the GBB complex in such a way as to enhance GABA function.[146–149] Benzodiazepines and ethanol decrease the firing rates of presumably noradrenergic cells in the rat locus coeruleus.[150–152] In addition, electrophysiological evidence suggests that a single ethanol dose can normalize the firing patterns of NOR cells that had been firing excessively in rats withdrawn from chronic ethanol exposure.[153]

The above studies suggest that elevated NOR turnover during withdrawal may result from a loss of GABA-ergic facilitation that had been present during ethanol exposure. If, as indicated above, ethanol enhances GABA function, then an approxpriate CNS adaptation to chronic ethanol exposure would be to attempt down-regulation of GABA function. This down-regulation would be revealed as an inadequacy of GABA function when ethanol is suddenly withdrawn. Therefore decreased brain GABA levels and elevated NOR turnover in withdrawing rats may be manifestations of inadequate GABA function.

An emphasis on diminished GABA activity in withdrawal pathophysiology would correctly predict that pharmacological enhancement of GABA function (i.e., administration of GABA agonists, barbituates, and benzodiazepines) would alleviate withdrawal. This conceptualization is consistent with the finding that rats genetically sensitive to alcohol withdrawal phenomena are cross-sensitive to barbituate and benzodiazepine after withdrawal.[154] In addition, there are differential enhancements of benzodiazepine binding by GABA in two strains of mice selectively bred for the sedative effect of alcohol.[155] Thus, a common mechanism (GABA inadequacy?) may underlie the symptoms of withdrawal from ethanol, barbituates, or benzodiazepines. The kindling theory is consistent with an emphasis on alcohol–GBB receptor interactions since elevating GABA transmission retards the development of kindling in rats.[156] Thus, the diminished GABA function proposed to occur during withdrawal would tend to enhance the possibility of kindling.

4. Conclusion

Individuals undergoing withdrawal from alcohol often experience anxiety, tremor, and marked dysphoria, and occasionally experience seizures and delirium tremens. The analogous syndrome in rodents is at least equally severe. Therefore, it is not surprising that CNS neurochemicals and CNS-regulated hormones manifest striking changes in humans and animals during alcohol withdrawal.

Evaluation of the studies reviewed in this chapter reveals that: (1) the measures with the greatest consistency are of CNS NOR turnover and HPA activity; (2) peptides have been used succesfully in studies of withdrawal (including corticotropin-releasing hormone, thyrotropin-releasing hormone, arginine vasopressin, and delta sleep-inducing peptide); (3) there are peptides with marked physiological activity that are known to interfere with actions of alcohol but have yet to be tested in studies of withdrawal (including cholecystokinin, bombesin, and neurotensin). On the negative side, the evaluation reveals that: (1) studies are often difficult to compare because of uncoordinated timing of samples; (2) there is frequent lack of prewithdrawal baseline samples for comparison to measures taken during withdrawal; (3) few studies extend the timing of samples out past acute withdrawal despite evidenced of sustained CNS hyperactivity after acute withdrawal[157] (see Chapter 13 by Gorelick and Wilkins).

The following suggestions are offered for consideration in future research: (1) employ perturbation measures in humans and animals in order to better distinguish subliminal dysfunction of CNS systems; (2) when performing perturbations studies consider the use of tropic peptides (including CRF with subsequent measures of ACTH and cortisol, and TRH with subsequent measures of TSH and Prl); (3) correlate biological measures in human subjects with drinking histories (including duration and amount of ethanol equivalency); (4) correlate withdrawal measures in humans with measures of medical complications including laboratory measures of liver function and glucose metabolism; (5) in animal studies employ, when possible, turnover measures of neurotransmitters or related neurochemicals and/or electrophysiological measures instead of measures of brain neurotransmitter levels or rates of neurotransmitter synthesis; (6) employ neurotransmitter agonists and antagonists either as CNS probes for perturbation tests or as a form of treatment; (7) use opiate agonists and antagonists as part of perturbation experiments or in treatment studies; (8) study the role of the GBB receptor complex in alcohol dependence and withdrawal; (8) study salsinol, a morphinelike product found in the brains of animals after receiving alcohol,[158] and (8) consider studies of alcohol withdrawal when performing family studies on alcoholism,[159] with a focus on the genetic influences on the severity of withdrawal and the speed of recovery following withdrawal.

References

1. Collier HOJ: A general theory of the genesis of drug dependence by induction of receptors. *Nature* 205:181–182, 1965.
2. Goldstein A, Goldstein DB: Wikler A (ed): *The Addictive States.* Baltimore, Williams and Wilkins, 1968, pp 265–267.
3. Hill NW, Bangham AD: General depressant drug dependency: A biophysical hypothesis. *Adv Exp Med Biol* 59:1–9, 1975.
4. Cicero TJ: Tolerance to and physical dependence on alcohol: Behavioral and neurobiological mechanisms, in Lipton MA, DiMascio A, Killam KF: *Psychopharmacology: A Generation of Progress.* New York, Raven Press, 1978, pp 1603–1617.
5. Littleton JM, John GR, Jones PA, Grieve SJ: The rapid onset of functional tolerance to ethanol-role of different neurotransmitters and synaptosomal membrane lipids. *Acta Psychiatr Scand (Suppl)* 286:137–51, 1980.
6. Post RM, Ballenger JC: Kindling models for the progressive development of psychopathology: Sensitization to electrical, pharmacological, and psychological stimuli, in Van Praag HM, Lader MH, Rafaelsen OJ, et al: *Handbook of Biological Psychiatry, Part IV.* New York, Marcel Dekker 1981, pp 609–651.
7. Girgis M: Kindling as a model for limbic epilepsy. *Neuroscience* 6:1695–1706, 1981.
8. Goddard GV: The kindling model of limbic epilepsy, Girgis M, Kiloh LG (eds): in *Limbic Epilepsy and the Dyscontrol Syndrome,* Amsterdam, Elsevier/North-Holland Biomedical Press, 1980, pp 107–116.
9. von Noorden GK: Experimental amblyopia in monkeys. Further behavioral observations and clinical correlations. *Invest Ophthalmol* 12.721–738, 1973.
10. Pinel JP: Alcohol withdrawal seizures: Implications of kindling. *Pharmacol Biochem Behav* 1(13):225–31, 1980.
11. Pinel JPJ, Cheung LF: Controlled demonstration of metrazol kindling. *Pharmacol Biochem Behav* 6:599–600, 1979.
12. Van Thiel DH: Alcohol and its effect on endocrine functioning. *Alcoholism* 4:44–49, 1980.
13. Morgan MY: Alcohol and the endocrine system. *Br Med Bull* 38:17–20, 1982.
14. Ellis FW: Adrenal cortical function in experimental alcoholism in dogs. *Proc Soc Exp Biol Med* 120:740, 1965.
15. Ellis FW: Effects of ethanol on plasma corticosterone levels. *J Pharmacol Exp Ther* 153:121–127, 1966.
16. Nolde EP: Ethanol and adrenocortical stimulation in inbred mouse strains, in: Mello NK, Mendelson JH (eds): *Recent Advances in Studies of Alcoholism.* Washington, D.C., U.S. Government Printing Office, 1971, pp 77–106.
17. Kakihana R, Butte JC, Hathaway A, et al: Adrenocortical response to ethanol in mice: Modification by chronic ethanol consumption. *Acta Endocrinol* 67:653–664, 1971.
18. Ratcliffe F: Hypothalamic sensitivity in rats following prolonged consumption of ethanol. *Arch Int Pharmacoldyn Ther* 197:306–316, 1972.

19. Kakihana R, Moore JA: Cireadian rhythm of corticosterone in mice: The effect of chronic consumption of alcohol. *Psychopharmacologia (Berlin)* 46:301–305, 1976.
20. Tabakoff B, Jaffe RC, Ritzman RF: Corticosterone concentrations in mice during ethanol drinking and withdrawal. *Pharm Pharmacol* 30:371–374, 1978.
21. Guaza C, Torrellas A, Borrell S: Adrenocortical response to acute and chronic ethanol administration in rats. *Psychopharmacology* 79:173–176, 1983.
22. Kissin B, Schenket V, Schenker AC: The acute effect of ethanol ingestion on plasma and urinary 17-hydroxy-corticoids in alcoholic subjects. *Am J Med Sci* 239:690–705, 1960.
23. Mendelson JH, Ogata M, Mello NK: Adrenal function and alcoholism. I. Serum cortisol. *Psychosom Med* 33:145–157, 1971.
24. Merry J, Marks V: The effect of alcohol barbituate and diazepam on hypothalamic/pituitary adrenol function in chronic alcoholics. *Lancet* 2:990–991, 1972.
25. Valimaki M, Pelkonen R, Harkonen M, et al: Hormonal changes in noncirrhotic male alcoholics during ethanol withdrawal. *Alcohol and Alcoholism* 19(3):235–242, 1984.
26. Keith LD, Crabbe JC, Robertson LM, et al: Ethanol dependence and the pituitary adrenal axis in mice. II. Temporal analysis of dependence and withdrawal. *Life Sci* 33:1889–1897, 1983.
27. Rivier C, Bruhn T, Vale W: Effect of ethanol on the hypothalamic-pituitary-adrenal axis in the rat: Role of corticotropin-releasing factor (CRF). *J Pharmacol Exp Ther* 229(1):127–131, 1983.
28. Smals AG, Kloppenborg PW, Njo KT, et al: Alcohol-induced Cushingoid Syndrome. *Br Med J* ii1298, 1976.
29. Rees LH, Besser GM, Jeffcoate WJ, et al: Alcohol-induced Pseudo-Cushing's Syndrome. *Lancet* 1:726–728, 1977.
30. Lamberts SWJ, Klun JGM, deJong HF, et al: Hormone secretion in alcohol-induced pseudo-Cushing's syndrome: Differential diagnosis with Cushing's disease. *JAMA* 242:1640–1643, 1979.
31. Merry J, Marks V: Plasma-hydrocortisone response to ethanol in chronic alcoholics. *Lancet* (Preliminary Communications):921–923, 1969.
32. Willenbring ML, Morley JE, Niewoehner CB, et al: Adrenocortical hyperactivity in newly admitted alcoholics: Prevalence, course and associated variables. *Psychoneuroendocrinology* 9:415–422, 1984.
33. Carroll BJ, Feinberg M, Greden JF, et al: A specific laboratory test for the diagnosis of melancholia. *Arch Gen Psychiatry* 38:15–22, 1981.
34. Edelstein CK, Roy-Byrne P, Fawzy FI, et al: Effects of weight loss on the dexamethasone suppression test. *Am J Psychiatry* 140:338–341, 1983.
35. Swartz CM, Dunner FJ: Dexamethasone suppression testing of alcoholics. *Arch Gen Psychiatry* 39:1309–1312, 1982.
36. Rihmer Z, Arato M: Depression and diabetes mellitus. *Neuropsychobiology* 8:315–318, 1982.
37. Wilkins JN, Carlson HE, Van Vunakis H, et al: Nicotine from cigarette smoking increases circulating levels of cortisol, growth hormone and prolactin in male chronic smokers. *Psychopharmacology* 78:305–308, 1982.
38. Targum SD, Wheadon DF, Chastek CT, et al: Dysregulation on hypothalamic-pituitary-adrenal function in depressed alcoholic patients. *J Affect Dis* 4:347–353, 1982.
39. Targum SD, Capodanno AE, Unger S, et al: Abnormal dexamethasone tests in withdrawing alcoholic patients. *Biol Psychiatry* 19(3):401–405, 1984.
40. Abou-Saleh MT, Merry J, Coppen A: Dexamethasone suppression test in alcoholism. *Acta Psychiatr Scand* 69:112–116, 1984.
41. Coopen A, Abou-Saleh M, Milln P, et al: Dexamethasone suppression test in depression and other psychiatric illness. *Br J Psychiatr* 142:498–504, 1983.
42. Newsom G, Murray N: Reversal of dexamethasone suppression test nonsuppression in alcohol abusers. *Am J Psychiatry* 140:3, 1983.
43. Ravi SD, Dorus W, Park YN, et al: The dexamethasone suppression test and depressive symptoms in early and late withdrawal from alcohol. *Am J Psychiatry* 141(11):1445–1448, 1984.

44. Dackis CA, Bailey J, Pottash ALC, et al: Specificity of the DST and the TRH test for major depression in alcoholics. *Am J Psychiatry* 141:680–683, 1984.
45. Borg S, Kvande H, Rydberg U, et al: Endorphin levels in human cerebrospinal fluid during alcohol intoxication and withdrawal. *Psychopharmacology* 78:101–103, 1982.
46. Savoldi F, Mazzella GL, Faccinetti F, et al: Beta endorphin, beta lipotropin and adrenocorticotropic hormone levels in cerebrospinal fluid, and brain damage in chronic alcoholics. *Eur Neurol* 22:265–271, 1983.
47. Berman RF, Lee JA, Olson KL, et al: Effects of naloxone on development of ethanol dependence in rats. *Soc Neurosci Abstr 10th Annual Meeting*. 10:49, 1980.
48. Blum K, Wallace JE, Schwerter HA, et al: Morphine suppression of ethanol withdrawal in mice. *Experientia* 32:79–82, 1976.
49. Blum K, Futterman S, Wallace JE, et al: Naloxone-induced inhibition of ethanol dependence in mice. *Nature* 265:49–51, 1977.
50. Hemmingsen R, Sorensen SC: Absence of an effect of naloxone on ethanol intoxication and withdrawal reactions. *Acta Pharmacol Toxicol* 46:62–65, 1980.
51. Jones MA, Spratto GR: Ethanol suppression of naloxone-induced withdrawal in morphine-dependent rats. *Life Sci* 20:1549–1556, 1977.
52. Markley HG, Mezey E: Induction of alcohol withdrawl symptoms by nalorphine in chronic alcoholic patients. *Int J Addict* 13(3):395–402, 1978.
53. Loosen PT, Prange AJ, Wilson IC: TRH (protirelin) in depressed alcoholic men. *Arch Gen Psychiatry* 36:540–547, 1979.
54. Extein I, Pottash ALC, Gold MS: Using the protirelin test to distinguish mania from schizophrenia. *Arch Gen Psychiatry* 39:77–81, 1982.
55. Loosen PT, Prange AJ: Thyrotropin releasing hormone (TRH): A useful tool for psychoneuroendocrine investigation. *Psychoneuroendocrinology* 5:63–80, 1980.
56. Majumdar SK: Serum prolactin concentrations during the hangover phase of ethanol withdrawal syndrome. *Neuroendocrinol Lett* 4(4):253–259, 1982.
57. Othmer E, Daughaday WH, Goodwin DW, et al: Sleep and growth hormone secretion in alcoholics. *J Clin Psychiatry* 43(10):411–414, 1982.
58. Prinz PN, Roehrs TA, Vitaliano PP, et al: Effect of alcohol on sleep and nighttime plasma growth hormone and cortisol concentrations. *J Clin Endocrinol Metab* 51(4):759–764, 1980.
59. Cicero TJ: Neuroendocrinological effects of alcohol. *Annu Rev Med* 32:123–142, 1981.
60. Chapin RE, Breese GR, Mueller RA: Possible mechanisms of reduction of plasma luteinizing hormone by ethanol. *J Pharmacol Exp Ther* 242:7–10, 1979.
61. Hoffman P, Ritzmann R, Tabakoff B: The influence of arginine vasopressin and oxytocin on ethanol dependence and tolerance, in Galanter M (ed): *Currents in Alcoholism*, vol 5. New York, Grune and Stratton, 1979, pp 5–16.
62. Crabbe JC, Rigter H: Hormones, peptides and ethanol responses, in Rigter H, Crabbe J (eds): *Alcohol Tolerance and Dependence*. New York, Elsevier/North-Holland Biomedical Press, 1980, pp 293–316.
63. Eisenhofer G, Whiteside E, Lambie D, et al: Brain water during alcohol withdrawal (letter). *Lancet* 1(8262):50, 1982.
64. Dick P, Grandjean ME, Tissot R: Successful treatment of withdrawal symptoms with delta sleep-inducing peptide, a neuropeptide with potential agonistic activity on opiate receptors. *Neuropsychobiology* 10:205–208, 1983.
65. Luttinger D, Nemeroff CB, Mason GA, et al: Enhancement of ethanol-induced sedation and hypothermia by centrally located administered neurotensin, β-endorphin and bombesin. *Neuropharmacology* 20:305–309, 1980.
66. McGivern RF, Harris JH, Yessaian N, et al: Antagonism of ethanol induced sleep-time by α-MSH, MSH/ACTH4-10 and naloxone. *Substance Alcohol Actions/Misuse* 1:335–342, 1980.
67. Ryder S, Straus E, Lieber CS, et al: Cholecystokinin and ankephalin levels following ethanol administration in rats. *Peptides* 2:223–226, 1981.
68. Horrobin DF: A biochemical basis for alcoholism and alcohol-induced damage including the fetal alcohol syndrome and cirrhosis: interface with essential fatty acid and prostaglandin and alcohol metabolism. *Med Hypotheses* 6:929–942, 1980.

69. Brown WA, Keitner G, Brandon Qualls C, et al: The dexamethasone suppression test and pituitary-adrenocortical function. *Arch Gen Psychiatry* 42:121–123, 1985.
70. Hong JS, Majchrowicz E, Hunt WA, et al: Reduction in cerebral methionine-enkephalin content during the ethanol withdrawal syndrome. *Substance Alcohol Actions/Misuse* 2:233–240, 1981.
71. Guaza C, Borrell S: Effect of naloxone administration upon responses of adrenal hormones to withdrawal from ethanol. *Psychopharmacology* 82:181–184, 1984.
72. Bliss EL, Ailion J, Zwanziger J: Metabolism of norepinephrine, serotonin and dopamine in rat brain with stress. *J Pharmacol Exp Ther* 164:122–134, 1968.
73. Bliss EL, Ailion J: Relationship of stress and activity to brain dopamine and homovanillac acid. *Life Sci* 10(1):1161–1169, 1971.
74. Thierry AM, Tassin JP, Blanc G, et al: Discovery of the mesocortical dopaminergic system: Some pharmacological and functional characteristics. *Adv Biochem Psychopharmacol* 16:5–12, 1977.
75. Blanc G, Herve D, Simon H, et al: Response to stress of mesocortico-frontal dopaminergic neurones in rats after long-term isolation. *Nature* 284:265–267, 1980.
76. Keller RW Jr, Stricker EM, Zigmond MJ: Environmental stimuli but not homeostatic challenges produce apparent increases in dopaminergic activity in the striatum: Analysis by the vivo voltammetry. *Brain Res* 279:159–170, 1983.
77. Dantzer R, Guilloneau D, Mormede P, et al: Influence of shock-induced fighting and social factors on dopamine turnover in cortical and limbic areas in the rat. *Pharmacol Biochem Behav* 20:331–335, 1984.
78. Herman JP, Stinus L, LeMoal M: Repeated stress increases locomotor response to amphetamine. *Psychopharmacology* 84:431–435, 1984.
79. Miller JD, Speciale SG, McMillen BA, et al: Naloxone antagonism of stress-induced augmentation of frontal cortex dopamine metabolism. *Eur J Pharmacol* 98:437–439, 1984.
80. Tabakoff B, Hoffman PL: Alcohol and neurotransmitters, in Righter H, Crabbe J (eds): *Alcohol Tolerance and Dependence*. Amsterdam, Elsevier/North-Holland Biomedical Press, 1980, pp 201–226.
81. Giacobini E, Izikowitz S, Wegmann A: Urinary norepinephrine and epinephrine excretion in delirium tremens. *Arch Gen Psychiatry* 3:289, 1960.
82. Hawley RJ, Major LF, Schulman EA, et al: CSF levels of norepinephrine during alcohol withdrawal. *Arch Neurol* 38:289, 1981.
83. Sjoquist B, Pardahl E, Winblad B: The effect of alcoholism on salsolinol and biogenic amines in human brain. *Drug Alcohol Depend* 12(1):15–23, 1983.
84. Fujimoto A, Nagao T, Ebara T, et al: Cerebrospinal fluid monoamine metabolites during alcohol withdrawal syndrome and recovered state. *Biol Psychiatry* 18(10):1141–1152, 1983.
85. Pohorecky LA: Effects of ethanol on the central and peripheral noradrenergic neurons. *J Pharmacol Exp Ther* 189:380, 1974.
86. Hunt WA, Majchrowicz E: Alterations in the turnover of brain norepinephrine and dopamine in alcohol-dependent rats. *J Neurochem* 23:549–552, 1974.
87. Rangaraj N, Kalant H: Effect of chronic ethanol treatment on temperature dependence and on norepinephrine sensitization of rat brain (Na+ + K+)-adenosine triphosphatase. *J Pharmacol Exp Ther* 223:536–539, 1982.
88. French SW, Palmer DS, Wiggers KD: Changes in receptor sensitivity of the cerebral cortex and liver during chronic ethanol ingestion and withdrawal. *Adv Exp Med Biol* 85A:515–538, 1977.
89. Banerjee SP, Sharma VK: Alterations in β-adrenergic receptor binding during ethanol withdrawal. *Nature* 276(5686):407–409, 1978.
90. Liljequist S, Anden NE, Engel J, et al: Noradrenergic receptor sensitization after chronic alcohol administration. *J Neural Transmission* 43:11–17, 1978.
91. Collier HOJ, Hammond MD, Schneider L: Biogenic amines and head twitches in mice during ethanol withdrawal. *Br J Pharmacol* 51:310–311, 1974.
92. Collier HOJ, Hammond MD, Schneider C: Effects of drugs affecting endogenous amines

or cyclic nucleotides on ethanol withdrawal head twitches in mice. *J Pharmacol* 58:9–16, 1976.
93. Kostowski W, Trzaskowska E: Effects of lesion of the locus coeruleus and clonidine treatment on ethanol withdrawal syndrome in rats. *Pol J Pharmacol Pharm* 32:617, 1980.
94. Walinder J, Balldin J, Bokstrom K, et al: Clonidine suppression of the alcohol withdrawal syndrome. *Drug Alcohol Depend* 8:345–348, 1981.
95. Nardoni A, Baldissera S, Iacono M, Copetti R, Cella R: La clonidina nel trattamento della sindrome da astinenza alcoolica. *Communicazione Preliminare 30:97(6):619–24, 1981.*
96. Gallant DM, Swanson WC, Guerrero-Faueroa R: A controlled evaluation of propranolol in chronic alcoholic patients presenting the symptomatology of anxiety and tension. *J Clin Pharm New Drugs* 13:41–43, 1973.
97. Rappolt RI: Treatment of ethanol withdrawal employing a beta-adrenergic blocking agent (propranolol). *Clin Toxicol* 6:293–294, 1973.
98. Teravainen H, Larsen A: Effect of propranolol on acute withdrawal tremor in alcoholic patients. *J Neurol Neurosurg Psychiatry* 39:607–612, 1976.
99. Goldstein DB: Alcohol withdrawal reactions in mice: Effects of drugs that modify neurotransmission. *J Pharm Exp Ther* 186:1–9, 1973.
100. Carlsso C, Johansson T: The psychological effects of propranolol in the abstinence phase of chronic alcoholics. *Br J Psychiatry* 119:605–608, 1971.
101. Ahtee L, Svartstrom-Fraser M: Effect of ethanol dependence and withdrawal on the catecholamines in rat brain and heart. *Acta Pharm Toxicol* 36:289–298, 1975.
102. Wajda IJ, Magnigault I, Hudick P: Dopamine levels in the striatum and the effect of alcohol and reserpine. *Biochem Pharmacol* 26:653–655, 1977.
103. Darden JH, Hunt WA: Reduction of striatal dopamine release during an ethanol withdrawal syndrome. *J Neurochem* 29:1143–1145, 1977.
104. Darden JH, Hunt WA: Depression of dopamine release during the ethanol withdrawal syndrome. *Pharmacologist* 17(2):240, 1975.
105. Blum K, Eubanks JD, Wallace JE, et al: Suppression of ethanol withdrawal by dopamine. *Experientia* 32:493–495, 1976.
106. Trzaskowska E, Pucilowski O, Kostowski W, et al: Effects of 6-hydroxydopamine-induced lesions of A10 dopaminergic neurons and neuroleptic or bromocriptine treatment on ethanol withdrawal syndrome in rats. *Pol J Pharmacol Pharm* 35:339–349, 1983.
107. Hunter B, Boast CA, Walker D, et al: Alcohol withdrawal syndrome in rats: neural and behavioral correlates. *Pharmacol Biochem Behav* 1:719–725, 1973.
108. Majchrowicz E: Induction of physical dependence upon ethanol and the associated behavioral change in rats. *Psychopharmacologia* 43:245–254, 1975.
109. Borg V, Weinholdt T: Bromocriptine in the treatment of the alcohol withdrawal syndrome. *Acta Psychiatry Scand* 65:101, 1982.
110. Karoum F, Wyatt RJ, Majchrowicz E: Brain concentrations of biogenic amine metabolites in acutely treated and ethanol-dependent rats. *Br J Pharmacol* 56:403–411, 1976.
111. Griffiths PJ, Littleton JM, Ortiz A: Changes in monoamine concentrations in mouse brain associated with ethanol dependence and withdrawal. *Br J Pharmacol* 50:489–498, 1974.
112. Gunne LM: Noradrenaline and adrenaline in the rat brain during acute and chronic morphine administration and during withdrawal. *Nature (London)* 184:1950–1951, 1951.
113. Bonnycastle D, Bonnycastle MFA, Anderson EG: The effect of a number of central depressant drugs upon brain 5-hydroxytryptamine levels in the rat. *J Pharm Exp Ther* 135:17–20, 1962.
114. Shen FH, Loh HH, Way EL: Brain serotonin turnover in morphine tolerant and dependent mice. *J Pharm Exp Ther* 175:427–434, 1970.
115. Hunt WA, Majchrowitz E: Alterations in the turnover of brain norepinephrine and dopamine in alcohol-dependent rats. *J Neurochem* 23:549–552, 1974.
116. Blum K, Wallace JE, Schwertner HA, et al: Enhancement of ethanol-induced withdrawal convulsions by blockade of 5-hydroxytryptamine receptors. *J Pharm Pharmacol* 28:832–835, 1976.

117. Roccatagliata G, Albano C, Maffini M, et al: Alcohol withdrawal syndrome: Treatment with trazadone. *Int Pharmacopsychiatry* 15:105–110, 1980.
118. Rawat AK: Brain levels and turnover rates of presumptive neurotransmitters as influenced by administration and withdrawal of ethanol in mice. *J Neurochem* 22:915–922, 1974.
119. Hunt WA, Dalton TK: Regional brain acetylcholine levels in rats acutely treated with ethanol or rendered ethanol dependent. *Brain Res* 109:628–631, 1976.
120. Major LF, Goyer PF, Murphy DL: Changes in platelet monoamine oxidase activity during abstinence. *J Stud Alcohol* 42:1052–1057, 1981.
121. Zimmer R, Cramer H, Athen D, et al: Changes in cerebrospinal fluid cyclic neucleotides in alcohol-dependent patients suffering from delirium tremens. *Biol Psychiatry* 17(7):837–843, 1982.
122. Askew WE, Charalampous KD: Chronic ethanol and neural cAMP. *Life Sci* 22:639–646, 1978.
123. Volicer L, Hurter BP: Effects of acute and chronic ethanol administation and withdrawal on adenosine-3′-5′monophosphate and guanosine3′-5′monophosphate levels in the rat brain. *J Pharmacol Exp Ther* 200:290–305, 1977.
124. Kuriyama K, Israel MA: Effect of ethanol administration on cyclic 3″5″ adenosine monophosphate metabolism in brain. *Biochem Pharmacol* 22:2919–2922, 1973.
125. French SW, Reid PE, Palmer DS, et al: Adrenergic subsensitivity of the rat brain during chronic ethanol ingestion. *Res Commun Chem Pathol Pharmacol* 9:575–578, 1974.
126. French SW, Palmer DS, Narod NE, et al: Noradrenergic sensitivity of the cerebral cortex after chronic ethanol ingestion and withdrawal. *J Pharmacol Exp Ther* 194:319–326, 1975.
127. Patel GL, Lal H: Reduction in brain gamma-aminobutryic acid and in barbital narcosis during ethanol withdrawal. *J Pharmacol Exp Ther* 186:625–629, 1973.
128. Leitch GL, Backes DJ, Siegman FS, et al: Possible role of GABA in the development of tolerance to alcohol. *Experientia* 33:496–497, 1977.
129. Sytinsky LA, Guzikov BM, Gomanko MV, et al: The gamma-aminobutyric acid (GABA) system in brain during acute and chronic ethanol intoxication. *J Neurochem* 25:43–48, 1975.
130. Cooper BR, Viik K, Ferris RM, et al: Antagonism of the enhanced susceptibility to audiogenic seizures during alcohol withdrawal in the rat by gamma-aminobutyric acid (GABA) and "GABA-mimetic" agents. *J Pharmacol Exp Ther* 209:396–403, 1979.
131. Noble EP, Gillies R, Vigran R, et al: The modification of the ethanol withdrawal syndrome in rats by di-n-propylacetate. *Psychopharmacologia (Berlin)* 46:127–131, 1976.
132. Gonzalez LP, Hettinger MK: Intranigral muscimol suppresses ethanol withdrawal seizures. *Brain Res* 298:163–166, 1984.
133. Abu-Murad C, Nordmann R: Effect of two iron-chelators, desferrioxamine and diethylenetriaminepentaacetic acid, on the development of tolerance to and physical dependence on ethanol in mice. *Drug Alcohol Depend* 12:371–379, 1983.
134. Valimaki M, Harkonen M, Ylikahri R: Serum ferritin and iron levels in chronic male alcoholics before and after ethanol withdrawal. *Alcohol Alcoholism,* 18(3):255–260, 1983.
135. Berglund M, Risberg J: Regional cerebral blood flow during alcohol withdrawal. *Arch Gen Psychiatry* 38:351–355, 1981.
136. Antelman SM, Cagguila AR: Norepinephrine-dopamine interactions and behavior. *Science* 195:646–653, 1977.
137. Renaud B, Buda M, Lewis BO, et al: Effects of 5,6-dihydroxytryptamine on tyrosine hydroxylase activity in central catecholaminergic neurons of the rat. *Biochem Pharmacol* 24:1739–1742, 1975.
138. Rochette L, Bralet J: Effect of the norepinephrine receptor stimulating agent clonidine in the turnover of 5-HTP in some areas of the rat brain. *J Neural Transm* 37:259–267, 1976.
139. Lewander T, Joliand TH, Reis. Prolonged activation of tyrosine hydroxylase in noradrenergic neurons of rat brain by cholinergic stimulation. *Nature* 258:440–441, 1975.
140. Erickson CK: Functional relationships among central neurotransmitters. *Rev Neurosci* 3:1–34, 1976.
141. Harris RA, Crabbe JC, McSwigan JD: Relationship of membrane physical properties to alcohol dependence in mice selected for genetic differences in alcohol withdrawal. *Life Sci* 35:2601–2608, 1984.

142. Ticku MK, Burch TP, Davis WC: The interactions of ethanol with the benzodiazepine-GABA receptor-ionophore complex. *Pharm Biochem Behav* 18:15–18, 1983.
143. Svensson TH, Bunney BS, Aghajanian GK: Inhibition of both noradrenergic and serotonergic neurons in brain by the alpha-adrenergic agonist clonidine. *Brain Res* 92:291–299, 1975.
144. Kellogg CK, Retell TM, Harary N: Benzodiazepine influence on norepinephrine release: Regional specificity. *Soc Neurosci Abstr 14th Annual Meeting* 10(2):972, 1984.
145. Suzdak PD, Granutsos G: Differential coupling of a GABA-A and GABA-B receptors to the noradrenergic system: Implications for a GABA-ergic role in depression. *Soc Neurosci Abstr 14th Annual Meeting* 10(2):889, 1984.
146. Nestoros JN: Ethanol specifically potentiates GABA-mediated neurotransmission in feline cerebral cortex. *Science* 209:708–710, 1980.
147. Squires RF, Saederup E: Diverse groups of psychotropic drugs interact with GABA/picrotoxin receptor complexes. *Soc Neurosci Abstr 13th Annual Meeting* 9(2):1039, 1983.
148. Dunwiddie TV, Worth TS: Enhancement of GABA-ergic inhibition by barbiturates and related depressant drugs in rat hypocampal slices. *Soc Neurosci Abstr 14th Annual Meeting* 10(2):966, 1984.
149. Ticku MK, Maksay G: Dissociation and equilibrium studies with {35S}T-bulylbicyclophosphorothionate and depressant drugs bind to different but coupled sites at the GABA receptor–ionophore couples. *Soc Neurosci Abstr 14th Annual Meeting* 10(1):389, 1984.
150. Grant SJ, Mayor B, Redmond DE Jr: Effects of alprazolam, a novel triazolobenzodiazepine, on locus coeruleus unit activity. Abstracts, 14th Annual Meeting, vol 10, part 2, p 952, 1984.
151. Shefner SA, Tabzkoff B: Ethanol-induced inhibition of spontaneous firing of locus coeruleus neurons is associated with an enhancement of the late afterhyperpolarization. *Soc Neurosci Abstr 14th Annual Meeting* 10(2):966, 1984.
152. Stone G, Skirboll L, Hommer DW: The effects of benzodiazepine antagonists on single unit activity in the locus coeruleus. *Soc Neurosci Abstr 14th Annual Meeting* 10(1):643, 1984.
153. Bloom FE, Siggins GR, Foote SL, et al: Noradrenergic involvement in the cellular actions of ethanol, Usdin E, Carlsson A, Dahlstrum A, et al: *Neurology and Neurobiology,* vol 8B. New York, Alan R Liss, 1984, pp 159–167.
154. Belknap JK, Crabbe JC, Danielson PW, et al: Genetic sensitivity to the ethanol withdrawal syndrome: Genetic cross-sensitivity to a barbiturate and a benzodiazepine in mice. *Soc Neurosci Abstr 14th Annual Meeting* 10(1):571, 1984.
155. Marley RJ, Wehner JM: Differential enhancement of benzodiazepine binding, by GABA, in mice selectively bred for sensitivity to ethanol. *Soc Neurosci Abstr 15th Annual Meeting* 11:291, 1985.
156. Shin S, Legg S, McNamara JO: Systemic gamma-vinyl GABA retards kindling development and suppresses kindled seizures. *Soc Neurosci Abstr 14th Annual Meeting* 10(1):343, 1984.
157. Begleiter H, Porjesz B: Persistence of brain hyperexcitability following chronic alcohol exposure in rats, in Gross MM (ed): *Alcohol Intoxication and Withdrawal,* vol 85B. New York, Plenum Press, 1977, pp 209–221.
158. Sjoquist B, Perolahl E, Winblad B: The effect of alcoholism on salsolinol and biogenic amines in human brain. *Drug Alcohol Depend* 12:15–23, 1983.
159. Goodwin DW: Alcoholism and genetics. *Arch Gen Psychiatry* 42:171–174, 1985.

12

Clinical Assessment and Pharmacotherapy of the Alcohol Withdrawal Syndrome

Claudio A. Naranjo and Edward M. Sellers

Abstract. All patients in alcohol withdrawal should have a full assessment for detecting medical complications. The Clinical Institute Withdrawal Assessment for Alcohol (CIWA-A) scale permits a quantitative assessment for following the clinical course and therapeutic response in patients in withdrawal. Most patients with mild withdrawal symptoms do not require hospitalization and respond to non-pharmacologic supportive care. Early initiation of treatment with supportive nursing care and, if necessary, benzodiazepines usually will prevent progression to serious withdrawal reactions and provide the patient with sufficient symptomatic relief. Pharmacotherapy can be considerably simplified by using the loading dose technique, i.e., giving diazepam every 1–2 hr initially until the patient shows signs of clinical improvement and/or mild sedation. If long half-life drugs (e.g., diazepam) are used, further therapy is rarely needed and complications are prevented. Short-acting benzodiazepines can also be given in a similar fashion in the milder clinical syndrome. Phenytoin should only be given to patients with a preexisting seizure disorder. Phenothiazines, barbiturates, paraldehyde, and antihistamines have no role in the treatment of withdrawal because of their toxicity or lack of efficacy. Haloperidol is effective in the control of hallucinations in patients also treated with a benzodiazepine. The treatment of alcoholic intoxication and withdrawal is only the first step toward full rehabilitation.

1. Introduction

Advances in the assessment and treatment of the alcohol withdrawal syndrome have led to substantial decreases in the development of serious morbidity and deaths. This progress has been associated with early recognition of the withdrawal, better methods of assessing patients, and optimization of the tactics for administering drug treatments. Advances are such that nowadays a treatment failure is almost certainly due to delay in therapy, an error

Claudio A. Naranjo • Clinical Pharmacology Program, Addiction Research Foundation Clinical Institute, and Departments of Pharmacology and Medicine, University of Toronto, Ontario M5S 2S1, Canada. **Edward M. Sellers** • Clinical Institute, Addiction Research Foundation, and Departments of Pharmacology and Medicine, University of Toronto, Ontario M5S 2S1, Canada. The views expressed in this publication are those of the authors and do not necessarily reflect those of the Addiction Research Foundation.

of omission or commission, or the severity of the concurrent illness, but not alcohol withdrawal per se.

We review recent developments in the clinical assessment and in the use of nonpharmacologic and pharmacologic treatments of the alcohol withdrawal syndrome. Other recent reviews have dealt with various aspects of the problem.[1–5]

2. Clinical Manifestations of the Alcohol Withdrawal Syndrome

Chronic exposure of excitable cells and tissues to ethanol results in adaptive changes that are temporarily correlated with, and presumably responsible for, the development of tolerance to ethanol.[1] Alcohol dependence is also produced by repeated exposure and usually, but not always, develops coincidentally with tolerance.[6] When alcohol consumption is abruptly stopped or rapidly decreased, the CNS, nonspecifically depressed by alcohol, undergoes "reequilibration" and the physical dependence on alcohol is manifested by the signs and symptoms of alcohol withdrawal. A major alcohol withdrawal also constitutes a severe physical stress that may add to or complicate the manifestations of the primary process of dependence on alcohol. In addition, reduction or cessation of alcohol is often the result of injury, intercurrent illness, or alcohol-related diseases, the manifestations of which are also present. The severity of alcohol withdrawal is related to the preceding alcohol intake; thus, the most severe reactions occur in patients exposed to highest doses over the longest time. All these factors may modify or complicate the clinical manifestations of the withdrawal reaction.

2.1. Usual Clinical Presentations (Table I and Fig. 1A)

It is customary to describe an "early or minor withdrawal" and a "late or major withdrawal" (delirium tremens), even though the validity of such a classification is not clearly documented. Some studies suggest that the various clinical manifestations of the alcohol withdrawal syndrome develop along a continuum ranging from common mild primary manifestations (e.g., tremulousness), which occur early, to the secondary manifestations or complications (seizures, hallucinations, arrhythmias and delirium), which occur later in only a few subjects.[7,8] Appropriate prospective studies for conclusively documenting the current natural history of this syndrome are needed. For lack of a better alternative, we will continue to describe the symptoms grouped in the traditional description, recognizing that this separation might not be entirely valid.

2.1.1. Early "Minor" Withdrawal. The severity of the early alcohol withdrawal reaction varies with both the intensity and duration of the preceding alcohol intake; hence it is quite variable among patients.[1,2,9,10] The earliest symptoms are insomnia, vivid dreaming, and "hangover." This symptomatology coincides with the rapid elimination of ethanol. Anxiety, mild

Table I. Usual Clinical Presentations of the Alcohol Withdrawal Syndrome

Clinical features	Early or minor withdrawal	Late or major withdrawal or delirium tremens
Symptoms or signs	Mild agitation Anxiety Restlessness Tremor Anorexia Insomnia	Extreme overactivity (speech, psychomotor, autonomic) Disorientation Confusion Disordered sensory perception
Timing Postethanol	0–48 hr	24–150 hr
Peak of symptoms	24–36 hr	72–96 hr
Severity	Mild	Potentially life-threatening
Seizures	Yes, 6–48 hr	No

agitation, anorexia, tremor, sleeplessness, mild tachycardia (<100), and hypertension (>150/90) appear a few hours after cessation of drinking and disappear after 48 hr. This syndrome indicates persistent ethanol consumption in excess of 150–200 g/day and usually requires no pharmacotherapy.

2.1.2. Late "Major" Withdrawal ("delirium tremens"). In severe reactions, however, these initial symptoms are gradually followed by increasing psychomotor, verbal and autonomic hyperactivity, disorientation, confusion, and auditory or visual hallucinations. Disorientation and confusion are the essential hallmarks of "delirium tremens." Seizures frequently precede such a reaction, although they may occur in patients who do not progress to a major withdrawal. The severity and risk of the syndrome are increased by delay in recognition, and the presence of concurrent medical or surgical illnesses (e.g., fever, infection, malnutrition, dehydration or hypovolemia, acid-base and electrolyte abnormalities, trauma, hemorrhage, cardiac disease, etc.). Fever over 104°F (40°C), malnutrition, and fluid and electrolyte disturbances are associated with a risk of developing major withdrawal signs (delirium tremens; DTs).

Less than 5% of hospitalized patients in alcohol withdrawal develop a major reaction. Early reports estimated the mortality of such a reaction at above 40%. More recently, an estimate of 2%[11] has been suggested. The lower estimate is possibly accurate in most centres nowadays, because of improved supportive therapy of the coexisting medical complications of alcohol withdrawal. The patients at greatest risk of severe or fatal withdrawal reactions are those over 45 years of age and those with serious medical complications. In the few deaths that still do occur, delayed diagnosis, inadequate initial therapy, inappropriate drug dose adjustment, and unrecognized concurrent disease are often apparent. Since these problems are amenable to careful clinical monitoring and standardization of pharmacotherapy, the mortality should be reducible to that of any coexistent medical or surgical problem.

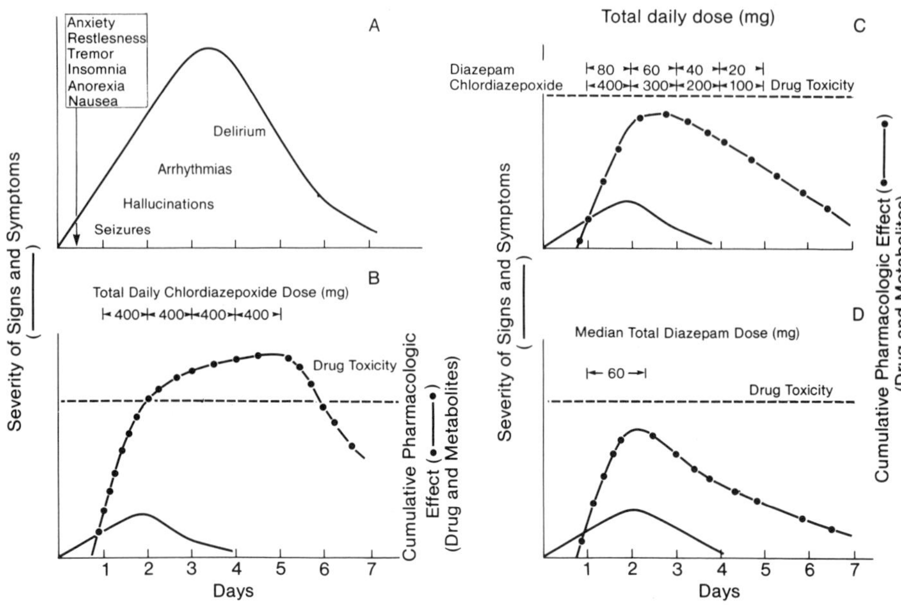

Figure 1. Effect of benzodiazepine therapy on the clinical course of alcohol withdrawal.

(A) Clinical features of the alcohol withdrawal syndrome.

(B) Cumulative pharmacologic effect of chlordiazepoxide and its active metabolite, desmethylchlordiazepoxide, during repeated daily administration of the same daily dose. Because of cumulation of parent drug and active metabolite, excessive sedation occurs.

(C) Cumulative pharmacologic effect of diazepam and/or chlordiazepoxide, during repeated administration of daily doses reduced gradually. This procedure is effective and avoids excessive sedation but requires administration of the drug for several days.

(D) Cumulative pharmacologic effect of diazepam and its active metabolite, desmethyldiazepam, when the loading dose technique is used. This procedure is simple and very effective and because total dose of drug are smaller and titrated to patient's response, excessive sedation is avoided.

2.1.3. Seizures in Alcohol Withdrawal. Seizures during alcohol withdrawal are relatively common. It is estimated that between 5% and 15% of alcoholics in withdrawal develop seizures, but the frequency may be higher in patients who will develop delirium tremens or in those with a prior history of withdrawal seizures.[12–15] More than 90% of seizures occur from 6 to 48 hr after discontinuation of ethanol and are usually grand mal type. Ten percent of subjects may present several seizures.[12,14]

The patient who has seizures for the first time in his life—even if it is likely a withdrawal seizure—should be investigated to rule out an organic disease or a structural lesion. Typical investigation should include routine hematology, blood sugar, BUN, serum electrolytes, serum Ca, serum Mg, skull X-rays, EEG, CT scan, and drug screening.

Patients having had one or more recent seizures suspected of being due to alcohol withdrawal require careful evaluation to rule out other causes of convulsions (CNS infections, trauma, electrolyte imbalances, tumor, etc.). These patients should have a full neurologic examination. Those patients with focal neurologic deficits need an evaluation with CT brain scanning.[16] Such a procedure increases the likelihood of detecting reversible focal lesions. In addition, the CT brain scanning might be helpful every time new focal deficits are detected by neurologic examination. This is particularly important in patients who had an acute head trauma. In the absence of either focal deficits on neurologic examination or signs of acute head trauma, the yield on CT brain scans is low and they do not improve the evaluation of patients with alcohol withdrawal seizures.

2.2. Unusual Clinical Presentations

While typically several components of the mild or severe reaction are present, occasional patients may present with only a single prominent clinical manifestation, e.g., seizure, severe tremor, cardiac arrhythmia, hallucination, internuclear opthalmoplegia, confusion, etc. Since, rarely, the symptomatology may be delayed for 7–14 days, accurate diagnosis may be difficult. Occurrence of these clinical features in isolation should always raise the possibility of alcohol as a primary or comorbid factor.

A protracted alcohol withdrawal can also occur.[17] For example, sleep EEG studies have demonstrated continued disturbance of sleep phases in alcoholics for 30 days or longer after the last ingestion of alcohol. In rats, studies of auditory evoked brainstem potentials and visually evoked cortical potentials have indicated persistence of hyperexcitability of the CNS for as long as 4–8 weeks after withdrawal of chronic ethanol intubation. These changes are suggestive of slow disappearance of physical dependence but they do not prove it conclusively. Since they are rather nonspecific, they might be produced by other factors. In humans, for example, sleep disturbances might reflect emotional and other problems related to drug-free existence, rather than physical dependence on ethanol. It has been suggested that relapse of drinking may occur because of withdrawallike symptoms in the absence of preceding drinking bouts.[18] However, the existence of a protracted alcohol withdrawal reaction remains controversial.

2.3. Assessment

All patients with severe withdrawal reactions or with medical or surgical complications should be hospitalized. Irrespective of whether the patient will be admitted or not, an appropriate history and physical and laboratory examination are mandatory because of the multisystem effects of alcohol.

In an effort to develop an instrument for systematically assessing the alcohol withdrawal syndrome, Gross *et al.*[7,8] identified disturbances in 30 clincial variables during experimental alcohol withdrawal studies. Using cluster analysis, they established that these symptoms constituted a single clinical syndrome that ranged in severity from mild tremulousness to delirium tremens. Two instruments were developed; a research battery designated Total Severity Assessment (TSA) and a clinical instrument named Selected Severity Scale (SSA). The TSA contained all of the original 30 clinical variables, while the SSA consisted of a short list of 11 items. The SSA correlated highly with the TSA.[7,8] In the SSA, a score was assigned to the following signs and symptoms: eating disturbances, sleep disturbances, agitation, hallucinations (auditory and/or visual), tremor, sweats, clouding of sensorium, quality of contact, temperature, pulse, and convulsions. This procedure has been further refined so that it can be applied hourly or more frequently to follow the clinical course of the withdrawal reaction. This modified 15-item scale is referred to as the Clinical Institute Withdrawal Assessment for Alcohol (CIWA-A).[19] This scale allows a quantitative rating (from zero to seven) of the following components of the withdrawal reaction: nausea and vomiting, tremor, paroxysmal sweats, tactile disturbances, auditory disturbances, visual disturbances, hallucinations, clouding of sensorium, quality of contact, anxiety, agitation, thought disturbances, convulsions, headache, and flushing of face (Table II). Heart rate, body temperature, and blood pressure were also recorded, but not included in the CIWA-A scoring.

Several studies have shown that the CIWA-A scale is a valid, reliable, and sensitive procedure for assessing the clinical course of the alcohol with-

Table II. Items Rated on the Clinical Institute Withdrawal Assessment Scale (CIWA-A)

Items	Score (range)
Tremor	0–7
Nausea and vomiting	0–7
Paroxysmal sweats	0–7
Tactile disturbances	0–6
Auditory disturbances	0–6
Visual disturbances	0–6
Hallucinations	0–3
Clouding of sensorium	0–4
Quality of contact	0–7
Anxiety	0–7
Agitation	0–7
Thought disturbances	0–3
Seizures	0–7
Headache	0–7
Flushing of face	0–2

drawal.[19–21] This scale has been successfully used for assessing therapeutic response in clinical trials and in the management of ambulatory and hospitalized patients in withdrawal.[19–21] One of the advantages of this standardized procedure is that the evaluators (e.g., nurses) become aware of the symptoms that make up the alcohol withdrawal syndrome, making it easier to assess and compare the effectiveness of treatments. Further studies have demonstrated that a shorter version of CIWA-A scale that includes only nine items (nausea, tremor, sweating, tactile disturbances, auditory disturbances, visual disturbances, hallucinations, anxiety, and agitation) correlates highly ($r = 0.95$) with the total CIWA-A scale. Thus it is possible for clinical simplicity to use this shorter version of the scale. The rating with either version by a trained observer usually takes less than 1 min.

3. Therapy of the Alcohol Withdrawal Syndrome

3.1. Goals of Treatment

The objectives of therapy are relief of subjective symptoms, prevention or treatment of the more serious complications (seizures, hallucinations, arrhythmias and delirium), and preparation for long-term rehabilitation with minimal hazard of a new drug dependence or direct drug-induced toxicity. In addition, optimal treatment should be standardized, humane, and as simple and economic as possible; it should have a pharmacokinetic and pharmacodynamic rationale, and its efficacy and safety should be established by methodologically sound studies. The need to adhere to a relatively well defined protocol has been clearly illustrated by a recent chart audit that confirmed the widely held impression that patients in withdrawal may have numerous changes in pharmacotherapy (with respect to drug, dose, interval, route, etc.) regardless of the severity of the withdrawal reaction.[19]

The treatment of withdrawal reactions involves non-pharmacologic and pharmacologic interventions.

3.2. Nonpharmacologic Interventions

3.2.1. Supportive Care. Uncontrolled studies showed that reassurance reality orientation, frequent monitoring of signs and symptoms, personal attention, and general nursing care were effective in over two thirds of patients in a mild alcohol withdrawal reaction.[22,23]

At the Addiction Research Foundation Clinical Institute, we developed a standardized supportive care package for treating alcohol withdrawal[19] (Table III). This procedure is aimed at satisfying the following patient needs: reduced sensory stimuli; maintenance of hydration; reality orientation; reassurance; nutrition; physical comfort; body temperature; sleep and rest; and positive encouragement toward long-term rehabilitation. Recent controlled

Table III. Components of Supportive Care for Treating Alcohol Withdrawal

Needs	Intervention
Environmental stimuli	Quiet, private room
	Control lighting
	Only one staff member in contact
	Use uniform or white lab coat
Foods and fluids	Offer fluids every 60 min
	Regular diet at meal time
	Record intake
Physical comfort	Change and/or support position with pillows
	Raise head of bed if necessary
Body temperature	Apply or remove blankets
Rest and sleep	Allow to rest or sleep between assessments
	Talk to patient only if he/she initiates conversation
Elimination	Assist to bathroom
	Record output
Reality orientation	With respect to time, place, and person
Reassurance	Positive encouragement
	Hourly contact
Rehabilitation	Discuss only if topic initiated by patient
	Agree with patient if he says he wants to quit drinking
Visitors	No visitors during supportive care
Smoking	Only if patients ask
	Limit to four cigarettes per hour

studies have confirmed the potency of such nonpharmacologic interventions. Eighty-five percent of emergency room patients[20] and 60% of inpatients responded to supportive care in less than 6–8 hr.[21]

The effectiveness of nonpharmacologic interventions have obvious major implications for design and interpretation of studies assessing drug therapies in alcohol withdrawal. Many drugs are claimed to be effective in treating alcohol withdrawal, but a major problem in the interpretation of data on the efficacy of drugs is that clinicians are reluctant, usually on ethical grounds, to use a placebo control.[20] In this context, it is notable that the frequency of placebo-controlled studies of alcohol withdrawal has declined markedly. Placebos were used in 11 of the 19 controlled studies published during the 1960s but in only 4 of the 19 in the 1970s.[9] Since our data indicate that to a substantial extent the efficacy of a drug may be due to the influence of nonpharmacologic interventions, it is essential to use a placebo control group.[20] Despite the effectiveness of nonpharmacologic interventions, drugs are still required by some patients. Since supportive care is not effective against hallucinations, seizures, or arrhythmias, and since patient characteristics do not predict responsiveness to supportive care, patients in moderate to severe withdrawal should also receive drugs (e.g., diazepam).[20,21]

3.3. Pharmacological Interventions

3.3.1. General Pharmacotherapy. Multivitamin preparations are commonly used, although their value is unproven.[1] Nevertheless, sixth cranial nerve paresis can be reversed dramatically by as little as 2 mg of thiamine i.v. Typically, doses of 50–100 mg are given i.m. or slowly i.v. In patients receiving intravenous glucose, thiamine should be given to avoid unmasking a relative thiamine deficiency.

Hydration may be required, although overhydration is more common in milder cases of withdrawal. Replacement of potassium is indicated in hypokalemic patients with weakness or cardiac arrhythmias and in those receiving digitalis gylcosides. Although intravenous or intramuscular magnesium may suppress withdrawal seizures, cardiac arrhythmias, and tremor, other drugs are also effective and probably less toxic.[2]

3.3.2. Specific Pharmacotherapy. More than 100 different drugs and drug combinations have been described for the treatment of alcohol withdrawal.[1,2,5,9,11] This profusion of drug treatments is unsupported by empirical evidence concerning their efficacy. Thus, a recent report has documented serious methodological problems in a large proportion of 81 therapeutic trials of alcohol withdrawal published since 1954.[24] Only 35.8% were randomized controlled trials, and a substantial proportion of those presented problems in the protocol design and in the statistical analysis of results. In addition, several of the studies were neither double-blind nor placebo-controlled, even though the effectiveness of nonpharmacologic interventions (e.g., supportive care) is well documented.[19,20] Thus, the evidence of efficacy for several of the drugs currently in use for treating alcohol withdrawal is questionnable and requires a more critical assessment.

The most widely used "treatment" for alcohol withdrawal is more alcohol, but this is inappropriate because alcohol has toxic effects on heart, liver, and brain, has a short duration of action, inhibits drug biotransformation, and perpetuates the many existing metabolic disturbances associated with the alcohol withdrawal syndrome.[1] The search for an ideal agent for treating alcohol withdrawal is pointless, since all agents can be ineffective or toxic in some circumstances. The pharmacologic properties of the drugs used in alcohol withdrawal are summarized in Table IV. Most of the drugs show cross-tolerance with alcohol and also have sedative, anxiolytic, or anticonvulsant therapy. Guidelines for the use of the most commonly prescribed drugs are summarized in Table V.

3.3.3. Benzodiazepines. The benzodiazepines are currently the drugs of choice.[1,2,5,11,21] The rationale for their use is their cross-tolerance with alcohol. Benzodiazepines do not cause enzyme induction and have a lower potential to produce physical dependence and tolerance than barbiturates.[25,26] They combine at least equal efficacy to other agents, with superior anticonvulsant activity and lesser toxicity than phenothiazines, barbiturates and par-

Table IV. Pharmacologic Properties of Drugs Used in the Treatment of Alcohol Withdrawal[a]

	Properties				
Drug class	Cross-tolerance with alcohol	Sedative effects	Antianxiety effects	Anticonvulsant effects	Safety/toxicity ratio
Benzodiazepines	×××	××	×××	×××	×××
Barbiturates	×××	×××	×	×××	×
Phenothiazines	×	××	×	0	×
Butyrophenones	×	××	×	0	××
Antihistamines	×	×	0	0	×××
Chloral hydrate	××	××	×	××	×
Thiazoles	×	××	×	×	×
β-adrenergic blockers	0	0	××	0	××
α_2-Agonists	0	×	×	0	×
Dopamine antagonists	0	×	×	0	×
Lithium	×	×	×	0	×
Anticonvulsants	××	×	0	×××	××

[a] ××× = very good or marked; ×× = moderate; × = mild or poor; 0 = absent.

Table V. Guidelines for Drug Therapy of Patients in Alcohol Withdrawal

Clinical Problem	Drug	Route	Dose	Interval	Comment
Withdrawal					
Moderate to severe	Diazepam	p.o.	20 mg	Every 1–2 hr	The initial dose can be repeated every 1–2 hr until patient shows signs of improvement or mild sedation; median dose is usually 60 mg of diazepam or 300 mg of chlordiazepoxide
	Chlordiazepoxide	p.o.	100 mg		
Extreme	Chlordiazepoxide	i.v.	12.5 mg/min	Slow infusion	Rarely needed; most patients respond to adequate dosing with oral diazepam. In those rare cases when needed, it should be given until patient is calm (subsequent dosages must be individualized on the basis of the clinical picture)
	Diazepam	i.v.	2.5 mg/min		
Hallucinations	Haloperidol	i.m.	0.5–5.0 mg	Every 2 hr	Until controlled or to maximum of five doses; appropriate doses of diazepam should be used concurrently
Seizure					
History of seizure disorder or previous withdrawal seizures	Phenytoin	p.o.	Diphenylhydantoin detected in blood, maintenance dose: 100 mg;	Every 8 hr	
			no diphenylhydantoin detected in blood, loading dose: 200–300 mg, maintenance dose: 100 mg	Every 8 hr	
Repeated seizures requiring acute therapy	Phenytoin	i.v.	Loading dose: 1 g	Infuse at 50 mg/min	Exact loading dose is 10 mg/kg; do not dilute in saline or dextrose solution
		p.o.	Maintenance dose: 100 mg	Every 8 hr	Diazepam i.v. should be used in the treatment of status epilepticus

aldehyde.[2] Numerous benzodiazepines, including alprazolam, bromazepam, chlordiazepoxide, chlorazepate, clobazam, diazepam, flurazepam, lorazepam, and oxazepam, have been used, and there is no evidence that any particular benzodiazepine is more effective.[2,11,24] Approximate equivalent doses relative to chlordiazepoxide 100 mg are diazepam 20 mg, oxazepam 120 mg, and lorazepam 5 mg. Most studies have been done with chlordiazepoxide, which is more effective than placebo or no drug therapy in decreasing anxiety, restlessness, tremor, seizure frequency, and development of DTs.[1,2] In effective dosages, chlordiazepoxide is at least as effective as promazine, chlorpromazine, pherphenazine, and paraldehyde-chloral hydrate in controlling various manifestations of alcohol withdrawal. Benzodiazepines are superior to phenothiazines in the prevention of seizures. Diazepam is effective in the control of continuous seizure activity during withdrawal.[11,21,25]

Since chlordiazepoxide is slowly and erratically absorbed from i.m. injection sites, p.o. or i.v. routes may be more appropriate.[27] Alternately, diazepam or lorazepam could be given intramuscularly. Sublingual lorazepam is rapidly absorbed and should be considered for nauseated patients.[20] Higher doses of benzodiazepines may be required in heavy smokers.[27] Lower doses might be anticipated in cirrhotics since chlordiazepoxide and diazepam are metabolized more slowly. In contrast, the metabolism of oxazepam and lorazepam is not affected.[27]

Both chlordiazepoxide and diazepam are long-acting drugs with pharmacologically active metabolites.[27] Repeated daily administration at a constant dosage results in cumulation of the parent compound and/or metabolites in the body[21] (Fig. 1). Therefore, desired therapeutic and unwanted toxic effects may not appear until several days of continuous therapy (Fig. 1B). Similar cumulation will occur with prazepam or chlorazepate, which are biotransformed to desmethyldiazepam, the pharmacologically active long half-life metabolite formed after diazepam administration.[27] If dosages are not adjusted carefully, excessive drowsiness, lethargy, ataxia, diplopia, and confusion may occur. Respiratory depression and increased risk of aspiration may occur after i.v. administration.[27]

3.3.4. Loading Benzodiazepine Dose Technique. In the past, to circumvent the consequences of cumulation kinetics, doses were reduced progressively (Fig. 1C). Larger doses of diazepam or chlordiazepoxide were given on the first day of treatment. Typically, multiple doses of diazepam 20–40 mg or chlordiazepoxide 100–400 mg were given until the patient was settled. Lower doses were given daily thereafter and were tapered at a rate of about 25–50% of the initial daily dose.[1,21] However, because of important variability both in the severity of withdrawal symptoms and in the metabolic disposition of the drugs, strict adherence to such dosage schedules may cause toxicity or ineffective treatment in some cases.[21] Recently, the effectiveness and simplicity of the tapering dose approach to treating alcohol withdrawal have been greatly improved.[21] This procedure consists of a loading dose of diazepam and takes advantage of the pharmacokinetic tapering afforded by diazepam's and *N*-desmethyldiazepam's long half-lives (Fig. 1D). Patients in moderate to severe withdrawal are assessed with the CIWA-A scale, and unit doses of 20 mg of diazepam p.o. are administered hourly until the patient shows clinical improvement (decrease in CIWA-A to $\leq$10) or becomes mildly sedated. In a recent double-blind controlled study, patients treated with diazepam using the loading dose approach, had a faster and greater improvement than those receiving placebo.[21] Fifty percent of patients responded to 60 mg of diazepam p.o. within 7.6 hr and most of the patients improved in less than 36 hr. More importantly, complications (seizures, hallucinations, arrhythmias) occurred exclusively in those treated with placebo, indicating that delay in therapy may be responsible for the appearance of complications in withdrawal.[21] We recommend that when using this procedure all patients should be loaded with at least 60 mg of diazepam. Diazepam has several advantages for treating alcohol withdrawal. Peak blood levels are reached quickly, ensuring a large amount of the drug is available when the clinical manifestations are more severe. Becaue of diazepam's (and metabolite's) long half-lives, a continued high drug level is maintained, making additional doses unnecessary when a large enough initial dose has been given. In addition, this procedure reduces the frequency of adverse reactions and the need for further pharmacotherapy.[21]

There is no evidence supporting the indiscriminate long-term use of benzodiazepines in alcoholics after the withdrawal symptoms are controlled.[18] However, benzodiazepines are still detected in 33% of alcoholics undergoing medical assessment.[28] These patients could be at a greater risk of developing dependence on benzodiazepines even though there is no data conclusively documenting such a relationship.

Other drugs such as β blockers, phenytoin, and haloperidol, are less commonly used or have specific indications.

3.3.5. β-Blockers. The hyperadrenergic manifestations of withdrawal reactions suggest that nonselective β-blockers, e.g., propranolol, might be a useful therapeutic agent in withdrawal. Propranolol can be used in patients with severe withdrawal tremor. In a randomized double-blind controlled trial, propranolol 10 mg every 6 hr and 40 mg every 6 hr decreased symptoms of tremor and urinary and plasma catecholamines during alcohol withdrawal to an equal extent to chlordiazepoxide 25 mg every 6 hr and significantly more than placebo.[29] Therefore, i.v. (0.5 mg) and p.o. (40 mg/day) propranolol can be used to decrease alcohol withdrawal tremor. Another study showed that propranolol 40 mg every 6 hr decreased arrhythmias in alcohol withdrawal.[30] It is important to note in this study that 33.3% of patients receiving propranolol developed parahallucinatory side effects.[31]

While propranolol can be used in patients with severe withdrawal tremor or cardiac arrhythmias associated with withdrawal, the limitation of the drug's use to patients without a history of bronchospasm, cardiomyopathy, or congestive failure, coupled with an apparent enhancement of the risk of hallucinations, limits the usefulness of the drug.

3.3.6. Haloperidol (Table V). The butyrophenone class of antipsychotic drugs cause less sedation or hypotension and are preferred to control hallucinations in withdrawal.[2] Benzodiazepines are not effective in this respect. Severe agitation, thought disorders, and hallucinatory and parahallucinatory problems are controlled with haloperidol (0.5 to 5 mg i.m.). Since haloperidol decreases seizure threshold, patients should also receive chlordiazepoxide or diazepam concurrently, to offset any increased risk of seizures.[2]

3.3.7. Chlormethiazole. This drug is widely used in Europe and elsewhere,[4] but it is not marketed in North America. Some controlled studies suggest that it is superior to placebo, chlordiazepoxide, trifluoperazine, and piracetam and equal to amobarbital. It has sedative-hypnotic properties of the alcohol–barbiturate type. The chemical similarity of the drug to thiamine (vitamin B1) apparently is unrelated to its clinical efficacy. Problems with this drug include death, addiction, and marked changes in pharmacokinetics in liver disease and by alcohol. It can also cause phlebitis and hemolysis when it is given intravenously or in large doses, respectively. Notwithstanding the popularity of this drug in some countries, its superiority on pharmacokinetic and safety grounds is not clear. Considering the efficacy and safety of other agents (e.g., benzodiazepines), its continued use is puzzling.

3.3.8. Treatment of Seizures in Alcohol Withdrawal. Seizures during alcohol withdrawal reactions are typically grand mal, nonfocal, and one or two in number are most likely to occur between 6 and 48 hr after cessation of drinking. They clearly require treatment if they are repeated, continuous, or life-threatening.

The optimal treatment of alcohol withdrawal seizures remains controversial.[2,5,32] The therapeutic and prophylactic value of diphenylhydantoin in alcohol withdrawal seizures is uncertain. The contradictory findings in the clinical studies possibly arise from the indiscriminate inclusion of patients with pre-existing convulsive disease, those with a previous history of withdrawal seizures only, and those with no previous seizures. In most patients without a previous history of seizures, benzodiazepines alone probably have sufficient anticonvulsant activity to prevent withdrawal seizures.[21] However, in patients with a previous history of withdrawal seizures a better result may be obtained when a benzodiazepine (e.g., chlordiazepoxide up to 400 mg daily) is combined with diphenylhydantoin 100 mg t.i.d. than with placebo. Some studies including some in laboratory animals, however, have indicated that phenytoin is relatively ineffective against alcohol withdrawal seizures.[3,4]

The efficacy of chlordiazepoxide alone, compared with chlordiazepoxide plus phenytoin, to prevent alcohol withdrawal seizures was compared in a randomized study in 200 patients.[33] Both groups included patients with and without history of withdrawal seizures. The dosage of phenytoin was 400 mg/day for 5 days, and the daily dosage of chlordiazepoxide was variable (up to 360 mg/day) but similar in both groups. No withdrawal seizures were observed in either group. The authors concluded that when adequate dosages of chlordiazepoxide are used, no additional phenytoin is required. In another study,[34,157] patients with history of alcohol withdrawal seizures were randomly assigned to receive either chlordiazepoxide plus placebo or chlordiazepoxide plus phenytoin (300 mg/day). The doses of chlordiazepoxide (up to 400 mg/day) were similar in both groups. Patients receiving phenytoin had a lower frequency of seizures than the control groups. These apparently contradictory results might be interpreted as indicating that phenytoin has no value as a routine treatment in detoxification; however, it may be valuable in patients at high risk for seizures.

Our clinical practice is to give phenytoin with diazepam only to patients with a history of epilepsy or recurrent multiple withdrawal seizures. Such patients are rare. When phenytoin is given the following guidelines should be followed (Table V). Since phenytoin is poorly absorbed after i.m. injection, it should be given p.o. or i.v. It is most effective when a loading dose of 10 mg/kg is infused i.v. at a rate of 50 mg/min and followed by maintenance doses of 300–400 mg daily. For simplicity, a total loading dose of 1.0 g can be given and will be effective and safe in most patients except those whose weight is less than 50 kg.[1]

Despite the fact that phenytoin has been reported to be effective at serum concentrations of only 3–5 mg/liter in alcohol withdrawal, concentrations of 10–20 mg/liter are required for optimal control of idiopathic epilepsy. Phenytoin disposition is highly variable in chronic alcoholics. Steady-state blood levels vary 9-fold and are low because drug clearance is increased in some of these patients. The estimated mean drug half-life is only 7.4 hr (cf. normals 20 hr). Therefore to achieve drug concentrations of 10–20 mg/liter the daily maintenance dose may need to be as high as 1000 mg.[35] Therapy should be continued for 5 days or as determined by underlying seizure disorder.

3.3.9. Sodium Valproate. Dipropylacetate is a C-8 branch chain fatty acid that increases brain gamma amino butyric acid levels. Since it has been postulated that abrupt cessation of the ingestion of a sedative substance (including alcohol) could lead to a period of reduced GABA transmission, restoration of GABA neurotransmission by using agonists could be a rational treatment of withdrawal reactions.[36,37] In animal studies, valproic acid decresed convulsions in alcohol dependent rats. Anecdotal and uncontrolled studies suggest the drug may be effective in decreasing withdrawal symptomatology, seizure frequency and progression to delirium tremens.[38] Hepatotoxicity that occasionally can lead to fatal hepatic failure has been reported.[39] More rigorous clinical trials are needed.

3.3.10. Other Drugs. Other time-honoured drugs are used very rarely nowadays.[1,2,5] They have been largely replaced by the benzodiazepines. Antihistamines should not be used because of no demonstrated efficacy. While the phenothiazines appear to be effective, they do not prevent the progression to delirium tremens, and their potential for serious side effects far outweigh their therapeutic benefit in alcohol withdrawal. Particularly important is the increased frequency of seizures which occur in patients receiving promazine or chlorpromazine.[2] In addition, a compilation of six studies reviewed by

Thompson[32] suggest that patients treated with phenothiazines are not only more likely to convulse, but the incidence of delirium tremens is greater than in patients receiving placebo.[40] In addition, phenothiazines might induce orthostatic hypotension blood dyscrasias, jaundice and other side effects. Paraldehyde is rarely used. The combination of chloral hydrate–paraldehyde has been advocated as effective against seizures, but chlordiazepoxide and diazepam are more easily administered in patients requiring parenteral medication since chloral hydrate cannot be given parenterally. Lithium is not used for treating alcohol withdrawal. Even though the barbiturates are effective, the abuse and dependence liability and narrow margin of safety of the shorter-acting barbiturates preclude their use.[2]

Adequate identification and early treatment of alcohol withdrawal is only the first step toward full rehabilitation. After the withdrawal reaction subsides, patients should be encouraged to enroll in a treatment for reducing alcohol intake and alcohol related problems.

References

1. Sellers EM, Kalant H: Drug Therapy: Alcohol intoxication and withdrawal. *New Engl J Med* 294:757–762, 1976.
2. Sellers EM, Kalant H: Alcohol withdrawal and delirium tremens, in Pattison EM, Kaufman E (eds): *Encyclopedic Handbook of Alcoholism.* New York, Gardner Press, 1982, pp 147–166.
3. Gessner PK: Failure of diphenylhydantoin to prevent alcohol withdrawal convulsions in mice. *Eur J Pharmacol* 27:120–129, 1974.
4. Shaw GK: Alcohol dependence and withdrawal. *Br Med Bull* 38(1):99–102, 1982.
5. Naranjo CA: Recent advances in the pharmacotherapy of alcoholism in Velasco M (ed): *Clinical Pharmacology anad Therapeutics.* Amsterdam, Excerpta Medica, 1983, pp 132–139.
6. Ritzmann RF, Tabakoff B: Dissociation of alcohol tolerance and dependence. *Nature* 263:418–420, 1976.
7. Gross MM, Lewis E, Nagarajan M: An improved quantiation system for assessing the acute alcoholic psychoses and related states (TSA and SSA), in Gross MM (ed): *Advances in Experimental Medicine and Biology,* vol. 35. *Alcohol Intoxication and Withdrawal: Experimental Studies.* New York, Plemum Press, 1973, pp 365–376.
8. Gross MM, Lewis E, Hastey J: Acute alcohol withdrawal syndrome, in Kissin B, Begleiter H (eds): *The Biology of Alcoholism,* vol 3. *Clinical Pathology.* New York, Plenum Press, 1974, pp 191–263.
9. Gessner PK: Drug therapy of the alcohol withdrawal syndrome, in Majchrowicz E, Noble E (eds): *Biochemistry and Pharmacology of Ethanol,* vol 2. New York, Plenum Press, 1979, pp 375–435.
10. Victor M: Treatment of alcoholic intoxication and the withdrawal syndrome: A critical analysis of the use of drugs and other forms of therapy. *Psychosom Med* 28:636–650, 1966.
11. Linnoila M, Martin PR: Benzodiazepines and alcoholism, in Trimble MR (ed): *Benzodiazepines Divided.* New York, John Wiley & Sons, 1983, pp 291–308.
12. Victor M, Adams RD: The effect of alcohol on the nervous system. *Res Pub Assoc Res Nerv Ment Dis* 32:526–623, 1953.
13. Victor M, Brausch C: The role of abstinence in the genesis of alcoholic epilepsy. *Epilepsia* 8:1–20, 1967.
14. Victor M: A study of epilepsy in the alcoholic patient, in Simmeon L (ed): *Modern Neurology.* Boston, Little Brown and Co., 1969, pp 555–576.

15. Josephson GW, Sabatier HS: Rational management of alcohol withdrawal seizures. *South Med J* 71:1095–1097, 1978.
16. Feussner JR, Linfors EW, Blessing CL, et al: Computed tomography brain scanning in alcohol withdrawal seizures. *Ann Intern Med* 94:519–522, 1981.
17. Kissin B: Biological investigations in alcohol research. *J Stud Alcohol (Suppl.)* 8:146–161, 1979.
18. Sellers EM, Naranjo CA, Peachey JE: Drugs to decrease alcohol consumption. *New Engl J Med* 305:1255–1262, 1981.
19. Shaw JM, Kolesar GS, Sellers EM et al: Development of optimal treatment tactics for alcohol withdrawal. I. Assessment and effectiveness of supportive care. *J Clin Psychopharmacol* 1:382–389, 1981.
20. Naranjo CA, Sellers EM, Chater K, et al: Nonpharmacologic intervention in acute alcohol withdrawal. *Clin Pharmacol Ther* 34(2):214–219, 1983.
21. Sellers EM, Naranjo CA, Harrison M, et al: Oral diazepam loading: Simplified treatment of alcohol withdrawal. *Clin Pharmacol Ther* 34(6):822–826, 1983.
22. Toshney J: An alcoholism and detoxication centre. *Nurs Times* 74:573–576, 1978.
23. Whitfield EL, Thompson G, Lamb A, et al: Detoxication of 1,024 alcoholic patients without psychoactive drugs. *JAMA* 293:1409–1410, 1978.
24. Moskowitz G, Chalmers TC, Sacks HS, Fagerstrom RM, Smith H: Deficiencies of clinical trials of alcohol withdrawal. *Alcoholism: Clin Exp Res* 7:42–46, 1983.
25. Greenblatt DJ, Shader RI, Abernethy DR: Current status of benzodiazepines. II. Clinical use of benzodiazepines. *New Engl J Med* 309:410–416, 1983.
26. Owen RT, Tyrer P: Benzodiazepine dependence: A review of the evidence. *Drugs* 25:385–398, 1983.
27. Greenblatt DJ, Shader RI, Abernethy DR: Current status of benzodiazepines. I. *New Engl J Med* 309:354–358, 1983.
28. Busto U, Simpkins J, Sellers EM, et al: Objective determination of benzodiazepine use and abuse in alcoholics. *Br J Addict* 78:429–435, 1983.
29. Zilm DH, Sellers EM, MacLeod SM, et al: Propranolol effect on tremor in alcoholic withdrawal. *Ann Int Med* 83:234–235, 1975.
30. Zilm DH, Jacob MS, MacLeod SM, et al: Propranolol and chlordiazepoxide effects on cardiac arrhythmias during alcohol withdrawal. *Alcoholism Clin Exp Res* 4:400–405, 1980.
31. Jacob MS, Zilm DH, MacLeod SM, et al: Propranolol-associated confused states during alcohol withdrawal. *J Clin Psychopharmacol* 3:185–187, 1982.
32. Thompson WL: Management of alcohol withdrawal syndrome. *Arch Intern Med* 138:278–283, 1978.
33. Rothstein E: Prevention of alcohol withdrawal seizures: The roles of diphenylhydantoin and chlordiazepoxide. *Am J Psychiatry* 130:1381–1382, 1973.
34. Sampliner R, Iber FL: Diphenylhydantoin control of alcohol withdrawal seizures. *JAMA* 230:1430–1432, 1974.
35. Sandor P, Sellers EM, Dumbrell M, et al: Effect of short-and long-term alcohol use on phenytoin kinetics in chronic alcoholics. *Clin Pharmacol Ther* 30(3):390–397, 1981.
36. Cowen P, Nutt DJ: Abstinence symptoms after withdrawal of tranquillising drugs: Is there a common neurochemical mechanism? *Lancet* 2:360–362, 1982.
37. Lloyd KG, Morselli L, Depoortere H, et al: The potential use of GABA agonists in psychiatric disorders: Evidence from studies with progabide in animal models and clinical trials. *Pharmacol Biochem Behav* 18:957–966, 1983.
38. Wilbur R, Kulik FA: Anticonvulsant drugs in alcohol withdrawal: Use of phenytoin, primidone, carbamazepine, valproic acid, and the sedative anticonvulsants. *Am J Hosp Pharm* 38:1138–1143, 1981.
39. Palm R, Silseth C, Alvan G: Phenytoin intoxication as the first symptom of fatal liver damage induced by sodium valproate. *Br J Clin Pharmacol* 17:597–599, 1984.
40. Thompson WL, Johnson AD, Maddrey WL, et al: Diazepam and paraldehyde for treatment of severe delirium tremens: A controlled trial. *Ann Intern Med* 82:175–180, 1975.

13

Special Aspects of Human Alcohol Withdrawal

David A. Gorelick and Jeffery N. Wilkins

Abstract. There are still surprising gaps in our knowledge of alcohol withdrawal. While quantitative alcohol consumption accounts for about one third of the variability in severity of acute withdrawal, there is little systematic knowledge about the other factors involved. Thus, we cannot precisely predict the severity of withdrawal in individual patients. Controversy exists as to the role of medical vs. social detoxification approaches to acute withdrawal, the influence of acute withdrawal and its treatment on the long-term outcome of alcoholism, and the importance (or even existence) of chronic withdrawal. There is little systematic data to guide withdrawal treatment in special clinical settings, e.g., with concurrent medical or psychiatric illness or with mixed substance dependence. This chapter reviews the published literature, tries to point out methodological and conceptual problems, and suggests areas for future research.

1. Introduction

Alcohol withdrawal is a clinically important phase of the long-term syndrome of alcohol dependence (alcoholism). It is during this phase that many alcoholic patients present for treatment, either because the physical and psychological discomforts associated with withdrawal have motivated them to seek help or because they have recently stopped drinking for other reasons. Even patients who have been drinking right up until entrance into treatment are likely to undergo withdrawal during the early part of treatment, since virtually all alcoholism treatment programs mandate immediate abstinence from alcohol. It is during this phase that patients are considered most susceptible to referral for the long-term rehabilitation that is considered esential to successful treatment of alcoholism.[1,2] Withdrawal is also the phase during which relapse rates tend to be highest, regardless of the type of treatment.[3,4] Furthermore,

David A. Gorelick • Alcohol and Drug Treatment Program, Behavioral Pharmacology Laboratory, Brentwood Division, West Los Angeles Veterans Administration Medical Center, Los Angeles, California 90073; and Department of Psychiatry, School of Medicine, University of California, Los Angeles, California 90024. **Jeffery N. Wilkins** • Crisis Oriented Psychiatric Evaluation Service, Clinical Psychopharmacology Unit, Brentwood Division, West Los Angeles Veterans Administration Medical Center, Los Angeles, California 90073; and Department of Psychiatry, School of Medicine, University of California, Los Angeles, California 90024.

some investigators believe that withdrawal plays a direct, etiological role in alcoholism, e.g., by stimulating craving for alcohol or by serving as a negative reinforcer for drinking (see Section 4).

Given the clinical and theoretical importance of the withdrawal syndrome, there are surprising gaps in our knowledge of it. It is now known that the signs and symptoms observed shortly after cessation of alcohol intake are manifestations of a true pharmacological withdrawal syndrome, rather than solely the effects of malnutrition or intercurrent illness secondary to chronic alcohol intake[5,6,7] (see Chapter 12). The phenomenology of this acute withdrawal syndrome has been well described on the basis of both systematic naturalistic observation of patients[7,8] and studies of experimental chronic intake and acute withdrawal in volunteers.[5,6,9] Effective pharmacological treatments for acute withdrawal have been developed and are widely used clinically.[10] However, it is still not possible to predict with much precision which alcoholic patients will undergo an acute withdrawal syndrome or how severe the withdrawal syndrome will be, nor is there a large systematic body of knowledge to guide the treatment of alcohol withdrawal in the context of complicating factors such as coexisting major psychiatric or medical disorders or other drug dependence. Furthermore, the issues of the existence and importance of withdrawal phenomena beyond the acute phase (so-called subacute, chronic, or persistent withdrawal) and the influence of withdrawal on the future course of alcoholism (including treatment outcome) have rarely been the object of systematic or controlled study.

This chapter will review what is known about these special aspects of human alcohol withdrawal, point out gaps in our present knowledge, and suggest areas we regard as important for future research. While the literature review does not pretend to be exhaustive, it is based on a computerized search (using the Medline/Medlars service of the U.S. National Library of Medicine) of literature on physical dependence and withdrawal syndromes from 1966 through May, 1984.

2. Acute Withdrawal in Special Clinical Contexts

2.1. Background

On strictly pharmacological grounds, it would be expected that the occurrence and severity of acute withdrawal would be determined largely or exclusively by total exposure to alcohol (i.e., quantity, frequency, and duration of alcohol intake). Animal studies find such a close correlation.[11] Naturalistic studies of alcoholic patients[12,13] and experimental human studies of chronic intake and acute withdrawal [5,6,9] also find a positive correlation between total alcohol consumption and severity of acute withdrawal, although the correlation is not as high as in animal studies. For example, among 100 male alcoholics attending a hospital outpatient alcohol clinic, the self-reported severity of physical withdrawal symptoms (e.g., tremor, nausea, sweating, palpitations, muscle cramps) was positively correlated with self-reported total alcohol consumption over the preceding 28 days ($r = 0.56$, $p < 0.001$) and with number of days drinking over the preceding 28 days ($r = 0.42$, $p < 0.001$)[14] A recent quantitive naturalistic study of 43 alcoholic inpatients found that total alcohol intake (and total intake/body weight) over the preceding 7 days correlated significantly with severity of acute withdrawal (over 3 days) ($r = 0.55$, $p < 0.01$), while duration of heavy drinking did not ($r = 0.16$, $p = 0.2$).[15] Furthermore, there was a significant correlation ($r = 0.8$, $p < 0.001$) between severity of withdrawal and the amount of benzodiazepine (diazepam + flurazepam) used in treatment, supporting the clinical validity of the withdrawal assessment. As expected on pharmacological grounds, volume of alcoholic beverage consumed (as opposed to amount of ethanol) and type of beverage do not influence the severity of acute withdrawal.[12,15]

Findings such as these suggest that only about one third of the variability in severity of human acute alcohol withdrawal is determined by the pharmacological factor of recent total alcohol consumption (i.e., variability accounted for = $r^2 = (.55)^2$ or $(.56)^2 = .30$). It is perhaps not surprising that this is a lower proportion than found in animal studies, since human subjects have variability in genetic makeup and biological and psychological condition not found among laboratory animals. Another possible source of variability in human alcohol withdrawal is circadian (or higher-order) variation in alcohol intake.[16] For example, in an experimental setting, alcoholics whose alcohol intake was fairly evenly distributed throughout the 24-hr day had less severe withdrawal than those who concentrated their intake at a particular time.[17]

Numerous biomedical and psychological factors have been proposed as influencing acute withdrawal, largely on the basis of anecdotal clinical impression, rather than on systematic studies that have controlled for patient differences in preceding alcohol intake or baseline withdrawal severity. No study has looked at more than a few factors simultaneously, so that the relative importance of various factors cannot be established. Few studies have systematically collected data on preceding alcohol consumption, so the relative contribution of the pharmacological factor *vis-à-vis* medical and psychological factors cannot be established. Most studies focus on only a few severe manifestations of withdrawal (e.g., seizures, delirium tremens) and do not broadly and systematically measure the withdrawal syndrome. Thus, there is little or no data on factors influencing milder or subtler withdrawal manifestations. Finally, different studies have focused on different factors, so there is less chance to replicate findings across studies. Even when the same factor is used in different studies, the results may be inconsistent. For example, despite the finding of a significant correlation between serum liver enzyme elevation and withdrawal severity,[18] another case series found no significant association between liver disease and occurrence of withdrawal seizures.[19] This inconsistency may arise from the use in the negative study of a single, extreme measure of withdrawal severity (withdrawal seizures),[19] while the positive study used a broad, sensitive 19-item withdrawal assessment rating.[18]

2.2. Withdrawal in the Setting of Medical Illness

It is generally considered that the presence of any concurrent serious medical (or surgical) illness tends to accelerate the course and increase the severity of the acute alcohol withdrawal syndrome.[10,16,20] (Some investigators also believe that concurrent illness may precipitate withdrawal in a patient who might not otherwise experience it.)[10,16] One recently published case series found that, among alcoholics referred to a British medical detoxification center, those referred by emergency rooms and physicians' offices tended to have severer withdrawal symptoms and to need more medication than did patients referred by police or the courts.[21] The former group had a greater history of alcohol-related medical problems, consistent with the above generalization. (However, the authors also noted that the former group tended to have a higher level of recent alcohol intake, which might by itself have accounted for the severer withdrawal. This highlights the pitfalls in drawing valid conclusions when the compared groups are not matched on important variables.) The presence of concurrent liver disease, pneumonia, or pancreatitis is associated with increased duration, severity, and mortality of delirium tremens ("DTs")[22,23] and increased requirements for sedative medication.[23] Other medical factors associated with increased withdrawal severity include dehydration,[24] fever,[25] electrolyte abnormalities (especially hypomagnesemia and hypokalemia),[24,26–29] and respiratory alkalosis.[27] Patients undergoing acute alcohol withdrawal are at increased risk for such medical conditions because they are highly likely to be chronic alcoholics, and alcoholics have a high incidence of major medical problems.[30] Thus, all withdrawal patients should have a thorough medical evaluation as part of their initial management, and any concurrent medical conditions should be appropriately treated, along with the withdrawal itself.[31,32]

The presence of a concurrent medical illness may also influence the treatment of acute alcohol withdrawal by dictating inpatient over outpatient treatment and by modifying the use of sedative medication.[31] Patients with serious liver disease (cirrhosis) should have sedatives given very cautiously in lower than usual doses, since sedatives can precipitate hepatic encephalopathy or coma, or worsen an existing encephalopathy.[20,31] Serious liver disease (hepatitis or cirrhosis) also impairs oxidative drug metabolism, contributing to drug accumulation and possible oversedation.[33] In these cases, it is probably safest to use an intermediate half-life benzodiazepine metabolized by glucuronide conjugation (e.g., oxazepam, lorazepam, temazepam), rather than a long half-life sedative metabolized by oxidation (e.g., chlordiazepoxide, diazepam, phenobarbital). There is no advantage to using paraldehyde in this situation, since metabolism in the liver is the major route of elimination (rather than exhalation via the lungs). In the presence of milder alcoholic liver disease (i.e., fatty liver, with no overt signs of cirrhosis or encephalopathy), it is the authors' experience that long half-life sedatives such as chlordiazepoxide and phenobarbital can be safely used in usual doses. Sedatives should also be given cautiously in the presence of chronic obstructive lung disease or head trauma.[31]

In the former case, oversedation may reduce the respiratory drive enough to precipitate carbon dioxide retention, narcosis, and coma. Hypoxia-induced agitation may be mistaken for withdrawal agitation and made worse by additional sedative medication. Arterial blood gas measurements can distinguish these respiratory problems from withdrawal or hepatic coma. In the case of head trauma, serial monitoring of level of consciousness may be important. Thus, sedatives should be given in doses and frequencies which avoid producing rapid or intense changes in level of consciousness.

Acute alcohol withdrawal may itself mimic, mask, or otherwise influence a concurrent medical disorder. Physiological abnormalities during withdrawal may produce signs and symptoms that can be mistaken for another medical condition or that may obscure the signs and symptoms of a preexisting primary medical condition. For example, withdrawal-related mental status changes may mimic or mask those produced by hypoxia, hepatic encephalopathy, intracranial bleeding, meningitis, or other causes of organic mental syndrome.[31] The transient electrocardiographic abnormalities often found during acute withdrawal may be mistaken for a primary cardiac arrhythmia and lead to unnecessary treatment with antiarrhythmic agents.[34] Thus, the diagnosis of a primary medical disorder should be made very cautiously in the setting of acute withdrawal; the definitive diagnosis and initiation of long-term treatment should be delayed until after the acute withdrawal syndrome has resolved.

Two major examples of this are hypertension and epilepsy. Elevated systolic and/or diastolic blood pressure (>140/90) is found in about one-quarter to one-half of patients during acute withdrawal.[35–38] Blood pressure elevation is highly correlated with withdrawal severity[37,38] and mean daily alcohol intake over the previous 3 months,[38] less correlated with degree of liver disease,[37,38] and not related at all to prior history of hypertension.[36–38] Blood pressure declines to normal levels in over 90% of patients as the acute withdrawal syndrome resolves (usually within 5–7 days).[35–38] Patients with persistent blood pressure elevation tend to be those 30 or older,[36,38] with signs of renovascular disease (e.g., proteinuria, elevated serum creatinine level), or signs of alcohol-induced Cushings' syndrome.[38]

A 1-year followup study found that blood pressure remained normal in those patients abstaining from alcohol (even if they had a prior history of hypertension) but was elevated again in those who resumed drinking.[38] These findings clearly suggest that in most patients (even those with a prior history of hypertension), elevated blood pressure during acute withdrawal is a manifestation of withdrawal, rather than of primary hypertension. Thus, the diagnosis of primary hypertension and initiation of antihypertensive medication are usually unwarranted. If such medication is started, there may be advantages to using an adrenergic agent such as clonidine or propranolol, rather than a thiazide diuretic. The former drugs have an immediate onset of action and also tend to alleviate autonomic symptoms of acute withdrawal,[39] while the latter have a delayed onset of action and their tendency to produce hypokalemia and hypomagnesemia may exacerbate the severity of withdrawal.[28,29]

A similar caution applies to the diagnosis and treatment of epilepsy during acute alcohol withdrawal. Seizures occur in up to 10% of severe acute withdrawal episodes, with up to one third of hospitalized alcoholics giving a history of seizures.[7,40,41] Such seizures are almost always generalized tonic-clonic (grand mal), nonfocal, and self-limited, i.e., one or two seizures without progression to status epilepticus. When occurring in the absence of other epileptogenic factors, they are a direct manifestation of withdrawal reflecting increased neuronal excitability (possibly related to adrenergic hyperactivity and GABA-ergic hypoactivity) (see Chapter 11), rather than a symptom of latent epilepsy activated by withdrawal.[42] This has been demonstrated by animal studies[43,44] and studies of experimental human chronic alcohol intake and acute withdrawal.[45] Patients with seizures occurring only during alcohol withdrawal (and without any epileptogenic factors) have normal interictal EEGs during withdrawal, similar to alcoholic patients with no history of seizures, but different from alcoholics with primary epilepsy.[46] (The latter group has a high proportion of focal abnormalities and generalized paroxysms, similar to nonalcoholic epileptics). Thus, the diagnosis of epilepsy and treatment with anti-convulsants is not indicated unless the patient has a history of prior seizures not associated with withdrawal.[31,32,47] Appropriate sedative treatment of the withdrawal syndrome itself is adequate prophylaxis against or treatment for withdrawal seizures. Those patients who do have a history of preexisting (primary) epilepsy should have their anticonvulsant medication continued (or restarted, with appropriate loading doses) during the withdrawal period, since the seizure threshold is lower during withdrawal.

More problematic is the treatment of patients with no history of seizures, but with epileptogenic factors, e.g., history of head injury, meningitis, encephalitis, or family history of epilepsy. Such patients have significantly fewer EEG abnormalities during acute withdrawal than do alcoholics with primary epilepsy but tend to have somewhat more focal abnormalities than alcoholics without any epileptogenic factors.[46] Retrospective case series suggest that alcoholics with a history of focal brain injury may have up to twice the risk of withdrawal seizures as patients without such a history.[41,48] However, some investigators recommend against using anticonvulsants even in such patients, out of concern that erratic use of medication by chronic alcoholics might actually increase the risk of seizures.[41] There is clearly a need for prospective, controlled studies of this issue to guide appropriate treatment decisions.

Acute withdrawal may also affect pharmacological aspects of treatment by altering drug pharmacokinetics. A recent study found significant changes in drug plasma protein binding over 1 week among 15 male alcoholics undergoing moderate to severe acute withdrawal.[49] Warfarin and propranolol binding decreased significantly during withdrawal, while diazepam binding increased. These changes were reflected in about 20% changes in serum drug free fractions, but no alteration in drug metabolism, per se. Since the free fraction is the pharmacologically active drug, these findings may be clinically relevant in affecting therapeutic or toxic blood and tissue drug levels.

2.3. Withdrawal in the Setting of Psychiatric Illness

Despite a voluminous literature on the relationship beween alcoholism and other major psychiatric disorders (e.g., schizophrenia,[50] depression, [51] biopolar disorder[52]), there are no published systematic or controlled studies on the effect of concurrent psychiatric illness on acute alcohol withdrawal or on the influence of acute withdrawal on preexisting psychiatric illness. However, the anecdotal and circumstantial data that do exist strongly suggest such influences.

Psychological factors undoubtedly influence acute alcohol withdrawal, as suggested by reports that the intensity of even severe withdrawal syndromes can often be reduced by close interpersonal monitoring and support, without pharmacotherapy.[18,35] Conversely, it seems likely that psychological symptoms associated with acute withdrawal might exacerbate a preexisting psychiatric illness; e.g., the depression, anxiety, and irritability so common during withdrawal might worsen a preexisting affective or anxiety disorder, especially if the presence of an acute withdrawal syndrome were overlooked. For example, acute withdrawal has been reported to increase the severity and frequency of panic attacks.[53] (A proposed neurophysiological mechanism for this is withdrawal-induced increased neuronal activity in the locus coeruleus, an area of the midbrain thought to mediate anxiety.)[54] Also, acute alcohol withdrawal may itself mimic a variety of other psychiatric disorders, with withdrawal-related psychological signs and symptoms mistaken for those of another psychiatric disorder. Thus, the diagnosis of a primary psychiatric disorder should be made very cautiously in the setting of acute withdrawal; the definitive diagnosis and initiation of long-term treatment should be delayed until after the acute withdrawal syndrome has resolved.

Two major examples of this are depression and hallucinations. Significantly depressed mood is present in up to 98% of alcoholic patients presenting for treatment [51] (whether or not they are in acute withdrawal). This is often associated with somatic complaints resembling the neurovegetative signs of depression, e.g., insomnia, anergia, anorexia.[55] Unless the history of recent alcohol intake is known, these patients could easily be misdiagnosed as having primary depressive disorder, and be unnecessarily treated with antidepressant medication. In fact, this secondary depression resolves spontaneously in at least three-quarters of patients,[56,57] often within the first week of sobriety.[51,56–58] Unfortunately, those remaining patients who will turn out to have primary or persistent depression (and thus require anti-depressant treatment) cannot currently be identified on the basis of initial symptomatology or past history.

Hallucinations with a clear sensorium (i.e., not associated with delirium tremens) occur in 3–10% of severe acute withdrawal episodes, [35,59,60] although about one quarter of alcoholics give a past history of hallucinations.[35,61] Withdrawal hallucinations may begin 12 hr to 7 days after cessation of (or decrease in) alcohol intake (usually within 2 days)[59] and last minutes to several weeks (usually 1-6 days).[59,62] They may be visual, auditory, or mixed, and are often accompanied by paranoid ideation.[59–61] These hallucinations are a direct manifestation of acute alcohol withdrawal, as shown by systematic study of alcoholic patients[59] and studies of experimental human chronic alcohol intake and acute withdrawal.[5,6,9] The content and intensity of withdrawal hallucinations are very similar to those of schizophrenic hallucinations, making cross-sectional diagnosis difficult, although there tends to be better insight and more external spatial localization with withdrawal hallucinations.[59,63,64] Unless the connection with alcohol withdrawal is recognized, such patients are often misdiagnosed as having schizophrenia or some other psychotic disorder. Thus, while symptomatic treatment of the hallucinations with a neuroleptic may be necessary in some patients, this should not replace complete treatment of the acute withdrawal syndrome by suppression with a sedative.

Many early authorities (including Bleuler himself) considered that withdrawal hallucinations were a symptom of underlying schizophrenia and only occurred in alcoholics with schizophrenia (or "latent" schizophrenia).[50,59] This belief was based on retrospective analysis of small, biased, case series with loose diagnostic criteria for schizophrenia. Larger, more representative case series found that 0–10% of patients with acute withdrawal hallucinations go on to develop schizophrenia,[59,65–68] consistent with the chance coexistence of two independent disorders. Schizophrenics are not overrepresented among large case series of alcoholics with hallucinosis,[59,61] and there is no increased family history of schizophrenia among alcoholics with a history of withdrawal hallucinations.[61,69] These findings further support the independence of acute withdrawal hallucinations and schizophrenia. In addition, preexisting schizophrenia does not seem to exacerbate withdrawal hallucinations, since their content, intensity, and duration are similar in schizophrenic and nonschizophrenic alcoholics.[59,63] Although relatively rare (probably less than 10–20% of all hallucinatory episodes[59,62,65]), chronic withdrawal hallucinations may have a closer relationship to schizophrenia. In two large case series, about half the patients with withdrawal hallucinations lasting more than 6 months went on to develop schizophrenia.[59,65] There may also be a tendency for patients with repeated episodes of withdrawal hallucinations to develop schizophrenia (although this is based on two very small case series of four and 16 patients).[59,70] Among patients with withdrawal hallucinations who continue drinking, about one third will have future hallucinatory episodes.[60]

Acute withdrawal can trigger a variety of extra-pyramidal movement abnormalities, consistent with the decreased dopaminergic activity reported during acute withdrawal.[71,72] (see Chapter 11). These include choreoathetosis,[73] Parkinsonism (resting tremor, cogwheel rigidity, bradykinesia),[74,75,76] dystonia,[76] and akathisia.[76] These abnormalities can occur in nonschizophrenic alcoholics who are not taking neuroleptics. This has obvious implications for a schizophrenic alcoholic who might be taking neuroleptics, with their own propensity for inducing extrapyramidal abnormalities.

2.4. Withdrawal in the Setting of Mixed Substance Dependence

Patients with mixed substance dependence disorders represent another complicated clinical context for alcohol withdrawal. Such mixed dependence can be considered in two categories: dependence on alcohol plus another (cross-tolerant) sedative-hypnotic and dependence on alcohol plus another (non-cross-tolerant) drug (opiate, stimulant). In the former case, the combined withdrawal syndrome will qualitatively resemble alcohol withdrawal alone (i.e., the typical sedative-hypnotic withdrawal syndrome). However, the time course may differ, depending on the pharmacokinetic characteristics of the second sedative. When this has a long half-life (e.g., benzodiazepine such as chlordiazepoxide or diazepam), withdrawal onset may be delayed and duration prolonged,[77,78] as would be expected for the benzodiazepine alone. This could be considered a case of the second sedative providing substitution pharmacotherapy for the acute alcohol withdrawal syndrome. Alternatively, there may be a bimodal withdrawal pattern, with signs and symptoms during the first 3–4 days after abstinence (presumably from alcohol withdrawal), then a period of improvement followed by the reappearance of withdrawal symptoms 1–3 weeks after abstinence (presumably from long-acting sedative withdrawal).[78] Unless the dual sedative dependence is recognized, both the patient and clinician may be surprised by the reemergence of withdrawal symptoms and may erroneously conclude that the patient has resumed drinking. When the second sedative has a relatively short half-life (e.g., meprobamate, methaqualone), the time course may follow that of alcohol withdrawal, but with increased severity requiring larger doses of detoxification medication.[78] In either case, the appropriate treatment for combined alcohol-sedative withdrawal would be the same as for alcohol withdrawal alone, i.e., tapering doses of a long-acting sedative such as phenobarbital or benzodiazepine.[77–79]

A recent study with mice concurrently administered alcohol and chlordiazepoxide reported an attenuation of acute withdrawal severity, as compared with mice given alcohol alone.[80] This effect appeared to be only partly accounted for by the presence of long half-life chlordiazepoxide metabolities in blood (or by changes in alcohol metabolism), leading the authors to raise the possibility that the benzodiazepine might have interfered with the development of physical dependence on alcohol. An opposite interaction has also been reported, with concurrent benzodiazepine use associated with increased frequency of alcohol withdrawal seizures in patients.[41] Because this effect occurred especially with intermittent benzodiazepine use, it may be related to a kindling response to repeated episodes of benzodiazepine withdrawal superimposed on alcohol dependence. Clearly, further research in both animals and humans is needed to clarify the withdrawal interactions between alcohol and other sedative drugs.

In the case of combined alcohol–nonsedative withdrawal, the clinical picture may be a mixture of alcohol and opiate or stimulant withdrawal syndromes.[81] Acute alcohol withdrawal has been reported to be severer in patients with previous physical dependence on opiates,[82] but this finding has not been replicated.[83] In neither study were the patient groups standardized and matched for variables such as prior alcohol consumption or baseline withdrawal severity. In one animal study, where such controls could be imposed, rats made physically dependent on alcohol had severer acute withdrawal syndromes if they had been previously treated with an opiate.[84]

The general treatment approach for mixed substance dependence is withdrawal first from the drug with the most potentially medically dangerous withdrawal syndrome, while maintaining dependence on the other drug(s) until detoxification from the first drug has been successfully completed.[81] In the case of combined alcohol–opiate dependence (or withdrawal), this means maintaining (or stabilizing) the patient on an opiate (usually methadone) while undergoing alcohol detoxification and then withdrawing the patient from the opiate.[32] Clonidine has also been suggested as treatment for such mixed drug withdrawal, since it can apparently suppress many of the symptoms of acute withdrawal regardless of drug type[85] (see Chapter 11). However, there are no systematic data on its efficacy in such a setting. Combined alcohol–stimulant withdrawal is usually satisfactorily handled by treatment for alcohol withdrawal alone.[81] Since alcoholics with mixed substance dependence tend to have more frequent and severer medical problems (e.g., trauma, malnutrition, gastritis, seizures) than do "pure" alcoholics,[86] such patients need a thorough medical evaluation as part of their initial management.

3. Chronic Alcohol Withdrawal Syndrome

The manifestations of an alcohol withdrawal syndrome can be operationally defined on the basis of the following criteria; (1) onset after cessation of alcohol intake, (2) disappearance after resumption of alcohol or other (cross-tolerant) sedative intake, and (3) inverted U-shaped curve of intensity over time, with initial increase to peak intensity after alcohol cessation, then a decrease in intensity over time. In addition, interpreting the signs and symptoms observed during the period of presumed withdrawal as being true withdrawal manifestations is strengthened by ruling out any other preexisting or concurrent disorders that might account for them. These criteria help distinguish true withdrawal from direct effects of alcohol that may persist during periods of abstinence or from chronic signs or symptoms that are actually unrelated to alcohol.

The existence of an acute alcohol withdrawal syndrome has been firmly established according to the above criteria, based on systematic studies of alcoholic patients and experimental studies of chronic human alcohol intake.[5–9] Manifestations of acute withdrawal include anxiety, depression, irritability, agitation, and fatigue, and signs of central and autonomic nervous system excitability and hyperactivity, such as tremors, diaphoresis, tachycardia, hypertension, lowered seizure threshold, increased amplitude of brain evoked potentials, and sleep disturbance. The acute syndrome begins 6–8 hr after cessation of alcohol intake (or substantial decline in blood alcohol level) and resolves within 5–10 days. Many clinicians consider that some manifestations of withdrawal persist beyond this period. This so-called chronic, prolonged, or protracted withdrawal syndrome is not well defined, but has been called "one of the most important areas in the biology of alcoholism.".[87] Some investigators consider that chronic withdrawal plays an important etiologic role in recovery and relapse (see Section 4 below). Unfortunately, the relatively few published studies on this topic tend to ignore the serious conceptual issues involved and have serious methodological flaws.

Anecdotal case series report chronic withdrawal symptoms such as anxiety, depression, irritability, emotional lability, restlessness, fatigue, and sleep disturbance lasting up to 2 years after the last alcohol intake.[40,88–90] The time course is either a progressive decrease in symptoms following the peak intensity reached during acute withdrawal or a fluctuating course with periods of intense symptoms for 3–5 weeks alternating with periods of weak or no symptoms. A cluster of more intense symptoms 1–3 months after drinking cessation has been associated with the "dry drunk" experience of recovering alcoholics.[89] More systematic cross-sectional studies (i.e., testing independent groups of subjects during acute and chronic withdrawal) have found persisting anxiety, fatigue, insomnia, and somatic complaints (especially pain) in patients tested 3–6 weeks after their last alcohol intake.[91,92] A Russian group tested patients 2–3 months after their last alcohol intake and reported a "protracted withdrawal" syndrome manifested in "emotional instability," mood shifts, irritability, apathy, insomnia, impaired concentration, and impaired cognitive function.[93]

The evidence of objective signs of chronic withdrawal is also based on a limited number of cross-sectional studies. Several studies found EEG-monitored sleep disturbances persisting 3–4 weeks after the last alcohol intake, reflected in decreased sleep time, increased sleep latency, decreased slow wave sleep (stages 3 and 4), increased REM sleep, and increased number of sleep stage shifts.[94–97] In general, abnormalities of sleep quality (i.e., initiation and maintenance of sleep) appeared to persist longer than abnormalities of sleep architecture (i.e., latency and duration of specific sleep stages). One study of patients after 12 weeks of abstinence found increased stage 3 sleep and decreased REM sleep,[95] somewhat the opposite of results after 3–4 weeks of abstinence. However, one study of patients abstinent for 1–2 years found decreased stage 4 sleep and increased number of sleep stage shifts,[98] similar to abnormalities reported after 3–4 weeks of abstinence. CNS hyperexcitability in the form of increased amplitude of visual or auditory evoked potentials has been found in patients 3–6 weeks after the last alcohol intake.[99–101]

Signs of autonomic nervous system dysfunction such as skin flushing, diaphoresis, sinus tachycardia, and hypotension have been reported in association with the psychological symptoms of chronic withdrawal.[89,102] More systematic cross-sectional studies have found evidence of increased muscle tension (reflected in handwriting pressure and respiratory irregularity),[103] decreased sympathetic nervous system activity (reflected in diastolic cold pressor response),[103,104] increased parasympathetic nervous system activity (reflected in IV glucose tolerance test, saliva flow, and saliva sodium concentration),[103] and (unspecified) "vasovegetative instability"[93] in patients abstinent for 3 weeks to 2 years. In one study, an alcohol challenge (1 ml/kg p.o.) normalized these abnormalities in a comparison group of "active alcoholics" (withdrawal state not defined).[103] Unfortunately, an alcohol challenge was not done in the chronic withdrawal patients, so that the reversibility of these abnormalities during withdrawal is not known.

These published studies on chronic alcohol withdrawal suggest that some psychological symptoms and signs of CNS hyperexcitability and autonomic nervous system dysfunction persist beyond the 5–10 day acute withdrawal period. The signs and symptoms appear to remain qualitatively similar over time, while their intensity declines, especially after 1–3 months of abstinence. The systematic time course data are too meager, especially for objective nervous system variables such as evoked potentials, to allow confident delineation of specific subacute (first 1–3 months) vs. chronic phases of withdrawal. More importantly, the published studies do not present data that satisfy operational criteria for a true withdrawal syndrome.

None of the published studies were longitudinal, i.e., none followed the same patients from a period of alcohol intake through acute withdrawal to chronic withdrawal. This means the studies do not specifically demonstrate the onset of symptoms after cessation of alcohol intake. This is particularly important to the argument that they are indeed withdrawal manifestations, since many of the proposed chronic withdrawal symptoms (e.g., anxiety, depression, irritability, fatigue, insomnia)[105] and signs (e.g., increased amplitude of sensory evoked potentials)[106] are also present during periods of active alcohol intake.

Many of these symptoms are also found in anxiety, affective, or adjustment disorders, which are common in active and recovering alcoholics. Some of the observed autonomic nervous system dysfunctions resemble those found in various neurological disorders and could be due to persisting damage from previous toxic effects of alcohol on the nervous system.[93,104] Thus, a thorough psychiatric and medical evaluation at the time of testing would be necessary to exclude the presence of a preexisting or concurrent psychiatric or neurologic disorder that might account for the observed symptoms and signs. This is something rarely done in the published studies. Furthermore, without longitudinal follow-up during the period of (presumed) abstinence that preceded testing, one cannot be confident that the subjects had not resumed some alcohol intake. Finally, none of the published studies provide data on what happens to chronic withdrawal manifestations after alcohol intake is resumed, so that their suppression by alcohol has never been demonstrated.

Future research on chronic alcohol withdrawal should include longitudinal studies that follow patients closely through the acute withdrawal period, as well as thereafter. Such studies should use systematic measures of proposed withdrawal symptoms, including standardized rating scales for subjective variables such as anxiety. Objective measures of proposed withdrawal signs should make use of newly developed sophisticated neurophysiological techniques (e.g., topographical EEG recording, neuroimaging), as well as dynamic probes of CNS function (e.g., neuroendocrine challenge tests; see Chapter 11). Based on the experience of animal withdrawal studies,[11] use of these sensitive techniques may detect subtle manifestations of chronic withdrawal that would be missed by conventional methods. Future studies should include thorough psychiatric and medical evaluations of subjects to rule out preexisting or concurrent disorders that might account for the observed symptoms and signs. They should also collect systematic data on alcohol consumption and severity of acute withdrawal, so that the influence of these factors on chronic withdrawal can be determined. (Published studies do not present any such data). Finally, when ethical and practical, future research studies should include an alcohol challenge procedure (or continue to follow subjects who spontaneously relapse back to drinking) to determine the suppressibility by alcohol of any proposed chronic withdrawal manifestation.

4. Influence of Withdrawal on Outcome

Most clinicians regard acute withdrawal as an important step on the road to long-term rehabilitation of the chronic disease of alcoholism.[107] Unfortunately, there are very little empirical data on how acute withdrawal or its treatment influence the prognosis of alcoholism. In the absence of data, there is a spectrum of clinical opinion as to the role of acute withdrawal and the implications for appropriate treatment. The opposite ends of this spectrum can be thought of as the medical detoxification model and the social detoxification model.

Proponents of medical detoxification advocate "controlling withdrawal symptomatology to the greatest possible extent" by use of cross-tolerant sedatives.[102] This treatment approach is proposed as having three advantages:

(1) all medically and psychiatrically serious manifestations of withdrawal (e.g., seizures, delirium tremens) are avoided; (2) attention to, and relief of, the patients' somatic complaints promotes a trusting, therapeutic relationship with the clinician, thus increasing the patients' motivation to enter rehabilitation; (3) by eliminating discomfort after drinking cessation, there is no opportunity for withdrawal to become conditioned as a negative reinforcer for further drinking, i.e., for patients to learn to resume drinking to avoid or escape the discomforts of withdrawal. Some medical detoxification proponents also advocate continuing medication beyond the period of acute withdrawal until all symptoms have resolved.[102] The rationale for this is to suppress the chronic withdrawal syndrome. The hypothesis is that this withdrawal state exists (perhaps mediating craving for alcohol or desire to drink during abstinence) and that alcoholics tend to relapse back to drinking out of a need to suppress this withdrawal state.[108] Thus, successful suppression of chronic withdrawal would promote recovery by removing an important contributor to relapse. An extension of this hypothesis is the postulated existence of a "subclinical conditioned withdrawal syndrome."[109] The hypothesis is that repeated episodes of drinking and withdrawal produce in the patient a conditioned association between subtle withdrawal symptoms and cues associated with abstinence. This conditioned withdrawal state then promotes craving for alcohol and relapse in the same manner as a true pharmacological withdrawal syndrome. A neurophysiological rationale for vigorously suppressing withdrawal with medication would be to avoid the development of kindling (see Chapter 11). Kindling refers to a phenomenon of repeated low level electrical (or chemical) stimulation of the limbic system lowering the seizure threshold for future stimulation.[110] Thus, a previously ineffective stimulus will later induce a seizure. Ballenger and Post [111] have proposed that repeated withdrawal episodes might activate the kindling process to lower the activation threshold of the limbic system, thus increasing vulnerability to, or the severity of, future withdrawal episodes.

Proponents of social detoxification advocate controlling withdrawal symptomatology without use of sedative medication, by psychological methods, e.g., the "3R's" of reality orientation, reassurance, and respect.[21] This avoids playing "addictive musical chairs"[112] between alcohol and the detoxification medication and avoids reinforcing the alcoholic's reliance on drugs to deal with dysphoria and discomfort. This is assumed to promote the patient's motivation to enter rehabilitation and his feeling of responsibility for his own recovery.[113] Critics of medical detoxification cite the possibility of sedation and impaired cognitive function from medication interfering with participation and learning during the initial phase of alcoholism therapy.[40,113] They also suggest that sedation from medication in a hospital environment with confinement to bed and other restrictions may cause relative sensory deprivation,[40] which may be a factor in increasing withdrawal severity.[114]

No firm answer to this difference of opinion can be given because the published data are so meager. What does seem clear is that the social detoxification approach without sedative medication is medically safe for the majority of patients in mild to moderate acute alcohol withdrawal, provided there is good screening for concurrent medical problems, close monitoring and support during withdrawal, and available medical backup. Two large case series of social detoxification patients found that less than 10% required transfer to a medical setting to complete acute withdrawal.[35,115] Even among inpatients undergoing moderate to severe alcohol withdrawal, the social detoxification approach ("supportive care" without sedative medication) has been found safe and effective for the majority of patients.[18,116,117]

The results of published studies are inconclusive as to whether medical or social detoxification provides a better resolution of the acute withdrawal syndrome. Whitfield[40] reported that patients undergoing social detoxification had a shorter duration of acute withdrawal (2 days) than patients receiving high dose benzodiazepines (3–5 days). However, this was a clinical impression not based on a systematic, controlled study. A double-blind, placebo-controlled study in outpatients undergoing mild to moderate acute withdrawal compared "supportive" nursing care (assessment, reassurance, and reality orientation for 10 minutes every hour for 7 hr) with or without medication (lorazepam, 2 mg s.l. every 2 hr for three doses).[118] Withdrawal severity was essentially the same in both groups over the 7-hr treatment period, and there was no significant severity difference between groups over the 5-day follow-up period.

Short-term outcome studies comparing benzodiazepine treatment with no sedative medication tend to show results favoring the latter approach. Three double-blind inpatient studies found that patients getting placebo showed greater self-care capability and social competence and less guilt, anger, tension, and dejection,[58] while patients getting chlordiazepoxide requested earlier hospital discharge[119] and showed a greater tendency towards alcohol use.[120] The interpretation of most other published studies is confounded by the sample bias created by the fact that patient assignment to treatment is usually made on clinical grounds, not at random. One study of 200 male alcoholics undergoing 7 days of treatment for acute withdrawal found that those patients undergoing social detoxification were significantly more likely to accept a (voluntary) referral for further alcoholism rehabilitation than those patients undergoing medical detoxification (with chlordiazepoxide) (67% vs. 50%).[113] Furthermore, among patients accepting a referral, 50% of social detoxification patients requested an inpatient program vs. 22% of the medical detoxification patients. To try to control for the nonrandom assignment of patients to the two detoxification settings (severer patients went to medical detoxification), the data were analyzed by analysis of covariance, using as covariates the admission data on physical condition, psychosocial status, alcoholism history, and motivation for change.

On the other hand, the few published long-term outcome studies suggest a better prognosis when acute withdrawal is treated with sedative medication. One open outpatient study compared patients treated with meprobamate + promazine (Prozine) for acute withdrawal with an historical control group treated only with vitamins (before the clinic began using sedative medication).[121] Patients getting medication during withdrawal had a significantly lower dropout rate (61% vs. 87%) and greater improvement rate (23% vs. 0%) over the 6-month follow-up period than did patients getting only vitamins. In fact, patients presenting in acute withdrawal who were treated with Prozine did better than patients who were not in withdrawal at admission, even though, among patients not receiving medication, those not in withdrawal did significantly better than those presenting in acute withdrawal. Smart *et al.*[122] did a multivariate analysis of factors that might predict dropout during the first year of treatment among 792 alcoholic outpatients followed at five different facilities in Ontario, Canada. The analysis found that treatment variables accounted for about 30% of the variance in dropout rates, with patients receiving medically oriented treatment and medication being most likely to stay in treatment.

There is little direct or systematic data on the possible relationship between withdrawal manifestations and conditioned withdrawal or craving for alcohol or on the possible role of withdrawal as a negative reinforcer for drinking. A survey of 349 alcoholic patients found many who reported craving for alcohol was associated with signs and symptoms (e.g., tension, depression, somatic complaints) similar to those occurring during alcohol withdrawal and that the strength of craving corresponded somewhat with recent withdrawal manifestations.[123] Another study found a significant correlation ($r = +.59$) between subjective craving for alcohol while sober and the reported severity of prior acute withdrawal episodes.[124] Many patients do anecdotally report resuming drinking shortly after stopping on their own, in order to escape or avoid the discomforts of withdrawal.[125] The results of open trials of chlordiazepoxide in the treatment of outpatient alcoholics are consistent with this, since patients getting the medication had decreased craving for alcohol,[126] greater abstinence,[127] better relationship with their psychotherapist,[126] and longer stay in treatment with lower dropout rate.[126–128] These patients may have benefitted from the substitution of one longer-acting sedative (chlordiazepoxide) for another shorter-acting sedative (alcohol), possibly via a process analagous to methadone maintenance treatment of heroin dependence. The actual factors mediating these beneficial effects of sedative treatment have never been explicitly studied. Animal studies suggest that acute or chronic benzodiazepine administration can decrease alcohol preference and consumption (probably by a CNS effect rather than a peripheral taste effect),[129,130] although one study found that diazepam given during acute withdrawal increased alcohol preference in rats.[131] A direct test of withdrawal (or conditioned withdrawal) as a negative reinforcer for drinking would be whether drinking increases significantly during withdrawal episodes as compared to other abstinent periods (all other factors being equal). Most (but not all) animal studies find no significant increase in alcohol intake during withdrawal episodes.[125] Furthermore, both animals and humans in experimental settings will voluntarily and spontaneously interrupt ongoing alcohol intake even when this behavior initiates a withdrawal episode.[108,125] Thus, withdrawal is clearly often neither a sufficient nor a necessary factor in initiating or maintaining drinking.

There are no adequate studies of a possible association between number and severity of prior withdrawal episodes and future withdrawal (while controlling for total alcohol intake). In both rodents and humans, the greater the number of prior episodes of alcohol intake and withdrawal, the quicker the development of physical dependence (i.e., the less alcohol intake needed to produce a withdrawal syndrome after cessation), the quicker the onset of acute withdrawal after alcohol cessation, and the severer the behavorial and neurophysiological manifestations of withdrawal[125,132,133] (although at least one negative animal study has been published[134]). However, all these studies confound the variable of number of prior withdrawal episodes with the variable of total prior alcohol intake; i.e., subjects with a greater number of withdrawal episodes are also those with the greater amount of alcohol intake and/ or duration of alcohol intake.

There are no human data directly bearing on the role of kindling in alcohol withdrawal. In rats, prior electrical kindling of the brain does increase the severity of acute alcohol withdrawal,[135,136] suggesting a connnection between the kindling process and withdrawal. In a direct test of this connection, it was found that acute withdrawal from chronic high blood alcohol levels (but not from low or moderate levels) did lower the threshold for electrically kindled seizures in rats.[137] However, there was no difference in the kindling effect between rats subjected to multiple withdrawal episodes and those subjected to a single withdrawal episode (both groups having the same total alcohol intake). The failure to find a differential effect of repeated withdrawal was considered by the authors' as possibly due to methodological factors such as the relatively short periods of alcohol intake (21–28 days) and use of suprathreshold electrical stimulation to test for kindling.

In summary, there is a large amount of theorizing based on unsystematic, anecdotal clinical data on the issue of the role of withdrawal and its treatment in the outcome of alcoholic patients. Unfortunately, there is much less direct evidence based on well-designed studies. It appears fairly well established that the type of treatment given for acute withdrawal (i.e., sedative medication vs. social detoxification) has little influence on short-term outcome for most patients; little else in this field is well established. Many published studies have serious methodological flaws: nonrandom assignment of patients to treatment groups, use of open treatments (rather than double-blind with placebo), use of subjective or vaguely defined outcome measures, and use of intervening variables (e.g., craving for alcohol, attitude toward therapist) as outcome measures (rather than directly studying outcome). Different studies have given inconsistent results. Thus, there is a great need for well designed, longitudinal studies using up-to-date measurement techniques to address the important hypotheses that have been put forth. Future research might profitably look into the following issues: (1) Are there specific, measurable factors that predict the severity of acute withdrawal, so that individual patients can be more confidently assigned to medical vs. social detoxification programs? (2) Does vigorous suppression of the acute withdrawal syndrome with sedatives improve long-term outcome? If it does, is this mediated by a decrease in chronic withdrawal or conditioned withdrawal (assuming they exist)? (3) If sedatives are used for treatment of alcohol withdrawal, what is the optimum duration of use? Is there a role for subacute or chronic sedative treatment? (4) What is the role of kindling in human alcohol withdrawal? (5) What is the relationship among craving for alcohol, chronic or conditioned withdrawal, and relapse to drinking? Are there objective manifestations of craving or withdrawal (e.g., neurophysiological, neuroendocrinological) that could serve as predictive markers for relapse?

References

1. Fox GP, Graham MB, Gill MJ: The therapeutic revolving door. *Arch Gen Psychiatry* 26:179–182, 1972.
2. Pisani VD: The detoxication of alcoholics—Aspects of myth, magic, or malpractice. *J Stud Alcohol* 38:927–985, 1977.
3. Norris JL: Prevention of chronicity in alcoholism. *Psychiatr Ann* 8:592–595, 1978.
4. Walker ND, Lightfoot CGL: An analysis of 1000 admissions to an alcohol treatment unit. *New Zealand Med J* 92:323–325, 1980.
5. Isbell H, Fraser HF, Wikler A, et al: An experimental study of the etiology of "rum fits" and delirium tremens. *Q J Stud Alcohol* 16:1–33, 1955.
6. Mendelson JH, LaDou L: Experimentally induced chronic intoxication and withdrawal in alcoholics. *Q J Stud Alcohol* (Suppl) 2:1–39, 1964.
7. Victor M, Adams RD: The effects of alcohol on the nervous system. *Proc Assoc Res Nerv Ment Dis* 32:525–573, 1953.
8. Mello NK, Mendelson JH: Clinical aspects of alcohol dependence, in Martin WR (ed): *Handbook of Experimental Pharmacology*, Part 1, Drug Addiction I. Berlin, Springer-Verlag, 45:613–666, 1977.
9. Gross MM, Lewis E, Best S, et al: Quantitative changes of signs and symptoms associated with acute alcohol withdrawal: incidence, severity, and circadian effects in experimental studies of alcoholics. *Adv Exp Biol Med* 59:615–631, 1975.
10. Sellers EM, Kalant H: Alcohol intoxication and withdrawal. *New Engl J Med* 294:757–762, 1976.
11. Freidman, HJ: Assessment of physical dependence on and withdrawal from ethanol in animals, in Rigter H, Crabbe, JC Jr. (eds): *Alcohol Tolerance and Dependence*. New York, Elsevier/North-Holland, 1980, pp 93–121.
12. Mello NK, Mendelson JH: The development of alcohol dependence: A clinical study. *McLean Hosp J* 1:64–88, 1976.
13. Turner TB, Mezey E, Kimball AW: Measurement of alcohol-related effects in man: chronic effects in relation to levels of alcohol consumption. Part B. *Johns Hopkins Med J* 141:273–286, 1977.
14. Herson HI: Alcohol withdrawal symptoms and drinking behavior. *J Stud Alcohol* 38:953–971, 1977.
15. Pristach CA, Smith CM, Whitney RB: Alcohol withdrawal syndromes—prediction from detailed medical and drinking histories. *Drug Alcohol Depend* 11:177–199, 1983.

16. Turner TB: Clinical aspects of ethanol tolerance and dependence, in Rigter H, Crabbe JC Jr (eds): *Alcohol Tolerance and Dependence*. New York, Elsevier/North-Holland, 1980, pp 393–424.
17. Mello NK, Mendelson JH: Experimentally induced intoxication in alcoholics: A comparison between programmed and spontaneous drinking. *J Pharmacol Exp Ther* 173:101–116, 1970.
18. Shaw JM, Kolesar GS, Sellers EM, et al: Development of optimal treatment tactics for alcohol withdrawal. I. Assessment and effectiveness of supportive care. *J Clin Psychopharmacol* 1:382–389, 1981.
19. Rhinehart JW: Factors determining "rum fits." *Am J Psychiatry* 118:251–252, 1961.
20. Baum R, Iber FL: Initial treatment of the alcoholic patient, in Gitlow SE, Peyser HS (eds): *Alcoholism: A Practical Treatment Guide*. New York, Grune and Stratton, 1980, pp 73–88.
21. Kessel N, Makenjuola JDA, Rossal CJ, et al: The Manchester detoxification serivce; description and evaluation. *Lancet* 2:839–842, 1984.
22. Tavel ME, Davidson W, Batterton TD: A critical analysis of mortality associated with delirium tremens. *Am J Med Sci* 242:18–29, 1961.
23. Thompson WL: Management of alcohol withdrawal syndromes. *Arch Intern Med* 138:288–283, 1978.
24. Johnson RM: The alcohol withdrawal syndrome. *Q J Stud Alcohol* (Suppl.) 1:66–76, 1961.
25. Gross MM, Rosenblatt SM, Chartoff S, et al: Evaluation of acute alcoholic psychoses and related states; the daily clinical course rating scale. *Q J Stud Alcohol* 32:611–619, 1971.
26. Tonnesen E: Delirium tremens and hypokalaemia. *Lancet* 2:97, 1982.
27. Victor M: The role of hypomagnesemia and respiratory alkalosis in the genesis of alcohol-withdrawal symptoms. *Ann NY Acad Sci* 215:235–248, 1973.
28. Wadstein J, Skude G: Does hypokalaemia precede delirium tremens? *Lancet* 2:549–550, 1978.
29. Sheehan JP: Alcohol and the heart. *Ann Intern Med* 98:1022, 1983.
30. Rydberg U, Skerfving S: The toxicity of ethanol. A tentative risk evaluation. *Adv Exp Biol Med* 85B:403–419, 1977.
31. Greenblatt DJ, Shader RI: Treatment of the alcohol withdrawal syndrome, in Shader RI (ed): *Manual of Psychiatric Therapeutics*. Boston, Little, Brown, 1975, pp 211–236.
32. Lewis DC, Femino J: Management of alcohol withdrawal. *Rational Drug Ther* 16(2):1–5, 1982.
33. Pelkonen O, Sotaniemi E: Drug metabolism in alcoholics. *Pharmacol Ther* 16:261–268, 1982.
34. Ballas M, Zoneraich S, Yunis M, et al: Noninvasive cardiac evaluation in chronic alcoholic patients with alcohol withdrawal syndrome. *Chest* 82:148–152, 1982.
35. Whitfield CL, Thompson G, Lamb A, et al: Detoxification of 1024 alcoholic patients without psychoactive drugs. *J Am Med Assoc*, 239:1409–1410, 1978.
36. Beckman H, Frank RR, Robertson RS, et al: Evaluation of blood pressure during early alcohol withdrawal. *Ann Emerg Med* 10:32–35, 1981.
37. Saunders JB, Beevers DG, Paton A: Factors influencing blood pressure in chronic alcoholics. *Clin Sci* 57:295s–298s, 1979.
38. Saunders JB, Beevers DG, Paton A: Alcohol induced hypertension. *Lancet* 2:653–656, 1981.
39. Wilkins AJ, Jenkins WJ, Steiner JA: Efficacy of clonidine in treatment of alcohol withdrawal state. *Psychopharmacol* 81:78–80, 1983.
40. Whitfield CL: Nondrug detoxification, in Fann WE, Karacan I, Pokorny AD, et al: (eds): *Phenomenology and Treatment of Alcoholism*. New York, Spectrum, 1980, pp 305–320.
41. Hillbom ME, Hjelm-Jager M: Should alcohol withdrawal seizures be treated with anti-epileptic drugs? *Acta Neurol Scand* 69:39–42, 1984.
42. Victor M, Braunsch C: The role of abstinence in the genesis of alcoholic epilepsy. *Epilepsia* 8:1–20, 1967.
43. Gibbins RJ, Kalant H, LeBlanc AE, et al: Sound induced seizures during ethanol withdrawal in mice. *Psychopharmacology* 22:24–49, 1971.
44. McQuarrie DG, Fingl E: Effects of single doses and chronic administration of ethanol on experimental seizures in mice. *J Pharmacol Exp Ther* 124:264–271, 1958.
45. Wikler A, Prescor FT, Fraser HF, et al: Electroencephalographic changes associated with chronic alcohol intoxication and the alcohol abstinence syndrome. *Am J Psychiatry* 113:106–114, 1956.

46. Deisenhammer E, Klinger D, Tragner H: Epileptic seizures in alcoholism and diagnostic value of EEG after sleep deprivation. *Epilepsia* 25:526–530, 1984.
47. Josephson GW, Sabatier HS Jr: Rational management of alcohol withdrawal seizures. *South Med J* 71:1095–1097, 1978.
48. Chu N-S: Periodic lateralized epileptiform discharges with preexisting focal brain lesions. Role of alcohol withdrawal and anoxic encephalopathy. *Arch Neurol* 37:551–554, 1980.
49. Sandor P, Naranjo CA, Khouw V, et al: Variations in drug free fraction during alcohol withdrawal. *Br J Clin Pharmacol* 15:481–486, 1983.
50. Freed EX: Alcoholism and schizophrenia: The search for perspectives. *Q J Stud Alcohol* 36:853–881, 1975.
51. Petty F, Nasrallah HA: Secondary depression in alcoholism: implications for future research. *Comp Psychiatry* 22:587–595, 1981.
52. Morrison JR: Bipolar affective disorder and alcoholism. *Am J Psychiatry* 131:1131–1133, 1974.
53. Dackis CA, Stuckey RF: Psychopharmacologic treatment of the alcoholic. *Psychiatry Lett* 2(7):1–4, 1984.
54. Redmond DE, Huang YH: New evidence for a locus coeruleus-norepinephrine connection with anxiety. *Life Sci* 25:2149–2162, 1979.
55. Gibson S, Becker J: Changes in alcoholics' self-reported depression. *Q J Stud Alcohol* 34:829–836, 1973.
56. Gorelick DA, Mintz JR, McKenna AM: Time course of depression in alcoholic inpatients. Paper presented at the 135th Annual Meeting, American Psychiatric Association, Toronto, 1982.
57. Nakamura MM, Overall JE, Hollister LE: Factors affecting outcome of depressive symptoms in alcoholics. *Alcoholism Clin Exp Res* 7:188–193, 1983.
58. Klett CJ, Hollister LE, Caffee EM, et al: Evaluating changes in symptoms during acute alcohol withdrawal. *Arch Gen Psychiatry* 74:174–178, 1971.
59. Victor M, Hope JM: The phenomenon of auditory hallucinations in chronic alcoholism. *J Nerv Ment Dis* 126:451–481, 1958.
60. Achte K, Seppala K, Girman L, et al: *Alcoholic Psychoses in Finland*. Helsinki, Finnish Foundation for Alcohol Studies, 1969.
61. Schuckit MA: The history of psychotic symptoms in alcoholics. *J Clin Psychiatry* 43:53–57, 1982.
62. Scott DF, Davies DL, Malherbe MEL: Alcoholic hallucinosis. *Int J Addict* 4:319–330, 1969.
63. Alpert M, Silvers KN: Perceptual characteristics distinguishing auditory hallucinations in schizophrenia and acute alcoholic psychoses. *Am J Psychiatry* 127:74–78, 1970.
64. Deikert T, Chambers HE: Structure and content of hallucinations in alcohol withdrawal and functional psychosis. *J Stud Alcohol* 39:1831–1840, 1978.
65. Benedetti G: *Die Alkoholhalluzinosen*. Stuttgart, Thieme, 1952.
66. Vorontsova GS: Ob atipichnykh alkogol'nykh psikhozakh. (On atypical alcoholic psychoses). *Zh Nevropat* 59:657–667, 1959.
67. Burton-Bradley BG: Aspects of alcoholic hallucinosis. *Med J Australia* 2:8–11, 1958.
68. Scott DF: Alcoholic hallucinosis—an aetiological study. *Br J Addict* 62:113–125, 1967.
69. Schuckit MA, Winokur G: Alcoholic hallucinosis and schizophrenia: A negative study. *Br J Psychiatry* 119:549–550, 1971.
70. Wolfensberger M: Der alkoholwahnsinn (akute Halluzinose der Trinker) und seine Beziehungen zu den Schizophrenien. *Z ges Neur* 82:385–418, 1923.
71. Darden JH, Hunt WA: Reduction of striatal dopamine release during an ethanol withdrawal syndrome. *J Neurochem* 29:1143–1145, 1977.
72. Tabakoff B, Hoffman PA: Alterations in receptors controlling dopamine synthesis after chronic ethanol ingestion. *J Neurochem* 31:1223–1229, 1978.
73. Mullin PJ, Kershaw PW, Bolt JMW: Choreoathetotic movement disorder in alcoholism. *Br Med J* 4:278–281, 1970.
74. Carlen PL, Lee MA, Jacob M, et al: Parkinsonism provoked by alcoholism. *Ann Neurol* 9:84–86, 1981.

75. Lang AE, Marsden CD, Obeso JA, et al: Alcohol and Parkinson disease. *Ann Neurol* 12:254–256, 1982.
76. Shen WW: Extrapyramidal symptoms associated with alcohol Withdrawal. *Biol Psychiatry* 19:1037–1043, 1984.
77. Benzer D, Cushman P: Alcohol and benzodiazepines: Withdrawal syndromes. *Alcoholism Clin Exp Res* 4:243–247, 1980.
78. Franken R, Seale FE: Withdrawal patterns in cross-addicted patients: Report of 100 cases. *Texas Med* 75:58–60, 1979.
79. Novick DM: Major medical problems and detoxification treatment of parenteral drug-abusing alcoholics. *Adv Alcohol Substance Abuse* 3(4):87–105, 1984.
80. Chan AWK, Leong FW, Schanley DL, et al: Alcohol withdrawal reactions after chronic intake of chlordiazepoxide and ethanol. *Pharmacol Biochem Behavior* 15:185–189, 1981.
81. Schuckit MA: *Drug and Alcohol Abuse: A Clinical Guide to Diagnosis and Treatment,* ed 2. New York, Plenum Press, 1984.
82. Bihari B: Alcoholism and methadone maintenance. *Am J Drug Alcohol Abuse* 1:79–87, 1974.
83. Gordis E, Sereny G: Effect of prior narcotic addiction on response to treatment of alcoholism. *Alcoholism Clin Exp Res* 4:34–39, 1980.
84. Ho AKS, Chem RCA, Morison JM: Interactions of narcotics, narcotics antagonists, and ethanol during acute, chronic and withdrawal states. *Ann NY Acad Sci* 281:297–310, 1976.
85. Glassman AH, Jackson WK, Walsh TB, et al: Cigarette craving, smoking withdrawal, and clonidine. *Science* 226:864–866, 1984.
86. Ashley MJ, le Riche WH, Olin JS, et al: 'Mixed' (drug abusing) and 'pure' alcoholics: A socio-medical comparison. *Br J Addict* 73:19–34, 1978.
87. Israel Y: Researching the biology of alcoholism; one way of seeing it. *J Stud Alcohol (Suppl.) 8:182–203, 1979.*
88. Shipley TE Jr: Alcohol withdrawal and its treatment: Some conjectures in the context of the opponent-process theory. *J Stud Alcohol* 43:548–569, 1982.
89. Wellman M: The late withdrawal symptoms of alcoholic addiction. *Can Med Assoc J* 70:526–529, 1954.
90. Worden M, Rossellini G: The dry drunk syndrome: a toximolecular interpretation. *Orthomol Psychiatry* 9:41–47, 1980.
91. Begleiter H, Porjesz B: Persistence of a "subacute withdrawal syndrome" following chronic ethanol intake. *Drug Alcohol Depend* 4:353–357, 1979.
92. Alling C, Balldin J, Bokstrom K, et al: Studies on duration of a late recovery period after chronic abuse of ethanol: A cross-sectional study of biochemical and psychiatric indicators. *Acta Psychiat Scand* 66:384–397, 1982.
93. Segal BM, Kushnarev VM, Urakov IG, et al: Alcoholism and disruption of the activity of deep cerebral structures: Clinical–laboratory research. *Q J Stud Alcohol* 31:587 601, 1970.
94. Lester BK, Rundell OH, Cowden LC, et al: Chronic alcoholism, alcohol, and sleep. *Adv Exp Biol Med* 35:261–279, 1973.
95. Rundell OH, Williams HL, Lester BK: Sleep in alcoholic patients: Longitudinal findings. *Adv Exp Med Biol* 85B:389–402, 1977.
96. Snyder S, Karacan I: Sleep patterns of sober chronic alcoholics. Paper presented at 135th Annual Meeting, American Psychiatric Association, Toronto, May 1982.
97. Wagman AM, Allen RP: Effects of alcohol ingestion and abstinence on slow wave sleep of alcoholics. *Adv Exp Biol Med* 59:453–466, 1975.
98. Adamson J, Burdick JA. Sleep of dry alcoholics. *Arch Gen Psychiatry* 28:146–149, 1973.
99. Coger RW, Dymond AM, Serafetinides EA: Alcoholism: Averaged visual evoked response amplitude—intensity, slope, and symmetry in withdrawal. *Biol Psychiatry* 11:435–443, 1976.
100. Pfefferbaum A, Horvath TB, Roth WT, et al: Event-related potential changes in chronic alcoholics. *EEG Clin Neurophysiol* 47:637–647, 1979.
101. Wagman AMI, Allen RP, Funderberk F, et al: EEG measures of functional tolerance to alcohol. *Biol Psychiatry* 13:719–728, 1978.
102. Kissin B: Theory and practice in the treatment of alcoholism, in Kissin B, Begleiter H (eds):

The Biology of Alcoholism, vol V. *Treatment and Rehabilitation of the Chronic Alcoholic*. New York, Plenum Press, pp 1–51, 1977.

103. Kissin B, Schenker V, Schenker A: The acute effects of ethyl alcohol and chlorpromazine on certain physiological functions in alcoholics. *Q J Stud Alcohol* 20:480–492, 1959.
104. Lovallo W, Parsons OA, Holloway FA: Autonomic arousal in normal, alcoholic, and brain-damaged subjects as measured by the plethysmograph response to cold pressor stimulation. *Psychophysiology* 10:166–176, 1973.
105. Gross MM, Lewis E: Observations on the prevalence of the signs and symptoms associated with withdrawal during continuous observation of experimental intoxication and withdrawal in humans. *Adv Exp Biol Med* 35:377–406, 1973.
106. Begleiter H, Porjesz B, Grubstein-Yerre C: Excitability cycle of somatosensory evoked potentials during experimental alcoholization and withdrawal. *Psychopharmacologia* 37:15–21, 1974.
107. Shulman GD, O'Connor RD: The rehabilitation of the alcoholic, in Gitlow SE, Peyser HS (eds): *Alcoholism: A Practical Treatment Guide*. New York, Grune and Stratton, 1980, pp 103–130.
108. Mello NK: A semantic aspect of alcoholism, in Cappell HD, and LeBlanc AE (eds): *Biological and Behavioral Approaches to Drug Dependence*. Toronto, Addiction Research Foundation, 1975, pp 73–87.
109. Ludwig AM, Wikler A: "Craving" and relapse to drink *Q J Stud Alcohol* 35:108–130, 1974.
110. Goddard GV, McIntyre DC, Leech CK: A permanent change in brain function resulting from daily electrical stimulation. *Exp Neurol* 25:295–330, 1969.
111. Ballenger JG, Post RM: Kindling as a model for alcohol withdrawal syndromes. *Br J Psychiatry* 133:1–14, 1978.
112. Cummings NA: Turning bread into stones. *Am Psychol* 34:1119–1129, 1979.
113. McGovern MP: Comparative evaluation of medical vs. social treatment of alcohol withdrawal syndrome. *J Clin Psychol* 39:791–803, 1983.
114. Simpson RK, Fitz E, Scott B, et al: Delirium tremens: A preventable iatrogenic and environmental phenomenon. *J Am Osteopath Assoc* 68:123, 1968.
115. Feldman DJ, Pattison EM, Sobell LC, et al: Outpatient alcohol detoxification: Initial findings on 564 patients. *Am J Psychiatry* 132:407–412, 1975.
116. Sellers EM, Naranjo CA, Harrison M, et al: Diazepam loading: Simplified treatment of alcohol withdrawal. *Clin Pharmacol Ther* 34:822–826, 1983.
117. Olbrich R: Alcohol withdrawal states and the need for treatment. *Br J Psychiatry* 134:466–469, 1979.
118. Naranjo CA, Sellers EM, Chater K, et al: Nonpharmacologic intervention in acute alcohol withdrawal. *Clin Pharmacol Ther* 34:214–219, 1983.
119. Rosenfeld JE, Bizzoco DH: A controlled study of alcohol withdrawal. *Q J Stud Alcohol (Suppl.) 4:77–84, 1961.*
120. Shaffer JW, Freinek WR, Wolf S, et al: A controlled evaluation of Chlordiazepoxide (Librium) in the treatment of convalescing alcoholics. *J Nerv Ment Dis* 137:494–507, 1963.
121. Haden HH, Fowler RD: Prozine as an adjunct to psychotherapy with alcoholic patients in the withdrawal stage. *Q J Stud Alcohol* 23:442–448, 1962.
122. Smart RG, Gray G: Multiple predictors of dropout from alcoholism treatment. *Arch Gen Psychiatry* 35:363–367, 1978.
123. Hore BD: Craving for alcohol. *Br J Addict* 69:137–140, 1974.
124. Ludwig AM, Wikler A, Stark LH: The first drink; psychobiological aspects of craving. *Arch Gen Psychiatry* 30:539–547, 1974.
125. Cicero TJ: Alcohol self-administration, tolerance and withdrawal in humans and animals: Theoretical and methodological issues, in Rigter H, Crabbe JC Jr (eds): *Alcohol Tolerance and Dependence*. New York, Elsevier/North-Holland, 1980, pp 1–51.
126. Lawrence FE: The outpatient management of the alcoholic. *Q J Stud Alcohol (Suppl.) 1:117–128, 1961.*

127. Hoff EC: The use of pharmacological adjuncts in the psychotherapy of alcoholics. *Q J Stud Alcohol (Suppl.) 1:138–150, 1961.*
128. Mooney HB, Ditman KS, Cohen S: Chlordiazepoxide in the treatment of alcoholics. *Dis Nerv Syst (Suppl.) 22:44–51, 1961.*
129. Chan AK, Leong FW, Schanley DL: Influence of chlordiazepoxide on alcohol consumption in mice. *Pharmacol Biochem Behav* 18:797–802, 1983.
130. Zakusov VV, Lyubimov I, Yavorsku AN, et al: Effect of phenazepam on ethanol intake in rats. *Bull Exp Biol Med* 88:708–711, 1979.
131. Deutsch JA, Walton NY: Diazepam maintenance of alcohol preference during alcohol withdrawal. *Science* 198:307–309, 1977.
132. LeBlanc AE, Cappell HD: Historical antecedents as determinants of tolerance and dependence upon psychoactive drugs, in Cappell HD, LeBlanc AE (eds): *Biological and Behaviorial Approaches to Drug Dependence.* Toronto, Addiction Research Foundation, 1975, pp 43–51.
133. Poldrugo F, Snead OC III: Electroencephalographic and behavioral correlates in rats during repeated ethanol withdrawal syndromes. *Psychopharmacology* 83:140–146, 1984.
134. Goldstein DB: Rates of onset and decay of alcohol physical dependence in mice. *J Pharmacol Exp Ther* 130:377–383, 1974.
135. Pinel JPJ, Van Oot PH, Mucha RF: Intensification of the alcohol withdrawal symptoms by repeated brain stimulation. *Nature* 254:510–511, 1975.
136. Carrington CD, Ellinwood EH Jr: Effects of alcohol withdrawal on kindling. *Alcoholism Clin Exp Res* 5:348, 1981.
137. Carrington CD, Ellinwood EH Jr, Krishnan RR: Effects of single and repeated alcohol withdrawal on kindling. *Biol Psychiatry* 19:525–537, 1984.

IV

Renal and Electrolyte Consequences of Alcohol Abuse

David H. Van Thiel, Section Editor

Overview

David H. Van Thiel

As a result of the considerable research of many individual investigators, each investigating the area defined by their own expertise, it has become recognized generally that ethyl alcohol is a pantissue toxin. Thus the tissue injurious consequences of alcohol abuse for such organs as the liver, brain, heart, bone marrow, skeletal muscles, and gonads have been identified over the last quarter of a century and are presently well known to most physicians and students of alcohol associated pathologies. The fact that alcohol abuse also adversely affects renal function and particularly salt and water balance is less well known. Therefore, this volume of *Recent Developments in Alcoholism* addresses the following topics:

1. Disorders of the serum electrolytes, acid–base balance and renal function;
2. Urinary tract infections and renal papillary necrosis;
3. Disorders of divalent ion and vitamin D metabolism;
4. Pathogenesis of renal sodium retention and ascites formation in Laennec's cirrhosis

The following four chapters by Pitts and Van Thiel provide an encyclopedic presentation of the currently available information relating to the perturbating effects of alcohol abuse, both direct and indirect, upon salt and water and acid–base balance, divalent mineral metabolism, and renal parenchymal function.

Chapter 14 discusses in detail the pathogenesis and therapy of hyponatremia. It also contains a discussion of hypokalemia and its pathogenesis and indications for therapy. Finally, the common and unusual causes of metabolic acidosis that occur in alcoholics are presented.

Chapter 15 discusses the clinically important issue of renal infection and papillary necrosis. Concepts concerning their pathogenesis in alcohol abusers and patients with liver disease are discussed.

In Chapter 16 an overview of vitamin D metabolism is followed by a

David H. Van Thiel • Division of Gastroenterology, Department of Medicine, University of Pittsburgh School of Medicine, Pittsburgh, Pennsylvania 15261.

discussion of the deficits in this system that occur as a consequence of alcoholism, liver disease, and the combination of the two conditions. In addition, the problems of hypomagnesemia and osteoporosis in these unique populations are discussed.

Chapter 17 addresses the problem of ascites formation, its progression and therapy. The pathophysiologic basis for each and the data available confirming or refuting common hypotheses about each are presented for the reader who is not an expert in this field.

Throughout the chapters, the authors have documented their presentation with current references wherever possible. In addition, they have provided useful headings for quick and easy reference for the busy reader. Finally, they have incorporated summary statements at the end of most sections to highlight the facts as they are currently known, separate from the speculation or controversy present in a given area. Controversial data are presented in detail within the individual presentations.

Clearly, the authors have learned much from the experience of preparing these chapters and hope that the reader will also benefit from them.

14

Disorders of the Serum Electrolytes, Acid–Base Balance, and Renal Function in Alcoholism

Thomas O. Pitts and David H. Van Thiel

Abstract. This chapter reviews the disturbances of the serum sodium and potassium concentrations, acid–base imbalances, and acute renal dysfunction that are seen frequently in alcoholic patients. The hyponatremia common in decompensated cirrhotics is caused by an impairment of renal free water clearance and concomitant water ingestion. Excessive proximal renal tubular sodium reabsorption and nonosmotic vasopressin release underlie the defect in renal water excretion in cirrhosis. Restriction of water intake is the principal therapeutic measure for hyponatremia. Hypokalemia is common in alcoholics but when observed does not always represent true potassium depletion. Although most cirrhotics have a diminished total body potassium content, intracellular potassium concentration is usually normal. In some patients gastrointestinal and renal potassium losses and nutritional potassium deficiency may cause true potassium depletion. Respiratory and metabolic alkalosis are the acid–base disturbances seen most frequently in alcoholics. Acidosis is relatively uncommon and is usually due to renal insufficiency, lactic acid or keto–acid accumulation. Toxin ingestion (methanol, ethylene glycol, or isopropanol) may also cause severe acidosis. Rhabdomyolysis, common in severe alcoholism, may produce various electrolyte disturbances and acute renal failure. The prognosis for recovery is good although temporary dialysis may be necessary.

1. Introduction

Alcoholic patients display a wide variety of metabolic disturbances including abnormalities of the serum electrolytes and acid–base balance and, occasionally, the development of acute renal failure. Most of these disorders occur not as a direct consequence of the action of ethanol on renal function but, rather, as a result of its effects on other systems. Certain disorders are particularly characteristic of acute alcoholism, whereas others arise more commonly in the cirrhotic individual. In addition, many of these consequences

Thomas O. Pitts • Renal–Electrolyte Division, Department of Medicine, University of Pittsburgh School of Medicine, Pittsburgh, Pennsylvania 15261. **David H. Van Thiel** • Division of Gastroenterology, Department of Medicine, University of Pittsburgh School of Medicine, Pittsburgh, Pennsylvania 15261.

of alcoholism occur with equal facility in both cirrhotic and noncirrhotic patients.

In this chapter we will examine abnormalities of the serum monovalent cations, sodium and potassium, and the derangements of acid–base balance that frequently occur in alcoholism. In addition, we will discuss toxin ingestions and myoglobinuric acute renal failure, problems that are particularly characteristic of the alcoholic patient.

2. Hyponatremia

2.1. Laennec's Cirrhosis

2.1.1. Frequency. Hyponatremia is a common feature of decompensated cirrhosis.[1,2] In the overwhelming majority of patients it occurs on a dilutional basis due to persistent water consumption in the face of impaired free water clearance.[2–4] Because of its chronicity, hyponatremia is usually asymptomatic. Therefore, it is difficult to estimate accurately the overall prevalence of this disorder in cirrhosis. Nonetheless, it would appear that as many as 40% of decompensated cirrhotics may manifest significant hyponatremia at the time of hospitalization.[2] In contrast, compensated cirrhotics usually have a normal serum sodium concentration.[1]

2.1.2. Water Excretion. The use of the water loading test has provided considerable insight into the prevalence of abnormalities of water excretion in cirrhosis. Decompensated cirrhotics have a mean free water clearance which is only fifty percent of that obtained from healthy controls.[5,6] In contrast, water excretion is normal in compensated patients.[7] However, not all decompensated subjects have compromised water excretion. Thus, the individual values of free water clearance seen in decompensated cirrhotics vary over a wide range from subnormal to normal.[8] In fact, water excretion is impaired in only 30–50% of decompensated cirrhotic patients,[9,10] similar to the apparent prevalence of hyponatremia seen in this same patient group.[2]

2.1.3. Pathogenesis of the Impaired Free Water Excretion in Cirrhosis.

2.1.3a. Elevated Plasma Arginine Vasopressin Levels. Plasma levels of arginine vasopressin are frequently elevated in cirrhotic patients,[11,12] particularly in those with ascites.[13] Although the presence of significant hyponatremia (serum sodium concentration less than 130 mEq/liter) does not necessarily correlate with the plasma vasopressin concentration, most patients with an elevated vasopressin level are hyponatremic.[11,13]

Non-osmotic vasopressin release is the primary cause of the elevations of the plasma vasopressin concentration seen in cirrhotics. In experimental models of cirrhosis, impaired water excretion is associated with non-osmotic vasopressin release.[14–16] Recently Bichet *et al.* have provided evidence for this same mechanism in humans with cirrhosis.[13] These investigators found impaired free water clearance in five of 12 cirrhotics subjected to a standard water loading test. Patients with impaired water excretion frequently have evidence for defective intravascular filling with a greater resting pulse, stimulation of the renin–angiotensin–aldosterone axis, lower creatinine clearances, and reduced urinary sodium excretion. When cirrhotics are subjected to head-out water immersion, the right atrial pressure increases and arginine vasopressin levels decrease as do the plasma renin activity and plasma aldosterone and norepinephrine concentrations.[17] Moreover, an increase in free water excretion observed during immersion correlates inversely with plasma arginine vasopressin levels and directly with right atrial pressure.[17] These data suggest that the elevated vasopressin levels seen in cirrhosis are due to an effective intravascular volume depletion.

Impaired hepatic degradation of vasopressin has frequently been cited as a factor possibly contributing to the elevation of plasma levels of this hormone in cirrhosis. Unfortunately, there are few data that bear on this question. Cirrhotics appear to metabolize radioiodine-labeled arginine vasopressin more slowly than do normal subjects.[18] However, the validity of this finding has been called into question as the iodine-labeled hormone apparently undergoes a different route of metabolism than does the natural hormone.[19,20] Recently it has been reported that the metabolic clearance rate of exogenously administered arginine vasopressin is greater in compensated cirrhotics than it is in decompensated subjects.[21] Because the mean serum creatinine values were roughly equivalent in the two patient groups studied in this investigation it was concluded that the diminished rate of vasopressin clearance was due to greater impairment in hepatic function present in the decompensated subjects.[21] However, there was no evidence other than the presence of ascites for more severe hepatic disease in the decompensated patients. Moreover, only the serum creatinine level was used as a measure of renal function. The serum creatinine is notoriously unreliable as an indicator of glomerular filtration rate in cirrhotics[22] and mild decrements in renal blood flow and in glomerular filtration rate are seen commonly in decompensated cirrhosis.[23,24] Thus, differences in the renal clearance of vasopressin may well have contributed to the findings (*vide infra*).

There is a significant body of evidence to suggest that impaired hepatic degradation of arginine vasopressin contributes little to the elevated hormone levels encountered in cirrhosis. Normally, the kidney is the major site of arginine vasopressin metabolism.[19,21,25] The liver may clear a percentage of the vasopressin present in the hepatic blood flow.[26] However, under certain conditions the hormone undergoes no degradation as it passes through the hepatic circulation.[27] Cirrhotics do not respond differently than do noncirrhotics in terms of the duration of their response to exogenously administered vasopressin preparations.[28] Because the rate of renal excretion of arginine vasopressin is related principally to the glomerular filtration rate and the peritubular vasopressin uptake,[19,25] a considerable impairment of the glomerular filtration rate and renal blood flow might contribute to retention of the hormone in some cirrhotics. However, if impaired metabolic clearance of arginine vasopressin induces an elevation of plasma vasopressin levels in cirrhosis, the subsequent hyponatremia should inhibit further vasopressin release and plasma levels would gradually return to normal. However, as this does not occur, excessive vasopressin secretion appears to be the major contributor to the elevated levels of this hormone seen in cirrhosis.

Although it is clear that vasopressin levels are often elevated in cirrhosis, considerable controversy exists regarding the contribution of this hormone to the water retention of cirrhosis. Acute portal venous hypertension in dogs results in an impairment of water excretion that is partially abolished by hypophysectomy.[14] Other experimental models of hepatic disease also have suggested a role for vasopressin in the generation of the water retention seen in cirrhosis.[29] The acute administration of ethanol to decompensated cirrhotic patients increases urinary water excretion due to the inhibitory effect of ethanol on vasopressin release.[30] Demeclocycline, an inhibitor of the renal tubular action of vasopressin, improves water excretion in cirrhosis despite the concomitant reduction it produces in the glomerular filtration rate and renal blood flow.[31,32]

Recently Perez-Ayuso *et al.* have provided additional evidence that increased vasopressin activity may contribute to the impaired water excretion seen in cirrhosis.[10] Prostaglandins appear to be physiologic antagonists of the renal action of vasopressin.[33–35] In addition, renal prostaglandin E_2 synthesis is stimulated by arginine vasopressin.[36] Both basal urinary PGE_2 excretion and plasma arginine vasopressin levels are often elevated in cirrhosis.[10] In cirrhotics, but not normal subjects, the inhibition of prostaglandin synthesis by salicylates results in an impairment in free water excretion that occurs independently of any changes in the glomerular filtration rate.[10]

2.1.3b. Decreased Distal Sodium Delivery. Despite the evidence favoring the role of vasopressin in the genesis of water retention, the major factor contributing to water retention in cirrhosis appears to be decreased delivery of filtrate to the renal tubular diluting segments, induced by avid proximal tubular sodium reabsorption. The key evidence supporting this concept is that various volume expansion maneuvers improve free water clearance in cirrhotics, presumably by augmenting distal sodium delivery.[37–39] In fact, the defect in distal delivery of sodium occurs early in cirrhosis, well before ascites is present.[40] In addition, in models of experimental liver disease, water retention occurs not only due to increased arginine vasopressin activity but also in conjunction with decreased distal solute delivery.[29]

Because in states of effective volume depletion nonosmotic stimulation of vasopressin secretion occurs simultaneously with decreased distal solute delivery, investigators have examined the relationship between changes in plasma vasopressin levels and the diuresis induced by expansion manuevers. Thus, Epstein *et al.* have demonstrated that head-out water immersion induces a diuresis and increases free water clearance in cirrhotics without suppressing endogenous arginine vasopressin levels.[41] Similarly, the placement of a peritoneovenous shunt acutely increases free water clearance independent of any change in plasma arginine vasopressin concentration.[42] These findings provide strong support for the importance of impaired distal solute delivery as the major cause of the water retention present in cirrhosis.

2.1.3c. Back-Diffusion of Tubular Water. Another cause of impaired free water excretion in cirrhosis is vasopressin-independent back-diffusion of water which occurs when the urinary flow rate is very low.[43] As many cirrhotics excrete small volumes of urine (less than 500 ml/day), this may be an important source of water retention. Unfortunately, in a clinical setting, it is not possible to examine this process directly. Indirect evidence for such a mechanism is that the administration of furosemide improves free water excretion of cirrhotics presumably by enhancing the distal tubular urine flow rate.[44] However, the same result is obtained when furosemide is given to cirrhotics receiving a simultaneous infusion of vasopressin, suggesting that the diuretic may antagonize the action of vasopressin.[44,45] Although it is not unreasonable to assume that flow dependent back-flux of water occurs in some cirrhotic patients and contributes to their water retention, there are no data that clearly demonstrate this phenomenon.

2.1.4. Therapy of Hyponatremia in the Cirrhotic. Because hyponatremia in cirrhotics is usually due to dilution, the standard therapeutic approach is fluid restriction. It is common clinical practice to limit fluid intake when the serum sodium concentration falls below 130 mEq/liter. In such a situation temporary withdrawal of diuretics is indicated also. Demeclocycline has been used successfully to correct hyponatremia in cirrhotics but is associated with an excessively high incidence of renal failure in such patients.[32] Peritoneal dialysis, which removes water more rapidly than it does sodium, has been employed successfully in end-stage cirrhosis to correct hyponatremia but should be considered only as a last resort.[46]

2.2. Water Handling in Noncirrhotic Alcoholic Patients

2.2.1. Acute Effects of Ethanol. The acute administration of ethanol to normal subjects produces little change in excretory parameters. There is a mild, transient decrease in urinary sodium excretion with no change in renal blood flow or glomerular filtration rate.[47,48] Ethanol acutely inhibits the release of vasopressin resulting in an increase in free water excretion.[30] However, this effect persists only while the blood ethanol level is rising. In subjects under 50 years of age, a rising blood ethanol concentration suppresses plasma immunoreactive arginine vasopressin levels despite a concomitant increase in the serum osmolality.[49] In contrast, subjects older than 50 years quickly escape the suppressive effect of the ethanol infusion and manifest sharp increases in their plasma arginine vasopressin levels. This escape occurs even though the increase in serum osmolality observed in the older subjects is similar to that encountered in the younger group. The difference in vasopressin response to ethanol between younger and older individuals may relate, in part, to an increase in osmoreceptor sensitivity with advancing age.[49]

Whether a similar variation of arginine vasopressin response to ethanol infusion occurs in chronic alcoholics is not know.

2.2.2. Chronic Effects of Ethanol. When normal nutrition is maintained, chronic ethanol administration usually produces no alteration in the serum sodium concentration. However, there is some evidence to suggest that water and solute retention may occur in alcoholism. Chronic ethanol administration (2–4 g/kg, enterally) to dogs over an 8-week period increases their total body water, extracellular volume, and plasma volume due to an isoosmotic renal water and solute retention.[50] In humans, withdrawal from chronic alcohol use is associated with declines in total body water and in intra- and extracellular volume that are accompanied by a solute diuresis, suggesting that chronic alcoholism may induce both solute and water retention.[51] These changes are not associated with alterations in the serum electrolytes and are not usually apparent. However, chronic volume expansion induced by ethanol use may contribute to the development of hypertension that is common in chronic alcoholism.[52–54]

2.2.3. Hyponatremia in Alcoholics without Cirrhosis. Chronic alcoholics can develop hyponatremia for any of the reasons that occur in nonalcoholics. However, from the preceding discussion it is apparent that acute or chronic ethanol use per se does not usually alter the serum sodium concentration. Therefore, hyponatremia in a noncirrhotic alcoholic is most often multifactoral in origin.

A hyponatremic syndrome peculiar to beer drinkers has been well described. Although the frequency of this syndrome is not clear, it may comprise a significant percentage of cases of symptomatic hyponatremia. Demanet *et al.* found that 12 of 67 patients admitted to the hospital with severe hyponatremia (serum sodium concentration $\leqslant$ 120 mEq/liter) had neurologic symptoms attributable solely to the electrolyte disorder.[55] Seven of these 12 individuals were heavy beer drinkers who consumed at least 4 liters of beer daily. Although there was no evidence of overt volume depletion in these alcoholics, vomiting and diarrhea or prehospital diuretic therapy was present in all and contributed to the sodium deficit, which was evidenced by a marked sodium retention during the 4 days subsequent to hospitalization. The excessive consumption of free water (as beer), however, was felt to have been the major factor leading to the development of the hyponatremia in these subjects.[55]

Hyponatremia also may occur in beer drinkers in the absence of any evidence of sodium depletion. Hilden and Svendsen observed hyponatremia in five patients who consumed at least 5 liters of beer daily with no additional form of nourishment.[56] The degree of hyponatremia and the severity of the associated symptoms were less prominent than in the patients reported by Demanet *et al.* Urinary osmolality was appropriately low in those patients in whom it was measured, confirming that vasopressin secretion was suppressed. The genesis of the hyponatremia in these patients appeared to be the consumption of free water in excess of solute sufficient to allow for excretion of the water. Because the minimum urinary osmolality is approximately 50–60 mOsm/kg water, roughly 300 mOsm of solute must be excreted to allow the elimination of 5 liters of water. Due to their poor protein intake and the low solute content of beer, these patients probably excrete less than 300 mOsm/day. Therefore, "beer-drinkers' hyponatremia" is a disorder of water overload per se and is not a direct consequence of ethanol ingestion.

3. Potassium Disorders in Alcoholism

3.1. Hypokalemia

3.1.1. Frequency of Hypokalemia. Hypokalemia occurs commonly in alcoholics. As is the case for nonalcoholics, the serum potassium concentration is a poor indicator of the total body stores.[57–59] Decreases in the serum potassium may arise due to total body potassium depletion or as a consequence of the movement of the ion into the intracellular compartment. Hypokalemia in alcoholism is most often associated with other electrolyte and acid–base disorders.[60] Therefore, the detection of hypokalemia in the alcoholic patient should prompt the physician to undertake a thorough search for other metabolic abnormalities.

Estimates of the frequency of hypokalemia in alcoholics have come largely from studies of hospitalized patients. Approximately 50% of patients hospitalized for Laennec's cirrhosis may be hypokalemic,[57–59,61,62] In the absence of ascites, however, cirrhotics usually have a normal serum potassium level.[57,59,63] In addition, hypokalemia is seen in approximately 50% of the chronic alcoholics who are hospitalized for acute alcohol withdrawal and usually develops after their hospitalization.[64,65]

3.1.2. Correlation of the Serum Potassium with Tissue Potassium Stores. Because the serum potassium level does not accurately reflect the state of potassium balance, efforts have been made to determine the total body potassium in alcoholics as a more sensitive measure of potassium depletion. In addition, many investigators have distinguished between true potassium depletion and states of pseudodepletion in which intracellular potassium is normal despite a reduction in total body potassium.[63]

Most patients with Laennec's cirrhosis have a total body potassium (or exchangeable potassium) content that is markedly decreased in comparison with that of healthy controls.[57,61,63] Although a diminished total body potassium is observed more frequently in ascitic patients,[59] it also is seen in the majority of compensated cirrhotics.[59,61,63] That the lower total body potassium content of cirrhotics may represent true potassium depletion is supported by the finding that oral potassium supplementation increases the total body potassium in some of these patients.[57,61] However, the majority of cirrhotics do not increase their total body potassium when given oral potassium supplements, suggesting either that no intracellular deficit is present or that some circumstance attributable to severe liver disease or its treatment (e.g. hyperaldosteronism, diuretic therapy) prevents the retention of the administered potassium.[59]

Other data suggest that the low total body potassium values seen in cirrhosis do not represent true potassium depletion or intracellular potassium deficits. Thus, the values of exchangeable potassium (corrected for total body weight) for alcoholic cirrhotic patients reported by Casey *et al.* are significantly lower than those of healthy subjects but are similar to those observed in hospitalized controls.[57] When an additional weight correction is made for the increased extracellular volume of the cirrhotics, the exchangeable potassium per kilogram of dry weight in ascitic and compensated cirrhotics is identical to that of hospitalized nonalcoholic controls.[66] In cirrhotics normal intracellular potassium levels are found in red blood cells,[67,68] muscle cells,[69,70] and leukocytes.[66,71] When lowered intracellular potassium values have been observed in the muscle cells of cirrhotics, there has been a concomitant loss of cellular nitrogen.[72] Additionally, the decrease in the calculated intracellular potassium level is due largely to an increase in intracellular water.[62,72] Therefore, in cirrhotics, the loss of muscle mass and an increase in the intracellular water content are responsible for the decreases observed in total body potassium.

In acute alcoholism without cirrhosis, muscle cell potassium levels may be low,[73,74] a finding which is consistent with depletion of the total body potassium stores.[75,76] The lack of correlation between the serum potassium concentration and the muscle cell potassium content in hospitalized withdrawing alcoholics emphasizes, however, that hypokalemia in these patients is often not associated with true potassium depletion.[74]

3.1.3. Causes of Potassium Deficiency.

3.1.3a. Urinary Potassium Loss. Renal potassium wastage may occur in the alcoholic in a number of ways. Metabolic alkalosis, which can arise as a consequence of vomiting or diuretic use, induces a shift of potassium into the cells that stimulates the secretion of potassium into the urine. Therapy with non-potassium-sparing diuretics augments urinary potassium excretion further by increasing the delivery of sodium to the distal tubular sodium–potassium exchange sites. Hyperaldosteronism is present in some decompensated cirrhotics[77,78] and occurs transiently in the 24 hr following acute alcohol administration.[79] Whereas the effect of hyperaldosteronism on potassium excretion in cirrhosis is not clear,[80,81] the rise in plasma aldosterone observed after acute alcohol administration correlates well with increases in urinary potassium excretion.[79] Although ethanol acutely has no significant effect on renal potassium excretion,[48,51] it produces excessive urinary magnesium losses,[48,82] which contribute to the development of hypomagnesemia. By an unknown mechanism, hypomagnesemia impairs renal tubular potassium reabsorption, promoting renal potassium wastage and, thus, hypokalemia.[83] Finally, excessive urinary potassium loss may occur in cirrhotics in association with renal tubular acidosis.[84]

3.1.3b. Nonrenal Potassium Losses and Deficient Intake. Hypokalemia can occur in the alcoholic by means other than excessive renal loss of the ion. Inadequate nutritional intake is common in alcoholics and is often associated with the development of a variety of vitamin and mineral deficiencies.[85,86] Severe potassium deficiency may result from gastrointestinal loss of the ion that occurs with vomiting and diarrhea. Often hypokalemic alcoholic patients have more than one source of potassium loss. Thus, for example, vomiting, which produces only minimal potassium loss from the gastrointestinal tract, stimulates renal potassium wastage secondary to the development of a metabolic alkalosis.

3.1.4. Hypokalemia without Potassium Deficiency. A well-recognized cause of abnormalities of the serum potassium concentration is a shift of the ion into or out of cells in response to alterations in acid–base status or the action of certain hormones.[87] In alcoholics several factors may induce hypokalemia by this mechanism.

3.1.4a. Respiratory Alkalosis. Respiratory alkalosis is seen with great frequency in patients with Laennec's cirrhosis[88–91] and in noncirrhotic chronic alcoholics.[92,93] The majority of these patients are mildly alkalemic (serum pH 7.44 or greater). The presence of alkalemia during acute alcohol withdrawal correlates well with the development of hypokalemia.[92] However, in many alcoholic subjects the occurence of hypokalemia or diminished total body potassium does not correlate with the serum pH or true potassium deficiency.[94] Thus, factors other than the alkalemia associated with respiratory alkalosis are often responsible for the development of hypokalemia in many alcoholics.

3.1.4b. Adrenergic Stimulation. Excessive sympathetic nervous system activity is a feature of alcohol withdrawal[95] and Laennec's cirrhosis.[96,97] Because β-adrenergic stimulation promotes entry of potassium into cells[98,99] the sympathetic nervous system hyperactivity seen in alcoholics may facilitate the development of hypokalemia by this mechanism.

3.1.4c. Effect of Insulin. Excessive insulin secretion also may contribute to the development of hypokalemia in alcoholics. An elevation of the plasma insulin concentration is frequently present in alcoholism.[100,101] Profound hypokalemia may develop following the intravenous administration of glucose to potassium-depleted patients, including alcoholics.[64,102] Insulin-induced cellular uptake of potassium appears to underlie this phenomenon.[103] In some alcoholics the concomitant presence of hypophosphatemia may contribute further to the excessive insulin secretion by augmenting glucose-stimulated insulin release.[104]

3.1.5. Consequences of Hypokalemia in Alcoholism. The manifestations of hypokalemia in alcoholics are similar to those occuring in nonalcoholics. Because of the concurrence of other electrolyte disorders, the treatment of hypokalemia in alcoholics may be difficult.[64] In addition, the presence of liver disease in many alcoholics increases the risk for serious sequelae of hypokalemia.

3.1.5a. Hepatic Encephalopathy. Hepatic encephalopathy may be precipitated by hypokalemia. Potassium depletion augments the renal generation of ammonia, which may further elevate the plasma ammonia levels of cirrhotics.[105] In addition, both hypokalemia and avid proximal sodium reabsorption impair urinary acidification,[106,107] which results in the back diffusion of ammonia from the urine into the blood and increases the plasma ammonia concentration.[84,108] Clinically, hypokalemia often, but not invariably, correlates with the development of hepatic encephalopathy.[94,109,110]

3.1.5b. Myopathy. In the alcoholic patient severe potassium depletion may result in the development of an acute myopathy.[111,112] This condition is characterized by painless muscle weakness and profound hypokalemia (serum potassium concentration less than 2.5 mEq/liter) and can lead to muscle cell necrosis.[111,112] In contrast, classical alcoholic myopathy, which causes severe weakness, muscle pain, and rhabdomyolysis, occurs in the absence of severe hypokalemia and most frequently is associated with hypophosphatemia.[70,74,113–115] Thus, although hypokalemia may cause acute paralysis or muscle necrosis it is not a common cause of myopathy in the alcoholic.[113]

3.1.5c. Delerium Tremens. It has been suggested that hypokalemia may be associated with the development of delerium tremens in patients hospitalized for acute alcohol withdrawal.[65] Support for this contention is derived from the observation that these patients are usually normokalemic on admission and develop delerium tremens subsequent to a spontaneous and rapid decline in the serum potassium that occurs despite oral potassium supplementation.[65] However, it is clear that hypokalemia per se does not cause delerium tremens. Alcoholics who undergo delerium tremens manifest multiple electrolyte disorders in addition to hypokalemia and have a more protracted history of alcohol abuse than do those who do not develop delerium tremens.[116]

3.2. Hyperkalemia in the Alcoholic Patient

Hyperkalemia is distinctly uncommon in alcoholics. When it occurs, it is usually associated with acidosis, acute renal failure, the hepatorenal syndrome, and/or the use of potassium-sparing diuretics or potassium supplements. Although hyperkalemia occurs in approximately one third of patients with cirrhosis and functional renal failure, it is not a frequent cause of mortality in these patients.[4] In contrast, the majority of cirrhotic patients given spironolactone develop hyperkalemic acidosis, which can occasionally preclude further therapy with this valuable agent.[117]

4. Acid–Base Disturbances in Alcoholism

Abnormalities of acid–base balance are quite common in alcoholic patients. Most acid–base disorders occur in cirrhotic and noncirrhotic patients with equal facility and by similar mechanisms. Not infrequently, alcoholic patients have a mixed acid–base disturbance, i.e., the concomitant presence of two or more simple acid–base disorders, which may not be readily apparent from an examination of the serum electrolytes alone. Moreover, some alcoholics develop an acid–base imbalance only after admission to the hospital. Therefore, it behooves the physician caring for such patients to be familiar with the various acid–base disorders that are particularly common to alcoholics.

Alkalosis is the acid–base disorder encountered most frequently in alcoholic patients. It occurs in a majority of the patients hospitalized for acute ethanol withdrawal and is most often either a simple respiratory alkalosis[118,119] or a mixed respiratory and metabolic alkalosis.[92] Thus, 50% of subjects with cirrhosis are alkalotic, with simple respiratory alkalosis accounting for the majority and metabolic alkalosis or combined respiratory and metabolic alkalosis comprising the remainder of cases.[94,120–123] In contrast, acidosis is uncommon in alcoholics, occurring most often in patients with preterminal cirrhosis.[123] Most cases of acidosis are due to renal insufficiency or lactate accumulation although respiratory acidosis may occur as a terminal event[123] or in association with muscle failure induced by coexistent phosphate depletion.[124]

4.1. Respiratory Alkalosis

The cause of the respiratory alkalosis associated with acute ethanol withdrawal is obscure. Acutely, ethanol depresses the central nervous system respiratory activity in a dose-dependent fashion in most subjects.[125,126] Within 8 hr following the cessation of ethanol intake, respiratory alkalosis may be detected.[119] Hypomagnesemia often accompanies the respiratory alkalosis and both disorders correlate with the presence of neuromuscular irritability.[118,119] It has been suggested that the hyperventilation that occurs during acute ethanol withdrawal represents a rebound increase in the sensitivity of the respiratory center to carbon dioxide following removal of the depressant effect of ethanol.[119]

Several factors may contribute to the development of respiratory alkalosis in cirrhotic patients. Arterial hypoxemia and diminished oxygen saturation, which occur as a consequence of arteriovenous shunts and ventilation perfusion imbalances, are present in many cirrhotics and correlate with the observed hyperventilation.[127,128] Although not all cirrhotics have resting hypoxemia,[129,130] many manifest respiratory alkalosis.[130] Increased sensitivity of the respiratory center to carbon dioxide has been demonstrated in some and is thought to be due to an intracellular acidosis.[91] A direct correlation between the blood ammonia concentration and hyperventilation has been reported by some investigators,[94] but not by others.[89] In dogs, infusion of the ammonium ion produces hyperventilation and a resultant respiratory alkalosis,[131] which correlates not with the blood ammonia content but, rather, with the cerebrospinal fluid ammonia levels.[132] This latter finding may explain the considerable variability in the reported observations on the correlation between blood ammonia concentration and hyperventilation.[89,94]

4.2. Metabolic Alkalosis

The development of metabolic alkalosis in alcoholics usually is preceded by vomiting or diuretic administration.[110,123] The pathogenesis of the metabolic alkalosis secondary to diuretic therapy is not completely understood. In the presence of volume contraction, potassium and/or chloride deficiency, or excessive mineralocorticoid hormone secretion, diuretic therapy may produce alkalosis by enhancing the delivery of sodium to the distal tubule hydrogen ion secretory sites.[27,76] However, chronic furosemide administration may produce excessive hydrogen ion excretion even in the absence of volume contraction, potassium or chloride depletion, or excessive mineralocorticoid hormone secretion.[133] In addition, some diuretics directly stimulate hydrogen ion secretion.[134]

4.3. Metabolic Acidosis

4.3.1. Renal Tubular Acidosis. Distal (type I) renal tubular acidosis is characterized classically by a hyperchloremic metabolic acidosis.[135] Affected patients are unable to lower their urine pH sufficiently to excrete the daily acid load and, if untreated, manifest overt acidemia. Patients with the incomplete form of distal renal tubular acidosis maintain acid balance and normal blood pH but are unable to maximally lower their urine pH following the administration of an acid load. The exact cause of the disorder has not been elucidated but may be the failure of the cells of the distal tubule to secrete hydrogen ion or the inability of the distal tubule to prevent back-flux of the secreted hydrogen ions into the blood. This disorder may arise spontaneously or may occur in concert with various systemic diseases.[135]

Distal renal tubular acidosis is a common finding in cirrhotics.[84,136] Although many investigators have not specified the cause of cirrhosis in their patients, it is clear from the more recent reports that 30–50% of patients with Laennec's cirrhosis may have distal renal tubular acidosis.[137,138] The great majority of these cases are of the incomplete variety. Indeed, the occurrence of complete distal renal tubular acidosis in Laennec's cirrhosis has not been described. In some, but not all, patients with this disorder there is an associated impairment in potassium conservation that may lead to hypokalemia and a predisposition to develop hepatic encephalopathy.[84]

The cause of the incomplete form of distal renal tubular acidosis in cirrhosis is not understood completely. Impaired delivery of sodium to the distal tubule has been implicated by some investigators.[106,137] Because of the excessive urinary alkalinity in distal renal tubular acidosis, the excretion of titratable acidity is diminished, and, in compensation, ammonium excretion is increased.[135] Protein malnutrition[139,140] and phosphate depletion[141–143] impair net acid excretion by further reducing titratable acidity and by producing renal bicarbonate wastage. Additionally, potassium deficiency impairs net acid excretion by suppressing aldosterone secretion.[107]

Because the incomplete distal renal tubular acidosis of cirrhosis produces no serious electrolyte abnormalities, therapy usually is not necessary. However, if hypokalemia occurs, potassium supplementation may be required.[84] In patients with hypokalemia and hyperchloremia the use of alkaline potassium salts (such as gluconate or citrate), rather than the chloride salt, is recommended.[135] There is no evidence that this renal tubular disorder predisposes the patient to the development of renal insufficiency, nor is the process related in any way to the alterations of renal hemodynamics or glomerular filtration rate observed in many cirrhotics.[138]

4.3.2. Lactic Acidosis in the Alcoholic. Huckabee first called attention to the clinical syndrome of lactic acidosis, including in his report several cases associated with severe hepatic disease or ethanol intoxication.[144] Although there is now a well-recognized association between alcoholism and the development of lactic acidosis, the appearance of this disorder in alcoholics is uncommon. Hyperlactatemia without acidosis occurs frequently in cirrhotics and is of little clinical significance.[145] In contrast, lactic acidosis is present in less than 5–10% of hospitalized cirrhotics and is often associated with major complicating conditions such as hypotension or sepsis.[146]

Pyruvate is a key intermediate of the glycolytic pathway. Normally it does not accumulate to any appreciable extent but enters other metabolic pathways such as the Krebs cycle or gluconeogenesis. Under anaerobic conditions pyruvate is converted to lactate by the enzyme lactate dehydrogenase, utilizing one reduced nicotinamide adenine dinucleotide (NADH) molecule. The production of lactate from pyruvate is directly proportional to the ratio of the concentration of oxidized nicotinamide adenine dinucleotide (NAD) to that of NADH. Normally the equilibrium of the reaction lies in the favor of lactate so that the ratio of blood lactate to pyruvate concentration is ten to one. Factors that influence pyruvate availability have qualitatively similar effects on lactate formation.[145,147]

In a normal adult lactate production is approximately 1000–1500 mmoles per day. The liver removes over one half of this amount while the kidneys metabolize an additional one third of the daily lactate load. These organs preferentially utilize lactate for gluconeogenesis in a reaction which consumes hydrogen ions, thereby balancing the hydrogen ions released when lactic acid is formed.[145,147]

Alcoholics may develop lactic acidosis through any of several mechanisms. Ethanol is metabolized by alcohol dehydrogenase to acetaldehyde which is subsequently converted to acetate by aldehyde dehydrogenase. Both enzymatic steps require the reduction of NAD and, therefore, decrease the

NAD/NADH ratio, increasing the formation of lactate from pyruvate.[148–150] Ethanol also increases hepatic lactate production[149,151] and decreases peripheral lactate utilization.[152]

The administration of ethanol moderately increases the blood lactate concentration by 1–4 mmoles/liter.[148] Usually, this degree of hyperlactatemia does not result in a significant acid–base disturbance. However, other factors may contribute to produce a more severe lactate accumulation. For example, hepatic dysfunction results in decreased hepatic clearance of lactate.[146,153,154] Mild hypotension and arterial hypoxemia are common features of advanced alcoholic liver disease and may impair peripheral oxygen delivery, thereby further increasing lactate production. Additionally, hypophosphatemia, which often occurs in alcoholics, decreases the red blood cell production of 2,3-diphosphoglycerate, which increases the affinity of hemoglobin for oxygen and, thus, impairs peripheral oxygen delivery.[155] Hyperventilation, another feature of alcoholism, decreases hepatic blood flow and causes the liver to produce rather than to utilize lactate.[156] In this regard respiratory alkalosis may evolve to lactic acidosis in cirrhotic patients.[120] Finally, the effects of ethanol on lactate accumulation may be particularly pronounced in patients with diabetes[157] or with chronic pulmonary disease[126] when the metabolism of lactate or the ability to compensate for its acid load is impaired.

The therapy of lactic acidosis in alcoholic patients depends on the magnitude of the disorder and its cause. Simple hyperlactatemia associated with ethanol intoxication usually resolves with abstention and the provision of adequate hydration.[154] In contrast, severe or progressive lactic acidosis associated with hepatic dysfunction and/or hypoperfusion is quite difficult to treat. Bicarbonate administration (often in massive amounts) has been the mainstay of the treatment of lactic acidosis but may increase lactate production in some patients[158] by enhancing glycolysis and, thereby, increasing pyruvate availability.[156] Moreover, the sodium load accompanying bicarbonate therapy may produce pulmonary edema or hypernatremia. The administration of glucose and insulin has been recommended by some investigators and may be of particular benefit in the diabetic patient.[146,147] Dialysis effectively removes lactate and occasionally has been employed in cases of drug induced lactic acidosis.[159] Additionally, vasodilator therapy has been advocated for idiopathic lactic acidosis[160] but probably is unsuitable for many patients with Laennec's cirrhosis due to their pre-existing hypotension and diminished peripheral vascular resistance.

4.3.3. Alcoholic Ketoacidosis. The most common form of metabolic acidosis associated with alcoholism is probably ketoacidosis. Although the condition is well described, its frequency is unclear. Some investigators feel that it is a rather rare condition,[161] whereas others have estimated that it accounts for approximately twenty percent of all cases of ketoacidosis, including those due to diabetes mellitus.[162] It is likely that the disorder occurs with greater frequency than is commonly reported because serum ketones usually are not measured immediately upon admission to the hospital and the condition is rapidly alleviated by hydration and the administration of glucose.

The clinical presentation of alcoholic ketoacidosis has several characteristic features.[162–169] Affected patients are usually chronic, heavy ethanol drinkers and recently have increased their ethanol use concurrently with a sharp reduction in their food intake. When severe nausea, vomiting, and abdominal pain develop, alcohol consumption is often stopped suddenly. The patient seeks medical attention, usually within 1–3 days, due to the persistent gastrointestinal complaints. The physical exam is often unremarkable but may reveal the odor of ketones on the patient's breath and evidence of alcoholic hepatitis and/or pancreatitis. The blood sugar can be low, normal, or slightly elevated. Ethanol is usually absent from the blood. The serum pH may be acidemic or alkalemic, often revealing the presence of a respiratory and/or metabolic alkalosis. The presence of ketoacidosis, however, is indicated by the elevated anion gap and excessive ketones in the blood. It may be helpful to determine blood levels of β-hydroxybutyrate as this compound is not detected by the standard nitroprusside test for ketone bodies. Mild to moderate lactic acidosis may be present also. Other electrolyte disorders, including hypomagnesemia, hyperphosphatemia, and hyperuricemia, are noted frequently.

The pathogenesis of alcoholic ketoacidosis is reasonably well understood.[170–173] Ethanol consumption decreases the NAD/NADH ratio, which inhibits gluconeogenesis. Hepatic glycogen stores are depleted as a result of the prolonged inadequate nutritional intake. In addition, hepatic ketogenesis and peripheral fatty acid mobilization are inhibited by ethanol. However, serum fatty acid levels may increase despite the presence of ethanol in the blood. With the decline of the blood ethanol levels the block to ketogenesis and lipolysis is removed and fatty acid mobilization increases and ketogenesis results. Plasma insulin levels are usually low, which impairs the metabolism of ketone bodies. In addition, the low NAD/NADH ratio favors the production of β hydroxybutyrate over acetoacetate. As long as the patient is unable to take normal nourishment the ketonemia will persist and acidosis may ensue.

The therapy of alcoholic ketoacidosis is usually very effective. Volume deficits must be corrected promptly, especially if hypotension is present. The infusion of glucose provides a nonketogenic calorie source, stimulates insulin secretion, and rapidly clears the ketosis. The use of insulin is rarely necessary and may potentially worsen preexisting hypokalemia or hypophosphatemia. In addition, bicarbonate therapy should be reserved for cases wtih life-threatening acidemia because a rebound metabolic alkalosis may ensue after the ketone bodies are metabolized or a sodium overload may occur.

4.3.4. Acidosis Due to Toxin Ingestion. Ethylene glycol, methanol, and isopropanol are intoxicants that alcoholics occasionally substitute for ethanol when the latter agent is unavailable. Each is metabolized by alcohol dehydrogenase. The common features of intoxication with these drugs are central nervous system depression and the presence of a metabolic acidosis, most often associated with a high anion gap. However, because the products of metabolism of these agents differ, the clinical syndromes produced by each have unique and characteristic features.

4.3.4a. Methanol. Methanol is probably the most common toxin consumed intentionally or accidentally by alcoholics. Epidemic methanol poisoning in chronic alcohol users has been described particularly well.[174–176] A characteristic feature of intoxication with methanol is a delay in the onset of adverse symptoms after ingestion, which may vary on an individual basis from a few hours up to 3 days.[176,177] The duration of this delay is influenced by the quantity of the toxin consumed, the concomitant ingestion of ethanol, and individual variability in the metabolism and excretion of the compound.[174,178,179] Following this latency period, the initial symptoms are somewhat variable but often include visual disturbances, headache, confusion, weakness, dyspnea, abdominal pain, and vomiting. Seizures, coma, hypotension, and respiratory arrest may follow. In surviving patients residual visual loss or complete blindness may occur. Permanent visual impairment appears not to correlate with the maximum serum methanol level attained or the degree of metabolic acidosis but, rather, with the duration of time between ingestion and treatment.[177]

Prominent among the laboratory findings in patients with methanol intoxication is a high anion gap metabolic acidosis. Although most patients are acidemic, a concomitant metabolic alkalosis due to vomiting may raise the serum pH to or above the normal range. The elevated anion gap persists, however, confirming the presence of a metabolic acidosis. An osmolal gap (i.e., a higher measured serum osmolality than that calculated from the serum electrolytes) is frequently observed and suggests the presence of a circulating toxin. Electrolyte disturbances often occur but are not directly related to methanol per se. Frequently, the hematocrit is elevated due to increased red blood cell size, and this correlates with the serum methanol levels and the clinical severity of the symptoms.[176] Acute renal failure has been reported in association with hypotension induced by methanol poisoning.[177]

The metabolism of methanol is well characterized.[178,179] The compound is highly water soluble and distributes throughout the total body water. A significant percent of ingested methanol can be eliminated by the lungs, but this process requires several days. Methanol is principally metabolized in the liver by the action of alcohol dehydrogenase to produce formaldehyde, which is rapidly converted to formic acid.[180] Methanol is a less avid substrate than ethanol for the enzyme and, thus, the metabolism of methanol is much slower.[181] This is responsible for the delay in the onset of clinical toxicity following methanol ingestion. Moreover, because it is the preferred enzyme substrate, ethanol will inhibit the metabolism of methanol by alcohol dehydrogenase. Formaldehyde is the principal toxic product of methanol degradation. The predisposition to retinal damage is explained by the presence of alcohol dehydrogenase in the retina and the marked inhibition of retinal metabolism by formaldehyde.[182,183] The metabolic acidosis of methanol intoxication does not arise as a result of formic acid production but, rather, is due to the inhibition of many oxidative enzyme systems and the resultant accumulation of various endogenous acids.[174]

The specific treatment principles of methanol toxicity include correction of the acidosis, inhibition of methanol degradation, and elimination of the compound from the body. Bicarbonate therapy should be used to correct the acidosis, with the goals of maintaining the serum bicarbonate concentration at or above 15 mEq/liter and the serum pH at approximately 7.30–7.35. Ethanol administration is essential to inhibit the rate of production of toxic methanol metabolites by alcohol dehydrogenase. Specific measures required to produce and maintain the serum ethanol level at 100 mg/dl in methanol-toxic patients have been provided by McCoy *et al.*[184] This ethanol concentration results in a maximal saturation of alcohol dehydrogenase catalytic sites with ethanol, thereby maximally inhibiting methanol metabolism. Hemodialysis should be employed when the ingestion exceeds the minimal lethal dose of 30 ml or when the blood methanol concentration is greater than 50 mg/dl.[176,177] Because rebound increases in the blood methanol concentration may occur after dialysis due to an internal redistribution of the compound, repeated episodes of dialysis may be necessary.[176] Peritoneal dialysis is much less efficient than hemodialysis in removing methanol and should be reserved only for situations in which hemodialysis cannot be employed.[185] Dialytic therapy may be stopped when the blood methanol concentration remains below 50 mg/dl but ethanol administration should continue until methanol is no longer detectable in the blood.

4.3.4b. Ethylene Glycol. Ethylene glycol poisoning is an infrequent cause of acidosis encountered in the alcoholic and usually follows the consumption of some form of antifreeze solution. Because of its easy availability and acceptable taste, ethylene glycol is occasionally used in suicide attempts. As the condition can be treated successfully, early recognition and prompt aggressive therapy are essential.

The clinical syndrome of acute ethylene glycol poisoning is distinctive.[186,188] In the initial 12 hr following ingestion, neurologic symptoms predominate. The patient appears to be intoxicated but there is no alcoholic fetor. The progression of neurologic abnormalities includes ophthalmoplegia, nystagmus, papilledema, depressed reflexes, generalized or focal seizures, and coma. In the next 12 hr the dominant findings are tachypnea, tachycardia, cyanosis, and, occasionally, cardiorespiratory failure. Acute renal failure appears 1–3 days after the ingestion and is accompanied by bilateral flank pain and severe oliguria or anuria.

The most remarkable laboratory finding encountered upon hospitalization of the patient is a profound metabolic acidosis with an anion gap above 20 and often over 30–40 mEq/liter. In addition, there is often a large osmolal gap. Serum lactate levels are moderately elevated but cannot account for the degree of acidosis present. Hypocalcemia is common and results from chelation of calcium by the oxalate formed form the metabolism of ethylene glycol.

Microscopic hematuria and excessive oxalate crystalluria are usually present. Confirmation of the diagnosis should be made by the analysis of blood for various toxins including both methanol and ethylene glycol.[187–189]

Ethylene glycol is metabolized via several enzymatic steps that include alcohol dehydrogenase and lactate dehydrogenase. These reactions produce NADH. The products of ethylene glycol degradation include glycoaldehyde, glycolate, glyoxylate, and oxalate. The depression of the NAD/NADH ratio by the metabolism of ethylene glycol increases lactate synthesis. Metabolic acidosis is, therefore, generated by the accumulation of the various products of ethylene glycol metabolism as well as the overproduction of endogenous acids such as lactic acid.[187–189]

The detrimental effects of ethylene glycol are due to the direct toxicity of its metabolites on the brain, heart, lungs, and kidneys. Deposition of calcium oxalate throughout various tissues, including the renal tubules, is a prominent histologic finding but is not required for the expression of tissue injury.[188]

Therapy of ethylene glycol poisoning must be aggressive. Bicarbonate is administered in quantities sufficient to correct the metabolic acidosis. Ethanol should be administered to maintain a serum ethanol level of approximately 100 mg/dl as long as ethylene glycol is detectable in the blood. This serves to completely inhibit the degradation of ethylene glycol by alcohol dehydrogenase. Peterson *et al.* have provided guidelines for this therapy.[190] Calcium infusion may be necessary if symptomatic hypocalcemia occurs. The administration of large doses of thiamine and pyridoxine has been recommended as these cofactors enhance the production of less toxic metabolites of ethylene glycol.[187] A high urinary flow rate should be sustained by the administration of fluid and diuretics to increase the urinary oxylate solubility and to enhance the urinary excretion of ethylene glycol.[186,187] Hemodialysis is a very effective method for removing ethylene glycol, with the rate of clearance of the toxin approaching that of urea when employing a hollow fiber dialyzer.[190,191] The use of a bicarbonate rather than acetate-based dialysis bath is recommended.[188] When conditions dictate, peritoneal dialysis rather than hemodialysis may be employed. With early diagnosis and prompt therapy most patients survive. However, a poor prognosis appears to accompany therapeutic delays or the ingestion of amounts greater than the estimated lethal dose of 100 ml.[189]

4.3.4c. Isopropanol Ingestion. Poisoning with isopropyl alcohol (rubbing alcohol) has been well described also.[192,193] The majority of these cases were chronic ethanol users who were unable to obtain ethanol. However, probably because of its disagreeable taste and its prompt and well-known adverse effects, isopropanol poisoning is very uncommon even in alcoholics.[193]

Isopropanol is absorbed rapidly from the gastrointestinal tract and distributed throughout total body water.[194] It is roughly twice as toxic as ethanol and undergoes a much slower metabolism.[195] Symptoms of toxicity appear soon after ingestion and their severity may be related to the quantity consumed, with 8 oz considered to be the lethal dose for an adult.[196] Mild toxicity may be manifested by an inebriation similar to that produced by ethanol. Profound coma, hypotension, hypothermia, cyanosis, and respiratory arrest often ensue rapidly.[193] Although no systematic evaluation of acid–base status in isopropyl alcohol poisoning has been reported, examination of various case reports reveals that the serum total carbon dioxide content is often depressed[193] and a normal anion gap metabolic acidosis may be present.[195] Acetone, the principal product of the metabolic degradation of isopropanol by alcohol dehydrogenase,[197] is present in high concentration in the blood and urine.[192,193,195] Lactic acid accumulation can also contribute to the acidosis. Acute renal failure has been reported following hypotension and rhabdomyolysis that occurs in some cases.[193,198]

No specific guidelines exist for the treatment of isopropanol ingestion. The toxicity principally relates not to the accumulation of acetone or other metabolic intermediates but to the effects of isopropanol itself. Thus, gastric lavage, may be useful to prevent the continued absorption of the alcohol from the stomach. Continuous gastric suction also aids by removing any isopropanol that, following its absorption, is secreted back into the stomach.[193] Hemodialysis is effective in the removal of isopropanol and should be employed if the blood levels are above 100 mg/dl.[199] Peritoneal dialysis appears to be a reasonable alternative if hemodialysis cannot be performed.[195]

5. Acute Renal Failure: Rhabdomyolysis

5.1. Frequency

Acute renal failure may complicate many medical and surgical conditions. Alcoholics may develop acute renal failure from any of the causes that arise in nonalcoholics, for example, drug-induced acute tubular necrosis. Rhabdomyolysis is implicated as a cause of approximately 5% of all cases of renal failure. Renal damage occurs in rhabdomyolysis because of the direct tubular toxicity of the myoglobin pigment as well as intratubular pigment deposition.[200] Of all cases of rhabdomyolysis approximately one third result in acute renal failure. Alcohol abuse is a contributing factor in up to 70% of episodes of rhabdomyolysis of all causes,[201] and in approximately 35% of cases of acute renal failure occurring with nontraumatic rhabdomyolysis.[202] Thus, the alcoholic patient displays a disproportionately high predisposition to develop acute renal failure from rhabdomyolysis.

5.2. The Clinical Syndrome

The clinical syndrome of atraumatic myoglobinuric acute renal failure has been well described.[114,201,203] Many patients have no muscular complaints,[115] while others may present with evidence of alcoholic myopathy including mild to moderate muscle weakness, pain or swelling.[204,205] Most often, rhabdomyolysis and acute renal failure follow a prolonged bout of heavy drinking.[114,115,200] However, the syndrome may occur in chronic alcoholics in the absence of recent ethanol use.[206] In some patients rhabdomyolysis may be related not to alcoholic myopathy but, rather, to the presence of acute severe hypokalemia[75,112] or hypophosphatemia.[207] Evidence of renal dysfunction is present upon hospital admission in most patients, with the serum creatinine concentration disproportionately higher than the blood urea nitrogen. Oliguria is present in the great majority of patients. Grossman *et al.* reported a characteristic triad of laboratory findings in rhadomyolysis and acute renal failure which included: (1) a strongly positive urine reaction to orthotolidin, (2) the presence of numerous pigmented granular casts on the urinalysis, and, (3) elevated serum creatine kinase levels.[200] However, a negative urine reaction to orthotolidin may be noted in a significant percentage of patients with myoglobinuric acute renal failure because the pigment is cleared rapidly from the blood.[201,202] The common electrolyte disturbances that follow rhabdomyolysis and acute renal failure include hyperphosphatemia, hyperuricemia, and, later, hypercalcemia, as these substances are released from the damaged muscle. A high anion gap metabolic acidosis and hypocalcemia are often present initially and are often of greater severity than that which is noted in acute renal failure due to other causes.[201]

The period of oliguria typically lasts 1–3 weeks.[200,202] Early in the course of renal failure, the serum creatinine and potassium levels rise rapidly. After the initial 3–5 days, however, the syndrome reverts to a pattern not different from that of other forms of acute renal failure. The return of renal function is heralded by the initiation of a diuresis, during which the serum creatinine begins to decline spontaneously. Concomitant with this diuretic phase of recovery, in approximately 20% of cases, the serum calcium concentration rises above the normal range. Hypercalcemia, occasionally severe enough to require therapy, may persist for 1–2 weeks before resolving spontaneously.[200,202,208] The prognosis for complete recovery of renal function is good.[200]

5.3. Abnormalities in Calcium Metabolism in Myoglobinuric Renal Failure

The alterations in calcium metabolism in acute renal failure due to rhabdomyolysis have received considerable attention. The hypocalcemia encountered during the oliguric phase of the syndrome has several causes.[209] Hyperphosphatemia and skeletal resistance to the calcemic action of parathyroid hormone have been well documented in acute renal failure.[210] Despite the concomitant presence of hyperparathyroidism, which normally stimulates renal 25-hydroxyvitamin D_3-1 hydroxylase activity, serum levels of 1,25-dihydroxyvitamin D_3 are low in patients with myoglobinuric acute renal failure.[211] This may be a consequence of the inhibition of renal 25-hydroxyvitamin

D_3-1 hydroxylase by hyperphosphatemia and/or the loss of the enzyme due to acute tubular necrosis. Gut calcium absorption is depressed when 1,25 dihydroxyvitamin D_3 levels are low.[212] In addition, significant amounts of calcium are deposited in damaged muscle tissue.[209]

The occurrence of hypercalcemia during recovery appears to result from a reversal of the processes noted above. As the uremia clears renal production of 1-25-dihydroxyvitamin D_3 increases, often producing abnormally high serum levels of the sterol due to the stimulation from persistently elevated serum parathyroid hormone levels.[211] The calcemic effect of parathyroid hormone on bone is restored and the calcium deposited in soft tissues is mobilized.[209] In the face of the persistent hypercalcemia the excessive parathyroid gland activity is eventually suppressed and normal calcium homeostasis is reestablished.[209]

5.4. Therapy

The therapeutic approach to myoglobinuric acute renal failure is not appreciably different from that of acute renal failure due to other causes. Some specific points are worthy of mention, however. Dehydration is a common finding in patients presenting with myoglobinuric renal failure and may enhance the nephrotoxicity of the myoglobin pigment.[202] Restoration of normal volume status will alleviate any additive renal insult from hypovolemia. The use of diuretics or mannitol has been recommended to increase the urine flow, thereby flushing out renal tubules occluded with pigment casts and converting the patient to a nonoliguric state.[213] Also, Knochel has cautioned against the overzealous use of calcium infusions in attempts to correct the hypocalcemia during the early course of rhabdomyolytic acute renal failure.[209] The serum calcium is raised only temporarily by this measure and, conceivably, the administered calcium may be sequestered in the damaged muscle and thereby exacerbate the muscle injury and the subsequent rebound hypercalcemia.

References

1. Eisenmenger WJ, Blondheim SH, Bongiovanni AM, et al: Electrolyte studies on patients with cirrhosis of the liver. *J Clin Invest* 29:1491–1499, 1950.
2. Arroyo V, Rodes J, Gutierrez-Lizarraga MA, et al: Prognostic value of spontaneous hyponatremia in cirrhosis with ascites. *Am J Dig Dis* 21:240–256, 1976.
3. Papper S, Saxon L: The diuretic response to administered water in patients with liver disease. II. Laennec's cirrhosis of the liver. *Arch Int Med* 103:750–757, 1959.
4. Shear L, Hall PW, Gabuzda GJ: Renal failure in patients with cirrhosis of the liver. II. Factors influencing maximal urinary flow rate. *Am J Med* 39:199–209, 1965.
5. Chiandussi L, Bartoli E, Arras S: Reabsorption of sodium in the proximal renal tubule in cirrhosis of the liver. *Gut* 19:497–503, 1978.
6. Wilkinson SP, Jowett TP, Slater DH, et al: Renal sodium retention in cirrhosis: Relation to aldosterone and nephron site. *Clin Sci* 56:169–177, 1979.

7. Vaamonde CA, Vaamonde LS, Presser JI, et al: The role of vasopressin and urea in the renal concentrating defect of patients with cirrhosis of the liver. *Clin Sci* 41:441–452, 1971.
8. Arroyo V, Rodes J: Treatment of ascites. A rational approach to the treatment of ascites. *Postgrad Med J* 51:558–562, 1975.
9. Klingler EL Jr, Vaamonde CA, Vaamonde LS, et al: Renal function changes in cirrhosis of the liver. *Arch Int Med* 125:1010–1015, 1970.
10. Perez-Ayuso RM, Arroyo V, Camps J, et al: Evidence that renal prostaglandins are involved in renal water metabolism in cirrhosis. *Kidney Int* 26:72–80, 1984.
11. Padfield PL, Morton JJ: Application of a sensitive radioimmunoassay for plasma arginine vasopressin to pathological conditions in man. *Clin Sci* 47: 16p–17p, 1974.
12. Wagner H, Maier V, Franz HE: Improved method and its clinical application of a radioimmunoassay of arginine vasopressin in human serum. *Horm Metabl Res* 9:223–227, 1977.
13. Bichet D, Szatalowicz V, Chaimovitz C, et al: Role of vasopressin in abnormal water excretion in cirrhotic patients. *Ann Int Med* 96:413–417, 1982.
14. Anderson RJ, Cronin RE, McDonald KM, et al: Mechanisms of portal hypertension-induced alterations in renal hemodynamics, renal water excretion, and renin secretion. *J Clin Invest* 58:964–970, 1976.
15. Better OS, Aisenbrey GA, Berl T, et al: Role of antidiuretic hormone in impaired urinary dilution associated with chronic bile-duct ligation. *Clin Sci* 58:493–500, 1980.
16. Linas SL, Anderson RJ, Guggenheim SJ, et al: Role of vasopressin in impaired water excretion in conscious rats with experimental cirrhosis. *Kidney Int* 20:173–180, 1981.
17. Bichet DG, Groves BM, Schrier RW: Mechanisms of improvement of water and sodium excretion by immersion in decompensated cirrhotic patients. *Kidney Int* 24:788–794, 1983.
18. Skowsky R, Riestra J, Martinez I, et al: Arginine vasopressin (AVP) kinetics in hepatic cirrhosis. *Clin Res* 24:101A, 1976.
19. Kelleher SP, Berl T, Schrier RW: Antidiuretic hormone, in Dunn M (ed): *Renal Endocrinology*. Baltimore/London, Williams and Wilkins, 1983, pp 224–268.
20. Shade RE, Share L: Metabolic clearance of immunoreactive vasopressin and immunoreactive (131 I) iodo vasopressin in the hypophysectomized dog. *Endocrinology* 99:1199–1206, 1976.
21. Ardaillou R, Benmansour M, Rondeau E, et al: Metabolism and secretion of antidiuretic hormone in patients with renal failure, cardiac insufficiency, and liver insufficiency, in Bach JF, Crosnier J, Funck-Brentano JL, et al: (eds): *Advances in Nephrology*, vol 13. Chicago, Yearbook Medical Publishers, 1984, pp 35–49.
22. Papper S, Belsky JL, Bleifer KH: Renal failure in Laennec's cirrhosis of the liver. I. Description of clinical and laboratory features. *Ann Int Med* 51:759–773, 1959.
23. Baldus WP, Feichter RN, Summerskill WH, et al: The kidney in cirrhosis II. Disorders of renal function. *Ann Int Med* 60:366–377, 1964.
24. Bosch J, Arroyo V, Betriu A, et al: Hepatic hemodynamics and the renin–angiotensin–aldosterone system in cirrhosis. *Gastroenterology* 78:92–99, 1980.
25. Lauson HD: Metabolism of antidiuretic hormones. *Am J Med* 42:713–744, 1967.
26. Rabkin R, Ghazeleh S, Share L, et al: Removal of immunoreactive arginine vasopressin by the perfused rat liver. *Endocrinology* 106:930–934, 1980.
27. Aziz O, Schmidt W: Elimination of vasopressin by the normal and the damaged liver. *Pflugers Arch* 367:165–168, 1976.
28. Bernstein SH, Weston RE, Ross G, et al: Studies on intravenous water diuresis and nicotine and pitressin antidiuresis in normal subjects and patients with liver disease. *J Clin Invest* 32:422–427, 1953.
29. Bichet DG, Schrier RW: Role of vasopressin in cardiac, pulmonary, hepatic, and adrenal disorders, in Bach JF, Crosnier J, Funck-Brentano JL, et al: *Advances in Nephrology*, vol 13. Chicago, Year Book Medical Publishers, 1984, pp 51–74.
30. Eggleton MG: The diuretic action of alcohol in man. *J Physiol* 101:172–191, 1942.
31. DeTroyer A, Pilloy W, Broeckaert I, et al: Demeclocycline treatment of water retention in cirrhosis. *Ann Int Med* 85:336–337, 1976.

32. Perez-Ayuso RM, Arroyo V, Camps J, et al: Effect of demeclocycline on renal function and urinary prostaglandin E_2 and kallikrein in hyponatremic cirrhotics. *Nephron* 36:30–37, 1984.
33. Anderson RJ, Berl T, McDonald KM, et al: Evidence for an in vivo antagonism between vasopressin and prostaglandin in the mammalian kidney. *J Clin Invest* 56:420–426, 1975.
34. Grantham JJ, Orloff J: Effect of prostaglandin E_1 on the permeability response of the isolated collecting tubule to vasopressin, adenosine 3′,5′-monophosphate, and theophylline. *J Clin Invest* 47:1154–1161, 1968.
35. Kramer HJ, Glanzer K, Dusing R: Role of prostaglandins in the regulation of renal water. *Kidney Int* 19:851–859, 1981.
36. Walker LA, Whorton AR, Smigel M, et al: Antidiuretic hormone increases renal prostaglandin synthesis in vivo. *Am J Physiol* 235:F180–F185, 1978.
37. Schedl HP, Bartter FC: An explanation for and experimental correction of the abnormal water diuresis in cirrhosis. *J Clin Invest* 39:248–261, 1960.
38. Vlahcevic ZR, Adham NF, Jick H, et al: Renal effects of acute expansion of plasma volume in cirrhosis. *N Engl J Med* 272:387–391, 1965.
39. Epstein M, Pins DS, Schneider N, et al: Determinants of deranged sodium and water homeostasis in decompensated cirrhosis. *J Lab Clin Med* 87:822–839, 1976.
40. Naccarato R, Messa P, D'Angelo A, et al: Renal handling of sodium and water in early chronic liver disease. *Gastroenterology* 81:205–210, 1981.
41. Epstein M, Weitzman RE, Preston S, et al: Relationship between plasma arginine vasopressin and renal water handling in decompensated cirrhosis. *Mineral Electrolyte Metab* 10:155–165, 1984.
42. Reznick RK, Langer B, Taylor BR, et al: Hyponatremia and arginine vasopressin secretion in patients with refractory hepatic ascites undergoing peritoneovenous shunting. *Gastroenterology* 84:713–718, 1983.
43. Berliner RW, Davidson DG: Production of hypertonic urine in the absence of pituitary antidiuretic hormone. *J Clin Invest* 36:1416–1427, 1957.
44. Schrier RW, Lehman D, Zacherle B, et al: Effect of furosemide on free water excretion in edematous patients with hyponatremia. *Kidney Int* 3:30–34, 1973.
45. Szatalowicz VL, Miller PD, Lacher JW, et al: Comparative effect of diuretics on renal water excretion in hyponatraemic oedematous disorders. *Clin Sci* 62:235–238, 1982.
46. Ring-Larsen H, Clausen E, Ranek L: Peritoneal dialysis in hyponatremia due to liver failure. *Scand J Gastroenterol* 8:33–40, 1973.
47. Rubini ME, Kleeman CR, Lamdin E: Studies on alcoholic diuresis. I. The effect of ethyl alcohol ingestion on water, electrolyte and acid-base metabolism. *J Clin Invest* 34:439–447, 1955.
48. Kalbfleisch JM, Lindeman RD, Ginn HE, et al: Effects of ethanol administration on urinary excretion of magnesium and other electrolytes in alcoholic and normal subjects. *J Clin Invest* 42:1471–1475, 1963.
49. Helderman JH, Vestal RE, Rowe JW, et al: The response of arginine vasopressin to intravenous ethanol and hypertonic saline in man: the impact of aging. *J Gerontol* 33:39–47, 1978.
50. Beard JD, Barlow G, Overman RR: Body fluids and blood electrolytes in dogs subjected to chronic ethanol administration. *J Pharm Exp Ther* 148:348–355, 1965.
51. Beard JD, Knott DH: Fluid and electrolyte balance during acute withdrawal in chronic alcoholic patients. *J Am Med Assoc* 204:133–139, 1968.
52. Klatsky AL, Friedman GD, Siegelaub AB, et al: Alcohol consumption and blood pressure. Kaiser-Permanente multiphasic health examination data. *N Engl J Med* 296:1194–1200, 1977.
53. Chan TCK, Sutter MC: Ethanol consumption and blood pressure. *Life Sci* 33:1965–1973, 1983.
54. Kaysen G, Noth RH: The effects of alcohol on blood pressure and electrolytes. *Med Clin N Am* 68:221–246, 1984.
55. Demanet JC, Bonnyns M, Bleiberg H, et al: Coma due to water intoxication in beer drinkers. *Lancet* 2:1115–1117, 1971.
56. Hilden T, Svendsen TL: Electrolyte disturbances in beer drinkers. A specific "hypo-osmolality syndrome." *Lancet* 2:245–246, 1975.

57. Casey TH, Summerskill WHJ, Orvis AL: Body and serum potassium in liver disease. 1. Relationship to hepatic function and associated factors. *Gastroenterology* 48:198–207, 1965.
58. Delwaide PA: Body potassium measurements by whole-body counting: screening of patient populations. *J Nucl Med* 14:40–48, 1973.
59. Soler NG, Jain S, James H, et al: Potassium status of patients with cirrhosis. *Gut* 17:152–157, 1976.
60. Knochel JP: Hypophosphatemia. *Clin Nephrol* 7:131–137, 1977.
61. Aikawa JK, Felts JH Jr, Harrell GT Jr: Alterations in the body potassium content in cirrhosis of the liver. *Gastroenterology* 24:437–443, 1953.
62. Schober O, Maris P, Schmidt FW, et al: Total body water, extracellular water, plasma volume, and total body potassium in cirrhosis of the liver. *Klin Wschr* 57:757–761, 1979.
63. DeDeuxchaisnes N, Collet RA, Busset R, et al: Exchangeable potassium in wasting, amyotrophy, heart-disease, and cirrhosis of the liver. *Lancet* 1:681–687, 1961.
64. Vetter WR, Cohn LH, Reichgott M: Hypokalemia and electrocardiographic abnormalities during acute alcohol withdrawal. *Arch Int Med* 120:536–541, 1967.
65. Wadstein J, Skude G: Does hypokalaemia precede delirium tremens? *Lancet* 2:549–550, 1978.
66. Mas A, Bosch J, Piera C, et al: Intracellular and exchangeable potassium in cirrhosis. Evidence against the occurrence of potassium depletion in cirrhosis with ascites. *Dig Dis Sci* 26:723–727, 1981.
67. Kessler E, Levy MR, Allen RL: Red cell electrolytes in patients with edema. *J Lab Clin Med* 57:32–41, 1961.
68. Astrup J, Prytz H, Thomsen AC, et al: Red cell sodium and potassium contents in liver cirrhosis. *Gastroenterology* 78:530–534, 1980.
69. Strub IH, Talso PJ, Kirsner JB: Intracellular and extracellular fluid and electrolyte alterations in cirrhosis of the liver with edema and ascites. *Gastroenterology* 28:163–175, 1955.
70. Knochel JP, Bilbrey GL, Fuller TJ, et al: The muscle cell in chronic alcoholism: the possible role of phosphate depletion in alcoholic myopathy. *Ann NY Acad Sci* 252:274–286, 1975.
71. Alam AN, Wheeler P, Wilkinson SP, et al: Changes in the electrolyte content of leucocytes at different clinical stages of cirrhosis. *Gut* 19:650–654, 1978.
72. Maschia G, D'Angelo A, Sirigu F, et al: Muscle biopsy studies in liver cirrhosis. *Scand J Gastroenterol* 6:363–368, 1971.
73. Kalant H, Mons W, Mahon MA: Acute effects of ethanol on tissue electrolytes in the rat. *Can J Physiol Pharmacol* 44:1–12, 1966.
74. Anderson R, Cohen M, Haller R, et al: Skeletal muscle phosphorus and magnesium deficiency in alcoholic myopathy. *Mineral Electrolyte Metab* 4:106–112, 1980.
75. Knochel JP, Schlein EM: On the mechanism of rhabdomyolysis in potassium depletion. *J Clin Invest* 51:1750–1758, 1972.
76. Cronin RE, Knochel JP: The consequences of potassium deficiency, in Brenner BM, Stein JH (eds): *Contemporary Issues in Nephrology*, vol 2. New York, Churchill Livingstone, 1978, pp 205–231.
77. Rosoff L Jr, Zia P, Reynolds T, et al: Studies of renin and aldosterone in cirrhotic patients with ascites. *Gastroenterology* 69:698–705, 1975.
78. Epstein M, Levinson R, Sancho J, et al: Characterization of the renin-aldosterone system in decompensated cirrhosis. *Circ Res* 41:818–829, 1977.
79. Linkola J, Fyhrquist F, Ylikahri R: Renin, aldosterone and cortisol during ethanol intoxication and hangover. *Acta Physiol Scand* 106:75–82, 1979.
80. Vesin P: Potassium metabolism and diuretic administration in liver cirrhosis. *Postgrad Med J* 51:545–548, 1975.
81. Epstein M: Aldosterone in liver disease, in Epstein M (ed): *The Kidney in Liver Disease*, ed 2. New York, Elsevier, 1983, pp 370–394.
82. McCollister R, Prasad AS, Doe RP, et al: Normal renal magnesium clearance and the effect of water loading, chlorothiazide and ethanol on magnesium excretion. *J Lab Clin Med* 52:928, 1958.

83. Whang R, Morosi HJ, Rodgers D, Reyes R: The influence of sustained magnesium deficiency on muscle potassium repletion. *J Lab Clin Med* 70:895–902, 1967.
84. Shear L, Bonkowsky HL, Gabuzda GJ: Renal tubular acidosis in cirrhosis. A determinant of susceptibility to recurrent hepatic precoma. *N Engl J Med* 280:1–7, 1969.
85. Lieber CS: General nutritional status in the alcoholic, including disorders of minerals and vitamins, in Smith LH, Jr (ed): *Major Problems in Internal Medicine*, vol 22: *Medical Disorders of Alcoholism, Pathogenesis and Treatment*. Philadelphia, WB Saunders, 1982, pp 551–568.
86. Thomson AD: Alcohol and nutrition. *Clin Endocrinol Metab* 7:405–428, 1978.
87. Schultze RG, Nissenson AR: Potassium: Physiology and pathophysiology, in Maxwell MH, Kleeman CR (eds): *Clinical Disorders of Fluid and Electrolyte Metabolism*, ed 3. New York, McGraw-Hill, 1980, pp 113–143.
88. Robin ED, Whaley RD, Crump CH, et al: The nature of the respiratory acidosis of sleep and of the respiratory alkalosis of hepatic coma. *J Clin Invest* 36:924, 1957.
89. Heinemann HD, Emirgil C, Mijnssen JP: Hyperventilation and arterial hypoxemia in cirrhosis of the liver. *Am J Med* 28:239–246, 1960.
90. Abelmann WH, Kramer GE, Verstraeten JM, et al: Cirrhosis of the liver and decreased arterial oxygen saturation. *Arch Int Med* 108:102–108, 1961.
91. Karetzky MS, Mithoefer JC: The cause of hyperventilation and arterial hypoxia in patients with cirrhosis of the liver. *Am J Med Sci* 244:797–804, 1967.
92. Sereny G, Rapoport A, Husdan H: The effect of alcohol withdrawal on electrolyte and acid–base balance. *Metabolism* 15:896–904, 1966.
93. Bellville JW, Swanson GD, Miyake T, et al: Respiratory stimulation observed following ethanol ingestion. *West J Med* 124:423–425, 1976.
94. Casey TH, Summerskill WHJ, Bickford RG, et al: Body and serum potassium in liver disease. II. Relationships to arterial ammonia, blood pH, and hepatic coma. *Gastroenterology* 48:208–215, 1965.
95. Mendelson JH: Biologic concomitants of alcoholism. *N Engl J Med* 283:71–81, 1970.
96. Ring-Larsen H, Hesse B, Henriksen JH, et al: Sympathetic nervous activity and renal and systemic hemodynamics in cirrhosis: Plasma norepinephrine concentration, hepatic extraction and renal release. *Hepatology* 2:304–310, 1982.
97. Keller U, Gerber PPG, Buhler FR, et al: Role of the splanchnic bed in extracting circulating adrenaline and noradrenaline in normal subjects and in patients with cirrhosis of the liver. *Clin Sci* 67:45–49, 1984.
98. Clausen T, Flatman JA: The effect of catecholamines on Na-K and membrane potential in rat soleus muscle. *J Physiol* 270:383–414, 1977.
99. Vick RL, Todd EP, Luedke DW: Epinephrine-induced hypokalemia: Relation to liver and skeletal muscle. *J Pharmacol Exp Ther* 181:139–146, 1972.
100. Conn HO: Cirrhosis and diabetes. IV. Effect of potassium chloride administration on glucose and insulin metabolism. *Am J Med Sci* 259:394–404, 1970.
101. Podolsky S, Zimmerman HJ, Burrows BA, et al: Potassium depletion in hepatic cirrhosis. A reversible cause of impaired growth-hormone and insulin response to stimulation. *N Engl J Med* 288:644–648, 1973.
102. Kunin AS, Surawicz B, Sims EAH: Decrease in potassium concentrations and appearance of cardiac arrhythmias during infusion of potassium with glucose in potassium-depleted patients. *N Engl J Med* 266:228–233, 1962.
103. Clausen T, Hansen O: Active Na-K transport and the rate of ouabain binding. The effect of insulin and other stimuli on skeletal muscle and adipocytes. *J Physiol* 270:415–430, 1977.
104. Harter HR, Santiago JV, Rutherford WE, et al: The relative roles of calcium, phosphorus, and parathyroid hormone in glucose- and tolbutamide-mediated insulin release. *J Clin Invest* 58:359–367, 1976.
105. Tannen RL: Relationship of renal ammonia production and potassium homeostasis. *Kidney Int* 11:453–465, 1977.
106. Better OS, Goldschmid Z, Chaimowitz C, et al: Defect in urinary acidification in cirrhosis.

The role of excessive tubular reabsorption of sodium in its etiology. *Arch Int Med* 130:77–83, 1972.
107. Hulter HN, Sebastian A, Sigala JF, et al: Pathogenesis of renal hyperchloremic acidosis resulting from dietary potassium restriction in the dog: Role of aldosterone. *Am J Physiol* 238:F79–F91, 1980.
108. Baertl JM, Sancetta SM, Gabuzda GJ: Relation of acute potassium depletion to renal ammonium metabolism in patients with cirrhosis. *J Clin Invest* 42:696–706, 1963.
109. Gabuzda GJ, Hall PW III: Relation of potassium depletion to renal ammonium metabolism and hepatic coma. *Medicine* 45:481–490, 1966.
110. Naranjo CA, Pontigo E, Valenegro C, et al: Furosemide-induced adverse reactions in cirrhosis of the liver. *Clin Pharmacol Ther* 25:154–160, 1979.
111. Martin JB, Craig JW, Eckel RE, et al: Hypokalemic myopathy in chronic alcoholism. *Neurology* 21:1160–1168, 1971.
112. Rubenstein AE, Wainapel SF: Acute hypokalemic myopathy in alcoholism. A clinical entity. *Arch Neurol* 34:553–555, 1977.
113. Haller RG, Knochel JP: Skeletal muscle disease in alcoholism. *Med Clin N Am* 68:91–103, 1984.
114. Hed R, Lundmark C, Fahlgren H, et al: Acute muscular syndrome in chronic alcoholism. *Acta Med Scand* 171: 585–599, 1962.
115. Perkoff GT, Dioso MM, Bleisch V, et al: A spectrum of myopathy associated with alcoholism. I. Clinical and laboratory features. *Ann Int Med* 67:481–492, 1967.
116. Ryback RS, Eckardt MJ, Pautler CP: Clinical relationships between serum phosphorus and other blood chemistry values in alcoholics. *Arch Int Med* 140:673–677, 1980.
117. Gabow PA, Moore S, Schrier RW: Sprionolactone-induced hyperchloremic acidosis in cirrhosis. *Ann Int Med* 90:338–340, 1979.
118. Wolfe SM, Victor M: The relationship of hypomagnesemia and alkalosis to alcohol withdrawal symptoms. *Ann NY Acad Sci* 162:973–984, 1969.
119. Victor M: The role of hypomagnesemia and respiratory alkalosis in the genesis of alcohol-withdrawal symptoms. *Ann NY Acad Sci* 215:235–248, 1973.
120. Mulhausen R, Eichenholz A, Blumentals A: Acid–base disturbances in patients with cirrhosis of the liver. *Medicine* 46:185–189, 1967.
121. Pande JN, Guleria JS: Acid–base and electrolyte disturbances in hepatic coma. *J Assoc Phys India* 17:17–23, 1969.
122. Record CO, Iles RA, Cohen RD, et al: Acid–base and metabolic disturbances in fulminant hepatic failure. *Gut* 16:144–149, 1975.
123. Prytz H, Thomsen AC: Acid–base status in liver cirrhosis. Disturbances in stable, terminal and porta-caval shunted patients. *Scand J Gastroenterol* 11:249–256, 1976.
124. Newman JH, Neff TA, Ziporin P: Acute respiratory failure associated with hypophosphatemia. *N Engl J Med* 296:1101–1103, 1977.
125. Johnstone RE, Reier CE: Acute respiratory effects of ethanol in man. *Clin Pharmacol Ther* 14:501–508, 1973.
126. Sahn SA, Lakshminarayan S, Pierson DJ, et al: Effect of ethanol on the ventilatory responses to oxygen and carbon dioxide in man. *Clin Sci* 49:33–38, 1975.
127. Williams MH Jr: Hypoxemia due to venous admixture in cirrhosis of the liver. *J Appl Physiol* 15:253–254, 1960.
128. Reinicke V, Friis T, Mullertz S: Respiratory alkalosis and decreased oxygen saturation of arterial blood in patients with acute and chronic hepatitis. *Scand J Clin Lab Invest* 15:29–36, 1963.
129. Kardel T, Rasmussen SN: Blood gases and acid–base disturbances of arterial blood in chronic liver disease. *Scand J Clin Lab Invest* 31:307–309, 1973.
130. Snell RE, Luchsinger PC: The relation of arterial hypoxemia to the hyperventilation of chronic liver disease. *Am J Med Sci* 245:289–292, 1963.
131. Roberts KE, Thompson EG III, Poppell JW, et al: Respiratory alkalosis accompanying ammonium toxicity. *J Appl Physiol* 9:367–370, 1956.

132. Wichser J, Kazemi H: Ammonia and ventilation: Site and mechanism of action. *Resp Physiol* 20:363–406, 1974.
133. Bosch JP, Goldstein MH, Levitt MF, et al: Effect of chronic furosemide administration on hydrogen and sodium excretion in the dog. *Am J Physiol* 232:F397–F404, 1977.
134. Lief PD, Mutz BF, Bank N: Diuretics stimulate H^+ secretion in turtle urinary bladder. *J Clin Invest* 65:1095–1103, 1980.
135. Narins RG, Goldberg M: Renal tubular acidosis: Pathophysiology, diagnosis and treatment. *DM*23:1–66, 1977.
136. Smith PM, Middleton JE, Williams R: Renal tubular acidosis and cirrhosis. *Postgrad Med J* 43:439–442, 1967.
137. Oster JR, Hotchkiss JL, Carbon M, et al: Abnormal renal acidification in alcoholic liver disease. *J Lab Clin Med* 85:987–1000, 1975.
138. Caregaro L, Lauro S, Ricci G, et al: Distal renal tubular acidosis in hepatic cirrhosis: Clinical and pathogenetic study. *Clin Nephrol* 15:143–147, 1981.
139. Klahr S, Tripathy K, Lotero H: Renal regulation of acid–base balance in malnourished man. *Am J Med* 48:325–331, 1970.
140. Kohaut EG, Klish WJ, Beachler CW, et al: Reduced renal acid excretion in malnutrition: a result of phosphate depletion. *Am J Clin Nutr* 30:861–867, 1977.
141. Gold LW, Massry SG, Arieff AI, et al: Renal bicarbonate wasting during phosphate depletion. *J Clin Invest* 52:2556–2562, 1973.
142. Emmett M, Goldfarb S, Agus ZS, et al: The pathophysiology of acid–base changes in chronically phosphate-depleted rats. *J Clin Invest* 59:294–298, 1977.
143. Hulter HN: Hypophosphatemia impairs the renal defense against metabolic acidosis. *Kidney Int* 26:302–307, 1984.
144. Huckabee WE: Abnormal resting blood lactate. I. The significance of hyperlactatemia in hospitalized patients. *Am J Med* 30:833–839, 1961.
145. Park R, Arieff AI: Lactic acidosis. *Adv Int Med* 25:33–68, 1980.
146. Heinig RE, Clarke EF, Waterhouse C: Lactic acidosis and liver disease. *Arch Intern Med* 139:1229–1232, 1979.
147. Alberti KGMM, Nattrass M: Lactic acidosis. *Lancet* 2:25–29, 1977.
148. Lieber CS, Jones DP, Losowsky MS, Davidson CS: Interrelation of uric acid and ethanol metabolism in man. *J Clin Invest* 41:1863–1870, 1962.
149. Lieber CS: Hepatic and metabolic effects of alcohol. *Gastroenterology* 50:119–133, 1966.
150. Krebs HA: The effects of ethanol on the metabolic activities of the liver, in Weber G (ed): *Advances in Enzyme Regulation*, vol 6. Oxford, Pergamon Press, 1968, pp 467–480.
151. Jorfeldt L, Juhlin-Donnfelt A: The influence of ethanol on splanchnic and skeletal muscle metabolism in man. *Metabolism* 27:97–106, 1978.
152. Kreisberg RA, Owen WC, Siegal AM: Ethanol-induced hyperlacticacidemia: inhibition of lactate utilization. *J Clin Invest* 50:166–174, 1971.
153. Berry MN: The liver and lactic acidosis. *Proc R Soc Med* 60:1260–1262, 1967.
154. Oliva PB: Lactic acidosis. *Am J Med* 48:209–225, 1970.
155. Lichtman MA, Miller DR, Cohen J, et al: Reduced red cell glycolysis, 2,3-diphosphoglycerate and adenosine triphosphate concentration, and increased hemoglobin-oxygen affinity caused by hypophosphatemia. *Ann Int Med* 74:562–568, 1971.
156. Berry MN, Scheuer J: Splanchnic lactic acid metabolism in hyperventilation, metabolic alkalosis and shock. *Metabolism* 16:537–547, 1967.
157. Doughaday WH, Lipicky RJ, Rasinski DC: Lactic acidosis as a cause of nonketotic acidosis in diabetic patients. *N Engl J Med* 267:1010–1014, 1962.
158. Fraley DS, Adler S, Bruns FJ, et al: Stimulation of lactate production by administration of bicarbonate in a patient with a solid neoplasm and lactic acidosis. *N Engl J Med* 303:1100–1102, 1980.
159. Misbin RI: Phenformin-associated lactic acidosis: Pathogenesis and treatment. *Ann Int Med* 87:591–595, 1977.
160. Taradash MR, Jacobson LB: Vasodilator therapy of idiopathic lactic acidosis. *N Engl J Med* 293:468–471, 1975.

161. Williams HE: Alcoholic hypoglycemia and ketoacidosis. *Med Clin N Am* 68:33–36, 1984.
162. Cooperman MT, Davidoff F, Spark R, et al: Clinical studies of alcoholic ketoacidosis. *Diabetes* 23:433–439, 1974.
163. Dillon ES, Dyer WW, Smelo LS: Ketone acidosis in nondiabetic adults. *Med Clin N Am* 24:1813–1822, 1940.
164. Jenkins DW, Eckel RE, Craig JW: Alcoholic ketoacidosis. *JAMA* 217:177–183, 1971.
165. Levy LJ, Duga J, Girgis M, et al: Ketoacidosis associated with alcoholism in nondiabetic subjects. *Ann Int Med* 78:213–219, 1973.
166. Fulop M, Hoberman HD: Alcoholic ketosis. *Diabetes* 24:785–790, 1975.
167. Miller PD, Heinig RE, Waterhouse C: Treatment of alcoholic acidosis. The role of dextrose and phosphorus. *Arch Int Med* 138:67–72, 1978.
168. Soffer A, Hamburger S: Alcoholic ketoacidosis: a review of 30 cases. *JAMWA* 37:106–110, 1982.
169. Halperin ML, Hammeke M, Josee RG, et al: Metabolic acidosis in the alcoholic: a pathophysiologic approach. *Metabolism* 32:308–315, 1983.
170. Lefevre A, Adler H, Lieber CS: Effect of ethanol on ketone metabolism. *J Clin Invest* 49:1775–1782, 1970.
171. Kreisberg RS: Diabetic ketoacidosis: new concepts and trends in pathogenesis and treatment. *Ann Int Med* 88:681–695, 1978.
172. Reichle FA, Owen OE, Golsorkhi M, Kreulen T: Hepatic metabolism in patients with alcoholic cirrhosis. *Surgery* 84:33–36, 1978.
173. Oster JR, Epstein M: Acid–base aspects of ketoacidosis. *Am J Nephrol* 4:137–151, 1984.
174. Bennett IL Jr, Cary FH, Mitchell GL Jr, et al: Acute methyl alcohol poisoning: a review based on experiences in an outbreak of 323 cases. *Medicine* 32:431–463, 1953.
175. Tonning DJ, Brooks DW, Harlow CM: Acute methyl alcohol poisoning in 49 naval ratings. *Can Med Assoc J* 74:20–27, 1956.
176. Schwartz RD, Milliman RP, Billi JE, et al: Epidemic methanol poisoning: clinical and biochemical analysis of a recent episode. *Medicine* 60:373–382, 1981.
177. Gonda A, Gault H, Churchill D, et al: Hemodialysis for methanol intoxication. *Am J Med* 64:749–758, 1978.
178. Roe O: The metabolism and toxicity of methanol. *Pharm Rev* 7:399–412, 1955.
179. Cooper JR, Kini MM: Biochemical aspects of methanol poisoning. *Biochem Pharmacol* 11:405–416, 1962.
180. Kini MM, Cooper JR: Biochemistry of methanol poisoning. III. The enzymatic pathway for the conversion of methanol to formaldehyde. *Biochem Pharmacol* 8:207–215, 1961.
181. Blair AH, Vallee BL: Some catalytic properties of human liver alcohol dehydrogenase. *Biochemistry* 5:2026–2034, 1966.
182. Kini MM, Cooper JR: Biochemistry of methanol poisoning. 4. The effect of methanol and its metabolites on retinal metabolism. *Biochem J* 82:164–172, 1962.
183. Martin-Amat G, McMartin KE, Hayreh SS, et al: Methanol poisoning: ocular toxicity produced by formate. *Toxicol Appl Pharmacol* 45:201–208, 1978.
184. McCoy HG, Cipolle RJ, Ehlers SM, et al: Severe methanol poisoning. Application of a pharmacokinetic model for ethanol therapy and hemodialysis. *Am J Med* 67:804–807, 1979.
185. Keyvan-Larijarni H, Tannenberg AM: Methanol intoxication. Comparison of peritoneal dialysis and hemodialysis treatment. *Arch Int Med* 134:293–296, 1974.
186. Underwood F, Bennett WM: Ethylene glycol intoxication. Prevention of renal failure by aggressive management. *JAMA* 226:1453–1454, 1973.
187. Parry MF, Wallach R: Ethylene glycol poisoning. *Am J Med* 57:143–150, 1974.
188. Frommer JP, Ayus JC: Acute ethylene glycol intoxication. *Am J Nephrol* 2:1–5, 1982.
189. Scully RE, Galdabini JJ, McNeely BU (eds): Case 38-1979. Case records of the Massachusetts General Hospital. *N Engl J Med* 301:650–657, 1979.
190. Peterson CD, Collins AJ, Himes JM, et al: Ethylene glycol poisoning. Pharmacokinetics during therapy with ethanol and hemodialysis. *N Engl J Med* 304:21–23, 1981.

191. Stokes JB III, Aueron F, Prevention of organ damage in massive ethylene glycol ingestion. *JAMA* 243:2065–2066, 1980.
192. McCord WM, Switzer PK, Brill HH Jr: Isopropyl alcohol intoxication. *South Med J* 41:639–642, 1948.
193. Adelson L: Fatal intoxication with isopropyl alcohol (rubbing alcohol). *Am J Clin Pathol* 38:144–151, 1962.
194. Wax J, Ellis FW, Lehman AJ: Absorption and distribution of isopropyl alcohol. *J Pharmacol Exp Ther* 97:229–237, 1949.
195. Mecikalski MB, Depner TA: Peritoneal dialysis for isopropanol poisoning. *West J Med* 137:322–325, 1982.
196. Freireich AW, Cinque TJ, Xanthaky G, et al: Hemodialysis for isopropanol poisoning. *N Engl J Med* 277:699–700, 1967.
197. Nordam R, Ribiere C, Rouach H, et al: Metabolic pathways involved in the oxidation of isopropanol into acetone by the intact rat. *Life Sci* 13:919–932, 1973.
198. Juncos L, Taguchi JT: Isopropyl alcohol intoxication. Report of a case associated with myopathy, renal failure, and hemolytic anemia. *JAMA* 204:186–188, 1968.
199. King LH Jr, Bradley KP, Shires DL: Hemodialysis for isopropyl alcohol poisoning. *JAMA* 211:1855, 1970.
200. Grossman RA, Hamilton RW, Morse BM, et al: Nontraumatic rhabdomyolysis and acute renal failure. *N Engl J Med* 291:807–811, 1974.
201. Gabow PA, Kaehny WD, Kelleher SP: The spectrum of rhabdomyolysis. *Medicine* 61:141–152, 1982.
202. Koffler A, Friedler RM, Massry SG: Acute renal failure due to nontraumatic rhabdomyolysis. *Ann Int Med* 85:23–28, 1976.
203. Rowland LP, Penn AS: Myoglobinuria. *Med Clin N Am* 56:1233–1256, 1972.
204. Perkoff GT, Hardy P, Velez-Garcia E: Reversible acute muscular syndrome in chronic alcoholism. *N Engl J Med* 274:1277–1285, 1966.
205. Martin FC, Slavin G, Levi AJ: Alcoholic muscle disease. *Br Med Bull* 38:53–56, 1982.
206. Saltissi D, Parfrey PS, Curtis JR, et al: Rhabdomyolysis and acute renal failure in chronic alcoholics with myopathy, unrelated to acute alcohol ingestion. *Clin Nephrol* 21:294–300, 1984.
207. Knochel JP: Skeletal muscle in hypophosphatemia in phosphorus deficiency, in Massry SG, Ritz E, Rapado A (eds): *Advances in Experimental Medicine and Biology,* vol 103. *Homeostasis of Phosphate and Other Minerals.* New York, Plenum Press, 1978, pp 357–366.
208. Segal AJ, Miller M, Moses AM: Hypercalcemia during the diuretic phase of acute renal failure. *Ann Int Med* 68:1066–1068, 1968.
209. Knochel JP: Serum calcium derangements in rhabdomyolysis. *N Engl J Med* 304:161–163, 1981.
210. Massry SG, Arieff AI, Coburn JW, et al: Divalent ion metabolism in patients with acute renal failure; studies on the mechanism of hypocalcemia. *Kidney Int* 5:437–445, 1974.
211. Llach F, Felsenfeld AJ, Haussler MR: The pathophysiology of altered calcium metabolism in rhabdomyolysis-induced acute renal failure. Interactions of parathyroid hormone, 25 hydroxycholecalciferol, and 1,25-dihydroxycholecalciferol. *N Engl J Med* 305:117–123, 1981.
212. Levine BS, Walling MW, Coburn JW: Intestinal absorption of calcium: its assessment, normal physiology, and alterations in various disease states, in Bronner F, Coburn JW (eds): *Disorders of Mineral Metabolism vol 2.* New York, Academic Press, 1982, pp 103–188.
213. Eneas JR, Schoenfeld PY, Humphreys MH: The effect of infusion of mannitol-sodium bicarbonate on the clinical course of myoglobinuria. *Arch Int Med* 139:801–805, 1979.

15

Urinary Tract Infections and Renal Papillary Necrosis in Alcoholism

Thomas O. Pitts and David H. Van Thiel

Abstract. An enhanced frequency and morbidity of urinary tract infections (UTI) have been observed in association with alcoholism and liver disease. The causes of these phenomena may relate, in part, to the defects in humoral and cellular immune mechanisms that occur in alcoholism. Urinary catheterization is the most common cause of UTI in hospitalized alcoholics. The severity of the sequelae of UTI in alcoholism is demonstrated by the unusually frequent occurrence of renal papillary necrosis (RPN) in conjunction with pyelonephritis in these patients. Indeed, in over 90% of the reported cases of RPN occuring with alcoholism or liver disease, pyelonephritis has been a contributing factor. The proclivity to medullary ischemia and RPN in this patient group may be, at least in part, a result of interstitial renal edema secondary both to infection and the effect of ethanol per se and to renal arterial vasoconstriction that occurs in cirrhosis. The frequency with which death due to sepsis or renal failure occurs in association with UTI in alcoholics obliges the physician to exercise caution in the prevention and treatment of UTI in these patients.

1. Introduction

An increased susceptibility to all types of infections is a well-recognized feature of chronic alcoholism. Although urinary tract infections (UTI) are among the most common infectious diseases, little attention has been given to their occurrence in alcoholics. The importance of such infections in alcoholic patients is exemplified, however, by the unusually frequent association of acute pyelonephritis and renal papillary necrosis (RPN) in alcoholics and cirrhotics. In this chapter we will review the effects of alcohol abuse on the immunologic defenses against UTI. In addition, we will examine the frequency, clinical syndrome and bacteriology of urinary tract infection both in alcoholism and liver disease.

Thomas O. Pitts • Renal–Electrolyte Division, Department of Medicine, University of Pittsburgh School of Medicine, Pittsburgh, Pennsylvania 15261. **David H. Van Thiel** • Division of Gastroenterology, Department of Medicine, University of Pittsburgh School of Medicine, Pittsburgh, Pennsylvania 15261.

2. The Effects of Alcoholism on the Immune System

A variety of alterations of the immune system occur in the alcoholic. The degree of impairment of immune function appears to relate directly to the extent and duration of alcoholism. Thus, in Laennec's cirrhosis or alcoholic hepatitis immune deficits occur more predictably and with greater severity than they do in acute ethanol intoxication. The extent to which associated nutritional deficiencies may contribute to the immune dysfunction in alcoholism has not been defined. In addition, the effect of these immune abnormalities in enhancing the individual's susceptibility to infection is not known. Immune dysfunction is, nonetheless, a systemic manifestion of alcoholism that is of considerable interest in view of its potential significance in the clinical setting of the urinary tract infection and sepsis.

2.1. Humoral Factors

2.1.1. Immunoglobulins. A well-described feature of alcoholic liver disease is hypergammaglobulinemia.[1,2] Characteristically serum levels of the three major immunoglobulin classes, IgA, IgM, and IgG, are elevated. Excessive antigenic stimulation is thought to be the principal cause of this disorder.[3–5] Normally, the hepatic Kupffer cells eliminate antigens that originate from the fecal flora in the intestinal lumen and enter the portal circulation. In the presence of cirrhosis and portal hypertension these antigens escape phagocytosis and enter the systemic circulation, which results in the excessive, persistent stimulation of the spleen and other immunoglobulin producing lymphoid tissues. Additionally, it has been suggested that a defect in suppressor T-cell function may be responsible, in part, for an exaggerated B-cell response to certain types of antigenic stimulation, thereby producing an uncontrolled gamma globulin synthesis.[6]

2.1.2. Serum Complement. Serum complement (C_3) levels are typically below normal in patients with advanced Laennec's cirrhosis.[7] Reduced hepatic synthesis of complement appears to cause this abnormality.[8] Although complement deficiency may affect chemotaxis adversely, no specific relationship between infection and depressed serum complement levels has been demonstrated in cirrhotic patients.

2.1.3. Serum Bactericidal Activity. Ethanol acutely depresses the normal bactericidal activity of human serum against several bacterial species.[9,10] A similar effect is produced by ethanol infusion in dogs[11] and is due to a depression by alcohol of the total hemolytic complement activity.[12] Of interest, the *in vitro* addition of ethanol to the serum of dogs is without such an effect, suggesting that ethanol impairs complement production *in vivo*. Approximately 90% of patients with Laennec's cirrhosis have deficient serum bactericidal activity due to a putative humoral inhibitor of bactericidal IgM activity.[13]

2.2. Cellular Factors

2.2.1. Granulocytopenia. In acute and chronic alcoholism leukopenia is a commonly recognized disorder.[14,15] Hypersplenism is a contributing factor in patients with cirrhosis. The inhibition of granulocytopoiesis by ethanol, directly[16] or through its inhibition of folate utilization[17] appears to be the major factor responsible for the leukopenia in noncirrhotic alcoholics. Compounding this problem is the high prevalence of dietary folate deficiency which is evident in this unique population.[15]

2.2.2. Inhibition of Chemotaxis. Defects in chemotaxis have been observed frequently in alcoholics. Acutely, ethanol, at normal pharmacologic serum concentration, has little effect on chemotaxis in humans,[18] although it does depress granulocyte adherence.[19] However, even in the absence of cirrhosis, chronic alcoholics frequently have impaired chemotaxis which appears to result from the presence of a humoral inhibitor of chemotaxis.[20] Acute systemic illness, including alcoholic hepatitis, produces a similar depression of chemotaxic activity that disappears when the acute hepatic dysfunction resolves.[21] The serum of patients with Laennec's cirrhosis profoundly inhibits chemotaxis by granulocytes harvested from both cirrhotics and normal subjects. In either case, replacement of the serum from the cirrhotic with normal serum restores chemotaxis.[22] The cause of this inhibition of chemotaxis observed in patients with active alcoholic liver disease may be the production of an IgA molecule that directly inhibits monocyte chemotaxis.[23]

2.2.3. Lymphocyte Alterations. Defects in cell-mediated immunity are common in patients with alcoholism. Skin anergy is encountered frequently in chronic alcoholics and may occur in as many as 40–50% of patients who have alcoholic hepatitis or Laennec's cirrhosis.[24–26] Lymphocyte responsiveness to phytohemagglutinin is inhibited by serum from some patients with Laennec's cirrhosis, although the same cells will respond in the presence of normal serum.[27] In Laennec's cirrhosis the development of an anamnestic response is impaired, possibly due to defective macrophage processing.[28–30] Lymphopenia is present frequently in alcoholics, with depletion of both T and B lymphocyte populations, although the T-cell deficiency is usually of greater magnitude.[26,31–34]

3. Immune Defenses against UTI: Relationship to Alcoholic Immune Dysfunction

3.1. Normal Bladder Defense Mechanisms

Although infections of the urinary tract may arise secondary to the hematogenous spread of bacteria from another source, most such infections are initiated by the entry of bacteria into the bladder through the urethera. Normally, the bladder is well defended against the retention of bacteria by the presence of a relatively brisk urine flow and periodic complete bladder emptying.[35] An acidic urine pH, the secretion of immunoglobulins into the urine, and the natural bactericidal activity of the bladder mucosal cells are also important defenses against the development of infection in the urinary tract. Clinically, UTI commonly arises in patients who have lost these physical or immunologic barriers, such as occurs with bladder catheterization, urinary tract obstruction, or anatomic or functional renal disease.[36] Although no studies have examined these questions, in alcoholics without overt renal or urinary tract disease, disruption of the normal immune mechanisms may conceivably alter the immunoglobulin response or the local bactericidal activity of the bladder and increase the susceptibility to urinary tract infection.

3.2. Bacterial Virulence Factors

Certain bacterial species may be particularly virulent in causing urinary tract infections. Several strains of *Escherichia coli* and *Klebsiella* are resistant to the bactericidal activity of serum and to macrophage phagocytosis and intracellular killing actions.[37,38] The capsular antigens of *E. coli* appear to be responsible, at least in part, for this unique virulence.[39] In addition, some strains of *E. coli* have surface pili that allow the organisms to bind avidly to the bladder mucosa.[40] The potential clinical importance of this phenomenon is demonstrated by the fact that the passive immunity conferred by the administration of anti-pili antibodies protects against the development of experimental ascending UTI in animals.[41]

3.3. Host Factors in the Development of UTI

3.3.1. Immunoglobulins. Systemic and local antibody synthesis is a well-recognized response to renal infection.[42,43] IgG and IgA are involved principally in the response,[44] which involves the lower urinary tract as well as the kidney.[45] The urinary mucosal cells of patients with recurrent UTI avidly bind *E. coli*.[46] This phenomenon has been shown to occur in oral and vaginal epithelial cells as well.[47] Normally secretory IgA and IgG bind to the surface of bacteria present in the urinary tract and prevent their attachment to the uroepithelium.[48] Thus, it has been proposed that impaired production of secretory IgA predisposes some patients to recurrent UTI.[49]

3.3.2. Cell-Mediated Immunity. The induction of experimental pyelonephritis in rats results in the proliferation of clones of T-lymphocytes that react specifically against antigens of the infecting bacteria. For 2–3 days following the onset of experimental pyelonephritis, T-lymphocytes harvested from infected kidneys are unresponsive to phytohemagglutinin stimulation. In contrast, B-cell proliferative response and antibody production are not impaired.[50] It has been speculated that this transient T-cell dysfunction observed in experimental conditions may be detrimental to the defense mechanisms that, under normal circumstances, prevent the initiation of infection.[50]

3.3.3. Differential Renal Susceptibility. Experimental studies of pyelonephritis have shown clearly that the renal medulla is much more susceptible to bacterial infection than is the renal cortex.[51] Thus, experimental infections can be induced by the innoculation of the renal medulla with ten bacteria whereas 10^3 organisms are required to produce a cortical infection.[52] The hypertonicity of the renal medulla appears to be the principal factor responsible for this phenomenon. Following experimental renal injury, granulocyte adherence and migration are markedly lower in the medulla than they are in the cortex.[53,54] This difference in granulocyte activity is abolished when the renal injury is induced during a water diuresis.[55] Hypertonicity also inhibits granulocyte phagocytosis,[56] depresses the serum bactericidal activity,[57] and augments the rate of bacterial multiplication in renal tissues.[58] To the extent that cirrhotic individuals have a concentrated urine chronically, excessive urinary and medullary hypertonicity may contribute to their increased susceptibility to renal medullary infections.

4. UTI in Alcoholism and Laennec's Cirrhosis

Alcoholism is considered to be a major factor which predisposes the individual to the development of infections. Indeed, Osler said of lobar pneumonia that "Alcoholism is perhaps the most potent predisposing factor."[59] Recent reviews have emphasized the alcoholic's predisposition to develop spontaneous bacterial peritonitis, spontaneous bacteremia, bacterial endocarditis and bacterial meningitis.[60,61] Despite the generalized phenomenon, the specific issue of UTI in alcoholics has received little attention. In fact, it has been said that there is no real evidence for an increased incidence of UTI in alcoholics.[62] However, although the data are few, recent reports suggest that UTI may indeed occur more often in alcoholics and in individuals with chronic liver disease and may impose significant morbidity and mortality in these populations.

4.1. Cirrhosis

4.1.1. Pyelonephritis in Alcoholic Liver Disease. It appears from an examination of retrospective studies, which utilized chart or autopsy review, that pyelonephritis is not unusually common in patients with cirrhosis. Ratnoff and Patek found chronic pyelonephritis in only 2 of 385 patients with Laennec's cirrhosis. In contrast, they noted pneumonia in 22 and peritonitis in 14.[63] Similarly, Edmondson *et al.* examined autopsy data from 2689 chronic alcoholics with cirrhosis or fatty liver and found that 105 had either acute or chronic pyelonephritis.[64] This frequency of pyelonephritis (3.5%) was not different from that encountered in the general population. However, RPN occurred in eighteen of these 105 patients during their first episode of acute pyelonephritis. This suggests that cirrhotics may be at high risk for the more severe sequelae of such infections.

The origin of the pyelonephritis observed in the patients with alcoholic liver disease examined by Edmondson *et al.* is not clear. Approximately half of the patients with pyelonephritis and RPN included in their report had evidence of cystitis at autopsy, and *E. coli* was the organism that was isolated most frequently from the renal tissues.[64] Thus, the lower urinary tract would appear to be the primary source of infection in many alcoholics with pyelonephritis.

4.1.2. Lower Urinary Tract Infection in Cirrhosis.

4.1.2a. Primary Biliary Cirrhosis. Burroughs *et al.* have examined the incidence of significant bacteriuria ($\geqslant 10^5$ colonies/ml) present in outpatients with primary biliary cirrhosis.[65] For comparative controls they determined the incidence of bacteriuria in outpatients with other causes of cirrhosis and in ambulatory outpatients with rheumatoid arthritis. Over a 3-month observation period, 19% of the patients with primary biliary cirrhosis had significant bacteriuria when examined using a single clean-catch mid-stream urine collection. In contrast, only 7% of the patients with cirrhosis due to other causes and 8% of the patients with rheumatoid arthritis had bacteriuria.

In a separate study, Burroughs *et al.* prospectively followed 144 outpatients with primary biliary cirrhosis for 1–2 years and obtained a clean-catch mid-stream urine collection from each patient at regular intervals.[65] Bacteriuria was found in 35% during the first year. Throughout the 2 years of follow-up, 47% of the patients with histologically advanced hepatic disease developed bacteriuria. In contrast, bacteriuria occurred in 23% of the patients with prefibrotic disease. Moreover, recurrent bacteriuria was more frequent in the patients with late-stage disease than in those with less severe disease. Thus, it appears that patients with advanced hepatic disease may be particularly susceptible to the development of UTI.

It should be noted, however, that the clinical and laboratory features of UTI of the patients studied by Burroughs *et al.* were not unusual. Of the bacteriuric episodes, 41% were symptomatic and 65% were accompanied by pyuria. *Escherichia coli* was the organism isolated most frequently, and accounted for 70% of the cases, while mixed infections were seen in 8% and the remainder of episodes were caused by gram negative organisms other than *E. coli*.[65]

No etiology for the increased frequency of UTI in the patients with primary biliary cirrhosis could be determined. The incidence of bacteriuria did not correlate with drug therapy, the serum bilirubin concentration, or patient age. Moreover, no urinary tract abnormalities were found in those patients who underwent intravenous pyelography to evaluate the cause of their recurrent UTI. The urinary pH was acidic in most samples and an alkaline urine did not correlate with the presence of bacteriuria. In contrast to the studies discussed earlier, the binding of *E. coli* to uroepithelial and buccal mucosal cells taken from patients with primary biliary cirrhosis was not increased.[65]

4.1.2b. Hospitalized Cirrhotics. Gomez *et al.* reviewed their experience over a 2-year period with infections in hospitalized cirrhotic patients.[66] The urinary tract was the most common site of infection, accounting for 22% of all infectious episodes in their patients. Both pulmonary infections and spontaneous bacterial peritonitis followed UTI in frequency. A total of 101 episodes of UTI occured in 85 patients, of whom 43% had a primary diagnosis of alcoholic cirrhosis. Ninety percent of the episodes of UTI arose after hospital admission. Catheterization of the bladder preceded the development of urinary tract infection in 60% of the episodes. Notably, only one patient who developed UTI following bladder catheterization had had prior UTI. In contrast, over one third of the patients who developed a spontaneous UTI in the hospital had a history of previous UTI. Thus, bladder catheterization was the chief factor predisposing to the development of UTI. A history of a prior UTI was a much less important contributing factor.[66]

The clinical features of UTI observed in these cirrhotic patients were similar to those seen in urinary tract infections occurring in the noncirrhotic population. The large majority of patients with UTI had fever and pyuria. Leukocytosis was observed in one third. Of note, however, men and women were affected equally. As expected, *E. coli* was the most frequently isolated organism while two organisms were isolated in 16% and *Streptococcus fecalis* was encountered in 12%.[66]

The potential for serious sequelae following UTI in cirrhotics is evidenced by the high death rate from urosepsis in these patients. Slightly over 15% of all patients who developed UTI died as a result of sepsis with the same organism that had been isolated from their urine. Moreover, urosepsis was responsible for nine (27%) of the 33 deaths which occurred in the 85 cirrhotic patients studied.[66]

4.2. Chronic Alcoholism and UTI

The only comparison of the incidence of bacteriuria in an alcoholic population with that observed in nonalcoholics has come from a group in Poland.[67] First morning-voided, clean-catch mid-stream urine specimens were obtained from 200 patients hospitalized for alcohol dependency and from 200 nonalcoholic patients hospitalized for noninfectious conditions. Neither group had a history of prior UTI, urinary symptoms, or recent antibiotic therapy. There were no age or sex differences between the two groups. Although the majority of the urine specimens contained some bacteria, significant bacteriuria ($\geq 10^5$ colonies/ml) was found in 46.5% of alcoholics and in only 11% of controls. *Escherichia coli* was the most frequently encountered organism in both groups. Staphylococcal species were isolated in one third of the episodes of bacteriuria in alcoholics while two organisms were isolated in 5% of the bacteriuric episodes of alcoholics and in none of the episodes of controls.[67]

4.3. Summary of UTI in Alcoholism and Liver Disease

Although the data are limited, some generalizations about UTI in alcoholism and cirrhosis may be made. The incidence of UTI appears to be increased in patients with advanced hepatic disease including Laennec's cirrhosis. Support for this is derived from the increased incidence of significant bacteriuria observed in hospitalized noncirrhotic alcoholics. Clinically important is the fact that hospitalized cirrhotic patients are at significant risk for death from sepsis caused by a UTI. The frequency with which bladder catheterization initiates this process should caution against the unnecessary use of such instrumentation in alcoholics.

The clinical and laboratory features of UTI in alcoholics and cirrhotics are similar to those observed in other patient groups. Uniformly, *E. coli* is the most common causative organism.

5. RPN in Alcoholics

5.1. Overview of Papillary Necrosis

RPN is a clinical and pathologic syndrome which occurs as a secondary phenomenon in a number of medical diseases. The most commonly recognized causes are analgesic abuse, diabetes mellitus, obstruction of the urinary tract, and sickle cell hemaglobinopathy. Urinary tract infection is a concomitant finding in the great majority of cases of RPN. On examination of the renal tissues, the damage may be widespread, involving the entire medullary tissue, or, more commonly, it is localized to one or more of the renal papillae.[68]

The clinical features of the syndrome are variable but usually include fever, pyuria, hematuria, low-grade proteinuria, and diminished urinary concentrating ability. The glomerular filtration rate is usually only mildly depressed and correlates inversely with the severity and extent of the necrotic process. In some asymptomatic patients, RPN is an incidental finding at autopsy or on excretory urography.[68]

5.2. Alcoholism and RPN

It appears that there is a slightly increased prevalence of RPN in patients with chronic alcoholism and liver disease. Edmonson *et al.* reviewed the data obtained from autopsies performed over a 20-year period.[64] RPN was found in 0.46% of all autopsies and in 0.74% of autopsies performed on alcoholic patients. The highest prevalence of RPN was encountered in patients with diabetes mellitus (5.5%) and in those with urinary tract obstruction (5.5%).

Although the prevalence of RPN is increased only slightly in alcoholics, a significant percentage of the reported cases of RPN have been associated with alcoholism or liver disease. Table I lists several reports of patients with

Table I. A Review of Reports of Renal Papillary Necrosis (RPN) and the Percentage of Cases Associated with Alcoholism and/or Hepatic Disease in the Absence of Diabetes Mellitus or Urinary Tract Obstruction

Reference	Cases of RPN	Cases of RPN in alcoholism/liver disease	
		No.	Percent
Knutsen *et al.*[69]	16	1	6
Schourup[70]	46	3	7
Lauler *et al.*[71]	6	1	17
Edmondson *et al.*[64]	195	20	10
Jungers *et al.*[72]	16	2	13
Eknoyan *et al.*[68]	27	1	4
Totals	306	28	9

RPN in whom alcoholism or liver disease was an identifiable coexistent problem without the concomitant presence of diabetes mellitus or urinary tract obstruction. One of 16 patients with RPN reported by Knutsen *et al.* had cirrhosis.[69] Of 46 cases of RPN reviewed by Schourup, two had cirrhosis and one had hepatitis.[70] One of six patients with RPN reported by Lauler *et al* had early alcoholic cirrhosis.[71] The 195 cases of RPN reported by Edmondson *et al.* included 20 alcoholics.[64] Jungers *et al.* observed 16 cases of RPN at the Necker hospital in Paris over a 10-year period. In two, cirrhosis was the only associated condition while an additional patient with RPN had both cirrhosis and diabetes mellitus.[72] Eknoyan *et al.* noted that hepatic disease was present in only one of 27 of their patients with RPN.[68] Thus, although Table I is not a comprehensive list of all of the reports of RPN, it appears from these data that approximately 5–10% of the cases of RPN may be associated with alcoholism or hepatic disease.

Despite an apparent frequent association with RPN, it appears that the presence of alcoholism or liver disease is rarely the only cause of RPN. UTI appears to be a frequent precipitating factor. Table II reviews the association of UTI with RPN occurring in alcoholism or liver disease. The alcoholic patient reported by Lauler *et al.* had sepsis and UTI with multiple organisms.[71] All of the cirrhotic patients with RPN reported by Edmondson *et al.* had acute pyelonephritis.[64] Longacre and Popky reviewed 102 autopsies of cirrhotic patients and found eleven cases with RPN.[73] Diabetes mellitus or urinary tract obstruction was also present in seven of these cirrhotic patients. Nine had a concurrent UTI and one patient had a past history of acute pyelonephritis. The patient with hepatic disease and RPN reported by Eknoyan *et al.* had acute pyelonephritis.[68] Jungers *et al.* found RPN in three cirrhotics in the absence of infection, however one of these patients also had diabetes mellitus.[72] Thus, over 90% of the reported cases of RPN associated with alcoholism or liver disease have been accompanied by UTI, which is usually acute pyelonephritis.

Table II. The Association of Renal Papillary Necrosis (RPN) in Alcoholism or Hepatic Disease with Urinary Tract Infection (UTI)

Reference	Cases of RPN in alcoholism or liver disease	Cases of RPN with UTI in alcoholism or liver disease	
		No.	Percent
Lauler *et al.*[71]	1	1	100
Edmondson *et al.*[64]	20	20	100
Longacre and Popky[73]	11[a]	10	91
Jungers *et al.*[72]	3[b]	0	0
Eknoyan *et al.*[68]	1	1	100
Totals	36	32	91

[a] Includes seven patients with concomitant diabetes mellitus or urinary tract obstruction.
[b] Includes one patient with coexistent diabetes mellitus.

Infection of the urinary tract is a common concomitant problem whenever RPN occurs. For example, 80% of the diabetics with RPN reported by Eknoyan *et al.* had UTI; overall, two thirds of the patients with RPN included in their report had UTI.[68] Similarly, infection rates of 70% and 95% have been reported in other reviews of RPN.[71,74] However, pyelonephritis alone is not a common cause of RPN. In an autopsy study by Edmondson *et al.*, RPN was found in only 21 of 1023 cases of acute pyelonephritis in nondiabetic patients.[75] Notably, however, 20 of these patients had obstruction of the urinary tract. Thus, in the absence of diabetes mellitus or urinary tract obstruction, RPN occurred in only 0.1% of cases of acute pyelonephritis. The contribution of alcoholism or hepatic disease to the development of RPN is exemplified further by the observation of Edmondson *et al.* that 20 of 105 (19%) alcoholics with acute pyelonephritis developed RPN.[64] The importance of alcoholism per se in this relationship is emphasized by the fact that twelve of these 20 patients did not have established Laennec's cirrhosis. Other case reports have also called attention to the association between alcoholism and bacterial or fungal pyelonephritis and the development of RPN.[76,77]

Of particular clinical concern is the observation that the occurrence of RPN in patients with alcoholism or liver disease appears to have a rather poor prognosis. Uremia was present in all of the patients reported by Edmondson *et al.* for whom sufficient data were available for analysis. Oliguria was noted in four of ten subjects who had their urinary output recorded.[64] Irreversible oliguric renal failure was present in both of the nondiabetic cirrhotics reported by Jungers *et al.*[72] Six of the 11 patients reported by Longacre and Popky died of causes related, at least in part, to the RPN.[73] However, three of the four cirrhotics, who had neither obstruction nor diabetes mellitus, survived their acute illness. These patients demonstrated only focal medullary necrotic lesions on intravenous pyelography.[73] Thus, it appears that the severity of the clinical syndrome of RPN in alcoholics is related to the extent of the renal necrosis.

The lethal nature of RPN complicating the course of a urinary tract infection in alcoholic patients underscores the need for aggressive therapy in this unique group of patients. This admonition is particularly true for those alcoholic patients who have concomitant diabetes mellitus or urinary tract obstruction. Interestingly, Edmondson *et al.* noted that antibiotic therapy appeared to improve renal function in several of the patients they studied despite their obligate fatal outcome required for inclusion in the study.[64] These authors emphasized the fact that many of these alcoholic patients had been placed on empiric antibiotic therapy which had been inadequate due either to insufficient dosage of the drug used or failure to properly identify the infecting organism.[64]

5.3. Cause of RPN in Alcoholism

The principal lesion leading to the development of RPN is thought to be medullary ischemia. Impaired medullary blood flow has been demonstrated in experimental animal models of RPN.[78,79] The putative medullary ischemia in patients with RPN is thought to result from postglomerular vasoconstriction. Such vasospasm, which has been demonstrated by angiographic studies, presumably decreases the blood flow to the vasa rectae that arise from the postglomerular vessels and supply the renal papillae.[80] Acute pyelonephritis contributes to the medullary ischemia induced by any other condition due to the compression of the highly compliant, thin-walled medullary blood vessels by the interstitial inflammatory response elicited by the infection.[71]

The association of RPN with alcoholism and chronic liver disease in the absence of infection has not been well explained. Under normal conditions medullary blood flow approximates only 4% of that present in the renal cortex.[81] In cirrhosis, particularly when ascites is present, renal blood flow is frequently decreased,[82,83] and severe renal arterial vasospasm accompanies the onset of functional renal failure in such patients.[84,85] Although a redistribution of renal blood flow to the medulla occurs,[86] the progressive decline in total renal blood flow can progress to tissue ischemia, as evidenced by the occasional development of acute tubular necrosis. Although this increase in the blood flow to the renal medulla relative to the cortex may protect against necrosis of medullary tissues, the interstitial edema associated with acute pyelonephritis may further reduce the medullary blood flow sufficient to induce RPN. An additional factor possibly contributing in alcoholics to the compression of the medullary vessels is the renal interstitial edema which has been observed in the tissues of alcohol fed rats.[86] Also, hyperbilirubinemia may contribute to the development of RPN in cirrhotics. Unconjugated bilirubin when present in high concentration in the blood has been shown to induce RPN in the Gunn rat.[88] In addition, this toxic effect of unconjugated bilirubin increases the frequency with which other factors such as analgesic administration cause RPN.[89] Finally, the intrinsic susceptibility of the renal medulla to infection may be worsened by the excessive urinary concentration and the immune deficits present in alcoholics.

References

1. Wilson ID, Onstad G, Williams RC Jr: Serum immunoglobulin concentrations in patients with alcoholic liver disease. *Gastroenterology* 57:59–67, 1969.
2. LoGrippo GA, Anselm K, Hayashi H: Serum immunoglobulins and five serum proteins in extrahepatic obstructive jaundice and alcoholic cirrhosis. *Am J Gastroenterol* 56:357–363, 1971.
3. Bjorneboe M, Pyrtz H, Orskov F: Antibodies to intestinal microbes in serum of patients with cirrhosis of the liver. *Lancet* 1:58–60, 1972.
4. Triger DR, Alp MH, Wright R: Bacterial and dietary antibodies in liver disease. *Lancet* 1:60–63, 1972.
5. Thomas HC, McSween RNM, White RG: Role of the liver in controlling the immunogenicity of commensal bacteria in the gut. *Lancet* 1:1288–1291, 1973.
6. Triger DR, Wright R: Hyperglobulinaemia in liver disease. *Lancet* 1:1494–1496, 1973.
7. Grieco MH, Capra JD, Paderon H: Reduced beta 1c/1a globulin levels in extrarenal disease. *Am J Med* 51:340–345, 1971.
8. Petz LD: Variable mechanisms for low serum complement in liver disease. *Lancet* 2:1033–1034, 1971.
9. Kaplan NM, Braude AI: Hemophilus influenzae infection in adults. Observations on the immune disturbance. *Arch Int Med* 101:515–523, 1958.
10. Johnson WD, Stokes P, Kaye D: The effect of intravenous ethanol on the bactericidal activity of human serum. *Yale J Biol Med* 42:71–85, 1969.
11. Marr JJ, Spilberg I: Depressant effect of ethanol on serum complement and serum bactericidal activity. *Clin Res* 22:35A, 1974.
12. Marr JJ, Spilberg I: A mechanism for infection by gram-negative bacteria in acute ethanol intoxication. *Clin Res* 22:449A, 1974.
13. Fierer J, Finley F: Deficient serum bactericidal activity against *Escherichia coli* in patients with cirrhosis of the liver. *J Clin Invest* 63:912–921, 1979.
14. McFarland W, Libre EP: Abnormal leukocyte response in alcoholism. *Ann Int Med* 59:865–877, 1963.
15. Liu YK: Leukopenia in alcoholics. *Am J Med* 54:605–610, 1973.
16. Tisman G, Herbert V: In vitro myelosuppression and immunosuppression by ethanol. *J Clin Invest* 52:1410–1414, 1973.
17. Sullivan LW, Herbert V: Suppression of hematopoiesis by ethanol. *J Clin Invest* 43:2048–2062, 1964.
18. Spagnuolo PJ, MacGregor RR: Acute ethanol effect on chemotaxis and other components of host defense. *J Lab Clin Med* 86:24–31, 1975.
19. Gluckman SJ, MacGregor RR: Effect of acute intoxication on granulocyte mobilization and kinetics. *Blood* 52:551–559, 1978.
20. MacGregor RR, Gluckman SJ, Senior JR: Granulocyte function and levels of immunoglobulins and complement in patients admitted for withdrawal from alcohol. *J Infect Dis* 138:747–753, 1978.
21. Van Epps DE, Palmer DL, Williams RC Jr: Characterization of serum inhibitors of neutrophil chemotaxis associated with anergy. *J Immunol* 113:189–200, 1974.
22. DeMeo AN, Andersen BR: Defective chemotaxis associated with a serum inhibitor in cirrhotic patients. *N Eng J Med* 286:735–740, 1972.

23. Van Epps DE, Strickland RG, Williams RC Jr: Inhibitors of leukocyte chemotaxis in alcoholic liver disease. *Am J Med* 59:200–207, 1975.
24. Berenyi MR, Straus B, Cruz D: In vitro and in vivo studies of cellular immunity in alcoholic cirrhosis. *Am J Dig Dis* 19:199–205, 1974.
25. Snyder N, Bessoff J, Dwyer JM, et al: Depressed delayed cutaneous hypersensitivity in alcoholic hepatitis. *Am J Dig Dis* 23:353–358, 1978.
26. Mills PR, Shenkin A, Anthony RS, et al: Assessment of nutritional status and in vivo immune responses in alcoholic liver disease. *Am J Clin Nutr* 38:849–859, 1983.
27. Hsu CCS, Leevy CM: Inhibition of PHA-stimulated lymphocyte transformation by plasma from patients with advanced alcoholic cirrhosis. *Clin Exp Immunol* 8:749–760, 1971.
28. Tennenbaum JI, Ruppert RD, St Pierre RL, et al: The effect of chronic alcohol administration on the immune responsiveness of rats. *J Allergy* 44:272–281, 1969.
29. Straus B, Berenyi MR, Huang JM, et al: Delayed hypersensitivity in alcoholic cirrhosis. *Am J Dig Dis* 16:509–516, 1971.
30. Gluckman SJ, Dvorak VC, MacGregor RR: Host defenses during prolonged alcohol consumption in a controlled environment. *Arch Int Med* 137:1539–1543, 1977.
31. Bernstein IM, Williams RC Jr, Webster KH, et al: Reduction in circulating T lymphocytes in alcoholic liver disease. *Lancet* 2:488–490, 1974.
32. Berenyi MR, Straus B, Avila L: T rosettes in alcoholic cirrhosis of the liver. JAMA 232:44–46, 1975.
33. Thomas HC, Freni M, Sanchez-Tapias J, et al: Peripheral blood lymphocyte populations in chronic liver disease. *Clin Exp Immunol* 26:222–227, 1976.
34. Lang JM, Ruscher H, Hasselmann JP, et al: Decreased autologons rosette-forming T lymphocytes in alcoholic cirrhosis. Absence of correlation with other T cell markers and with delayed cutaneous hypersensitivity. *Int Arch Allergy Appl Immun* 61:337–343, 1980.
35. Cox CE, Hinman F Jr: Factors in resistance to infection in the bladder. I. The eradication of bacteria by vesical emptying and intrinsic defense mechanisms, in Kass EH (ed): *Progress in Pyelonephritis*. Philadelphia, F A Davis Co, 1965, pp 563–570.
36. Cotran RS, Pennington JE: Urinary tract infection, pyelonephritis, and reflux nephropathy, in Brenner BM, Rector FC Jr: *The Kidney*, ed 2. Philadelphia, WB Saunders, 1981, pp 1571–1632.
37. Kimball H, Garcia M, Petersdorf RG: The epidemiology of nonenteric *Escherichia coli* infections. II. Relationship of prevalence of E. Coli in urinary infections to the bactericidal effect of human serum. *J Lab Clin Med* 63:901–913, 1964.
38. Weinstein RJ, Young LS: Neutrophil function in gram-negative rod bacteremia. The interaction between phagocytic cells, infecting organisms, and humoral factors. *J Clin Invest* 58:190–199, 1976.
39. Howard CJ, Glynn AA: The virulence for mice of strains of *Escherichia coli* related to the effects of K antigens on their resistance to phagocytosis and killing by complement. *Immunology* 20:767–777, 1971.
40. Svanborg-Eden C, Hansson HA: *Escherichia coli* pili as possible mediators of attachment to human urinary tract epithelial cells. *Infect Immun* 21:229–237, 1978.
41. Silverblatt FJ, Cohen LS: Antipili antibody affords protection against experimental ascending pyelonephritis. *J Clin Invest* 64:333–336, 1979.
42. Hanson LH, Ahlstedt S, Fasth A, et al: Antigens of *Escherichia coli*, human immune response, and the pathogenesis of urinary tract infections. *J Inf Dis* 136 (suppl):S144–S149, 1977.
43. Kaijser B, Larsson P, Olling S: Protection against ascending *Escherichia coli* pyelonephritis in rats and significance of local immunity. *Infect Immun* 20:78–81, 1978.
44. Smith J, Holmgren J, Ahlstedt S, et al: Local antibody production in experimental pyelonephritis: amount, avidity, and immunoglobulin class. *Infect Immun* 10:411–415, 1974.
45. Darwish ME, Staubitz WJ, Neter E: Antibody response of dogs to experimental infection of bladder pouch with different serogroups of Escherichia coli. *Invest Urol* 8:412–416, 1971.

46. Svanborg-Eden C, Jodal U: Attachment of Escherichia coli to urinary sediment epithelial cells from urinary tract infection-prone and healthy children. *Infect Immun* 26:837–840, 1979.
47. Schaeffer AJ, Jones JM, Dunn JK: Association of in vitro Escherichia coli adherence to vaginal and buccal epithelial cells with susceptibility of women to recurrent urinary-tract infections. *N Engl J Med* 304:1062–1066, 1981.
48. Svanborg-Eden C, Svennerholm AM: Secretory immunoglobulin A and G antibodies prevent adhesion of Escherichia coli to human urinary tract epithelial cells. *Infect Immun* 22:790–797, 1978.
49. Stamey TA, Wehner N, Mihara G, et al: The immunologic basis of recurrent bacteriuria: role of cervicovaginal antibody in enterobacterial colonization of the introital mucosa. *Medicine* 57:47–56, 1978.
50. Miller TE, Stewart E, North JDK: Immunobacteriological aspects of pyelonephritis. *Contrib Nephrol* 16:11–15, 1979.
51. Rocha H, Guze LB, Freedman LR, et al: Experimental pyelonephritis. III. The influence of localized injury in different parts of the kidney on susceptibility to bacillary infection. *Yale J Biol Med* 30:341–354, 1958.
52. Freedman LR, Beeson PB: Experimental pyelonephritis. IV. Observations on infections resulting from direct innoculation of bacteria in different zones of the kidney. *Yale J Biol Med* 30:406–414, 1958.
53. Rocha H, Fekety FR Jr: Acute inflammation in the renal cortex and medulla following thermal injury. *J Exp Med* 119:131–138, 1964.
54. Rocha H, Fekety FR Jr: Delayed granulocyte mobilization in the renal medulla, in Kass EH (ed): *Progress in Pyelonephritis*. Philadelphia, FA Davis Co, 1965, pp 211–220.
55. Andriole VT: Acceleration of the inflammatory response of the renal medulla by water diuresis. *J Clin Invest* 45:847–854, 1966.
56. Chernew I, Braude AI: Depression of phagocytosis by solutes in concentrations found in the kidney and urine. *J Clin Invest* 41:1945–1953, 1962.
57. Hubert EG, Montgonerie JZ, Kalmanson GM, Guze LB: Effect of renal physicochemical milieu on serum bactericidal activity. *Am J Med Sci* 253:225–229, 1967.
58. Delucchi C, Kass EH: Effect of osmolality in regional bacterial multiplication in the kidney, in Kass EH (ed): *Progress in Pyelonephritis*. Philadelphia, FA Davis Co, 1965, pp 280–283.
59. Osler W: *The Principles and Practice of Medicine,* ed. 7. New York, D. Appleton & Co, 1910, pp 166.
60. Tapper ML: Infections complicating the alcoholic host, in Grieco MH (ed): *Infections in the Abnormal Host*. New York, Yorke Medical Books, 1980, pp 474–507.
61. Adams HG, Jordan C: Infections in the alcoholic. *Med Clin N Am* 68:179–200, 1984.
62. Smith FE, Palmer DL: Alcoholism, infection and altered host defenses: A review of clinical and experimental observations. *J Chron Dis* 29:35–49, 1976.
63. Ratnoff OD, Patek AJ Jr: The natural history of Laennec's cirrhosis of the liver. An analysis of 386 cases. *Medicine* 21:207–268, 1942.
64. Edmondson HA, Reynolds TB, Jacobson HG: Renal papillary necrosis with special reference to chronic alcoholism. A report of 20 cases. *Arch Int Med* 118:255–264, 1966.
65. Burroughs AK, Rosenstein IJ, Epstein O, et al: Bacteriuria and primary biliary cirrhosis. *Gut* 25:133–137, 1984.
66. Gomez J, Vilardell F, Casais L, et al: Infecciones urinarias del cirrotico. *Rev Esp Enf Ap Digest* 56:321–326, 1979.
67. Pawliszyn W, Telesnicki S: Urinary tract infections in chronic alcoholics. Bacteriological investigations. *Pol Tyg Lek* 29:1831–1834, 1974.
68. Eknoyan G, Qunibi WY, Grissom RT, et al: Renal papillary necrosis: An update. *Medicine* 61:55–73, 1982.
69. Knutsen A, Jennings ER, Brines OA, et al: Renal papillary necrosis. *Am J Clin Pathol* 22:327–336, 1952.
70. Schourup K: Necrosis of the renal papillae. Post-mortem series. *Acta Pathol Microbiol Scand* 41:462–478, 1957.

71. Lauler DP, Schreiner GE, David A: Renal medullary necrosis. *Am J Med* 29:132–156, 1960.
72. Jungers P, Kleinknecht D, Grunfeld JP, et al: Necrose medullaire renale et cirrhose hepatique. *Ann Med Interne* 121:639–643, 1970.
73. Longacre AM, Popky GL: Papillary necrosis in patients with cirrhosis: A study of 102 patients. *J Urol* 99:391–395, 1968.
74. Simon HB, Bennett WA, Emmett JL: Renal papillary necrosis: A clincopathologic study of 42 cases. *J Urol* 77:557–567, 1957.
75. Edmondson HA, Martin HE, Evans N: Necrosis of renal papillae and acute pyelonephritis in diabetes mellitus. *Arch Int Med* 79:148–175, 1947.
76. Case records of the Massachusetts General Hospital (Case 33-1970). *N Engl J Med* 283:305–313, 1970.
77. Madge GE, Lomvardias S: Chronic liver disease and renal papillary necrosis with Aspergillus. *South Med J* 66:486–488, 1973.
78. Kincaid-Smith P, Saker BM, McKenzie IFC: Lesions of the vasa recta in experimental analgesic nephropathy. *Lancet* 1:24, 1968.
79. Wyllie RG, Hill GS, Murray G, et al: Experimental papillary necrosis of the kidney. III. Effects of reserpine and other pharmacologic agents on the lesion. *Am J Pathol* 68:235–254, 1972.
80. Lagergren C, Ljunquist A: The intrarenal arterial pattern in renal papillary necrosis. A microangiographic and histologic study. *Am J Pathol* 41:633–644, 1962.
81. Thorburn GD, Kopald HH, Herd JA, et al: Intrarenal distribution of nutrient blood flow determined with Krypton^{85} in the unanesthetized dog. *Circ Res* 13:290–307, 1963.
82. Baldus WP, Feichter RN, Summerskill WHJ, et al: The kidney in cirrhosis. II. Disorders of renal function. *Ann Int Med* 60:366–377, 1964.
83. Baldus WP, Summerskill WHJ, Hunt JC, et al: Renal circulation in cirrhosis: observations based on catheterization of the renal vein. *J Clin Invest* 43:1090–1097, 1964.
84. Epstein M, Berk DP, Hollenberg NK, et al: Renal failure in the patient with cirrhosis. The role of active vasoconstriction. *Am J Med* 49:175–185, 1970.
85. Baldus WP: Etiology and management of renal failure in cirrhosis and portal hypertension. *Ann NY Acad Sci* 170:267–279, 1970.
86. Kew MC, Varma RR, Williams HS, et al: Renal and intrarenal blood-flow in cirrhosis of the liver. *Lancet* 2:504–510, 1971.
87. Van Thiel DH, Gavaler JS, Little JM, et al: Alcohol: its effect on the kidney. *Metabolism* 26:857–866, 1977.
88. Axelsen RA, Burry AF: Bilirubin-associated renal papillary necrosis in the homozygous Gunn rat: light- and electron-microscopic observations. *J Pathol* 120:165–175, 1976.
89. Axelsen RA, Burry AF: Papillary necrosis in the Gunn rat: rapid induction by analgesics. *Pathology* 4:225–229, 1972.

16

Disorders of Divalent Ions and Vitamin D Metabolism in Chronic Alcoholism

Thomas O. Pitts and David H. Van Thiel

Abstract. This chapter reviews the pathogenesis of disordered divalent mineral and bone metabolism in alcoholism, emphasizing the role of impaired vitamin D physiology. Normally, vitamin D metabolites are derived principally from cholecalciferol, which is synthesized in the skin via the energy of sunlight. Most alcoholics have subnormal levels of 25-hydroxyvitamin D [25(OH)D]. Those with Laennec's cirrhosis also have low levels of vitamin D binding protein due to impaired hepatic protein synthesis and as a result, have low serum concentrations of total, but not free, 1,25-dihydroxyvitamin D. The causes of 25(OH)D deficiency in alcoholics include reduced hepatic 25-hydroxylase activity, lack of sun exposure, inadequate dietary intake, and malabsorption. Hypomagnesemia and hypophosphatemia, which are very common in hospitalized alcoholics, result from deficient intake, malabsorption, excessive renal losses, and cellular uptake of both ions. Hypocalcemia in alcoholics is caused primarily by hypoalbuminemia but can result also from deficient intake, malabsorption, hypomagnesemia, and renal calcium wastage. Low vitamin D activity may contribute significantly to the calcium and phosphate deficiencies. Osteoporosis is extremely common in alcoholics whereas osteomalacia is exceptional. However, both bone disorders respond well to vitamin D therapy. Thus, alcoholics should be screened periodically for vitamin D deficiency and osteopenia, and when either is detected they should receive vitamin D supplements.

1. Introduction

It is well recognized that alcoholics often manifest derangements of divalent mineral metabolism. However, details of the pathogenesis of these problems have remained incomplete. Over the last decade much new information has been acquired regarding both the normal aspects of vitamin D physiology and the effects of alcoholism on the vitamin D endocrine system. In this chapter we will review the recent developments in vitamin D pathophysiology

Thomas O. Pitts • Renal–Electrolyte Division, Department of Medicine, University of Pittsburgh School of Medicine, Pittsburgh, Pennsylvania 15261. **David H. Van Thiel** • Division of Gastroenterology, Department of Medicine, University of Pittsburgh School of Medicine, Pittsburgh, Pennsylvania 15261.

as they pertain to the problem of alcoholism. In addition, we will examine the frequency, characteristics, and causes of bone disease, hypocalcemia, hypomagnesemia, and hypophosphatemia and their relationship to the impairments of vitamin D metabolism present in alcoholics.

2. Vitamin D: Normal Physiology

2.1. Metabolism

Derived from plant sources, ergocalciferol, vitamin D_2, is the dietary form of vitamin D. It constitutes 10–30% of the total vitamin D pool in normal humans. Cholecalciferol, vitamin D_3, is the principal form of vitamin D in Europeans and North Americans. It is synthesized in the skin by the photoconversion of 7-dehydrocholesterol to pre-vitamin D, which is slowly converted by a temperature-dependent reaction to vitamin D_3. Vitamin D metabolites are transported in the blood by vitamin D binding protein (DBP), an α-globulin synthesized in the liver and having a molecular weight of approximately 53,000 daltons. Identical to the human group specific protein, G_C, DBP is present normally in the serum at a molar concentration approximately 100-fold greater than that of the sum of the various metabolites of vitamin D. Conjugated in the liver and secreted into bile, vitamin D metabolites undergo an enterohepatic circulation. Nonetheless, the major route of excretion of vitamin D and its metabolites is via the feces.[1–3]

Vitamin D_3 is a prohormone which must be converted to its active metabolites (Fig. 1). The initial step in this pathway is the conversion of vitamin D_3 to 25-hydroxyvitamin D_3 [25(OH)D], by the hepatic microsomal exzyme, vitamin D-25-hydroxylase. This reaction is not tightly regulated and the production of 25(OH)D depends primarily on the availability of substrate cholecalciferol. Thus, serum 25(OH)D levels show a seasonal variation, varying directly with the individual's exposure to sunlight.[1–3]

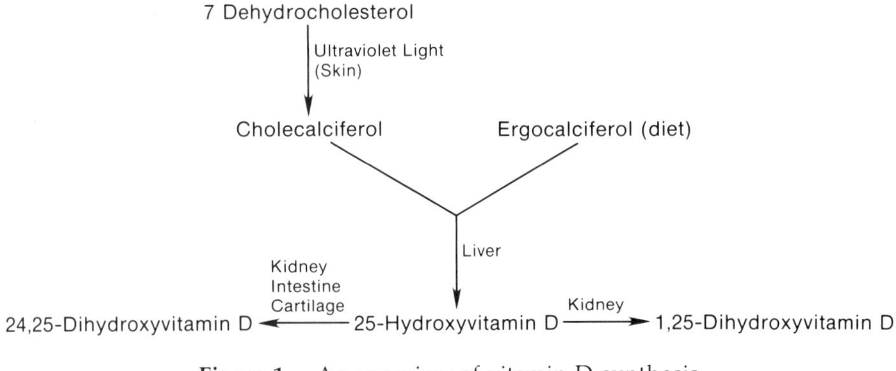

Figure 1. An overview of vitamin D synthesis.

Although 25(OH)D has some physiological effects, the most active form of vitamin D is 1,25-dihydroxyvitamin D_3 [1,25$(OH)_2$D]. This metabolite is formed in the proximal renal tubules from 25(OH)D by the action of 25(OH)D-1α-hydroxylase, a mitochondrial mixed function monooxidase. Also present primarily in the renal proximal tubule cells (but also in cartilage and intestine), is 25(OH)D-24-hydroxylase, which produces 24,25-dihydroxyvitamin D [24,25$(OH)_2$D]. The activities of these two enzymes are tightly regulated in a reciprocal fashion such that factors activating the 1-hydroxylase inhibit the 24-hydroxylase and vice versa. Production of 1,25$(OH)_2$D is stimulated by dietary calcium or phosphate deficiency, hypocalcemia, hypophosphatemia, vitamin D deficiency, and various hormones, including parathyroid hormone (PTH), estrogens, prolactin, insulin, and human growth hormone. In contrast, 24,25$(OH)_2$D is the predominant metabolite formed in the presence of calcium and phosphate surfeit and in the vitamin D replete state.[1–3]

2.2. Actions of Vitamin D Metabolites

The physiologic actions of vitamin D metabolites are necessary for the maintenance of calcium and phosphate homeostasis. 1,25$(OH)_2$D stimulates the intestinal absorption of calcium and phosphate and acts with parathyroid hormone to mobilize calcium from bone. In addition to the effect of increasing calcium availability through its actions on gut absorption, 1,25$(OH)_2$D appears to stimulate bone mineralization by a direct effect on bone cells. 24(OH)D and 24,25$(OH)_2$D also may act on bone and cartilage to promote mineralization. In states of vitamin D or phosphate deficiency, 1,25$(OH)_2$D and 25(OH)D augment the renal reabsorption of phosphate. Both 1,25$(OH)_2$D and 24,25$(OH)_2$D appear to diminish the secretion of PTH, possibly by augmenting the entry of calcium into the cells of the parathyroid gland.[1–3]

3. Alterations of Vitamin D Metabolism in Alcoholism

3.1. 25(OH)D Levels in Cirrhosis

Table I summarizes the available data on serum or plasma levels of 25(OH)D in alcoholic patients.[4–18] Two groups of investigators have found no significant difference in the 25(OH)D concentrations between patients with Laennec's cirrhosis and control subjects.[8,10] However, in the great majority of studies a significant reduction in the 25(OH)D concentration has been reported in alcoholics with cirrhosis. Of particular note are the observations that 25(OH)D levels are subnormal in patients with Laennec's cirrhosis who are abstinent[9] as well as in those who have alcoholic hepatitis and/or fatty liver.[5,12,13,17] Sonnenberg *et al.* found that the serum concentration of 25(OH)D in alcoholics declines progressively as the histologic liver disease worsens.[17] Moreover, alcoholics without evidence of liver disease have lower 25(OH)D concentra-

Table I. Plasma or Serum Concentration of 25-Hydroxyvitamin D in Alcoholics and Healthy Controls.[a]

Reference	Patients (No.)	Plasma or serum 25(OH)D levels (ng/ml)		$P < 0.05$, patients vs. controls?
		Patients	Controls	
Barragry *et al.*[4]	Chronic liver disease (45) (including alcoholics)	13.1 ± 1.7	20.4 ± 5.4	Yes
Barragry *et al.*[5]	Alcoholic liver disease (5)	4.4 ± 1.6	40.7 ± 6.6	Yes
Bikle *et al.*[6]	Alcoholic liver disease (25)	9.7 ± 4.5	19.2 ± 6.6	Yes
Bouillon *et al.*[7]	Alcoholic cirrhosis (11)	11.4 ± 5.2	14.4 ± 4	No
Garcia-Pascual *et al.*[8]	Alcoholic cirrhosis (12)	19.4 ± 13.1 (spring)	35.6 ± 10.3	Yes
	Noncirrhotic alcoholics (13)	18.0 ± 8.4		
	Alcoholic cirrhosis (15)	23.7 ± 18.5 (autumn)	57.2 ± 22.5	Yes
	Noncirrhotic alcoholics (15)	35.2 ± 21.8		
Hepner *et al.*[9]	Inactive alcoholic cirrhosis (31)	20 ± 11	35 ± 12	Yes
	Active alcoholic cirrhosis (8)	12 ± 9		Yes
	Noncirrhotic alcoholics (15)	28 ± 12		Yes
Jung *et al.*[10]	Alcoholic cirrhosis (8)	8.7 ± 4.0	10.4 ± 3.8	No
Long[11]	Alcoholic cirrhosis (25)	8.6 ± 4.9	9–44	Yes
	Alcoholic hepatitis (9)	9.8 ± 5.3		Yes
Long *et al.*[12]	Alcoholic liver disease (6)	8.6 + 5	26 ± 8	Not reported
Long *et al.*[13]	Alcoholic liver disease (6) and cryptogenic cirrhosis (1)	5.1 ± 3.9	9–44	Not reported
Meyer *et al.*[14]	Alcoholic and postnecrotic cirrhosis (23)	11.3 ± 3.2	21.4 ± 4.3	Yes
Posner *et al.*[15]	Alcoholic cirrhosis (32)	40 ± 6	55 ± 3	Not reported
Roginski *et al.*[16]	Alcoholic cirrhosis (18)	12.3 ± 6.9	29.9 ± 9.9	Not reported
	Noncirrhotic alcoholics (12)	26.6 ± 11.5		No
Sonnenberg *et al.*[17]	Alcoholic liver disease (23)	10.0 ± 6.5	26.5 ± 12.1	Yes
Velentzas *et al.*[18]	Noncirrhotic alcoholics (13)	15.0 ± 7.6	23.6 ± 9.8	Yes

[a] Values shown represent mean ± S.D., except references 4, 5, 14 and 15 which report standard error.

tions than do control subjects.[8,9,18] Thus, although some alcoholics may have a normal blood 25(OH)D concentration, the majority have subnormal levels even in the absence of active liver disease.

3.2. Vitamin D Binding Protein in Liver Disease

Table II reviews the published data on the alterations of the serum concentration of vitamin D binding protein in patients with liver disease. The DBP concentrations of patients with Laennec's cirrhosis, as well as other types of cirrhosis, are depressed in comparison to those observed in healthy controls.[4,6,7,10,19,20] Impaired hepatic protein synthesis appears to be the principal cause of this phenomenon as exemplified by the finding of a direct correlation between the levels of DBP and serum albumin.[7,19,20] In addition, in patients with acute infectious hepatitis, serum DBP levels correlate inversely with serum transaminase and bilirubin concentrations.[20]

3.3. Serum 1,25(OH)$_2$D Concentrations in Alcoholic Cirrhosis

Alterations of the serum concentrations of the dihydroxylated vitamin D metabolites in patients with liver disease have received little attention. No data regarding 24,25(OH)$_2$D levels in cirrhosis have been reported and only two groups have examined 1,25(OH)$_2$D concentrations in these patients. The mean serum 1,25(OH)$_2$D concentration observed by Bouillon *et al.* in 11 patients with Laennec's cirrhosis was 31 ± 18 (S.D.) ng/liter, a value which was

Table II. Serum or Plasma Concentration of Vitamin D Binding Protein in Chronic Liver Disease.

Reference	Patients/No.	Blood Vitamin D binding protein concentration (mg/liter)[a]	
		Patients	Controls
Barragry *et al.*[4]	Alcoholic cirrhosis (14)	219 ± 14	276 ± 10
	Chronic liver disease (15)	216 ± 9	
Bikle *et al.*[6]	Alcoholic liver disease (25)	188 ± 21	404 ± 29
Bouillon *et al.*[7]	Alcoholic cirrhosis (11)	289 ± 29	325 ± 7
Brown *et al.*[19]	Chronic liver disease (44) (includes 11 alcoholics)	224 ± 6	292 ± 3
Imawari *et al.*[20]	Postinfectious/cryptogenic cirrhosis (14)	230 ± 16	370 ± 9
	Chronic hepatitis, nonalcoholics (13)	290 ± 14	
Jung *et al.*[10]	Alcoholic (8) and cryptogenic (2) cirrhosis	298 ± 23	300 – 550

[a] Mean ± S.E.

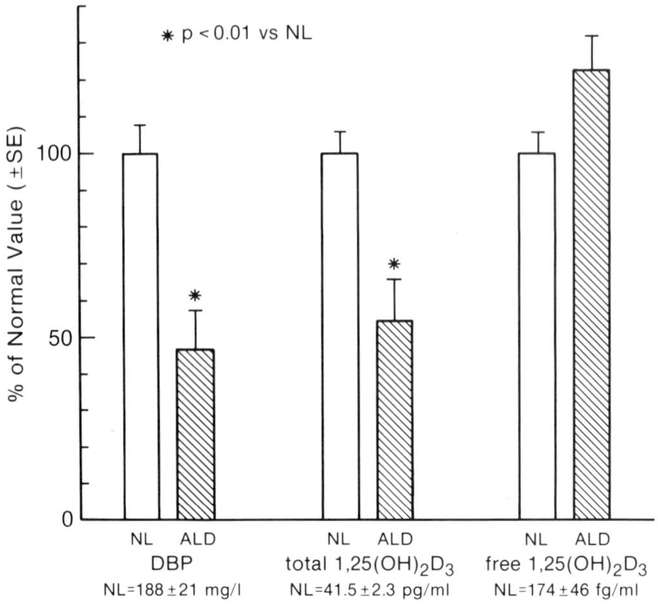

Figure 2. Serum concentrations of vitamin D binding protein (DBP) and total and free 1,25-dihydroxycholecalciferol [1,25$(OH)_2D_3$] in normal subjects (NL) and patients with alcoholic liver disease (ALD). Adapted from Bikle *et al.*[6]

significantly lower than that obtained in healthy subjects, 42 ± 13 ng/liter, ($P < 0.05$).[7] However, the estimated free 1,25$(OH)_2$D concentration was normal in patients with alcoholic cirrhosis, and the total 1,25$(OH)_2$D levels were noted to correlate with the DBP concentrations. Similarly, Bikle *et al.* (see Fig. 2) found a reduced concentration of 1,25$(OH)_2$D in the serum of patients with alcoholic liver disease.[6] However, the serum concentration of free 1,25$(OH)_2$D was not reduced. Moreover, the percent of total 1,25$(OH)_2$D present in the serum in the unbound form was actually elevated in the cirrhotic patients as compared to the controls and correlated inversely with the serum DBP concentration. Thus, the depression in the total serum 1,25$(OH)_2$D concentration observed in alcoholic cirrhotics appears to be due to a reduction of DBP rather than to a primary defect in 1- or 25-hydroxylation.

3.4. Causes of Diminished 25(OH)D Concentration in Alcoholics

Because the 25-hydroxylation of vitamin D occurs in the liver, it is not surprising that patients with alcoholic cirrhosis have subnormal levels of 25(OH)D. However, even in the absence of histologic evidence of hepatic disease alcoholics have low levels of 25(OH)D suggesting that the deficiency of this sterol is multifactoral. Indeed, several factors may contribute to the reduction in circulating 25(OH)D in alcoholic patients.

3.4.1. 25-Hydroxylation in Alcoholics. Impaired 25-hydroxylation of vitamin D is present in some patients with alcoholic liver disease. Hepner *et al.* observed a significant increase in the serum 25(OH)D concentration 25 hrs after the parenteral injection of 120 μg of vitamin D_3 in subjects without liver disease but not in patients with Laennec's cirrhosis.[9] In their cirrhotic patients, the serum 25(OH)D level correlated directly with measures of hepatic function such as the serum albumin concentration and the results of the aminopyrine breath test.[9] Similarly, Jung *et al.* found a delayed appearance of [^{3}H]-25(OH)D_3 in the serum of cirrhotics compared with that seen in normal subjects four hours after the injection of [^{3}H]-cholecalciferol.[10] However, this difference was not apparent at 8, 12, or 24 hrs following the injection, demonstrating that 25-hydroxylation, although delayed, does occur in cirrhosis. The importance of hepatocellular dysfunction to 25-hydroxylation is further evidenced by the findings of Lund *et al.* that in patients with alcoholic liver disease the elevation of 25(OH)D concentration produced by the chronic administration of cholecalciferol was only 50% that of normal subjects given the same dose of cholecalciferol.[21]

In contrast to the results of Jung *et al.* other investigators have found a normal appearance of ^{3}H-25(OH)D_3 in the serum of patients with alcoholic liver disease following the administration of [^{3}H]-cholecalciferol.[5,22] Thus, 25-hydroxylation of vitamin D is not defective in all subjects with alcoholic liver disease. Indeed, when adequate supplementation is provided, serum 25(OH)D levels can be normalized even in patients with Laennec's cirrhosis.[15] These findings suggest therefore that impaired 25-hydroxylation of vitamin D has only a permissive role in the 25(OH)D deficiency observed in patients with alcoholic liver disease.

3.4.2. Reduced Sun Exposure. In most alcoholics diminished substrate availability due to inadequate exposure to sunlight appears to contribute significantly to the deficiency of 25(OH)D. Jung *et al.* found no difference in plasma 25(OH)D concentration between normal subjects and patients with alcoholic cirrhosis studied during the winter.[10] Moreover, Lund *et al.* noted that the normal seasonal variations in serum 25(OH)D concentration were absent in alcoholic patients.[21] In addition, the serum 25(OH)D concentrations in their alcoholic subjects were below normal only in the summer months.[21] Garcia-Pascual *et al.* (see Table I) observed a similar blunting of the normal seasonal increase in 25(OH)D levels in alcoholics with cirrhosis but not in noncirrhotic alcoholics.[8] Notably however, when seasonal variations have been observed in alcoholics, the serum 25(OH)D concentrations of alcoholics have always been lower than those of healthy controls.[8,23] This observation suggests that decreased sun exposure, although important, is not the only factor causing a depression of the 25(OH)D concentration in alcoholics.

3.4.3. Reduced Dietary Vitamin D Intake. In the absence of adequate sunlight exposure, normal serum vitamin D levels can be maintained in alcoholics if adequate oral vitamin D intake is achieved. However, malnutrition is a common feature of alcoholism.[24] In alcoholics and in patients with cirrhosis of other causes, the depression of the serum 25(OH)D concentration is often accompanied by deficiencies of other vitamins including folic acid, ascorbic acid, vitamins A and E, and carotene.[9,23,25] Although no systematic analysis of the vitamin D intake of alcoholics has been undertaken, several authors have observed an apparent dietary vitamin D deficiency in their alcoholic patients.[9,15,25,26]

3.4.4. Malabsorption of Vitamin D. Malabsorption of vitamin D in patients with liver disease may occur in association with steatorrhea and/or the lack of intraluminal bile salts. Meyer *et al.* demonstrated impaired intestinal absorption of orally administered cholecalciferol in rats with experimentally induced cirrhosis[27] and in patients with postnecrotic and alcoholic cirrhosis.[22] In contrast, Lund *et al.* observed similar increases in the serum 25(OH)D concentration when patients with alcoholic liver disease were given cholecalciferol either orally or via intramuscular injection.[21] Moreover, Posner *et al.* found no correlation between the fecal fat excretion and deficient serum 25(OH)D levels in patients with Laennec's cirrhosis.[15] Despite the presence of mild steatorrhea, supranormal serum 25(OH)D concentrations have been achieved in such patients by chronic oral administration of ergocalciferol.[15] Thus, in subjects with alcoholic cirrhosis the detrimental effects of malabsorption of vitamin D can be avoided if oral vitamin D intake is increased sufficiently.

3.4.5. Deficient DBP Concentration. Theoretically, the decrease in circulating DBP observed in cirrhosis can contribute to the lower levels of 25(OH)D. However, Barragry *et al.* found no correlation between the serum concentrations of DBP and 25(OH)D in alcoholic cirrhotics.[4] In contrast, others have observed a direct correlation between these parameters in cirrhosis.[7,20] It is not clear whether this correlation relates primarily to depressed hepatic synthesis of both DBP and 25(OH)D or to an effect of DBP availability on the 25(OH)D concentration. Because DBP is normally only 3–5% saturated with vitamin D metabolites, it is unlikely that a low DBP concentration contributes significantly to the decreased levels of 25(OH)D in cirrhosis.

3.4.6. Increased Breakdown of Vitamin D. Jung *et al.* observed a shortened half-life of intravenously administered [^{3}H]-cholecalciferol in patients with alcoholic cirrhosis suggesting that the rate of metabolism of vitamin D is increased in such subjects.[10] However, others have found a normal [22] or delayed [28] cholecalciferol half-life in patients with alcoholic cirrhosis. Thus, an accelerated metabolism of vitamin D cannot be implicated as a major cause of the 25(OH)D deficiency seen in alcoholics.

4. Hypomagnesemia in Alcoholism

4.1. Frequency

Alcoholism is the most commonly recognized cause of disturbed magnesium balance. Although the serum magnesium concentration is normal in most alcoholics, particularly when adequate nutritional intake is maintained,[23,29–34] approximately 25–50% of the patients hospitalized for alcohol related problems are hypomagnesemic.[35–40] However, because less than 1% of the total body magnesium is present in the serum, significant deficits of magnesium can occur in the absence of any overt change in the serum magnesium concentration.[41] That the great majority of hospitalized alcoholics are magnesium deficient, regardless of their magnesium concentration, has been demonstrated by the observations that alcoholic subjects retain a greater percentage of a parenterally administered magnesium load than do paired controls[31,42,43] and that they remain in positive magnesium balance for several days following hospital admission.[42,44] In addition, hospitalized alcoholics have a reduced exchangeable ^{28}Mg content[42,45] and depressed muscle magnesium concentration.[30,31,42,46] This latter finding may be due to a coexistent potassium depletion rather than to magnesium depletion per se.[47]

4.2. Causes of Magnesium Deficiency and Hypomagnesemia in Alcoholics

Malnutrition often accompanies alcoholism and, certainly, inadequate magnesium intake can contribute significantly to the development of magnesium deficiency in many chronic alcoholics.[23,34,48] However, because magnesium is present in most foods, is readily absorbed from the gastrointestinal tract, and is avidly conserved by the kidneys during periods of dietary magnesium deficiency, the production of a total body magnesium deficit in normal volunteers by dietary means alone is quite difficult to achieve and requires the consumption of a rigidly controlled and monotonous diet for several weeks.[41,49,50] Thus, inadequate dietary intake of magnesium is rarely the only cause of magnesium deficiency in alcoholics.

Impaired gastrointestinal magnesium absorption may contribute to the development of a magnesium deficit in alcoholism in a number of ways. Chronic diarrhea of any cause leads to magnesium deficiency. Thus steatorrhea [51] and other malabsorption syndromes[52,53] have been associated with magnesium deficit due to the formation of nonabsorbable magnesium fatty acid complexes in the gut. Similarly hypomagnesemia often accompanies acute and chronic pancreatitis.[54] In addition, gut magnesium absorption is dependent, in part, on the action of vitamin D[55,56] and the presence of hypomagnesemia in alcoholics has been shown to correlate with the serum concentrations of 25(OH)D.[15]

Nonetheless, renal magnesium wastage appears to be a major factor contributing to the development of magnesium deficiency in alcoholism. Ethanol inhibits the renal tubular reabsorption of magnesium and ethanol ingestion acutely produces a profound magnesuria.[35,57–59] This effect is most prominent when the blood ethanol concentration is rising[60] and is absent when magnesium-depleted nonalcoholics are given ethanol.[41] The potential mechanisms for this phenomenon include a direct effect of ethanol on the renal tubular magnesium transport systems and the ethanol-induced increased production and excretion of lactate and ketones which bind magnesium and prevent its reabsorption from the renal tubule.[57,61,62] Several additional factors that increase urinary magnesium excretion and that are present frequently in chronic alcoholism include phosphate depletion,[63,64] therapy with thiazides or loop-blocking diuretics,[65–67] secondary hyperaldosteronism,[68] chronic volume expansion,[69,70] and renal tubular acidosis.[52,62,66]

Transient hypomagnesemia may occur in the alcoholic patient due to the acute movement of magnesium ions out of the extracellular fluid. This is observed most commonly in alcoholics hospitalized for withdrawal symptoms, and is associated with an acute respiratory alkalosis.[71] As insulin increases cellular Mg uptake,[72] the provision of calories by dextrose infusions or the resumption of dietary intake in withdrawing alcoholics may produce transient hypomagnesemia. In addition, the increase in lipolysis that accompanies alcohol withdrawal apparently results in the formation of magnesium-fatty acid complexes that are removed from the circulation, producing an acute decrease in the extracellular magnesium concentration.[73]

4.3. Consequences of Magnesium Deficiency

The consequences of magnesium deficiency, recently reviewed elsewhere,[74,75] involve predominately the neuromuscular and cardiovascular systems and are not unique to the alcoholic patient. Of particular interest, however, are certain biochemical disturbances caused by hypomagnesemia which may compound preexisting derangements common to alcoholism.

Thiamine deficiency is present frequently in severe alcoholism and has been related to the development of many of the neurologic disturbances observed in alcoholics.[76] Magnesium deficit increases the effects of thiamine deficiency and both deficiencies must be corrected to restore the biochemical actions of thiamine to normal.[77]

Hypokalemia, decreased intracellular potassium content, and renal potassium wasting are encountered frequently in magnesium deficiency.[41,49,78,79] Impaired activity of Na/K-ATPase, induced by hypomagnesemia, is the cause of these disturbances. Clinically, restoration of the potassium deficit cannot be accomplished unless the magnesium deficiency also is corrected.[79]

Magnesium deficiency produces a state of hypocalcemia and pseudohypoparathyroidism[80–82] that is resistant to the action of vitamin D.[80,83] The causes of this disorder include end-organ resistance to the calcemic actions of PTH[80,81] and impaired glandular release of PTH.[81,82,84] The resistance to PTH seen in magnesium deficiency is demonstrated by the failure of exogenously administered parathyroid extract to increase the urinary excretion of both cyclic AMP[81] and phosphate[80] and to release calcium from bone.[85,86] An impairment in adenylate cyclase activity by hypomagnesemia appears to be a cause of both PTH resistance and failure to release PTH.[75] An additional stimulus to hypocalcemia may be a PTH-independent reduction in bone matrix solubility induced by the decrease in the magnesium content of bone.[87] Correction of the magnesium deficiency rapidly ameliorates the associated hypocalcemia by restoring the parathyroid gland activity and end-organ PTH responsiveness.[80–83]

Much attention has been given to the potential role of hypomagnesemia in the symptoms of alcohol withdrawal.[38,71,88] Indeed many of the symptoms of alcohol withdrawal are similar to those observed in subjects with experimental Mg deficiency and may improve with magnesium infusions.[50,71] However, it has been shown clearly that patients can experience alcohol withdrawal symptoms in the absence of hypomagnesemia[36,42] and that delirium tremens may resolve despite the persistence of hypomagnesemia.[89] Therefore, although magnesium deficiency may worsen the neurologic picture of alcohol withdrawal, it does not have a causal role in the genesis of the condition.

5. Hypocalcemia in Alcoholism

5.1. Frequency

The majority of stable, chronic alcoholics appear to have normal total and ionized serum calcium concentrations.[5,7,15,23,32,36,90] However, approximately 20–50% of individuals admitted to the hospital for alcohol withdrawal or Laennec's cirrhosis have been found to be hypocalcemic,[5,14,33,36,40,91] and severe, symptomatic hypocalcemia is often seen in the seriously ill alcoholic.[89]

5.2. Causes of Hypocalcemia in the Alcoholic

5.2.1. Hypoalbuminemia. The serum albumin concentration is a principal determinant of the total serum calcium concentration.[91] Thus, it has been found that in alcoholic cirrhosis the total calcium concentration correlates directly with the serum albumin concentration. Moreover, the ionized calcium concentration is often normal and is unrelated to the albumin concentration.[7,32,91] However, in some alcoholics the degree of hypocalcemia observed is excessive relative to the depression of the serum albumin concentration[14,92] and, thus, cannot be explained by the hypoalbuminemia alone.

5.2.2. Hypocalcemia in Alcoholic-Related Gastrointestinal Diseases. Hypocalcemia may occur in chronic alcoholism associated with gastrointestinal diseases for a number of reasons. Steatorrhea and chronic diarrhea occur in many alcoholics and led to malabsorption of calcium.[93] In addition, in both cirrhotic and noncirrhotic alcoholics, depressed intestinal calcium absorption has been observed to correlate with low serum concentrations of vitamin D.[8] In rats, ethanol ingestion results in the inhibition of intestinal calcium absorption which is not reversible by the administration of vitamin D, $25(OH)D_3$, or $1,25(OH)_2D_3$.[94,95] Finally, hypocalcemía occurs more often in acute alcoholic pancreatitis than in pancreatitis of other etiologies and this increased frequency may be a consequence of the concomitant nutritional and electrolyte disturbances frequently present in alcoholics.[96]

5.2.3. Direct Effect of Ethanol on the Serum Calcium Concentration. Whether ethanol ingestion per se actually causes hypocalcemia in humans has been a subject of controversy. In experimental animals, the oral administration of ethanol produces a modest hypocalcemia that appears to result from the movement of calcium out of the extracellular compartment.[97–99] In humans, however, the acute ingestion of ethanol usually is without effect on the serum calcium concentration.[57,100] Recently, Avery *et al.* reported a very mild but sustained hypocalcemic effect of ethanol consumption in both alcoholics and nonalcoholic volunteers.[101] However, the lack of a nonalcohol control drinking session and the minimal degree of the depression of the calcium concentrations observed cast some doubt on the reliability of this study.

5.2.4. Urinary Calcium Excretion. An increase in urinary calcium excretion following ethanol ingestion has been observed in both alcoholic and nonalcoholic subjects.[57,102,103] Although PTH secretion increases after ethanol ingestion,[99,100] the urinary excretion of cyclic AMP is suppressed [103] and calciuria persists despite increased PTH secretion. These observations suggest that ethanol directly inhibits the end-organ response to PTH, independent of the effects of hypomagnesemia discussed earlier and, thereby, prevents the anticalciuric action of PTH.

6. Hypophosphatemia in the Alcoholic

6.1. Frequency

Alcoholism is the most commonly recognized cause of severe hypophosphatemia in hospitalized patients.[104,105] In the majority of alcoholics, hypophosphatemia is present upon admission to the hospital, or occurs within 1–4 days thereafter.[33,34,106] Evidence suggests that phosphate depletion is present even in alcoholics who maintain a normal serum phosphate concentration. Thus, the muscle phosphorus content is depressed independent of the serum phosphate concentration in virtually all alcoholic patients in whom it has been examined, as well as in chronic ethanol-fed experimental animals.[107–109]

6.2. Causes of Hypophosphatemia and Phosphate Depletion in Alcoholics

As is the case for both calcium and magnesium deficiencies discussed earlier, phosphate deficiency can occur in the alcoholic, at least in part, as a consequence of a poor diet and gastrointestinal disturbances such as malabsorption. In addition, antacids, which are frequently administered to hospitalized alcoholic patients, bind phosphorus in the gut and prevent its absorption. The malabsorption of phosphate seen in some alcoholics correlates with vitamin D deficiency[12] and responds well to adequate vitamin D supplementation.[110]

Magnesium deficiency produces excessive urinary phosphate loss in experimental animals.[111] Although urinary phosphate wasting is a somewhat variable and less prominent finding in humans during experimental magnesium depletion,[41,49,112,113] mild to moderate hypophosphatemia often occurs despite an adequate dietary phosphate intake.[49,50] Recently, Adler *et al.* demonstrated a low renal phosphate threshold, despite the coexistance of hypophosphatemia, in patients with Laennec's cirrhosis.[114] Although the cause of this finding was not clear, the lack of the antiphosphaturic effect of vitamin D[115,116] due to the deficiency of 25(OH)D often present in alcoholics may be a contributing factor.

Hypophosphatemia may also develop in alcoholics as a consequence of cellular phosphate uptake. Respiratory alkalosis is a highly predictable feature of alcohol withdrawal[117] and, by stimulating glycolysis, increases the entry of phosphate into cells, often resulting in profound hypophosphatemia.[118] Similarly, the infusion of dextrose and the resumption of dietary intake during alcohol withdrawal results in an intracellular shift of phosphate ions.[119,120] Although the transient decline in the serum phosphate concentration associated with these phenomena may have no detrimental effects in otherwise healthy subjects, the coexistant phosphate depletion often present in chronic alcoholics predisposes them to the development of serious consequences of hypophosphatemia such as hemolysis or rhabdomyolysis.[119]

7. Bone Disease in Alcoholism

7.1. Types of Bone Disease Observed in Alcoholics

A well-known feature of chronic alcoholism is an increased incidence of skeletal fractures. Although trauma is probably the most common precipitating factor, metabolic bone disease often contributes.[121,122] Given the high frequency of vitamin D and mineral deficiencies seen in alcoholics, it is not surprising that the skeleton is affected adversely. The bone disorders which occur in alcoholics are osteoporosis, osteomalacia, avascular necrosis,[123] neuropathic arthropathy,[124] and periostitis.[125]

7.2. Osteoporosis in Alcoholism

Clearly, osteoporosis is the skeletal disorder seen most often in alcoholics. Using postmortem iliac crest bone biopsies, Saville found decreased bone density in alcoholics of both sexes that correlated well with the roentenographic evidence of decreased cortical bone thickness in the peripheral skeleton.[126] In addition, other workers, using specialized radiographic techniques, have shown decreased bone mineral content in alcoholics,[122,127] which is particularly prominent in those who previously have undergone gastric resection.[122,128] In a prospective study, Dalen and Lamke observed that the annual loss of bone mineral, as measured by X-ray spectrophotometry, is 2% higher in alcoholics than it is in controls,[129] a finding that is consistent with other, static, observations suggesting the presence of accelerated age-related bone mineral loss in alcoholics.[122,126]

The causes of the bone mineral loss observed in alcoholic patients have not been elucidated completely. The nutritional and metabolic disturbances discussed earlier may play an important role. Thus, chronic ethanol administration to experimental animals given an adequate diet, failed to produce either metabolic derangements or osteoporosis.[130] Recently, Mobarhan *et al.* observed osteoporosis and low serum levels of 25(OH)D in 18 patients with Laennec's cirrhosis.[131] Treatment of several of these patients with vitamin D_2 or 25(OH)D for up to a year produced a significant increase in their bone density that was not observed in those patients who served as controls and were untreated. Notably, the serum 25(OH)D levels rose only slightly in the control patients while a 10- to 15-fold increase was observed in those receiving a vitamin D preparation. There were no changes in the ionized calcium concentration in either group. Over the follow-up period, the serum phosphorus concentration fell dramatically in the untreated patients while it remained unchanged in the vitamin D-treated group. Although urinary phosphate excretion was not examined, it is possible that a lack of the antiphosphaturic action of 25(OH)D may have contributed to the phosphate deficiency observed in the untreated patients.

7.3. Osteomalacia in Alcoholism

The occurrence of osteomalacia in alcoholics appears to be quite infrequent when adequate histologic studies of bone biopsy specimens have been performed. For example, Long *et al.* diagnosed osteomalacia in four of six alcoholics on whom they performed transiliac bone biopsy.[13] However, they did not directly examine the calcification fronts in these patients. In contrast, using double tetracycline labeling to examine the calcification fronts, other workers found no evidence for osteomalacia in alcoholics despite the concomitant presence of low serum levels of 25(OH)D.[131] When osteomalacia has been observed in alcoholics, coexistent malnutrition, in addition to vitamin D depletion, appears to be an important contributing factor.[25] In this clinical setting, a bone biopsy with appropriate histologic examination is the most reliable means of diagnosis, because bone pain and serologic tests and X-ray findings have a rather poor predictive value for osteomalacia. A good therapeutic response to the provision of an adequate diet and vitamin D supplementation should be expected.

8. Therapeutic Considerations

It is clear that most alcoholics have a reduced production of 25(OH)D independent of their hepatic functional status. In patients with alcoholic liver disease, synthesis of DBP is impaired and is responsible, at least in part, for a decrease in the total plasma 1,25$(OH)_2D_3$ concentration. Armed with this knowledge and, considering the potential roles for the impairment of vitamin D metabolism in the genesis of bone and mineral disturbances in the alcoholic, the physician caring for such patients must decide when to administer vitamin D supplements and which of the several available metabolites to use.

The most obvious indication for therapy with vitamin D in the alcoholic is the presence of osteomalacia and/or hypovitaminosis D. Previously, bone biopsy has been used to differentiate between osteomalacia and osteoporosis because X-rays and serologic biochemical tests are inadequate for this task. Vitamin D therapy has been reserved for those patients found to have osteomalacia, as osteoporosis was not thought to respond to any form of therapy.[132] However, the recent work of Mobarhan *et al.*[131] has provided evidence that osteoporosis in alcoholics improves with treatment with vitamin D. Therefore, use of the bone biopsy appears to be less important in the uncomplicated alcoholic patient, although it may still be particularly useful for those with bone pain or pathologic fractures.

Currently we recommend that alcoholics be screened periodically with X-rays and determination of the serum 25(OH)D concentration. Vitamin D supplementation is indicated for those with radiologic evidence of osteopenia and subnormal serum 25(OH)D levels. Ergocalciferol is an effective and economical agent and should be initiated at a dose of 50,000 I.U. orally once each week. If steatorrhea is present a three-times-per-week dosing schedule is reasonable. Dosage should be monitored with serial determinations of the serum calcium, phosphate, and 25(OH)D concentrations, and adjusted as necessary to normalize these parameters. A few patients may require calcium or phosphate supplementation. In those patients with documented, symptomatic osteomalacia, 1,25$(OH)_2D_3$ may be an appropriate initial agent because of its more rapid onset of action and greater potency. After symptoms have improved the patient may be switched to ergocalciferol.

Hypocalcemia, hypophosphatemia, and hypomagnesemia occurring in the hospitalized alcoholic are of multifactoral etiologies and are often unrelated to disturbances in vitamin D metabolism. Each patient must be evaluated individually to determine the causes of their disorders. Vitamin D deficiency, as evidenced by a low serum 25(OH)D concentration, can occasionally be implicated as a contributing factor in the pathogenesis of hypocalcemia and hypophosphatemia, and in such cases vitamin D therapy is indicated. In contrast, hypomagnesemia is unlikely to result from vitamin D deficiency per se, and, thus, is not an indication for treatment with vitamin D.

References

1. Haussler MR, Brickman AS: Vitamin D: metabolism, actions, and disease states, in Bronner F, Coburn JW (eds): *Disorders of Mineral Metabolism*, vol 2. *Calcium Physiology*. New York, Academic Press, 1982, pp 359–431.

2. Holick M: Synthesis, metabolism, and actions of vitamin D, in Brenner BM, Stein JH (eds): *Contemporary Issues in Nephrology*, vol 11. *Divalent Ion Homeostasis*. New York, Churchill Livingstone, 1983, pp 83–106.
3. Lemmann J Jr, Gray RW: Vitamin D metabolism and the kidney, in Dunn MJ (ed): *Renal Endocrinology*. Baltimore/London, Williams and Wilkins, 1983, pp 114–141.
4. Barragry JM, Corless D, Auton J, et al: Plasma vitamin D-binding globulin in vitamin D deficiency, pregnancy and chronic liver disease. *Clin Chim Acta* 87:359–365, 1978.
5. Barragry JM, Long RG, France MW, et al: Intestinal absorption of cholecalciferol in alcoholic liver disease and primary biliary cirrhosis. *Gut* 20:559–564, 1979.
6. Bikle DD, Gee E, Halloran B, et al: Free 1,25-dihydroxyvitamin D levels in serum from normal subjects, pregnant subjects, and subjects with liver disease. *J Clin Invest* 74:1966–1971, 1984.
7. Bouillon R, Auwerx J, Dekeyser L, et al: Serum vitamin D metabolites and their binding protein in patients with liver cirrhosis. *J Clin Endocrinol Metab* 59:86–89, 1984.
8. Garcia-Pascual B, Donath A, Courvoisier B: Plasma 250HD, bone mass densitometry and ^{47}CA intestinal absorption deficiency in chronic alcoholism, in Norman AW, Schaefer K, Coburn JW, et al (eds): *Vitamin D Biochemical, Chemical and Clinical Aspects Related to Calcium Metabolism*. Berlin/New York, deGruyter, 1977, pp 819–821.
9. Hepner GW, Roginsky M, Moo HF: Abnormal vitamin D metabolism in patients with cirrhosis. *Am J Dig Dis* 21:527–532, 1976.
10. Jung RT, Davie M, Hunter JO, et al: Abnormal vitamin D metabolism in cirrhosis. *Gut* 19:290–293, 1978.
11. Long RG, Wills MR, Skinner RK, et al: Serum-25-hydroxy-vitamin-D in untreated parenchymal and cholestatic liver disease. *Lancet* 2:650–652, 1976.
12. Long RG, Varghese Z, Skinner RK, et al: Phosphate metabolism in chronic liver disease. *Clin Chim Acta* 87:353–358, 1978.
13. Long RG, Meinhard E, Skinner RK, et al: Clinical, biochemical, and histological studies of osteomalacia, osteoporosis, and parathyroid function in chronic liver disease. *Gut* 19:85–90, 1978.
14. Meyer MS, Wexler S, Jedvab M, et al: Low levels of serum calcium, phosphorus and plasma 25-hydroxy vitamin D in cirrhosis of the liver. *Isr J Med Sci* 14:725–730, 1978.
15. Posner DB, Russell RM, Absood S, et al: Effective 25-hydroxylation of vitamin D_2 in alcoholic cirrhosis. *Gastroenterology* 74:866–870, 1978.
16. Roginsky MS, Zanzi I, Cohn SH: Skeletal and lean body mass in alcoholics with and without cirrhosis. *Calcif Tis Res* 21 (Suppl.):386–391, 1976.
17. Sonnenberg A, vonLifienfeld-Toal H, Sonnenberg GE, et al: Serum 25—hydroxyvitamin D_3 levels in patients with liver disease. *Acta Hepato-Gastroenterol* 24:256–258, 1977.
18. Velentzas C, Oreopoulos DG, Brandes L, et al: Abnormal vitamin-D levels. *Ann Int Med* 86:198, 1977.
19. Brown IRF, Carter ND, Sood A: Vitamin D binding globulin phenotypes in liver disease. *Clin Chim Acta* 95:75–82, 1979.
20. Imawari M, Akanuma Y, Itakura H, et al: The effects of diseases of the liver on serum 25-hydroxyvitamin D and on the serum binding protein for vitamin D and its metabolites. *J Lab Clin Med* 93:171–180, 1979.
21. Lund B, Sørensen OH, Hilden M, et al: The hepatic conversion of vitamin D in alcoholics with varying degrees of liver affection. *Acta Med Scand* 202:221–224, 1977.
22. Meyer M, Wechsler S, Shibolet S, et al: Malabsorption of vitamin D in patients and rat with liver cirrhosis, in Norman AW, Schaeffer K, Coburn JW, DeLuca HF, et al (eds): *Vitamin D Biochemical, Chemical and Clinical Aspects Related to Calcium Metabolism*. Berlin/New York, deGruyter, 1977, pp 831–833.
23. Devgun MS, Fiabane A, Paterson CR, et al: Vitamin and mineral nutrition in chronic alcoholics including patients with Korsakoff's psychosis. *Br J Nutr* 45:469–473, 1981.

24. Leevy CM, Thompson A, Baker H: Vitamins and liver injury. *Am J Clin Nutr* 23:493–499, 1970.
25. Dibble JB, Sheridan P, Hampshire R, et al: Osteomalacia, vitamin D deficiency and cholestasis in chronic liver disease. *Q J Med* 51:89–103, 1982.
26. Long RG, Sherlock S: Vitamin D in chronic liver disease, in Popper H, Schaffner F: *Progress in Liver Diseases*, vol 6. New York, Grune & Stratton, 1979, pp 539–555.
27. Meyer MS, Edelstein S, Peled M, et al: Intestinal loss of vitamin D_3 metabolites in rats with cirrhosis of the liver. *Isr J Med Sci* 18:1027–1031, 1982.
28. Avioli LV, Lee SW, McDonald JE, et al: Metabolism of vitamin D_3–^3H in human subjects: distribution in blood, bile, feces, and urine. *J Clin Invest* 46:983–992, 1967.
29. Beard JD, Knott DH: Fluid and electrolyte balance during acute withdrawal in chronic alcoholic patients. *JAMA* 204:133–139, 1968.
30. Lim P, Jacob E: Magnesium deficiency in liver cirrhosis. *Q J Med* 41:291–300, 1972.
31. Lim P, Jacob E: Magnesium status of alcoholic patients. *Metabolism* 21:1045–1051, 1972.
32. Long RG, Varghese Z, Wills MR, et al: Plasma calcium and magnesium fractions in liver disease. *Clin Chim Acta* 84:239–245, 1978.
33. Ryback RS, Eckardt MJ, Pautler CP: Clinical relationships between serum phosphorus and other blood chemistry values in alcoholics. *Arch Int Med* 140:673–677, 1980.
34. Mills PR, Shenkin A, Anthony RS, et al: Assessment of nutritional status and in vivo immune responses in alcoholic liver disease. *Am J Clin Nutr* 38:849–859, 1983.
35. Stutzman FL, Amatuzio DS: Blood serum magnesium in portal cirrhosis and diabetes mellitus. *J Lab Clin Med* 41:215–219, 1953.
36. Martin HE, McCuskey C Jr, Tupikova N: Electrolyte disturbance in acute alcoholism. *Am J Clin Nutr* 7:191–196, 1959.
37. Heaton FW, Pyrah LN, Beresford CC, et al: Hypomagnesaemia in chronic alcoholism. *Lancet* 2:802–805, 1962.
38. Sullivan JF, Wolpert PW, Williams R, et al: Serum magnesium in chronic alcoholism. *Ann NY Acad Sci* 162:947–962, 1969.
39. Chatterjea MN, Saran A: Serum magnesium in hepatic diseases. *J Assoc Phys Ind* 24:507–510, 1976.
40. Sullivan JF, Blotcky AJ, Jetton MM, et al: Serum levels of selenium, calcium, copper, magnesium, manganese and zinc in various human diseases. *J Nutr* 109:1432–1437, 1979.
41. Dunn MJ, Walser M: Magnesium depletion in normal man. *Metabolism 15:884–895, 1966.*
42. Jones JE, Shane SR, Jacobs WH, et al: Magnesium balance studies in chronic alcoholism. *Ann NY Acad Sci* 162:934–946, 1969.
43. Bøhmer T, Mathiesen B: Magnesium deficiency in chronic alcoholic patients uncovered by an intravenous loading test. *Scand J Clin Lab Invest* 42:633–636, 1982.
44. McCollister RJ, Flink EB, Doe RP: Magnesium balance studies in chronic alcoholism. *J Lab Clin Med* 55:98–104, 1960.
45. Mendelson JH, Barnes B, Mayman C, et al: The determination of exchangeable magnesium in alcoholic patients. *Metabolism* 14:88–97, 1965.
46. Stendig-Lindberg G, Bergstrom J, Hultman E: Hypomagnesaemia and muscle electrolytes and metabolites. *Acta Med Scand* 201:273–280, 1977.
47. Alfrey AC, Miller NL, Butkus D: Evaluation of body magnesium stores. *J Lab Clin Med* 84:153–162, 1974.
48. Thomson AD; Alcohol and nutrition. *Clin Endocrinol Metab* 7:405–428, 1978.
49. Shils ME: Experimental human magnesium depletion. *Medicine* 48:61–85, 1969.
50. Shils ME: Experimental production of magnesium deficiency in man. Ann NY Acad Sci 162:847–855, 1969.
51. Booth CC, Babouris N, Hanna S, et al: Incidence of hypomagnesaemia in intestinal malabsorption. *Br Med J* 2:141–144, 1963.
52. Hanna S: Plasma magnesium in health and disease. *J Clin Pathol* 14:410–414, 1961.

53. Caddell JL: Magnesium deficiency in protein-calorie malnutrition: a follow-up study. *Ann NY Acad Sci* 162:874–890, 1969.
54. Hersh T, Siddiqui DA: Magnesium and the pancreas. *Am J Clin Nutr* 26:362–366, 1973.
55. Hodgkinson A, Marshall DH, Nordin BEC: Vitamin D and magnesium absorption in man. *Clin Sci* 57:121–123, 1979.
56. Levine BS, Brautbar N, Walling MW, et al: Effects of vitamin D and diet magnesium on magnesium metabolism. *Am J Physiol* 239:E515–E523, 1980.
57. Kalbfleisch JM, Lindeman RD, Ginn HE, et al: Effects of ethanol administration on urinary excretion of magnesium and other electrolytes in alcoholic and normal subjects. *J Clin Invest* 42:1471–1475, 1963.
58. McCollister RJ, Flink EB, Lewis MD: Urinary excretion of magnesium in man following the ingestion of ethanol. *Am J Clin Nutr* 12:415–420, 1963.
59. Dick M, Evans RA, Watson L: Effect of ethanol on magnesium excretion. *J Clin Pathol* 22:152–153, 1969.
60. Mendelson JH, Ogata M, Mello NK: Effects of alcohol ingestion and withdrawal on magnesium states of alcoholics: clinical and experimental findings. *Ann NY Acad Sci* 162:918–933, 1969.
61. Drenick EJ, Hunt IF, Swendseid ME: Magnesium depletion during prolonged fasting of obese males. *J Clin Endocrinol Metab* 29:1341–1348, 1969.
62. Anast CS, Gardner DW: Magnesium metabolism, in Bronner F, Coburn JW (eds): *Disorders of Mineral Metabolism,* vol 3. *Pathophysiology of Calcium, Phosphorus, and Magnesium.* New York, Academic Press, 1981, pp 423–506.
63. Dominguez JH, Gray RW, Lemann J Jr: Dietary phosphate deprivation in women and men: Effects on mineral and acid balances, parathyroid hormone and the metabolism of 25-OH-vitamin D. *J Clin Endocrinol Metab* 43:1056–1068, 1976.
64. Kreusser W, Kurakawa K, Aznar E, et al: Effect of phosphate depletion on magnesium homeostasis in rats. *J Clin Invest* 61:573–581, 1978.
65. Jackson CE, Meier DW: Routine serum magnesium analysis. Correlation with clinical state in 5,100 patients. *Ann Int Med* 69:743–748, 1968.
66. Martin HE: Clinical magnesium deficiency. *Ann NY Acad Sci* 162:891–900, 1969.
67. Wheeler PG, Smith T, Golindano C, et al: Postassium and magnesium depletion in patients with cirrhosis on maintenance diuretic regimes. *Gut* 18:683–687, 1977.
68. Cohen MI, McNamara H, Finberg L: Serum magnesium in children with cirrhosis. *J Pediatr* 76:453–455, 1970.
69. Massry SG, Coburn JW, Chapman LW, et al: The effect of NaCl infusion on urinary Ca^{++} and Mg^{++} during reduction in their filtered loads. *Am J Physiol* 213:1218–1224, 1967.
70. Massry SG, Coburn JW, Kleeman CR: Renal handling of magnesium in the dog. *Am J Physiol* 216:1460–1467, 1969.
71. Wolfe SM, Victor M: The relationship of hypomagnesemia and alkalosis to alcohol withdrawal symptoms. *Ann NY Acad Sci* 162:973–984, 1969.
72. Lostroh AJ, Krahl ME: Magnesium, a second messenger for insulin: ion translocation coupled to transport activity. *Adv Enz Reg* 12:73–81, 1973.
73. Flink EB, Shane SR, Scobbo RR, et al: Relationship of free fatty acids and magnesium in ethanol withdrawal in dogs. *Metabolism* 28:858–865, 1979.
74. Ebel H, Gunther T: Magnesium metabolism: A review. *J Clin Chem Clin Biochem* 18:257–270, 1980.
75. Rude RK, Singer FR: Magnesium deficiency and excess. *Ann Rev Med* 32:245–259, 1981.
76. Lieber CS: General nutritional status in the alcoholic, includng disorders of minerals and vitamins, in Smith LH Jr (ed): *Major Problems in Internal Medicine,* vol 22. *Medical Disorders of Alcoholism: Pathogenesis and Treatment.* Philadelphia, WB Saunders, 1982, pp 551–568.
77. Zieve L: Influence of magnesium deficiency on the utilization of thiamine. *Ann NY Acad Sci* 162:732–743, 1969.

78. MacIntyre I, Davidsson D: The production of secondary potassium depletion, sodium retention, nephrocalcinosis and hypercalcaemia by magnesium deficiency. *Biochem J* 70:456–462, 1958.
79. Whang R, Morosi HJ, Rodgers D, et al: The influence of sustained magnesium deficiency on muscle potassium repletion. *J Lab Clin Med* 70:895–902, 1967.
80. Estep H, Shaw WA, Watlington C, et al: Hypocalcemia due to hypomagnesemia and reversible parathyroid hormone unresponsiveness. *J Clin Endocrinol Metab* 29:842–848, 1969.
81. Rude RK, Oldham SB, Singer FR: Functional hypoparathyroidism and parathyroid hormone end-organ resistance in human magnesium deficiency. *Clin Endocrinol* 5:209–224, 1976.
82. Rude RK, Oldham SB, Sharp CF Jr, et al: Parathyroid hormone secretion in magnesium deficiency. *J Clin Endocrinol Metab* 47:800–806, 1978.
83. Medalle R, Waterhouse C, Hahn TJ: Vitamin D resistance in magnesium deficiency. *Am J Clin Nutr* 29:854–858, 1976.
84. Anast CS, Winnacker JL, Forte LR, et al: Impaired release of parathyroid hormone in magnesium deficiency. *J Clin Endocrinol Metab* 42:707–717, 1976.
85. MacManus J, Heaton FW, Lucas PW: A decreased response to parathyroid hormone in magnesium deficiency. *J Endocrinol* 49:253–258, 1971.
86. Freitag JJ, Martin KJ, Conrades MB, et al: Evidence for skeletal resistance to parathyroid hormone in magnesium deficiency. *J Clin Invest* 64:1238–1244, 1979.
87. MacManus J, Heaton FW: The influence of magnesium on calcium release from bone in vitro. *Biochim Biophys Acta* 215:360–367, 1970.
88. Victor M: The role of hypomagnesemia and respiratory alkalosis in the genesis of alcohol-withdrawal symptoms. *Ann NY Acad Sci* 215:235–248, 1973.
89. Fankushen D, Rasin D, Dimich A, et al: The significance of hypo-magnesemia in alcoholic patients. *Am J Med* 37:802–812, 1964.
90. Bogden JD, Troiano RA; Plasma calcium, copper, magnesium, and zinc concentrations in patients with the alcohol withdrawal syndrome. *Clin Chem* 24:1553–1556, 1978.
91. Moore, EW: Studies with ion exchange calcium electrodes. III. The state of serum calcium in patients with cirrhosis. *Gastroenterology* 60:43–54, 1971.
92. Knochel JP: Renal disease, water, and electrolyte metabolism in the alcoholic, in Suki W, Eknoyan G (eds): *The Kidney in Systemic Disease*, ed 2. New York, Wiley, 1981, pp 347–357.
93. Levine BS, Walling MW, Coburn JW: Intestinal absorption of calcium: its assessment, normal physiology, and alterations in various disease states, in Bronner F, Coburn JW (eds): *Disorders of Mineral metabolism*, vol 2. *Calcium Physiology*. New York, Academic Press, 1982, pp 103–188.
94. Krawitt EL: Effect of ethanol ingestion on duodenal calcium transport. *J Lab Clin Med* 85:665–671, 1975
95. Krawitt EL, Sampson HW, Katagiri CA: Effect of 1,25-dihydroxycholecalciferol on ethanol mediated suppression of calcium absorption. *Calcif Tiss Res* 18:119–124, 1975.
96. Decaux G, Hallemans R, Mockel J, et al: Chronic alcoholism: A predisposing factor for hypocalcemia in acute pancreatitis. *Digestion* 20:175–179, 1980.
97. Peng TC, Cooper CW, Munson PL: The hypocalcemic effect of ethyl alcohol in rats and dogs. *Endocrinology* 91:586–593, 1972.
98. Peng TC, Gitelman HJ: Ethanol-induced hypocalcemia, hypermagnesemia and inhibition of the serum calcium-raising effect of parathyroid hormone in rats. *Endocrinology* 94:608–611, 1974.
99. Shah JH, Bowser EN, Hargis GK, et al: Effect of ethanol on parathyroid hormone secretion in the rat. *Metabolism* 27:257–260, 1978.
100. Williams GA, Bowser EN, Hargis GK, et al: Effect of ethanol on parathyroid hormone and calcitonin secretion in man. *Proc Soc Exp Biol Med* 159:187–191, 1978.
101. Avery DH, Overall JE, Calil HM, et al: Plasma calcium and phosphate during alcohol intoxication. Alcoholics versus non-alcoholics. *J Stud alcohol* 44:205–214, 1983.

102. Markkanen T, Nanto V: The effect of ethanol infusion on the calcium-phosphorus balance in man. *Experientia* 22:753–754, 1966.
103. Linkola J, Fyhrquist F, Ylikahri R: Adenosine 3′,5′ cyclinc monophosphate, calcium and magnesium excretion in ethanol intoxication and hangover. *Acta Physiol Scand* 107:333–337, 1979.
104. Territo MC, Tanaka KR: Hypophosphatemia in chronic alcoholism. *Arch Int Med* 134:445–447, 1974.
105. Larsson L, Rebel K, Sorbo B: Severe hypophosphatemia—a hospital survey. *Acta Med Scand* 214:221–223, 1983.
106. Stein JH, Smith WO, Ginn HE: Hypophosphatemia in acute alcoholism. *Am J Med Sci* 252:78–83, 1966.
107. Knochel JP, Bilbrey GL, Fuller TJ, et al: The muscle cell in chronic alcoholism: the possible role of phosphate depletion in alcoholic myopathy. *Ann NY Acad Sci* 252:274–286, 1975.
108. Anderson R, Cohen M, Haller R, et al: Skeletal muscle phosphorus and magnesium deficiency in alcoholic myopathy. *Mineral electrolyte Metab* 4:106–112, 1980.
109. Blachley JD, Ferguson ER, Carter NW, et al: Chronic alcohol ingestion induces phosphorus deficiency and myopathy in the dog. *Trans Assoc Am Phys* 93:110–122, 1980.
110. Caniggia A, Gennari C: Intestinal absorption of radiophosphate after physiological doses of $25(OH)D_3$ in normals, liver cirrhosis and chronic renal failure patients, in Normal AW, Schaefer K, Coburn JW, et al (eds): *Vitamin D Biochemical, Chemical and Clinical Aspects Related to Calcium Metabolism.* Berlin/New York, deGruyter, 1977, pp 755–757.
111. Clark I: Effects of magnesium ions on calcium and phosphorus metabolism. *Am J Physiol* 214:348–356, 1968.
112. Petersen VP: Metabolic studies in clinical magnesium deficiency. *Acta Med Scand* 173:285–298, 1963.
113. Whang R, Welt LG: Observations in experimental magnesium depletion. *J Clin Invest* 42:305–313, 1963.
114. Adler AJ, Gudis S, Berlyne GM: Reduced renal phosphate threshold concentration in alcoholic cirrhosis. *Mineral Electrolyte Metab* 10:63–66, 1984.
115. Puschett JB, Moranz J, Kurnick WS: Evidence for a direct action of cholecalciferol and 25-hydroxycholecalciferol on the renal transport of phosphate, sodium, and calcium. *J Clin Invest* 51:373–385, 1972.
116. Winaver J, Sylk DB, Robertson JS, et al: Micropuncture study of the acute renal tubular transport effects of 25-hydroxyvitamin D_3 in the dog. *Mineral Electrolyte Metab* 4:178–188, 1980.
117. Wolfe SM, Mendelson J, Ogata M, et al: Respiratory alkalosis and alcohol withdrawal. *Trans Assoc Am Phys* 82:344–352, 1969.
118. Mostellar ME, Tuttle EP Jr: The effects of alkalosis on plasma concentration and urinary excretion of inorganic phosphate in man. *J Clin Invest* 43:138–149, 1964.
119. Knochel JP: The pathophysiology and clinical characteristics of severe hypophosphatemia. *Arch Int Med* 137:203–220, 1977.
120. Miller PD, Heinig RE, Waterhouse C: Treatment of alcoholic acidosis. The role of dextrose and phosphorus. *Arch Int Med* 138:67–72, 1978.
121. Nilsson BE: Conditions contributing to fracture of the femoral neck. *Acta Chir Scand* 136:383–384, 1970.
122. Johnell O, Nilsson BE, Wiklund PE: Bone morphometry in alcoholics. *Clin Orthop* 165:253–258, 1982.
123. Saville PD: Alcohol-related skeletal disorders. *Ann NY Acad Sci* 252:287–291, 1975.
124. Thornhill HL, Richter RW, Shelton ML, et al: Neuropathic arthropathy (Charcot forefeet) in alcoholics. *Orthop Clin N Am* 4:7–20, 1973.
125. Epstein O, Dick R, Sherlock S: Prospective study of periostitis and finger clubbing in primary biliary cirrhosis and other forms of chronic liver disease. *Gut* 22:203–206, 1981.
126. Saville PD: Changes in bone mass with age and alcoholism. *J Bone Joint Surg* 47-A:492–499, 1965.

127. Nilsson BE, Westlin NE: Changes in bone mass in alcoholics. *Clin Orthop* 90:229–232, 1973.
128. Nilsson BE, Westlin NE: Femur density in alcoholism and after gastrectomy. *Calcif Tiss Res* 10:167–170, 1972.
129. Dalen N, Lamke B: One mineral losses in alcoholics. *Acta Orthop Scand* 47:469–471, 1976.
130. Mezey E, Potter JJ, Merchant CR: Effect of ethanol feeding on bone composition in the rat. *J Clin Nutr* 32:25–29, 1979.
131. Mobarhan SA, Russell RM, Recker RR, et al: Metabolic bone disease in alcoholic cirrhosis: a comparison of the effect of vitamin D_2, 25-hydroxyvitamin D, or supportive treatment. *Hepatology* 4:266–273, 1984.
132. Long RG, Wills MR: Hepatic osteodystrophy. *Br J Hosp Med* 20:312–321, 1978.

17

The Pathogenesis of Renal Sodium Retention and Ascites Formation in Laennec's Cirrhosis

Thomas O. Pitts and David H. Van Thiel

Abstract This chapter critically reviews our current understanding of the pathogenesis, clinical syndrome, and therapy of the disturbances of renal sodium handling, renal perfusion, and glomerular filtration rate that occur in patients with Laennec's cirrhosis. Avid renal sodium reabsorption, a characteristic feature of cirrhosis, occurs independent of moderate changes in renal function and precedes the onset of ascites. The initiation of sodium retention may be a direct consequence of the hepatic disease process and may also result from defective intravascular filling. In the presence of ascites the most important sodium retaining signal is a defective intravascular volume. The principal effectors of renal sodium retention and vasoconstriction are stimulation of the renin–angiotensin–aldosterone axis and augmentation of renal sympathetic nerve activity. Deficient production of natriuretic hormone(s) and endogenous renal vasodilators, such as prostaglandins and kinins, also contributes to the sodium retention and renal hypoperfusion seen in cirrhosis. The hepatorenal syndrome is an extreme imbalance in these renal vasoconstrictor and vasodilator forces. In the therapy of ascites in Laennec's cirrhosis, abstention from alcohol, sodium restriction, and cautious diuresis are the principal therapeutic measures. A grave prognosis accompanies the diagnosis of the hepatorenal syndrome although recoveries have been reported.

1. Introduction

Laennec's cirrhosis is a major cause of morbidity and mortality in adult males.[1] Ascites, a common complication of alcoholic cirrhosis, is recognized as a difficult management problem and is generally associated with a poor prognosis.[2] Although an association between oliguric renal failure and advanced Laennec's cirrhosis was described well over a century ago,[3] the importance of the kidneys in the avid sodium and fluid retention of this disorder has become clear only in the last four decades.[4] Investigation of the mechanisms

Thomas O. Pitts • Renal–Electrolyte Division, Department of Medicine, University of Pittsburgh School of Medicine, Pittsburgh, Pennsylvania 15261. **David H. Van Thiel** • Division of Gastroenterology, Department of Medicine, University of Pittsburgh School of Medicine, Pittsburgh, Pennsylvania 15261.

underlying the initiation and maintenance of ascites and the occasional deterioration of the condition to oliguric renal insufficiency has implicated a number of factors that include circulatory imbalances, altered neural pathways, abnormalities in various hormonal systems, and retention of metabolic products. Much debate exists as to whether the kidneys are primarily at fault or are unwitting participants in the initiation of ascites. Interestingly, despite a proliferation of data bearing on the renal abnormalities of cirrhosis, relatively few changes have been introduced into the standard medical management of the condition over the last decade.

In this chapter we will examine the current concepts regarding the role of the kidneys in the disturbed sodium and volume homeostasis of alcoholic cirrhosis. We will provide a description of the factors involved in the initiation and maintenance of ascites and the onset of the hepatorenal syndrome. A brief review of current trends in the medical therapy of these conditions is also provided. We will restrict our discussion as much as possible to Laennec's cirrhosis, which is the most common form of cirrhosis in the United States as well as in other developed countries. Of necessity, findings from experimental models of cirrhosis and nonalcoholic cirrhosis will be included.

2. Clinical Features

2.1. Presentation

The clinical presentation of patients with Laennec's cirrhosis encompasses a broad spectrum ranging from the asymptomatic (compensated) state to sodium retention with overt ascites (decompensated) to the oliguric functional renal failure commonly referred to as the hepatorenal syndrome. Patients may change from a compensated to a decompensated state with relative ease.[5,6] Roughly 30% of decompensated cirrhotics will undergo a spontaneous diuresis with bed rest and sodium restriction.[7] The development of ascites is often seen in conjunction with a deterioration in previously stable hepatic function, but sodium loading (e.g., dietary indiscretion), in the absence of new hepatic functional loss, may induce decompensation. The progression to oliguric renal failure is usually seen in patients with the most advanced hepatic disease and, indeed, may occur in a majority of patients with end-stage cirrhosis as a preterminal event.[8] Although some patients with oliguric renal failure and decompensated cirrhosis may have a reversible component to their renal failure, cirrhotics with the hepatorenal syndrome rarely undergo spontaneous remission.[9]

2.2. Renal Function in Cirrhosis

Glomerular filtration rate as determined by inulin or endogenous creatinine clearance is usually normal in compensated cirrhotic patients[10,11] but may be mildly depressed.[12] Renal plasma flow, estimated from para-aminohippurate clearance, is also normal in these subjects.[10,11,13] The serum creatinine correlates poorly with renal function due to the muscle wasting that is common in alcoholics[14] and usually does not rise above the normal range until the glomerular filtation rate falls below 30–50 ml/min.[5,10,11]

Glomerular filtration rate and renal plasma flow are quite variable when ascites is present. Baldus *et al.* reported that these parameters are usually normal in patients whose ascites responds rapidly to dietary sodium restriction and diuretics, while subnormal values occur in the presence of more resistant ascites.[10,11] Others have confirmed that mild decrements in glomerular filtration rate and renal plasma flow are common with decompensated cirrhosis.[15,16]

In contrast, a prospective study of 17 patients with Laennec's cirrhosis revealed no correlation between glomerular filtration rate or renal plasma flow and degree of compensation.[5] This emphasizes that the clinical status of an individual may vary independently of renal function, unless hepatorenal syndrome supervenes.

2.3. Renal Sodium Handling

Avid renal sodium retention is a prominent feature of the decompensated cirrhotic patient.[17,18] Compensated cirrhotic individuals excrete a greater percentage of their filtered sodium than do ascitic patients.[10] However, despite the fact that cirrhotic patients may maintain sodium balance while in the compensated state, these individuals have a persistent defect in their ability to excrete sodium. Naccarato *et al.* produced isotonic volume expansion in eight biopsy-proven cirrhotic patients with no history of ascites or edema and compared the resultant changes in sodium excretion with those obtained in a group of normal subjects. Both fractional sodium excretion and the rate of sodium excretion were significantly higher in normals than in the compensated cirrhotics following volume expansion.[19] There were no changes in endogenous creatinine clearance in either group. Thus, renal sodium handling is abnormal early in the course of cirrhosis before decompensation is evident or measurable alterations in renal function occur.

2.4. Segmental Sites of Sodium Reabsorption

Several lines of evidence have implicated the proximal tubule as a major site of augmented sodium reabsorption in cirrhosis. As compensated patients spontaneously develop ascites the glomerular filtration rate and renal blood flow often decrease slightly.[10,11] In many subjects the renal blood flow may decline out of proportion or independent of the glomerular filtration rate, resulting in an increase in the filtration fraction, i.e., that percentage of renal plasma flow filtered across the glomerulus.[5,11] The increase in filtration fraction raises the protein concentration in the peritubular capillaries, which favors proximal tubular reabsorption. Micropuncture studies in experimental cirrhosis in rats and dogs have provided support for this concept.[20–23]

Because the renal generation of free water depends on sodium reabsorption in the diluting segment of the distal renal tubule, water excretion is impaired if avid proximal tubular sodium reabsorption diminishes distal sodium delivery. Hyponatremia and diminished free water clearance are common features of cirrhotics. Enhancement of distal sodium delivery using the osmotic diuertic mannitol[24,25] or by volume expansion[26,27] often improves water excretion in cirrhotics, suggesting that avid proximal sodium reabsorption is present in these patients.

Somewhat variable results have been found using the technique of water loading, which allows investigators to estimate the relative contributions of proximal and distal sodium transport to overall sodium reabsorption. In compensated cirrhotics isotonic volume expansion during maximal water diuresis produces a smaller increment in proximal fractional sodium excretion than is seen in normal controls, while distal sodium handling remains normal.[19] In contrast, some decompensated cirrhotics have normal sodium delivery out of the proximal tubule and elevated distal sodium reabsorption during hypotonic saline diuresis.[28] Wilkinson *et al.* have compared the segmental sodium handling of cirrhotics in sodium balance with that of cirrhotics during sodium retention. The sodium avid state was associated with increased reabsorption at both the proximal and the distal tubular sites.[29] The latter observations are in agreement with micropuncture findings.[23]

Finally, since sodium and phosphate are reabsorbed in parallel in the proximal tubules, segmental sodium handling has been examined inferentially by comparing changes in sodium and phosphate excretion induced by volume expansion. Phosphaturia occurs uniformly in cirrhotics following volume expansion regardless of the state of compensation, whereas the natriuresis may be normal, blunted or absent.[30,31]

Taken as a whole the available data suggest that while proximal reabsorption of sodium is increased frequently in cirrhotics, distal tubular sites also play an important role in sodium retention. Whether proximal or distal reabsorption predominates at any point in time depends on the prevailing pathophysiologic factors.

2.5. Circulatory Alterations in Cirrhosis

A variety of circulator disturbances of relevance to renal function occur in cirrhotics. Plasma volume and whole blood volume are both generally elevated or normal and appear to be independent of the state of compensation.[32,33] Similarly the cardiac output is usually normal or elevated in cirrhotic patients.[32,34,35] This results in part from the opening of systemic anteriovenous shunts, decreased peripheral vascular resistance and an expanded blood volume.[32,36,37] In addition to the elevated cardiac output, cirrhotic subjects appear to have an impaired response to cardiotropic agents.[38] Moreover, the presence of tense ascites may impair cardiac output further by diminishing venous return.[39] In the nonazotemic patient, a change from a compensated to a decompensated state or vice versa does not appear to correlate with any obvious change in the cardiac output. In patients who progress to oliguria with diminished renal function, renal blood flow falls and renal vascular resistance rises well above the normal range.[35,40] Some patients develop lowered arterial blood pressure and cardiac output but the response to volume replacement is variable.[41]

2.6. Summary of Clinical Features

Cirrhotics may present to the physician either in a compensated state, i.e., free of ascites, or in a decompensated condition manifesting avid sodium retention and ascites. Advanced hepatic cirrhosis is associated often with progression to functional renal failure. Nonetheless, most cirrhotic subjects have normal renal function, particularly so when in the compensated state. Avid sodium retention appears to occur independent of the glomerular filtration rate and renal blood flow. The kidneys appear to reabsorb sodium in excess both in the proximal and distal tubules and the prevailing sites of sodium reabsorption depend on the current pathophysiology. Cirrhotics demonstrate a wide range of circulatory alterations. Blood volumes usually are elevated early in cirrhosis. Moreover, the cardiac output is usually increased. The heart rate is usually higher in cirrhotic patients than it is in normals. Thus, cirrhotic individuals are characterized by a decrease in peripheral vascular resistance and the opening of a wide array of arteriovenous shunts within the systemic circuit.

3. Consequences of Hepatic Cell Destruction Favoring Ascites Formation

The repetitive pattern of cell destruction, nodular regeneration, and fibrosis characteristic of alcoholic liver disease ultimately leads to permanent physical alterations of the hepatic architecture and intrahepatic hemodynamics. In addition, many synthetic and degradative functions of the liver are impaired as the hepatic pathology progresses. Several pathologic processes occurring in the liver play major roles in the pathogenesis of ascites both independent of and in concert with the previously identified renal functional changes. Although a detailed review of the physiologic and hemodynamic consequences of the alterations in hepatic cellular architecture in Laennec's cirrhosis is beyond the scope of this chapter, it is appropriate to examine certain of these factors in terms of their effects on renal function. The reader is referred to any of several recent reviews for a more thorough description of these abnormalities.[42–46]

3.1. Hepatic Venous Outflow Obstruction

The *sine qua non* for ascites formation is obstruction of hepatic venous outflow.[46] Obstruction of the hepatic veins experimentally[47,48] or clinically (as in the Budd–Chiari Syndrome) results in ascites, whereas hepatic inflow obstruction does not.[49] Radiologic studies as well as postmorten histologic and gross anatomic evaluations of cirrhotics have demonstrated the uniform presence of extensive fibrotic compression of hepatic outflow tracks with a relative increase in inflow volume.[50–53] Hepatic venous outflow block has several effects which result in ascites.

3.1.1. Lymphatic Flow. The most important cause of hepatic venous outflow block is intrasinusoidal hypertension. This occurs because hepatic inflow from the portal veins and hepatic artery is not diminished in proportion to outflow obstruction. Under normal conditions hepatic sinusoidal pressure favors transudation of fluid from the sinusoids to the space of Disse from where it reenters the circulation via the regional lymphatics and the thoracic duct. In the normal liver and early in cirrhosis, the hepatic sinusoids are freely permeable to protein. Thus, there is no oncotic gradient retarding flow out of the sinusoids, and intrasinusoidal hydrostatic pressure is the primary force driving the formation of hepatic lymph. When cirrhosis is present, the progressive elevation of sinusoidal pressure induces a tremendous increase in lymph flow through the thoracic duct.[54] When the rate of lymph formation exceeds the capacity of the lymphatics to return it to the circulation, the excess lymph exudes from the surface of the liver as ascitic fluid. Clinically detectable ascites occurs when ascitic fluid formation exceeds its reabsorption from the peritoneal cavity.[43,45]

3.1.2. Sodium Retention. Hepatic venous outflow block may eventuate in renal sodium retention in a number of ways. In a series of experiments in dogs, Orloff *et al.* have demonstrated that elevated intrahepatic pressure activates the renin–angiotensin system independently of any measurable hemodynamic changes produced by the maneuver. Relatively small increases in intrahepatic pressure produced by mechanical partial venous outflow obstruction result in a stimulation of aldosterone synthesis.[55] Bilateral nephrectomy obviates the aldosterone response, suggesting that the renal production of renin is the mediator of this reflex.[56] When blood is cross-circulated from a nephrectomized animal undergoing graded hepatic venous outflow occlusion to an intact animal, aldosterone, but not cortisol or corticosterone secretion, is stimulated in the recipient animal in proportion to the degree of hepatic venous occlusion produced in the donor.[57] Thus, it has been suggested that a humoral agent, possibly of hepatic origin, released in response to sinusoidal hypertension produces renal renin release and subsequent hypersecretion of aldosterone.[46,57]

Although the putative humoral mediator of renin secretion in cirrhosis has not been described, recent work by Kostreva *et al.* has demonstrated an activation of the renal afferent nerve fibers in response to an increase in hepatic sinusoidal pressure.[58] Moreover, renal nerve stimulation may reduce sodium excretion directly and induce renin secretion.[59] These observations are in agreement with those of Orloff *et al.*[55–57] in an experimental model of ascites.

Hepatic venous outflow block may blunt urinary sodium excretion without stimulating aldosterone. Levy produced hepatic venous outflow block in dogs by the infusion of histamine into the portal vein.[60] In contrast to the studies of Orloff *et al.*, this technique results in decrements of both central venous pressure and renal perfusion. However, when the potential contributions of aldosterone, central hypovolemia, renal nerve stimulation, portal hypertension, and increased filtration fraction are each eliminated, a defect in renal sodium excretion persists. Hepatic release of a putative antinaturetic factor acting directly on the renal tubules may explain, at least in part, the sodium retention seen with this model.[60]

Other possible mechanisms by which hepatic venous outflow block may result in sodium retention include decreased hepatic clearance of renin and aldosterone occurring as a result of impaired hepatic blood flow[61] and reflex renal nervous stimulation due to diminished effective intravascular volume induced by the sequestration of blood in the portal circulation.[42,60]

3.2. Portal Hypertension

Portal venous hypertension occurs as a consequence of hepatic venous outflow block. While obstruction of the portal vein flow is not itself the initial cause of ascites in the laboratory animal, it may exacerbate ascites formation in cirrhotic individuals in a number of ways.

3.2.1. Lymph Formation. Under normal conditions intestinal capillary hydrostatic pressure exceeds the local blood-lymph oncotic pressure gradient, thereby favoring the formation of gut lymph. When the portal venous pressure is elevated, fluid is extruded into the tissues in a greater proportion than is plasma protein, resulting in a hypotonic lymph fluid.[62] Eventually the oncotic pressure gradient retards further lymph formation. With extreme, chronic elevation of portal vein pressure, oncotic inhibition of lymph formation is overcome and the excessive lymph weeps from the mesentery and bowel surface increasing the ascites.[63,64] Patients with advanced hepatic disease not only have severe hepatic venous outflow block but also have a presinusoidal obstruction to portal inflow,[63] which results in a sizeable increase in the contribution of gut lymph to the production of ascites.

3.2.2. Portasystemic Shunting. Portal venous hypertension results in the formation of a network of collateral veins that shunt portal venous blood into the systemic circulation. This results in abnormal sodium handling due to alterations in the delivery of absorbed products to the liver. For example, if sodium is ingested orally[65] or infused into the portal vein,[66] there is a more rapid natriuresis than when it is infused into the systemic circuit. Interesting as these findings are, it should be noted that others have been unable to duplicate them.[42,67]

Some evidence suggests that portasystemic shunting may be a protective factor in cirrhotic patients. Lebrec *et al.* have compared systemic and splanchnic hemodynamic observations in a group of cirrhotics with refractory ascites with those obtained from patients with medically responsive ascites.[68] Both groups had similar degrees of hepatic dysfunction, arterial blood pressure, hepatic venous outflow block, portal hypertension, and hepatic blood flow. The group with refractory ascites had a lower mean cardiac output and greater systemic vascular resistance. There was *less* portasystemic shunting in the refractory group than in the responsive subjects. The intrahepatic resistance was slightly higher in the refractory group although this difference was not statistically significant. Unfortunately, the study was carried out when the responsive patients had cleared most of their ascites such that the effects of the ascites could not be examined. Nevertheless, in some patients, ascites formation may be exacerbated when portal collateral resistance is high.[68]

3.2.3. Renal Effects of Portal Venous Hypertension. There is considerable controversy as to the role of portal venous hypertension in the development of abnormal renal sodium handling. In addition, all the data that bear on the issue have been obtained in animals subjected to acute rather than chronic changes in portal venous pressure. In the patient with alcoholic cirrhosis, portal venous hypertension develops very slowly and, thus, is not pathophysiologically well represented by an acute animal model. All experimental findings in animals must be judged with this limitation in mind.

Levy studied the effects of graded elevations of portal venous pressure in normal dogs on systemic and renal hemodynamics and renal sodium handling.[69] With increases in portal venous pressure roughly three times over baseline, there were no changes in glomerular filtration rate, renal blood flow or urinary sodium excretion. All three parameters fell when further portal venous pressure increases resulted in hypotension. Similar declines were noted in these parameters when the renal perfusion pressure was lowered by arterial clamping in dogs free of portal hypertension. In addition, renal denervation did not alter the response to acute portal venous hypertension. These findings suggest that portal venous hypertension does not modify renal function unless hypotension supervenes.

Anderson *et al.* more recently have provided data which are in contrast to those of Levy.[70] These investigators produced acute portal venous constriction in dogs achieving approximately threefold increments over baseline in portal venous pressure, and observed the effect on hemodynamics, renal functional parameters, and renin secretion. In all these studies, renal perfusion was maintained at a constant level by partial clamping of the renal arteries. Acute portal venous hypertension slightly reduced the arterial blood pressure (less than 10%) and the cardiac output (less than 20%). The glomerular filtration rate and renal blood flow fell while renal vascular resistance rose by approximately 25% each. Filtration fraction did not change. In addition, free water clearance was impaired by portal venous hypertension as was solute excretion. Prior renal denervation prevented the changes observed in glomerular filtration rate, renal blood flow, renal resistance, and solute excretion. Previous hypophysectomy partially, but incompletely, prevented the impairment in free water clearance induced by portal venous hypertension. The renin secretory rate, augmented sharply by acute portal venous hypertension, did not change when renal denervation preceded the portal venous constriction. Similar decrements in blood pressure and cardiac output produced in another group of animals by occlusion of the thoracic vena cava produced no changes in renal hemodynamics. Thus, in this animal model acute portal venous hypertension activates an adrenergic portorenal reflex that induces afferent renal arteriolar constriction, renin production, and decrements in glomerular filtration rate, renal blood flow, and sodium excretion.[70]

It is presently impossible to reconcile the conflicting findings of Levy with those of Anderson *et al.* While portal venous hypertension may contribute to the alterations in sodium handling and renal function seen in cirrhotic patients, other factors are apparently more important in the initiation of ascites. Levy and Wexler[71] constructed an end-to-side portacaval fistula in dogs in which they subsequently produced cirrhosis by the administration of dimethylnitrosamine. Despite the presence of normal venous pressure, the cirrhotic dogs developed sodium retention and ascites. These findings underscore the concept that the many factors that favor ascites formation in cirrhosis may vary in their relative contribution to the overall clinical status throughout the course of the disease.

3.2.4. Mesenteric Blood Sequestration. Another mechanism through which portal venous hypertension may produce sodium retention is the mesenteric sequestration of blood with a resultant decrease in effective vascular volume. Very small changes in filling volume, unmeasureable by conventional monitoring techniques, may be detectable by thoracic or cardiac baroreceptors.[72] Sodium retention may occur as a consequence of the reflex stimulation of the afferent renal nerves which results in augmented proximal sodium reabsorption and the stimulation of renin secretion.[73] With the restoration of effective blood volume, sodium retention should cease. The combination of hepatic mesenteric sequestration that results from hepatic venous outflow obstruction and portal venous hypertension, both of which are usually present in cirrhotics, may conceivably have an additive effect on the reduction of effective intravascular volume, particularly if acute hepatic inflammation (e.g., alcoholic hepatitis) is present.

3.3. Defective Albumin Synthesis

Progressive hepatocellular loss is characterized by diminished hepatic synthesis of several proteins, including albumin, which can result in hypoalbuminemia. Early in the course of cirrhosis, the serum oncotic pressure is not a factor in ascites formation because the hepatic sinusoids are highly permeable to protein. However, with chronic intrahepatic hypertension, the sinusoidal endothelium forms a basement membrane that reduces its permeability to protein to a level similar to that of normal capillaries.[74] Moreover, alcoholic liver disease is characterized by sinusoidal fibrosis and a reduction in the number and size of the pores within the sinusoidal membrane. Thus, as liver disease progresses the serum oncotic pressure becomes a more important factor in ascites formation, with hypoalbuminemia further facilitating intestinal and mesenteric lymph flow. Indeed, a major portion of the ascitic fluid may come from this source when advanced liver disease results in obstruction to portal venous inflow and severe portal venous hypertension.[63]

4. Genesis of Sodium Retention and Ascites in Laennec's Cirrhosis

A practical approach to explain the various abnormalities resulting in defective volume regulation in cirrhotic patients is to examine first those factors signaling the kidneys to retain sodium, often referred to as afferent events, and subsequently to describe the mechanisms whereby sodium is retained, i.e., the efferent events. In this section we shall analyze the afferent factors.

4.1. Limitations to Data Interpretation

Unfortunately, it is impossible to study human subjects in a prolonged, prospective fashion as alcoholic liver disease begins and eventually progresses to frank cirrhosis with disordered volume homeostasis. Much of the available data comes from studies in which the cirrhotic subjects examined were in a decompensated condition, which is not pathophysiologically identical to compensated, early cirrhosis. Data relevant to early cirrhosis come largely from animal studies in which cirrhosis is produced by feeding the animal dimethylnitrosamine. Again, this is a model which does not represent completely the clinical features of human alcoholic cirrhosis. The shortcomings in such experimental data limit our ability to draw firm conclusions.

4.2. The Underfill Theory

Traditionally, sodium retention in hepatic cirrhosis has been viewed to be the result of a diminished intravascular volume[75] (Fig. 1). As hepatic venous outflow obstruction produces a displacement of plasma fluid from the intravascular space into the lymphatics, a decrease in central volume activates control mechanisms that serve to retain sodium and restore the volume deficit. Other factors, such as decreased oncotic pressure and portal hypertension, contribute also to a progressive displacement of the increased plasma volume out of the vascular space with further stimulation of the volume receptors. Ascites results when the formation of lymph fluid outstrips its reabsorption from the peritoneal space and return to the circulation via the thoracic duct. The key factors in this "underfill theory" are that sodium retention is secondary to intravascular volume depletion and that the accelerated splanchnic lymph and ascitic fluid formation generates the volume deficit.

This theory may appear to be in conflict with the well-described increases in blood volume seen in both human and experimental cirrhosis in animals.

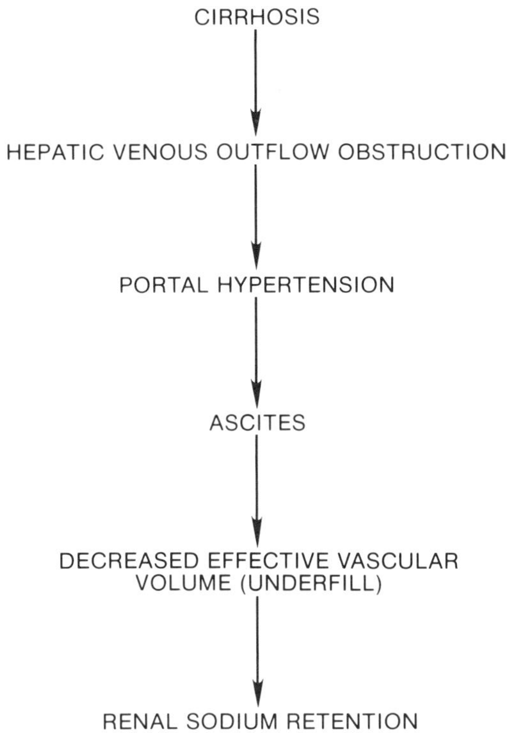

Figure 1. The traditional underfill concept of the sequence of events leading to renal sodium retention and ascites formation in cirrhosis.

However, the concept of an "effective" intravascular volume is consistent with these findings. An increase in splanchnic plasma volume, at the expense of the nonsplanchnic volume, produces an increase in the total plasma volume but may not stimulate the intracardiac and intrathoracic mechano-baroreceptors.[72,73] Thus, this volume expansion is hemodynamically ineffective. Therefore, defective central venous or arterial filling may occur while fluid is being sequestered in a vascular bed of greatly expanded capacity (the portal circulation) associated with an increased total blood volume.

Several factors in addition to ascites formation may reduce the effective intravascular volume in cirrhosis. These include an expanded splanchnic volume,[33] hypoalbuminemia and peripheral edema, impaired cardiac responsiveness,[38] an extensive network of systemic and splanchnic arteriovenous shunts,[32,36,37,68] and impaired autonomic responsiveness due to excessive circulating weak neurotransmitters.[76] Some cirrhotic patients have the added insult of overt volume loss due to gastrointestinal bleeding, vomiting, diarrhea, or diuretic therapy.

Because it is not possible to directly evaluate volume receptor stimulation in cirrhotic patients, most efforts to test the underfill theory have examined the response of hemodynamics and/or volume correlates (e.g., cardiac output, renal function, plasma aldosterone, vasopressin, and norepinephrine levels) to augmentation of the intravascular volume. Expansion with an isotonic saline–albumin[26] or dextran solution,[41] or by reinfusion of ascitic fluid[77–79] increases the urine flow, glomerular filtration rate, sodium excretion, and renal blood flow in these patients. The infusion of pressor agents increases the renal blood flow, decreases the plasma renin activity and increases urinary solute excretion in cirrhotics, but not normal subjects.[80,81] Moreover, implantation of a peritoneovenous shunt increases cardiac output, renal blood flow, creatinine clearance, sodium excretion, and urine volume, and inhibits renin and aldosterone secretion.[82–84] These beneficial effects of shunting, including abolition of ascites, usually persist in patients who survive shunt placement.[84,85]

The data that most strongly support the underfill theory have come from studies employing head-out water immersion of cirrhotic patients. This technique generates a potent central volume stimulus that is equivalent to approximately 2 liters of saline infusion but has the unique advantages that it produces no change in serum chemistry, is rapidly reversible, and may be sustained for several hours while actually diminishing the patients' total body sodium stores.[86]

Epstein *et al.*[27] have examined the responses to water immersion in eleven cirrhotic patients including three individuals without clinically detectable ascites. Immersion produces a prompt and sustained increase in mean urine flow, urinary sodium and potassium excretion, percent excretion of sodium, and free water clearance. The mean creatinine clearance did not change although some individuals showed an increase in this measurement. The three patients without ascites manifested increases in sodium excretion similar to those seen in normal subjects. However, two of these three had greater than normal increases in free water excretion suggesting that (1) proximal tubular sodium reabsorption was diminished and/or (2) nonosmotic stimulation of vasopressin had ceased. In another study of 16 cirrhotics,[87] immersion augmented the creatinine clearance and the fractional and absolute sodium excretion and suppressed both plasma renin activity and plasma aldosterone levels.

In a recent study by Bichet *et al.*, eight ascitic patients with Laennec's cirrhosis were hemodynamically monitored during head-out water immersion and their response to water loading before and during immersion was examined.[88] Cardiac index and right atrial and wedged pulmonary capillary pressures were increased and plasma renin activity, aldosterone, arginine-vasopressin, and norepinephrine levels were decreased by immersion. Furthermore, immersion produced a natriuresis and restored the suppressibility of arginine-vasopressin secretion by a water load. The augmentation of right atrial pressure appeared to be the factor primarily responsible for the improvement in renal water handling and sodium excretion induced by immersion. The reduction of plasma norepinephrine levels by immersion cor-

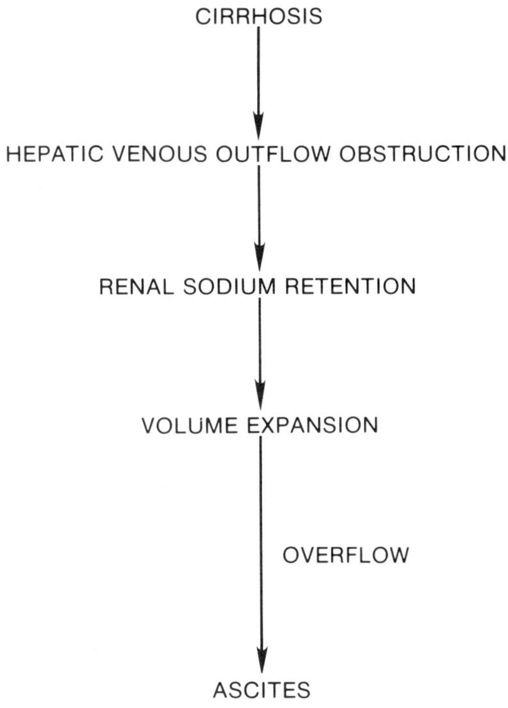

Figure 2. The "overflow" theory of the genesis of sodium retention in cirrhosis.

related directly with the increase in right atrial pressure and inversely with the increase in urinary sodium excretion. These findings clearly implicate the role of a diminished effective intravascular volume in the pathogenesis of the sodium and water retention of patients with established ascites.

Ironically, just as the volume expansion data cited above provide strong support of the underfill theory, they also point out some of the shortcomings of this concept. Close scrutiny of the individual responses to water immersion published by Epstein *et al.*[27] reveals that roughly one half of these patients did *not* undergo a natriuresis even though the renin–aldosterone axis was suppressed by the volume stimulus. In many, if not most, patients diuresis does not occur after peritoneovenous shunt placement until furosemide or another diuretic agent is administered.[83,84] Moreover, marked restriction of sodium intake and, occasionally, diuretic use are required on a chronic basis to prevent the formation of edema and ascites after successful shunt placement.[85] Most patients have a persistent defect in their excretory response to an oral sodium load despite the presence of a functioning peritoneovenous shunt. In some individuals this may be due to persistently elevated renin and aldosterone secretion, but it is also seen in subjects with normal aldosterone levels.[85] Additionally, in patients studied hemodynamically, shunt placement produces a reduction in intrasinusoidal pressure that correlates with the increase in urinary sodium excretion.[85] While it has been implied that this relationship suggests a role of portal hypertension to the pathogenesis of sodium retention, the data do not confirm this concept. Nevertheless, these observations, which are at odds with the underfill theory, demonstrate that factors other than the effective intravascular volume status participate in the abnormal sodium handling of cirrhosis.

4.3. The Overflow Theory

Following a series of very detailed experiments examining the components of blood volume in cirrhotic patients, Lieberman and his colleagues proposed an alternative hypothesis for the generation of ascites[33,89,90] (Fig. 2). This theory holds that cirrhosis induces a primary renal retention of sodium resulting in an expanded splanchnic and nonsplanchnic blood volume. Ascites forms on an "overflow" basis, when the retained fluid and sodium exacerbate the preexisting intrahepatic hypertension and further increase the rate of splanchnic lymph formation. Thus, by this "overflow" theory, renal sodium retention is the primary abnormality in the formation of ascites.

Supporters of the underfill theory explain the elevated blood volume of cirrhotics as being a consequence of a greatly expanded splanchnic capacity in the presence of a diminished nonportal volume. In addition, leakage of the isotope used to perform these measurements, into the ascitic fluid and the expanded lymph pool, could have conceivably resulted in an overestimation of the measured splanchnic blood volume. Lieberman and Reynolds measured the plasma and red blood cell volumes in a large group of normal subjects and cirrhotics.[33] The appearance of radiolabel in the thoracic duct lymph and ascitic fluid was negligible during the time required for the volume determination. Cirrhotics, regardless of their state of compensation, had elevated mean plasma and whole blood volumes and slightly decreased red blood cell volumes. There was a direct correlation between wedged hepatic vein pressure and plasma volume in those cirrhotics studied by venous catheterization. Decompression of portal hypertension by portacaval anastamosis decreased the plasma volume in a majority of patients studied before and 6 months after surgery. The authors concluded that the elevated blood volume in cirrhosis is a consequence of portal hypertension per se.[33]

According to the underfill theory, the total plasma volume should increase as ascites resolves in cirrhotic patients providing the splanchnic volume is unchanged.[89] To test the validity of this prediction, Lieberman *et al.* measured the plasma volume and red cell mass in cirrhotics before and after diuretic therapy had resolved their ascites. Red blood cell mass increased, but the plasma volume was unchanged when ascites was eliminated. In addition, wedged hepatic vein pressure, which was thought to reflect the splanchnic blood volume, did not change. These findings support the contention that a decrease in effective intravascular volume was not present. An additional study revealed that paracentesis of approximately 2 liters of ascitic

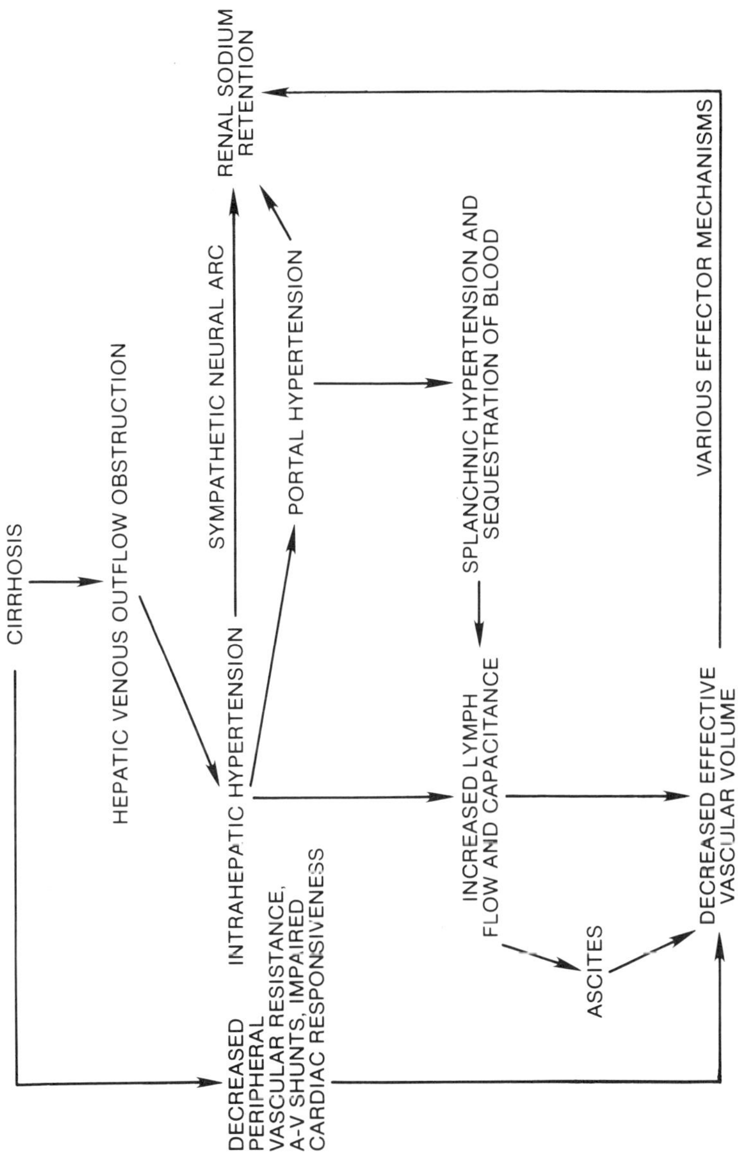

Figure 3. The interaction of the pathophysiologic forces resulting in sodium retention in cirrhosis.

fluid does not change the plasma volume and does not increase the rate of transudation of systemically administered radioisotope into ascitic fluid. These results are inconsistent with the underfill theory, which predicts the rapid reformation of ascitic fluid at the expense of a contracted intravascular volume. These investigators also induced renal sodium retention and subsequent decompensation in nonascitic cirrhotic patients by the administration of the mineralocorticoid, 9-α-fluorohydrocortisone, clearly demonstrating that ascites can occur as an overload phenomenon.[46,91]

A considerable body of data supporting the overflow theory has come from studies by Levy and his colleagues employing an experimental model of canine cirrhosis produced by the intermittent feeding of dimethylnitrosamine. This toxin-induced cirrhosis histologically resembles alcoholic cirrhosis and produces many biochemical and clinical abnormalities seen in the human disease. The cirrhosis is induced over a period of 6–8 weeks, and the animals can be monitored prospectively with serial measurements of sodium balance, plasma volume (including its splanchnic and nonsplanchnic components), renal function, cardiac output, blood pressure, and peripheral vascular resistance.[92,93] Such serial studies reveal that, after cirrhosis is established, sodium retention occurs before any other abnormalities are present. Subsequently, total plasma volume rises as do both splanchnic and nonsplanchnic volumes. There is a selective increase in the splanchnic volume, as the nonsplanchic volume (as a percentage of total plasma volume) declines. Portal venous pressure increases when cirrhosis is present but does not correlate with the observed sodium retention. Ascites appears only after sodium retention is well established, and does not reform after paracentesis if dietary sodium intake is precluded. Arterial blood pressure and glomerular filtration rate are unchanged with progression from the noncirrhotic to the decompensated cirrhotic state. Cardiac output rises and peripheral vascular resistance falls only after ascites is present. Micropuncture studies[94] have revealed that glomerular filtration rate and distal delivery of filtrate are normal throughout the progression of the disease, suggesting that the sodium retention producing ascites is primarily a distal tubular phenomonon. Because renal denervation and sympathetic blockade have no effect on sodium handling, and because plasma renin activity and aldosterone levels are normal until cirrhosis is present, neither sympathetic nerve activity nor activation of the renin–angiotensin–aldosterone axis is responsible for the initiation of sodium retention.[94] Placement of an end-to-side portacaval fistula prior to the induction of cirrhosis does not prevent the previously documented sequence of events leading to ascites but maintains a normal distribution of the expanded plasma volume between the splanchic and nonsplanchnic compartments and obviates the development of portal hypertension.[71] Similar to other studies,[85] the placement of a peritoneovenous shunt ameliorates ascites in these cirrhotic animals but does not abolish the inability to excrete a sodium load.[95] Thus, in this animal model of cirrhosis, sodium retention apparently is initiated by factors other than a decrement in effective or nonsplanchnic vascular volume. Based on these data and the previously cited report demonstrating the sodium retaining effects of hepatic outflow blockage,[60] Levy has suggested that hepatic vein or sinusoidal hypertension, perhaps by acting on intrahepatic baroreceptors, generates the sodium retaining stimulus in cirrhosis. The effector mechanism activated by this stimulus may be a humoral factor or a reflex neural pathway.[45]

Although the overflow theory explains several of the features of cirrhosis that are inconsistent with the underfill concept, it, too, has a number of shortcomings. The exaggerated natriuretic response to volume expansion cannot be explained by the overflow theory unless one postulates impaired baroreceptors in the systemic circuit that respond inappropriately to a diminished effective intravascular volume. Similarly, this theory cannot account for the elevated plasma renin, aldosterone, vasopressin, and norepinephrine levels encountered in many cirrhotics or the suppression of these levels by various volume expansion maneuvers. However, it is wise to exercise caution in forming generalizations based on the dimethylnitrosamine-induced model of cirrhosis. Glomerular filtration rate does not decline in these cirrhotic dogs even after ascites is present.[93] In contrast, human cirrhotics often manifest mildly impaired renal function once ascites is established.[10,11,15] Additionally, although the change is not statistically significant, arterial blood pressure declines slightly during the period when sodium retention occurs in dogs with experimental dimethylnitrosamine cirrhosis.[93] It is not unreasonable to assume that volume control sensors respond to subtle changes in filling. Furthermore, whereas peritoneovenous shunt placement does not alter renal function in cirrhotic dogs, it increases cardiac output and blood volume and decreases plasma renin and aldosterone levels. These changes suggest the presence of decreased effective vascular filling prior to shunting, despite the preshunt elevation of the nonsplanchnic vascular volume.

4.4. Resolution of the Conflicting Theories

From the data currently available it is impossible to pinpoint the factor(s) responsible for the initiation of sodium retention in cirrhosis. While many studies in experimental animals have provided evidence that a hepatorenal reflex may be active early in cirrhosis, the preponderance of findings in human subjects implicate a decline in effective intravascular volume as the major mechanism causing the sodium retention. Indeed, most clinicians are all too familiar with the classic presentation of cirrhotics with emaciation, tense ascites, and a tendency toward arterial hypotension. Nevertheless, because we recognize most cirrhotics only when they present in this decompensated fashion we must be cautious not to let this experience unduly influence our interpretation of the potential early events. Figure 3 represents a scheme whereby sodium retention may result from cirrhosis. Hepatic venous outflow block initiates a series of events that directly and indirectly stimulate renal sodium reabsorption. Because ascites formation is a gradual process and does not occur until fluid is sequestered in various beds, sodium retention may logically be expected to precede the onset of clinically detectable ascites. If renal sodium retention is primary, when a state of positive sodium balance occurs the expanded volume may drive ascites formation until other factors, such as decreased venous return from tense ascites, convert the status to one of underfilling. In contrast, in the compensated state a decreased natriuretic response to volume expansion or oral salt load may occur due to (1) a persistent primary stimulus to the kidney by the diseased liver and/or (2) a rapid dispersal of the administered sodium into lymphatic and vascular systems of increased capacitance, resulting in an ineffective volume receptor stimulation. The prevailing factors promoting sodium reabsorption most likely vary with the stage of the disease. Thus, the two theories are not mutually exclusive and neither theory should be rejected outright in favor of the other.

5. The Effectors of Renal Sodium Retention in Cirrhosis

5.1. Renin–Angiotensin–Aldosterone Axis

5.1.1. Aldosterone.

5.1.1a. Normal Physiology. Aldosterone is the most extensively studied of the hormonal mediators of renal sodium handling. This hormone is synthesized and secreted by the zona glomerulosa of the adrenal cortex. The dominant factors controlling its release are the state of activitation of the renin–angiotensin system and the serum potassium concentration. The serum sodium concentration and adrenocorticotrophic hormone level may influence aldosterone secretion but are of lesser importance. Aldosterone degradation occurs principally in the liver and is dependent partly upon hepatic blood flow. The principal physiologic action of aldosterone is to promote distal renal tubular sodium reabsorption in exchange for potassium and hydrogen ions.

5.1.1b. Aldosterone Levels in Cirrhosis. Early studies demonstrating enhanced urinary secretion of aldosterone in cirrhotics have fostered the widely held view that these patients frequently have secondary hyperaldosteronism.[96,97] With the advent of radioimmunoassay methods for determination of serum aldosterone levels investigators have examined this relationship more accurately.

Rosoff *et al.* found an approximately fourfold elevation of plasma aldosterone in cirrhotics with refractory ascites.[98] The increase in plasma aldosterone normally produced in response to standing was blunted when compared with that of normal controls on an identical sodium intake, which suggests that in the cirrhotic subjects the baseline aldosterone secretion is near the maximal level possible. In contrast, Epstein *et al.* found elevated plasma aldosterone levels in only four of 16 cirrhotic subjects, most of whom were in a decompensated state.[87] Two recent studies demonstrated that the mean plasma aldosterone level of cirrhotic patients is elevated when compared with that of normals, regardless of the state of compensation.[61,99] However, a review of the individual plasma aldosterone values in these reports reveals that 20 of a total of 33 patients had levels that were within two standard deviations of the mean of their respective controls. A number of other studies have now confirmed that the majority of patients with cirrhosis do *not* have elevated plasma aldosterone levels.[16,29,100–102] With regard to clinical status, most compensated cirrhotics have normal or suppressed plasma aldosterone levels,[15,100–102] whereas untreated decompensated patients exhibit normal or elevated plasma aldosterone levels.[15,100,102] Diuretic therapy frequently produces or worsens hyperaldosteronism in the latter group of patients.[101]

5.1.1.c. Control of Aldosterone Secretion in Cirrhosis. Activation of the renin–angiotensin system is the primary factor controlling aldosterone secretion in cirrhosis. A close correlation exists between plasma aldosterone and plasma renin activity,[15,16,61,87,101,102] and between plasma aldosterone and angiotensin II levels[101,103] in cirrhotics. In addition, measures such as immersion and salt loading, which suppress renin secretion, reduce plasma aldosterone levels in parallel with the plasma renin activity.[87,88,104] Pharmacologic blockade of angiotensin II with saralasin, diminishes plasma aldosterone levels in cirrhotic patients.[105–107] However, attempts to suppress renin production with β-adrenergic blockade have produced conflicting results,[108,109] probably because of the many complex actions of these drugs on renal hemodynamics.

Hyponatremia has been cited as a possible cause of the elevated plasma aldosterone levels seen in cirrhotics.[67] An inverse correlation between serum sodium concentration and plasma aldosterone levels has been observed by some authors,[101,110] but not by others.[15,16,61] This may be a coincidental relationship as diminished free water clearance and elevated plasma aldosterone levels are features encountered in patients with more advanced stages of cirrhosis. Moreover, a direct stimulation of aldosterone secretion by hyponatremia has not been demonstrated in cirrhotics.

5.1.1.d. Altered Hepatic Metabolism of Aldosterone. Following the observation of reduced hepatic clearance of aldosterone in cirrhotics,[97] it was suggested that hyperaldosteronism occurs primarily as a result of diminished hepatic degradation in these subjects rather than excessive secretion of the hormone.[111] Rosoff *et al.*, in normal subjects and in cirrhotic patients, examined the clearance rate of intravenously administered, radiolabeled aldosterone and simultaneously estimated the aldosterone secretion rate as the product of the plasma concentration and the metabolic clearance rate of the hormone.[98] In cirrhotics, the clearance of aldosterone was decreased by roughly 20% whereas the secretion rate was increased greater than tenfold. Mitch *et al.* directly measured hepatic extraction of renin and aldosterone by hepatic vein catheterization in a large number of cirrhotic and normal subjects.[61] Aldosterone clearance was depressed in cirrhotics by approximately one third, similar to the findings of other workers.[98,111] In addition, hepatic renin clearance was decreased by 50% and was related to the impairment in hepatic blood flow. However, plasma renin activity was elevated more than 12-fold and levels of plasma aldosterone were found to correlate directly with the plasma renin activity. Based on these findings it appears that renin secretion rather than decreased hepatic renin and aldosterone clearance is responsible for the elevation of plasma aldosterone seen in cirrhotics.[61] Further consideration of the abnormal renin metabolism present in cirrhosis will be discussed in a subsequent section.

5.1.1e. Role of Aldosterone in the Sodium Retention of Cirrhosis. A number of observations have shown a dissociation of sodium handling in the individual cirrhotic from the plasma level of aldosterone. Thus, the plasma aldosterone concentration may be normal in decompensated as well as in compensated patients.[15,61,101] Individual patients may undergo spontaneous changes in their clinical status without a corresponding change in the plasma aldosterone concentration.[98] In addition, measures which inhibit aldosterone secretion (as documented by decreasing plasma aldosterone levels), are not always associated with an improvement in renal sodium excretion.[87,98,104] Epstein *et al.* have compared the effects of chronic spironolactone administration and head-out water immersion on sodium excretion in a small group of cirrhotic patients.[27] Spironolactone induces a mild increase in the rate of sodium excretion although the total sodium excretion during the 4-hr study is not significantly greater than that seen without spironolactone therapy. Water immersion of cirrhotic subjects taking spironlactone induces a highly significant increase in both the rate of sodium excretion and the cumulative 4-hr sodium excretion. These authors maintain that aldosterone plays only a permissive role in the sodium retention of cirrhosis.[27,87]

Such a conclusion may not be completely justifiable, however, as other studies have underscored the importance of aldosterone in the sodium retention of cirrhosis. Adrenalectomy improves sodium excretion in cirrhosis,[112,113] although this is not a reasonable therapeutic approach. A randomized study of 40 cirrhotic patients with normal renal function has demonstrated that spironolactone, a less potent natriuretic agent than furosemide, is more effective than the latter drug in the treatment of ascites.[114] In this investigation, the response to diuretic therapy was influenced by the state of activation of the renin–angiotensin system in that failure to respond to furosemide occurred in those individuals with higher mean plasma aldosterone and plasma renin activity levels. Since roughly half of the patients randomized to furosemide failed to resolve their ascites with this therapy and later responded to spironolactone, aldosterone apparently plays an important role in sodium retention in many patients.[114] This conclusion receives support from the observations of several groups that the rate of sodium excretion correlates inversely with plasma aldosterone levels in cirrhotic individuals.[15,16,29,103,115] It has been suggested that the distal tubule is "supersensitive" to the effect of aldosterone such that sodium retention may occur with low or normal plasma aldosterone levels.[29,102] Whereas other factors may be of greater importance to sodium retention, the contribution of aldosterone is often significant, particularly so in patients with ascites.

5.1.2. Renin-Angiotensin Axis.

5.1.2a. Normal Physiology. The normal biochemistry and physiology of the renin–angiotensin system have been reviewed extensively in several recent publications[116–119] and will be considered only briefly here. Renin, a protein of molecular weight in the range of 40,000–44,000 Daltons is produced and stored principally in the juxtaglomerular cells of the renal cortex. These cells are in contact with the afferent glomerular arterioles and the macula densa of the distal tubules, forming the juxtaglomerular apparatus. Renin acts locally within the kidney or enters the systemic circulation. In the plasma, renin acts on angiotensinogen, an hepatically produced α-globulin, to form the inactive decapeptide, angiontensin I. Angiotensin I-converting enzyme, located predominately in the lung but present also in the serum and various other tissues, including the juxtaglomerular apparatus of the renal cortex, cleaves angiotensin I to form angiotensin II. Angiotensin II is the most potent vasoconstrictor substance known and stimulates aldosterone production by the adrenal glands. Angiotensinases degrade angiotensin II, producing at least one product, angiotensin III, which has a metabolic activity as a stimulator of aldosterone secretion. Figure 4 summarizes the various components of the renin-angiotensin system.

Control of renal renin release is affected through three principal mechanisms: (1) the level of stimulation of stretch or pressure receptors in the afferent renal arterioles; (2) sodium delivery to the macula densa of the distal tubule; and (3) stimulation of the β-1-adrenergic receptors of the juxtaglomerular apparatus by sympathetic renal nerve fibers or circulating catecholamines. Most factors that alter renin production act via one or more of these mechanisms. Thus, effective vascular volume depletion stimulates renin secretion by decreased arterial pressure, by diminished distal tubular delivery of sodium, and as a result of sympathetic stimulation due to alterations in central baroreceptor activity. Angiotensin II is a direct inhibitor of renin release in a feedback loop that is independent of its hemodynamic effects. Prostaglandin synthesis and renal renin release are mutually stimulatory. Age, race, posture, and sodium intake are also determinants of plasma renin activity that must be considered when examining clinical data.

Angiotensin II is the primary effector agent of the renin–angiotensin system. It produces vascular smooth muscle contraction, stimulates aldosterone and catecholamine secretion by the adrenal gland, acts in the central nervous system to induce thirst and increase blood pressure via activation of the autonomic nervous system, and stimulates secretion of vasopressin and adrenocorticotropic hormone. The renin–angiotensin system participates in the regulation of intrarenal hemodynamics, possibly through local production of angiotensin II, as renal tissue and vessels contain all of the individual components of the system. Although the details of angiotensin II action within the kidney are not understood fully, most studies suggest that systemically administered or intrarenally produced angiotensin II diminishes the renal blood flow and to a lesser degree the glomerular filtration rate, thereby in-

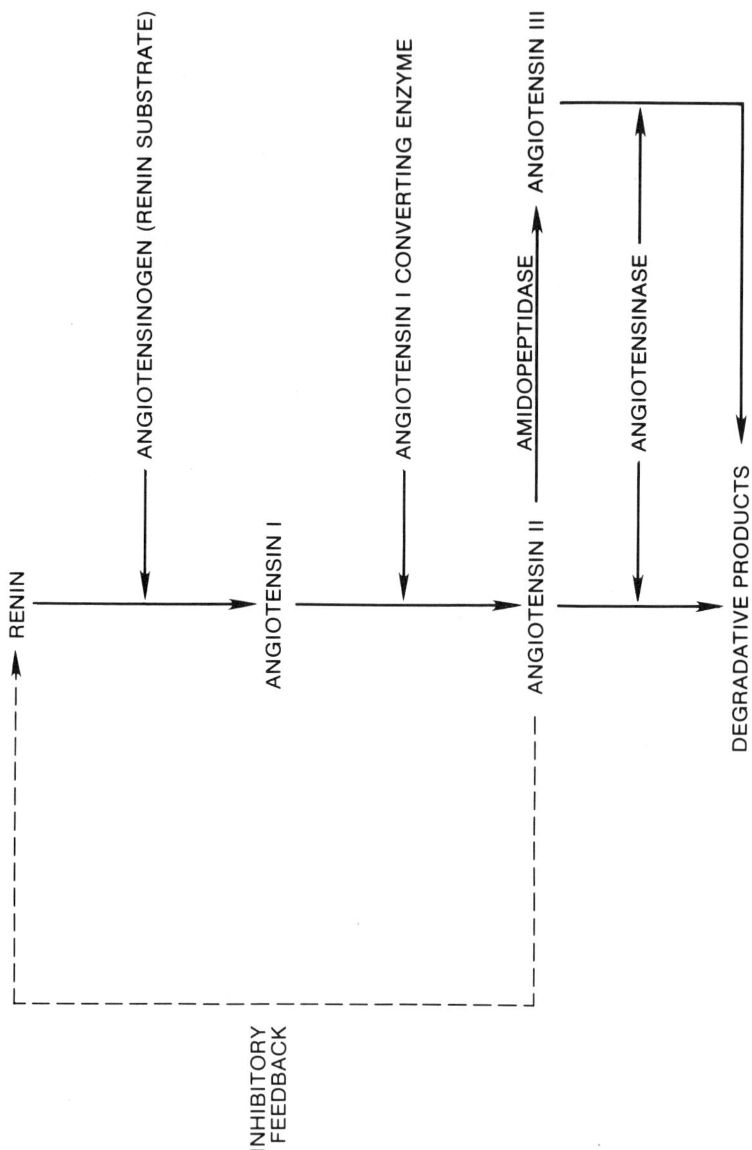

Figure 4. The renin–angiotensin system.

creasing the filtration fraction. Angiotensin II may decrease the outer cortical blood flow also, but this finding has not been a consistent observation. Intrarenal prostaglandin synthesis, stimulated by angiotensin II, has local vasodilatory effects that may balance the vasoconstrictor properties of the peptide.

5.1.2b. Renin–Angiotensin Levels in Cirrhosis. Plasma levels of renin substrate (angiotensinogen) in cirrhotic patients usually are depressed regardless of the state of compensation.[101,103,120] This occurs partly as a consequence of diminished hepatic synthesis. Decreases of renin substrate in cirrhotics correlate with decrements in the serum cholesterol, which is also a product of hepatic synthesis. That plasma renin activity correlates inversely with renin substrate in cirrhotics suggests that increased substrate consumption may contribute to its deficiency.[121] In advanced cirrhosis renin substrate levels correlate inversely with the serum creatinine. A popular thesis holds that depletion of renin substrate may result in deficient intrarenal production of angiotensin II.[122] This impairment of angiotensin II synthesis is thought to induce disproportionate vasoconstriction between pre- and postglomerular arterioles, causing a diminished glomerular filtration rate and renal blood flow. In addition, excessive cortical afferent arteriolar vasoconstriction may result in a shift of blood flow to the inner juxtamedullary nephrons. Because measures that increase renin substrate concentration do not improve renal function consistently in patients with the hepatorenal syndrome,[122] it appears that factors other than renin substrate depletion are primarily responsible for the development of renal hypoperfusion in advanced cirrhosis.

Two techniques may be used to measure plasma renin levels. The plasma renin "activity" measures the amount of angiotensin I produced by the patient's plasma under controlled conditions. The plasma renin "concentration" determines the amount of angiotensin I produced by the patient's plasma with the addition of renin substrate in excess. Thus, plasma renin activity is a measure of the endogenous activity of the renin–angiotensin system, whereas plasma renin concentration reflects the actual renin content of the blood. These measures may not correlate in the presence of advanced, decompensated cirrhosis, presumably due to renin substrate deficiency.[103,120] Plasma renin concentration has been felt by some to provide a more accurate assessment of renin activation in cirrhotics.[98,120] However, plasma renin activity and plasma renin concentration usually correlate with plasma aldosterone levels in cirrhotics.[15,16,61,87,101,102] In addition, plasma renin activity has been shown to correlate directly with plasma renin concentrations in these patients.[18] Therefore, plasma renin activity generally is considered a reliable measure of activation of the renin–angiotensin system in cirrhosis and is the method most often utilized.

Determination of plasma renin levels in cirrhotics has resulted in controversy. Early studies revealed that plasma renin concentration and plasma renin activity are often but not invariably elevated in decompensated cirrhotics.[87,98,120] Particularly high renin values have been encountered in patients with severe resistant ascites and functional renal failure.[80,120,123] Some investigators find no correlation between the degree of compensation and elevations of plasma renin activity in cirrhosis.[61,99] However, the majority of studies demonstrate that compensated patients usually have suppressed or normal plasma renin activity whereas decompensated patients often have elevated renin levels.[15,16,80,102,121,123]

The discrepancy in the results of measurements of plasma renin activity in compensated and decompensated patients may relate to prior diuretic therapy in the patients studied. In this regard, Wernze *et al.* have examined plasma renin activity in cirrhotic patients segregated into groups according to the presence or absence of diuretic therapy.[101] Untreated, compensated cirrhotics and decompensated ascitic cirrhotics, not taking diuretics for 2–4 weeks prior to study, have normal plasma renin activity values. In contrast, cirrhotics undergoing diuretic therapy to reach or to maintain compensation have markedly elevated plasma renin activity. Many investigators of the renin–angiotensin activation state in cirrhosis either have not commented on the prior use of diuretics or have withheld diuretics only briefly before the measures of plasma renin activity were determined. If diuretics are stopped and a sodium restricted diet is instituted when patients are hospitalized for metabolic study, diuretic-induced hyperreninemia may persist for several days. Thus, from an examination of the studies that have taken measures to exclude the contributions of previous diuretic therapy on renin levels it is clear that elevated plasma renin levels are uncommon in early cirrhosis, including those subjects with previously untreated ascites.

A recent study by Arroyo *et al.* underscores the validity of the thesis that elevated renin levels only appear late in the course of cirrhosis.[115] These workers examined the activation of the renin–angiotensin system in 75 ascitic cirrhotics and correlated their findings with patient survival rate. Thirty-four cirrhotic patients had normal plasma renin activity while 41 had high levels. The two groups were otherwise indistinguishable on clinical grounds. Inulin and para-aminohippuric acid clearances were normal in both groups. In contrast, urinary sodium excretion was eightfold greater in the patients with normal renin values than in those with high renin levels. Moreover, wedged hepatic venous pressure was much higher in the latter group, suggesting that these individuals had more severe hepatic disease. A 50% survival rate was observed at 28 months in the patients with normal renin levels but less than 6 months in those with elevated plasma renin activity. Similarly, a urinary sodium greater than 10 mEq/day correlated positively with survival rate.[115]

Few investigators have measured the changes in angiotensin II levels induced by cirrhosis. Because of a deficient synthesis of renin substrate in cirrhotics, the levels of angiotensin II might not be expected to correlate directly with plasma renin activity. However, examinations of plasma renin activity (or concentration) and angiotensin II levels in cirrhotics disclose a linear relationship between both renin and plasma angiotensin II levels and angiotensin II and plasma aldosterone levels.[101,103] Therefore, deficiency of renin substrate in cirrhosis usually does not alter the relation between renin production and secretion of the end products of the system. Similarly, changes of plasma renin activity reflect concomitant changes in angiotensin II and plasma aldosterone levels. Thus, on an individual basis previously untreated cirrhotics with or without ascites, usually have normal plasma angiotensin II levels which increase with diuretic therapy.[101]

Increased serum activity of both major enzyme components of the renin–angiotensin system, angiotensin-converting enzyme[124] and angiotensinase[125,126] have been observed in cirrhotics. The importance of either of these changes in serum enzyme activity is obscure as both enzymes act locally. Moreover, there is no evidence to suggest that a change in the serum activity of either enzyme accurately reflects an alteration in the tissue levels of enzyme activity. It has been suggested that the increase in serum angiotensin-converting enzyme activity observed in cirrhotics may be due, at least in part, to increased activity of the enzyme in the pulmonary vasculature induced by arterial hypoxemia.[124,127] Any future examination of the activity of these enzymes in cirrhosis should be directed toward determination of their activity in tissue rather than in serum or plasma.

5.1.2c. Causes of Activation of the Renin–Angiotensin Axis. The importance of the liver in the clearance of renin and aldosterone has been mentioned previously. Indeed, the hepatic clearance of renin is the principal mechanism contributing to the total metabolic clearance of renin.[128] Because the main determinants of the hepatic clearance of renin are its hepatic extraction and hepatic blood flow,[128] it is not surprising that cirrhotics have an impaired clearance of renin.[61,129] However, as renin is excreted in the bile,[130] a diminished biliary excretion of renin occuring in advanced cirrhosis may contribute also to the overall decreased hepatic clearance of renin. In addition, systemic arterial renin may be lower than hepatic venous renin in some cirrhotics,[120,131] suggesting that there may be a splanchnic source of renin production.[131] Thus, a reduced hepatic clearance of renin in cirrhosis contributes importantly to systemic elevations.

Nevertheless, increased renin secretion is the primary mechanism responsible for the increased plasma level of renin activity present in cirrhosis. Autopsy specimens of renal tissue obtained from cirrhotic patients show evidence of markedly increased juxtaglomerular cell activity when compared with tissues obtained from normal subjects.[103] Plasma renin activity in cirrhotics is directly proportional to the rate of renal renin secretion.[16] In addition, Mitch *et al.*[61] observed a 12-fold increase in plasma renin activity in decompensated ascitic cirrhotics despite only a 50% reduction in hepatic renin extraction.

Of the many factors that may be responsible for the stimulation of renin secretion observed in cirrhosis, effective volume depletion has been demonstrated most clearly. Head-out water immersion of cirrhotic patients promptly decreases the mean plasma renin activity, which remains low throughout the immersion period and returns to preimmersion values within an hour of cessation of immersion.[87] The decreases in plasma renin activity associated with water immersion correlate closely with the right atrial pressure, which is elevated consistently by the maneuver.[88]

Several animal studies have indicated that increasing hepatic sinusoidal pressure may increase renin release. One group of investigators has observed a correlation between wedged hepatic venous pressure and plasma renin activity in human cirrhosis.[15,115] In cirrhotics, the wedged hepatic vein pressure, when correlated for inferior vena cava pressure, strongly and directly correlates with plasma renin levels. Further, the hepatic wedge pressure is highest in decompensated cirrhotics who avidly retain sodium, and is lowest in compensated patients.[15] Moreover, higher venous pressures are encountered in those patients with the shortest survival.[115] In contrast, Mitch *et al.* did not observe a correlation between the corrected hepatic venous wedge pressure and plasma renin activity.[61] Thus, it is not clear that increases in wedged hepatic venous pressure are related causally to the increased activity of plasma renin. In contrast, the apparent correlation between these two factors may result from the simultaneous occurrence of two phenomena that independently are related to the severity of the hepatic disease. In addition, the infusion of angiotensin II into cirrhotic patients decreases hepatic blood flow and increases the hepatic venous pressure.[132,133] Therefore, the elevated angiotensin II levels observed in cirrhosis might cause, rather than result from, the increased hepatic venous pressure. Data presently available do not support a role for elevated hepatic venous pressure in the stimulation of renin secretion in humans.

Renal hypoperfusion is often cited as a potential cause of renin hypersecretion in cirrhosis. Several studies have examined the relationship between renal hemodynamics and plasma renin activity. Barnardo *et al.* observed an inverse correlation between plasma renin activity and the clearances of para-aminohippurate and creatinine in a group of decompensated cirrhotics that included several subjects with significantly impaired renal function.[80] Infusion of subpressor doses of dopamine (1–3 mg/kg/min) increased the clearance of para-aminohippuric acid and decreased plasma renin activity in cirrhotics.[80] This finding prompted the authors to attribute the elevated plasma renin activity to decreased renal perfusion.[80] Other investigators have confirmed the presence of an inverse relationship between renal function and plasma renin activity in decompensated cirrhotics when subjects with renal insufficiency are included in the analysis.[123] However, when subjects with glomerular filtration rates below 50 ml/min are excluded no correlation exists between renal hemodynamics and plasma renin activity.[15,16]

Recently, Bernardi *et al.* examined this problem in greater detail.[102] Compensated cirrhotics with no history of ascites had suppressed plasma renin activity levels that did not correlate with any of the measured renal hemodynamic variables. In contrast, decompensated cirrhotics who had not received prior diuretic therapy had mildly elevated plasma renin activity and normal renal function, and an inverse correlation was observed between both renal plasma flow and glomerular filtration rate and the plasma renin activity. When the decompensated cirrhotics were separated into two groups with elevated and normal plasma renin activity, glomerular filtration rate and renal plasma flow were found to be within the normal range for all the subjects studied but were significantly lower in the subjects with elevated renin levels. Importantly, there were no differences between these two subgroups in blood volume, serum potassium, or arterial blood pressure. Therefore, whereas most studies demonstrate no correlation between renal functional parameters and the activation of the renin–angiotensin system until late in cirrhosis, well after the onset of functional renal failure, these findings show that a relationship does indeed exist between renal hypoperfusion and elevated plasma renin activity in the initial stages of decompensation.

A shift of intrarenal blood flow from the outer cortical to the inner juxtamedullary nephrons may produce a relative cortical ischemia and, thereby, stimulate the renin–angiotensin system in decompensated cirrhosis. Studies employing the ^{133}xenon washout technique have shown that the outer renal cortical blood flow, both as an absolute flow and as a percentage of total renal blood flow, is diminished in cirrhotics with well-preserved glomerular filtration rates[12,134] and may be severely depressed in patients with functional renal failure.[135] Because the ^{133}xenon washout technique has been criticized as a poor indicator of regional blood flow,[136] recent studies have utilized the radiolabeled iodohippurate renogram to examine the cortical and medullary components of renal blood flow in cirrhotic subjects. Decompensated cirrhotics with preserved renal function frequently have diminished renal cortical blood flow by this technique and demonstrate an inverse correlation between outer cortical blood flow and plasma renin activity.[99,137] Thus, redistribution of intrarenal blood flow to the deeper juxtamedullary nephrons is observed in cirrhotics and may be related to the increased renin secretion in such subjects. Pharmacologic β-blockade with propranolol reduces or abolishes the hyperreninemia seen in cirrhotics but does not consistently change outer renal cortical blood flow.[108] It has been suggested that the reduction in outer cortical blood flow observed in cirrhotics is the cause of elevated plasma renin activity. This conclusion is not justifiable, however, because propranolol produces direct renal vasoconstriction[138] via blockade of the renal vascular β-receptors and subsequent, unopposed α-adrenergic stimulation.[139] Moreover, because angiotensin II reduces outer cortical blood flow to a greater degree than it does inner cortical flow,[140] stimulation of the renin–angiotensin axis may be a cause rather than a consequence of the altered intrarenal blood flow. Available data do not answer the question of cause and effect for these phenomena.

Evidence has been accumulated to suggest that mild arterial hypotension may activate the renin–angiotensin system in some cirrhotic subjects. Infusion of the angiotensin II antagonist, saralasin, to sodium-restricted, decompensated cirrhotics produces significantly greater decreases in arterial blood pressure than those observed in normal subjects who are on an identical sodium restriction.[105] When subjects consume a diet high in sodium, saralasin infusion induces only mild decrements in mean arterial pressure in cirrhotics and increases the mean pressure of normals only slightly. In compensated cirrhotics the blood pressure response to saralasin infusion is identical to that of normal subjects.[105] Other investigators have administered a different angiotensin II antagonist to ascitic cirrhotics who were on a high sodium diet and observed a decline in mean arterial pressure in only one of eight patients.[141] These conflicting findings may relate to differences in sodium balance, the degree of hepatic disease, and the preexisting level of renin secretion in the subjects studied. It is probable that for many cirrhotics, activation of the renin–angiotensin system provides an important support for systemic arterial blood pressure.

The role of hyponatremia in the stimulation of aldosterone has been discussed earlier. Although hyponatremia is not known to stimulate aldosterone release directly, it may do so through renin release, occuring as a consequence of decreased distal tubular delivery of sodium chloride.[142,143] Plasma renin activity inversely correlates with the serum sodium in cirrhotics[101,102,110] but a causal relationship between these two factors has not been demonstrated clearly.

5.1.2d. Consequences of Activation of the Renin–Angiotensin System. The most obvious result of the activation of the renin–angiotensin system is the stimulation of aldosterone secretion by angiotensin II. As discussed earlier, a direct correlation exists between plasma renin activity and plasma aldosterone in cirrhotics. Similarly, levels of angiotensin II correlate directly with plasma aldosterone levels.

The contribution of the renin–angiotensin system to the maintenance of blood pressure is well known. Clinically, hypotension does not occur in liver disease until cirrhosis is advanced. However, cirrhotics may have an abnormal hemodynamic response to postural changes earlier in the course of their disease when the renin–angiotensin system is activated excessively by upright tilting, possibly in order to support the systemic blood pressure in the face of an impaired sympathetic nervous responsiveness.[76,144]

In addition, activation of the renin–angiotensin system may decrease the renal blood flow and the glomerular filtration rate in cirrhotic patients. It is not surprising, therefore, that the highest plasma renin levels encountered are in cirrhotic subjects with functional renal failure. Relative cortical ischemia may contribute further to the increased renin secretion observed in these subjects.

Sodium retention may result also from activation of the renin angiotensin system. A direct relationship between plasma renin activity or plasma renin concentration and plasma aldosterone in cirrhosis has been mentioned. In addition, in cirrhotic subjects, all three parameters correlate inversely with urinary sodium excretion.[15] A shift in intrarenal blood flow from the cortical to the juxtamedullary nephrons also may result in sodium retention. Plasma renin activity has been shown to correlate inversely with outer cortical blood flow.[137] Furthermore, outer cortical blood flow, as a percentage of the total renal blood flow, correlates inversely with the urinary sodium excretion.[99]

Finally, when renal function is compromised, sodium retention occurs due to decreased filtration of sodium at the level of the glomerulus.

5.1.3. Summary of the Alterations of the Renin–Angiotensin–Aldosterone Axis in Cirrhosis. Despite the widely held view that cirrhosis is associated with secondary hyperaldosteronism, the majority of cirrhotic patients have normal plasma aldosterone levels and plasma renin activity. When these parameters become elevated, it is most often in decompensated subjects, particularly those receiving diuretic therapy. Defective hepatic clearance of both renin and aldosterone contributes to this process. However, plasma levels of these substances are predominately a function of their respective rates of release. Activation of the renin–angiotensin axis is the key stimulus to aldosterone release in cirrhotics. Renin release in these patients may occur as a result of a decreased intravascular volume, arterial hypotension, alterations in renal perfusion including a redistribution of intrarenal blood flow, and intrahepatic hypertension. In many individuals, the observed changes in the level of activation of the renin–angiotensin–aldosterone axis are not associated with the clinical status, particularly with respect to sodium retention and ascites formation. Nevertheless, there is a significant inverse correlation between both the plasma renin activity and plasma aldosterone level and the rate of sodium excretion. Although activation of the renin–angiotensin–aldosterone system does not appear to be an event initiating the accumulation of ascites, it may become a prominent feature of the syndrome when therapy is instituted. It is now apparent that avid sodium retention and elevated plasma renin activity are both associated with an accelerated mortality in cirrhotic patients. It is not clear, however, whether correction of these abnormalities increases survival. It is more likely that both phenomena are merely manifestations of end-stage hepatic disease.

5.2. The Sympathetic Nervous System in Cirrhosis

Over the last decade it has become evident that the sympathetic nervous system plays a major role in the regulation of sodium and volume homeostasis in man. A good deal of evidence has been accumulated to suggest that alterations in the activity of the sympathetic nervous system may, in part, mediate the avid sodium retention characteristic of hepatic cirrhosis. Indeed, many references have been made already to an activation of the sympathetic nervous system reflex arcs, such as the hepatorenal and the cardiorenal reflexes, which stimulate renin release by β-1-afferent renal nerves. The role of the sympathetic nervous system in the regulation of normal renal function and renal tubular sodium handling has been reviewed recently[73,145–147] and will be presented only briefly here prior to a discussion of the alterations of this system encountered in cirrhosis.

5.2.1. Normal Anatomy and Physiology of the Renal Sympathetic Nervous System. The kidneys are innervated by a diffuse system of renal nerves including the greater the lesser splanchnic nerves which contain both efferent and afferent fibers. The efferent nerves are postganglionic fibers with adrenergic terminals. Norepinephrine release produces the postsynaptic responses. In addition, there are adrenergic nerve terminals in direct contact with the basement membrane of both proximal and distal renal tubular cells, and it is through action at these junctions that the sympathetic nervous system influences renal sodium reabsorption.[145,147]

Mention has been made previously of the extensive network of sensory endings which are located in the cardiac and pulmonary circuits, and which respond to changes in intravascular filling.[72] These sensors monitor not only changes in blood volume but also the heart rate, pulmonary interstitial volume, and the oncotic pressure. The afferent fibers from these sensors travel in the vagus nerve and terminate in the vasomotor center of the central nervous system. The carotid baroreceptor afferents provide additional input to this center. The efferent fibers alter renin secretion, vasopressin release, resistance in peripheral capillary beds, and effect changes in the activity of the efferent renal sympathetic nerves. Vagal afferent fibers from the cardiopulmonary circuit exert a continuous input to the efferent renal sympathetic nerve activity as well. Maneuvers that expand the blood volume decrease renal efferent sympathetic nerve activity. Conversely, decreasing left atrial filling pressure increases the efferent sympathetic renal nerve activity. These changes are part of an integrated response to changes in volume status.

Low level stimulation of the efferent renal sympathetic nerves, either directly or by activation of reflex arcs, results in a decrease in urinary sodium excretion with no concomitant change in glomerular filtration rate, renal blood flow or intrarenal blood flow.[148–150] This antinatriuresis is accomplished largely by augmented proximal tubular sodium reabsorption,[151–152] although distal sites also may be involved.[153] The antinatriuretic action of sympathetic nerve stimulation is mediated by β-1-adrenoreceptors[59] and is independent of the renin–angiotensin system[154] and prostaglandin synthesis.[155] The acute interruption of renal efferent innervation by surgical or pharmacologic means increases urinary sodium excretion[151] and prevents the antinatriuretic response to reflex activation.[150]

Whether the sympathetic nervous system participates in the day-to-day regulation of plasma volume and sodium homeostasis in humans and non-anesthetized animals has been a subject of considerable debate. However, some evidence exists to support this position. Human subjects with adrenergic insufficiency due to the Shy–Drager syndrome[156] or pharmacologic blockade[157] are unable to adequately suppress urinary sodium excretion to maintain sodium balance. Similar observations have been made in animals chronically denervated by pharmacological or surgical means.[145,158]

5.2.2. Evidence of Increased Sympathetic Nervous System Activity in Cirrhosis.

5.2.2a. Plasma Norepinephrine Levels in Cirrhosis. The demonstration of renal vasoconstriction[10,41] and a subnormal response to pressor agents[159] in cirrhotic subjects has produced an interest in the potential contribution of an enhanced activity of the sympathetic nervous system in the generation of these abnormalities. Early investigators found no elevation of urinary catecholamine excretion[80] or plasma catecholamines[160] in cirrhotics. However, several recent studies, using more precise techniques to measure norepinephrine, have documented that cirrhotics frequently have systemic plasma norepinephrine levels which are greater than those of normal subjects.[76,123,161–164]

5.2.2b. Causes of Elevation of Plasma Norepinephrine Levels. It has been suggested that systemic norepinephrine levels are not a reliable indicator of regional sympathetic nervous system activity.[165] Furthermore, decreased hepatic extraction of norepinephrine conceivably might contribute to elevated systemic norepinephrine levels in the absence of any real increase in renal sympathetic nervous system activity. In this regard, Kopp *et al.* have demonstrated that low-level stimulation of the efferent renal nerves in the anesthetized dog significantly increases the renal vein to renal artery plasma norepinephrine ratio, from 0.89 to 2.01, but does not alter the arterial plasma norepinephrine concentration or the urinary norepinephrine excretion rate.[166] Ring-Larsen *et al.*[161] catheterized ten cirrhotics under local anesthesia and found a renal vein to renal artery plasma norepinephrine concentration ratio of 1.34. Because normal subjects at rest have nearly equivalent systemic arterial and renal vein plasma norepinephrine concentrations,[167] it was concluded that cirrhotics have an increased sympathetic renal stimulation.[161] In the patients studied by Ring-Larsen *et al.* there did not appear to be a diminished hepatic extraction of norepinephrine.[161] Moreover, other investigators have confirmed that an impaired hepatic norepinephrine extraction does not contribute to the elevated plasma levels of this neurotransmitter agent in cirrhosis.[162,163] Therefore, elevated plasma norepinephrine levels in cirrhosis apparently reflect, at least in part, increased renal sympathetic nerve activity.

5.2.2c. Relationship to Renal Vasoconstriction. The contribution of the sympathetic nervous system to renal vasoconstriction in cirrhosis has been less easy to characterize. Epstein *et al.* have demonstrated severe renal arterial vasospasm and cortical hypoperfusion by the xenon wash-out technique in a group of cirrhotic patients with impaired renal function.[135] Infusion of phentolamine, an α-adrenergic blocker, into the renal artery of four such subjects did not alter intrarenal blood flow. However, marked hypotension occurred and may have prevented increases in renal perfusion from occurring.[135] In contrast, Baldus administered another α-blocker, dibenzyline, to a volume-expanded cirrhotic patient with functional renal failure and observed a doubling of the clearance of para-aminohippuric acid and a mild increase in the glomerular filtration rate.[40] Gatta *et al.* infused dihydroergocristine into the renal artery in cirrhotic individuals with a wide range of renal function and observed similar changes in glomerular filtration rate and renal blood flow.[168] The baseline mean cortical blood flow and total renal blood flow of the cirrhotics studied was significantly below the normal range. Infusion of the α-blocker produced no change in systemic hemodynamics but significantly increased mean total and renal cortical blood flow although the values achieved still remained below those observed in normals. Nonetheless, there was no change in urine flow or urinary sodium excretion. Moreover, the glomerular filtration rate fell with drug infusion. These findings suggest that α-adrenergic mediated vasospasm accounts for the increased renal vascular resistance and hypoperfusion seen in cirrhotics. (The fall in the glomerular filtration rate observed during dihydroergocristine infusion may be the result of preferential vasorelaxation at the postglomerular capillary, which decreases the glomerular filtration pressure and, hence, the glomerular filtration rate). Since most of the patients of this study were in a compensated state, these findings suggest a role for increased sympathetic nervous system activity in promoting the renal vasoconstriction seen in the absence of ascites. Unfortunately, the authors give no specific information concerning the previous or concurrent diuretic therapy for the patients studied, so no inferences about the prevailing afferent events can be made.[168]

Cirrhotics often manifest impaired responsiveness of the cardiovascular system to sympathetic stimulation associated with the accumulation of weak neurotransmitter amines.[144] Ring-Larsen *et al.* examined the systemic and renal hemodynamic responsiveness to postural changes of normals and cirrhotics.[161] The cirrhotic patients had a greater baseline cardiac index and renal vascular resistance and lower renal blood flow and mean arterial blood pressure than did the normal subjects. In cirrhotics, these parameters change in parallel with the changes observed in normal subjects to head-up or head-down tilting. Thus, at all levels of tilt, the renal vascular resistance is elevated in cirrhotics. In addition, plasma norepinephrine levels are higher in cirrhotic patients than normals in both the recumbant and the upright positions. These data support the suggestion that excessive renal sympathetic nervous activity may be, in part, responsible for the active renal vasoconstriction seen with cirrhosis. Additional support for this conclusion has come from the recent observations that the mean renal blood flow and glomerular filtration rate in cirrhotics correlate inversely with the plasma norepinephrine concentration.[169,170]

5.2.2d. Relationship to Renal Sodium Retention. Recently investigators have examined the relationship between urinary sodium excretion and plasma norepinephrine levels. Bichet *et al.* administered a water load to 26 cirrhotic patients and segregated them into two groups based on their free water excretion.[171] Nineteen subjects, all with ascites, had markedly impaired free water excretion while seven subjects, including two with ascites, were able to excrete the administered water load normally. In comparison with patients who excreted water normally, those with abnormal water excretion had significantly higher plasma levels of norepinephrine, aldosterone, plasma renin activity, and arginine-vasopressin, and lower sodium excretion, serum sodium concentration, and creatinine clearances. When all the patients were considered, plasma norepinephrine concentration correlated directly with plasma renin activity, plasma aldosterone, and arginine vasopressin levels, factors that the authors considered to be volume correlates. There was a strong inverse correlation between urinary sodium and water excretion and the plasma norepinephrine levels. No casual relationship between increased sympathetic nervous system activity (as evidenced by the elevated plasma norepinephrine levels) and impaired sodium and water excretion was obvious from this study. However, the findings suggest that activation of the sympathetic nervous system induced by defective intravascular filling may participate with other volume-protective reflexes in the renal retention of sodium observed in decompensated cirrhotics.

Studies using head-out water immersion of cirrhotics to examine the relationship between norepinephrine levels and urinary sodium excretion have produced conflicting results. Bichet *et al.* subjected eight decompensated cirrhotics to immersion and observed a decline in plasma norepinephrine levels which correlated directly with the observed increases in right atrial pressure induced by water immersion.[88] Fractional sodium excretion increased with the increases produced in right atrial pressure and correlated inversely with plasma norepinephrine levels. In contrast, in fifteen decompensated cirrhotic patients, Epstein[172] observed elevated baseline norepinephrine levels which were suppressed by immersion in only six. In these decompensated subjects, no correlation between sodium excretion and suppression of the plasma norepinephrine levels was observed.[172] The reasons for the discrepancy between these two investigations is obscure. The patients studied were clinically similar and the immersion techniques and the assays of plasma norepinephrine levels employed by each group did not differ appreciably.

Because it is impossible at present to separate the individual contributions of the various effectors of sodium retention in human cirrhotic subjects, it would be quite a challenge to demonstrate a direct participation of the sympathetic nervous system in this process. Pharmacologic blockade of the renin–angiotensin–aldosterone axis and subsequent immersion of cirrhotic patients in studies similar to those of Epstein *et al.* may facilitate further examination of the relationship between the sympathetic nervous system and renal sodium retention. Concomitant determinations of the arterial to renal vein plasma norepinephrine ratios in such studies would add validity to any such approach.

5.2.3. Summary of the Contribution of the Sympathetic Nervous System to Altered Renal Function in Cirrhosis. Afferent arcs that contribute to the level of activity in the efferent renal sympathetic nerves include volume receptors in the cardiovascular tree and hepatic venous baroreceptors. Efferent renal nerve fibers terminate directly on the tubular basement membranes as well as the peritubular structures such as the juxtaglomerular apparatus. Volume depletion increases, whereas volume expansion decreases, the efferent renal sympathetic nerve activity. Increases in renal nerve discharge act directly on the renal tubule to augument sodium reabsorption and, also, may induce renin secretion. In cirrhotics, increased sympathetic nervous activity may be produced by volume depletion and, possibly, by intrahepatic or portal hypertension. Cirrhotics often have elevated plasma norepinephrine levels, which probably reflect enhanced norepinephrine secretion due to circulatory unresponsiveness. Renal release of norepinephrine may be responsible for the elevations of serum norepinephrine. Excessive renal sympathetic nerve activity in cirrhosis is apparently associated with renal arteriolar vasoconstriction. It is not clear that augmented renal sympathetic nervous activity is responsible for the sodium retention seen in cirrhosis, but some studies support this concept.

5.3. Role of Altered Prostaglandin Metabolism in Cirrhosis

Abnormalities of prostaglandin metabolism recently have received a good deal of attention as potential effectors of renal vasoconstriction and sodium retention in cirrhosis. Much of the available data have been derived from studies employing systemic or intrarenal infusion of prostaglandins or the administration of inhibitors of prostaglandin synthesis. Unfortunately, both of these techniques have been of more pharmacologic than physiologic interest, as prostaglandins are locally synthesized and active agents. In addition, the physiologic role of prostaglandins in the regulation of renal function and sodium balance is not well understood. Thus, it is appropriate to review briefly the features of normal prostaglandin physiology that are pertinent to a subsequent discussion of the alterations of prostaglandin metabolism encountered in cirrhosis. Renal prostaglandin physiology and biochemistry has been extensively reviewed elsewhere.[173–175]

5.3.1. Normal Biochemistry and Physiology of Prostaglandins. Prostaglandin synthesis is initiated when a cell surface receptor is activated leading to the release of archidonic acid from cellular phospholipids by the enzyme phospholipase A_2 (see Fig. 5). Prostaglandin synthetase, which has cyclooxygenase and peroxidase components, converts arachidonic acid to PGG_2 and PGH_2. Salicylates and nonsteroidal antiinflammatory agents block prostaglandin synthesis by inhibiting the cyclooxygenase component of this enzyme. PGG_2 and PGH_2 are converted to other prostaglandin metabolites including PGE_2, PGI_2 (prostacyclin), PGD_2, and TXA_2 (thromboxane A_2). Each cell type synthesizes predominately one prostaglandin metabolite. Thus, renal arterioles produce PGI_2 whereas glomerular and distal renal tubular cells synthesize mainly PGE_2. PGE_2 and other metabolites may enter the circulation but are removed almost totally in a single transit through the pulmonary vasculature. Prostaglandins exert their function within the cells of their origin or in nearby cells. Renal prostaglandin excretion represents renal prostaglandin synthesis, although it is not clear whether the prostaglandins excreted are of vascular or interstitial origin.[175] The physiologic functions of renal prostaglandin are less well understood. While TXA_2 is a vasoconstrictor, PGE_2 and PGI_2 are vasodilator agents that appear to preserve renal blood flow in the presence of vasoconstrictor influences. For example, prostaglandin synthesis inhibitors augment renal vasoconstriction in response to angiotensin II infusion[176] or hemorrhage.[177] In sodium-deprived, but not sodium-replete,

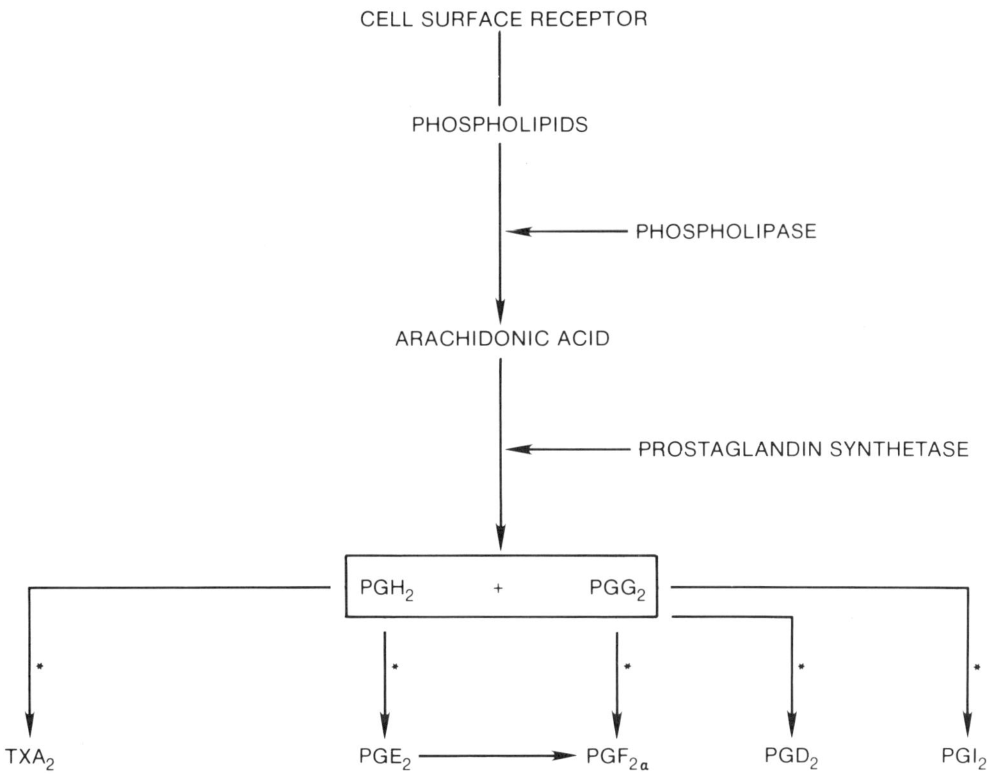

Figure 5. Prostaglandin synthesis pathways. PG denotes prostaglandins. TX represents thromboxane. Asterisk indicates the action of specific PG synthesis enzymes.

animals, inhibition of prostaglandin synthesis sharply diminishes renal blood flow and glomerular filtration rate.[178] The vasoconstrictor agents angiotensin II and norepinephrine stimulate renal prostaglandin synthesis.[179,180] Presumably this serves to attenuate the vasoconstrictive response and preserve renal blood flow.

The actions of prostaglandins on sodium excretion are somewhat obscure. Intrarenal infusion of vasodilator prostaglandins produces a natriuresis[181] which may occur independent of renal vasodilatation.[182] PGE_2 inhibits sodium reabsorption in isolated perfused proximal and distal tubule segments.[183,184] In contrast, others have reported an increase in sodium excretion in the dog during inhibition of prostaglandin synthesis.[185] However, in the sodium-depleted state in humans, prostaglandin synthesis inhibition blunts sodium excretion.[186] Whether the apparent natriuretic actions of prostaglandins are direct (tubular) or indirect (hemodynamic) in origin is a subject of considerable controversy.[187,188] However, a reasonable viewpoint holds that, whereas other factors are of more importance, renal prostaglandins may participate in regulating sodium balance when other such mechanisms are stressed.[174]

5.3.2. Alterations of Prostaglandins in Cirrhosis. The best evidence supporting the role of prostaglandins in the preservation of the renal blood flow and glomerular filtration rate in cirrhosis has come from studies employing prostaglandin synthesis inhibitors. The administration of indomethacin to cirrhotics produces sharp decrements in both renal blood flow and glomerular filtration rate in most subjects with ascites, but no, or minimal, declines in these parameters in compensated patients.[189] Other investigators using salicylates[123,190,191] and indomethacin and/or ibuprofen[192,193] have confirmed these effects of prostaglandin synthesis inhibition in cirrhosis and the predisposition of sodium-avid ascitic patients to experience these untoward consequences.

The effects of prostaglandin synthesis inhibitors on sodium excretion have been characterized less well. Arroyo *et al.* administered lysine acetylsalicylate to normal and cirrhotic individuals who were on a 50 mM sodium diet.[123] Both the normals and compensated cirrhotics showed no change in glomerular filtration rate, urinary volume, or sodium excretion. In contrast, the decompensated cirrhotics could be separated into two groups: those who developed renal insufficiency during salicylate infusion and those whose glomerular filtration rate was not altered by salicylate therapy. (Although it was not measured, renal plasma flow probably fell in conjunction with the decline in glomerular filtration rate[190]). Despite the different effects on glomerular filtration rate and renal plasma flow observed, prostaglandin synthesis inhibition induced a similar, marked decrease in urinary sodium excretion as well as urinary PGE_2 excretion in both groups of decompensated cirrhotics. Basal values of glomerular filtration rate, plasma renin activity, and urinary PGE_2 were similar for the two groups, but the basal plasma norepinephrine levels were significantly greater in subjects who developed impaired renal function. These findings suggest that in the latter patients, basal sympathetic nervous system activity was greater, implying an important role for renal prostaglandins in maintaining renal perfusion in the vasoconstricted state. Furthermore, it appears that prostaglandins support renal sodium excretion independent of any actions they might have on renal hemodynamics in cirrhosis.[123] Additional support for this conclusion has been provided by work from the same laboratory demonstrating that cirrhotics receiving intravenous salicylates have a blunted natriuresis in response to furosemide despite well preserved renal blood flow and glomerular filtration.[190]

Studies that have examined basal urinary PGE excretion in cirrhotics have produced conflicting results. Kramer reported that basal urinary PGE_2 excretion determined by radioimmunoassay was lower in decompensated cirrhotics than in healthy controls.[194] However, the relevance of this observation is limited as dietary sodium and renal function were not reported for either group of subjects. Studies that controlled dietary sodium have revealed the decompensated cirrhotics with well-preserved renal function have elevated mean basal urinary PGE_2 excretion.[123,191,192] In contrast, when functional renal failure is present, urinary PGE_2 excretion is lower than that observed for either normal subjects or decompensated cirrhotics with preserved renal function.[123] Impaired urinary PGE_2 excretion in the functional renal failure of cirrhosis is associated with more avid sodium retention and impaired free water secretion.[123,191] The relevance of urinary prostaglandin excretion to sodium excretion is called into question by the observation that urinary PGE_2 excretion in compensated patients is not different from that of decompensated cirrhotics despite the fact that the latter group has a markedly reduced urine sodium excretion with only a minor depression in glomerular filtration rate.[123] Nevertheless, the majority of studies have shown elevated urinary PGE_2 excretion in decompensated cirrhotics.

In contrast, Epstein *et al.* found normal basal urinary PGE excretion in a group of 13 cirrhotic patients, twelve of whom were decompensated at the time of study.[195] When these patients were subjected to head-out water immersion, seven exhibited a brisk "supranormal" natriuresis, whereas six had a minimal or subnormal response. The group as a whole exhibited a marked rise in urinary PGE excretion to levels much greater than those of normal controls. Unfortunately, the authors did not give the individual responses or separate their patients into groups based on their natriuretic response. Thus, it is not possible to determine if the subjects who did not respond to immersion with a natriuresis were able to increase their urinary PGE production. From the data shown for one patient it appears that there may well be a dissociation of natriuresis and PGE excretion, i.e., that natriuresis does not necessarily accompany increased PGE excretion.[195] This study does, however, reveal that cirrhotics can augment their urinary PGE excretion in the face of a volume load similar to the responses previously observed in normal subjects.[186]

The infusion of prostaglandins into cirrhotics has not been of any therapeutic value. Similarly, the intravenous infusion of PGA_1, a synthetic vasodilatory prostaglandin, has failed to augment renal plasma flow in patients with depressed renal function.[196] It did however restore perfusion after the administration of indomethacin in a group of cirrhotics with well-preserved renal function.[196] Infusion of graded doses of PGE_1 into the renal artery of three subjects with functional renal failure produced no change in the level of renal vasoconstriction or urinary sodium or volume output.[197] Interestingly, plasma levels of PGE_1 rose markedly during the intrarenal infusion of this agent, a phenomenon not seen when normal subjects are infused with PGE_1. Presumably this occurred because the extensive pulmonary shunts characteristic of cirrhosis allowed the prostaglandin to escape degradation. This finding suggests a mechanism whereby prostaglandins may accumulate in the circulation of cirrhotics and, conceivably, produce systemic effects such as vasodilatation. No reliable data on systemic levels of prostaglandins are available currently, but more sensitive radioimmunoassay techniques should provide the tools for such a study.

There is some evidence to suggest that nonrenal prostaglandins may participate in the resistance to pressor agents encountered in cirrhosis. Although the administration of prostaglandin synthesis inhibitors to cirrhotics does not change the mean basal blood pressure, it reduces by 50% the dose of intravenous angiotensin II required to produce a defined pressor response in cirrhotics.[192] Because inhibition of prostaglandin synthesis in normal man increases the vasoconstrictor response to exogeneous angiotensin II, it is not clear that altered systemic vascular prostaglandin synthesis underlies the peripheral vasodilatation of cirrhosis. In addition, other workers have not been able to reproduce these findings.[193]

Increased urinary excretion of thromboxane B_2, the degradation product of TXA_2, has been encountered in patients with functional renal failure.[198] This suggests that augmented TXA_2 and decreased PGE_2 synthesis may account, at least in part, for the excessive renal vasoconstriction observed. However, the concomitant presence of factors such as neural stimulation and elevated angiotensin II levels make it impossible to assign a causative role for such a prostglandin imbalance per se in the vasoconstriction of functional renal failure.

Diminished arachidonate availability might account for the impaired renal prostaglandin synthesis and the low levels of urinary prostaglandin excretion seen in the hepatorenal syndrome. Perez-Ayuso *et al.* reported that cirrhotic patients have a lesser proportion of total plasma lipids as arachidonic acid than do normal subjects.[191] Further studies are required to examine the issue of arachidonate availability.

5.3.3. Summary of Prostaglandin Abnormalities in Cirrhosis. Prostaglandins apparently have a role in modulating the vasoconstrictor forces encountered in pathophysiologic conditions. Participation of these agents in normal sodium and volume homeostasis is not yet clear. They may contribute to the maintenance of sodium and volume status when other mechanisms are inadequate. In cirrhosis, renal prostaglandin synthesis protects the renal circulation from a plethora of vasoconstrictor forces. It also is likely that renal prostaglandins contribute to sodium excretion independently of their hemodynamic effects. The use of urinary prostaglandin excretion as an index of renal prostaglandin synthesis has not produced consistent data. It appears from immersion studies that the level of sodium excretion may not always be related to renal prostaglandin synthesis in cirrhosis. Furthermore, cirrhotics increase their renal prostaglandin synthesis appropriately in the face of a volume load. Implicit in these observations is the fact that abnormalities, other than impaired prostaglandin synthesis, underlie the avid retention of sodium seen in most cirrhotics. In the syndrome of functional renal failure, deficiencies in the production of vasodilator prostaglandins may contribute to the renal vasoconstriction, although probably not in a major way.

5.4. Role of the Renal Kallikrein–Kinin System in Cirrhosis

Because of the well-known vasodilatory actions of kinins there has been considerable interest in the possibility that alterations of the kallikrein–kinin

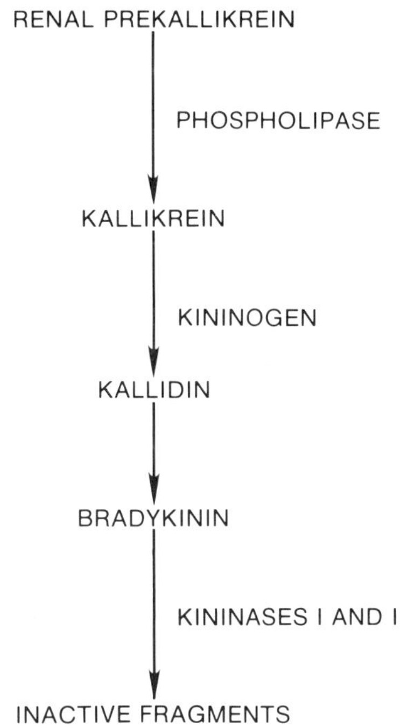

Figure 6. The renal kallikrein–kinin system.

system might account for the renal vasoconstriction or sodium retention seen in cirrhosis. This enzyme system (see Fig. 6) is not well understood, although knowledge of its biochemistry has been enhanced in the last several years.[199,200]

5.4.1. Normal Biochemistry and Physiology. Renal kallikrein is produced in the renal cortical distal tubular cells and acts on its substrate kininogen to produce kallidin, a decapeptide, which is converted to the nonapeptide, bradykinin. These peptides, the active components of the system, are catabolized by kininases. Kininase II is also known as angiotensin-converting enzyme. Since all kinins filtered at the glomerulus are catabolized completely by proximal tubular cell kininases, urinary kinins are of distal tubular origin. In practice, urinary kallikrein excretion is usually assessed as a measure of renal kallikrein–kinin activity.

Kinins, like prostaglandins, are vasodilatory. Although the function of the renal kallikrein–kinin system is not known, many studies suggest that it plays a role in the local regulation of renal blood flow. Kinins apparently interact with the renin–angiotensin–aldosterone axis, antagonizing the vasoconstrictor actions of this latter system. Kinins stimulate renal prostaglandin synthesis which may, in part, mediate kinin-induced vasodilation in the whole animal. Whether renal kinins have any physiologic action on sodium excretion is not known.

5.4.2. Plasma Kallikrein System in Cirrhosis. Early investigations focused on the plasma kallikrein system rather than on the renal system. The plasma kallikrein is distinctly different from its renal counterpart. It primarily produces bradykinin and is an important component of the coagulation–fibrinolysis pathways. It has been suggested but not proven that the system also plays a role in blood pressure regulation.

Wong *et al.* examined the plasma levels of various components of the plasma kallikrein system in cirrhosis.[201] All of the cirrhotics studied had impaired bradykinin production which was due to a decreased synthesis of the prekallikrein component of plasma by the liver.[201,202] The lowest levels of plasma prekallikrein and bradykinin occurred in individuals who had the hepatorenal syndrome. This finding of a markedly depressed plasma bradykinin level and elevated angiotensin II levels in patients with functional renal failure led these investigators to propose that an imbalance in the circulating levels of these two agents might have precipitated the hepatorenal syndrome.[203]

5.4.3. Renal Kallikrein–Kinin System in Cirrhosis. More recently investigators have assessed the activity of the renal kinin system in cirrhosis. Greco *et al.* found increased urinary kallikrein excretion in cirrhosis regardless of the state of compensation.[204] In contrast, Zipser *et al.* reported depressed urinary kallikrein excretion and elevated plasma renin activity and aldosterone levels in cirrhotic patients.[205] Administration of spironolactone to cirrhotics did not suppress the urinary kallikrein secretion further, as occurs in normal subjects. This suggests that the renal kallikrein system is resistant to the stimulatory effect of the elevated plasma levels of aldosterone. Moreover, differences in the methodology of assessment of kallikrein activity, between the two studies may explain the conflicting results of these studies.[204,205]

In the largest and most detailed study of this problem yet published, Perez-Ayuso *et al.* measured insulin and para-aminohippuric acid clearances and urinary kallikrein excretion in a large group of cirrhotics, including individuals with functional renal failure.[170] Ascitic cirrhotics with well preserved renal function had mildly elevated urinary kallikrein excretion. Urinary PGE_2 excretion was elevated also. In contrast, the excretion of both agents was subnormal in the presence of functional renal failure. Cirrhotics consistently displayed elevated plasma norepinephrine levels and plasma renin activity, which were increased further in the patients with functional renal failure. When all cirrhotics were considered as a whole, the glomerular filtration rate and renal plasma flow correlated with the urinary PGE_2 and kallikrein excretion and indirectly with plasma norepinephrine levels and plasma renin activity.[170] These findings suggest that renal kinin production, perhaps through stimulation of prostaglandin synthesis, antagonizes the renal vasoconstrictive actions of angiotensin and sympathetic nerve activity in cirrhosis.

These same authors have provided additional evidence that renal kinins may regulate renal vasodilatation independent of their actions on local prostaglandin production. The administration of demeclocycline to cirrhotics in an attempt to improve their hyponatremia, results in a marked impairment of glomerular filtration rate in the majority.[206] Those patients who develop renal dysfunction during such drug therapy have a sharp decline in their urinary kallikrein excretion associated with an increased urinary PGE_2 excretion. Subjects who do not develop renal insufficiency have no change in their urinary kallikrein excretion attendant with either an increase or no change in urinary PGE_2 excretion. Thus, deficient renal kallikrein activity appears to be associated with impairment of renal function in cirrhotics, independent of any renal prostaglandin synthesis inhibition.[206]

5.4.4. Summary of Renal Kallikrein–Kinin System in Cirrhosis. In summary, the renal kallikrein–kinin system functions at a local level, interacting with vasoconstrictor forces and renal prostaglandins to regulate renal blood flow. The plasma kallikrein–kinin system is important in hemostasis but has no proven role in the control of systemic blood pressure or renal blood flow. The plasma enzyme system is deficient in severe cirrhosis but the relevance of this finding to the development of renal dysfunction in cirrhosis is probably minimal. More recently, investigators have demonstrated an increased activity of renal kallikrein–kinin system in cirrhotics with well-preserved renal plasma flow and glomerular filtration rate despite the presence of augmented vasoconstrictor forces. When renal hemodynamics are impaired in cirrhotics as a result of increasing stimulation of the renin–angiotensin axis and renal nerve activity, renal kallikrein activity is found to be diminished. The renal kallikrein system apparently acts as a local vasodilatory mechanism to maintain renal blood flow in decompensated cirrhosis. Therefore, a deficiency of renal kallikrein activity attendant to severe hepatic cirrhosis probably contributes to the development of functional renal failure in such patients. There is no apparent role for the observed abnormalities of the renal kallikrein system in the development of sodium retention seen early in cirrhosis.

5.5. Role of Natriuretic Hormone in the Sodium Retention of Cirrhosis

A considerable body of data indicates that a putative circulating natriuretic hormone plays an important role in the physiologic response to sodium and volume loading. Recently investigators have considered whether abnormalities in the production or release of this hormone might contribute to the sodium retention seen in cirrhosis. At the present time, however, we are just beginning to understand the physiology of natriuretic hormone and, thus, there are few data regarding its alterations in cirrhosis.

5.5.1. Normal Chemistry and Physiology of Natriuretic Hormone. It is clear from cross-circulation studies in animals that volume expansion results in the appearance of a natriuretic factor in the blood and urine. Recent findings have suggested that there are probably several natriuretic hormones. The best described is a low molecular weight substance (<500 Daltons), possibly a polypeptide,[207] which is natriuretic, inhibits sodium transport in anuran membranes *in vitro* (i.e., has antinatriferic activity), and inhibits Na–K-adenosinetriphosphatase. Another agent, of molecular weight of 20,000–50,000 Daltons, has delayed natriuretic action. It is without antinatriferic activity and may be a precurser to another, less well defined, low-molecular-weight natriuretic hormone.[207] In addition, left atrial tissue contains at least two peptides (atriopeptins) that are natriuretic and may induce changes in renal hemodynamics.[208,209]

The sites of origin of the noncardiac natriuretic hormones have not been determined as yet. However it is certain that the central nervous system is a component of the natriuretic hormone release mechanism if not its site of synthesis. There also is evidence that the liver may produce a natriuretic hormone.[210] The role of the natriuretic hormones in the maintenance of sodium and volume homeostasis in man in not clear. However, the finding of natriuretic activity in the urine in proportion to dietary sodium intake supports a physiologic role for such a factor in the maintenance of sodium balance.[211] It has been suggested that putative natriuretic hormones such as atriopeptins are released into the circulation by increases in central filling occurring as a consequence of stimulation of cardiothoracic volume receptors.[208] Such a theory is supported by the data obtained in immersion studies performed with normal subjects.[212]

5.5.2. Altered Natriuretic Hormone Activity in Cirrhosis. That production of one or more natriuretic hormones may be deficient in cirrhosis is suggested by the observation that many cirrhotic subjects progressively retain sodium when treated with mineralocorticoid agents.[91,213] In contrast, normal individuals given mineralocorticoids retain sodium only for a brief period, then undergo a spontaneous natriuresis.[214] This phenomonon of mineralocorticoid "escape" is associated, in the dog model, with the appearance in both blood[215] and urine[216] of a natriuretic hormone activity. Wilkinson has demonstrated that a natriuretic hormone activity is present in the urine of mineralocorticoid-treated cirrhotics who undergo mineralocorticoid "escape" but is absent in those cirrhotics who fail to achieve escape.[217] Even though total extracellular fluid volume, estimated by a radioisotopic technique, is elevated in such patients, it is not clear whether effective plasma volume is different between those patients who undergo escape and those who do not.[217] Thus, failure to "escape" the sodium retaining effects of mineralocorticoid therapy could either be the result of defective synthesis of natriuretic hormone or a failure to expand the effective vascular volume.

Other investigators have demonstrated the absence of any natriuretic hormone activity in cirrhotic patients who have ascites. For example, Kramer found no natriuretic of antinatriferic activity in the plasma of such cirrhotics.[218] Similarly, Favre found no basal urinary natriuretic factor activity in eight similiar cirrhotics.[211] When he subsequently volume expanded these patients with a hyperoncotic solution, only four manifested a natriuresis. Moreover, urinary natriuretic factor activity increased only in the four who exhibited a diuresis. Importantly, all eight had a depression of aldosterone excretion indicating that the volume expansion produced was adequate. In addition, Favre has observed that two decompensated patients whom he studied during a spontaneous diuresis had over a fourfold increase in their urinary natriuretic factor activity during their diuretic period.[211]

Recently, Naccarato *et al.* have provided additional evidence for impaired natriuretic hormone release in cirrhotics.[19] They demonstrated that compensated cirrhotics have a subnormal natriuresis in response to acute volume expansion with isotonic saline. The urine of the expanded normal control subjects had threefold greater low-molecular-weight natriuretic hormone activity than did that of the volume-expanded cirrhotics. The defect in sodium excretion observed in the cirrhotics appeared to localize predominately to the proximal tubule. Because no volume expansion-induced changes in endogenous creatinine clearance occurred, and because compensated cirrhotics are known to be hypervolemic in the basal state, it was suggested that the lack of urinary natriuretic factor activity observed in the cirrhotics was due to failure to produce a hormone rather than failure to stimulate volume receptors.[19]

Although cirrhotics may not respond to acute volume expansion with release of a natriuretic hormone, there remain many unanswered questions concerning such a possibility. Primary among these is whether depressed or defective synthesis of such a putative natriuretic hormone or ineffective stimulation of volume receptors is at fault. In addition, there are as yet no techniques to identify and quantitate natriuretic agents either in the blood or urine. Moreover, more than one circulating natriuretic factor may be involved. Finally, chronic volume expansion as seen frequently in cirrhosis may not be well represented by the model of acute volume expansion that usually has been employed to evaluate natriuretic hormone release. The head-out water immersion technique probably represents the best model for evaluating natriuretic hormone release in cirrhotics as it produces sustained volume expansion and can be combined with hemodynamic monitoring.

5.6. Additional Factors Influencing Renal Function in Cirrhosis

Several additional factors possibly may contribute to sodium retention or diminished renal perfusion in individuals with cirrhosis. Although these abnormalities have been mentioned frequently in reviews of the topic there are few data to support a major contribution by any of these disturbances in the altered renal function or sodium handling found in cirrhosis.[194,219–222]

5.6.1. Endotoxin. The presence of bacterial endotoxins in the venous blood of cirrhotic individuals or patients with hepatic failure has been well documented.[223,224] The observation that endotoxinemia occurs with greater frequency in cirrhotic patients with hepatorenal syndrome as compared to cirrhotics with normal renal function[223–225] has led to the speculation that it may contribute to the renal hypoperfusion observed in the hepatorenal syndrome.[226,227] It is not surprising that aseptic endotoxinemia should occur in advanced hepatic disease. In normal subjects endotoxins released from intestinal flora and transported across the intestinal epithelium appear in the portal blood and are cleared by the Kupffer cells in the liver.[228,229] Extensive portasystemic shunting and decreased hepatic blood flow, both of which are common in advanced cirrhosis, probably account for hepatic escape of endotoxins and the appearance of such materials in the systemic circulation. Such endotoxinemia may have systemic side effects in cirrhosis.[226] Indeed, infusion of ascitic fluid high in endotoxin content[230] may contribute to the development of disseminated intravascular coagulation which occasionally follows the placement of a peritoneovenous shunt.

The specific actions of endotoxins on renal function are not well characterized. The acute injection of endotoxin into animals results in an impairment of renal function and severe renal arteriolar vasoconstriction. However, this renal response occurs secondarily to the systemic hypotension induced by the endotoxin.[231] The consequences of chronic low-level endotoxinemia on renal function are unknown. In cirrhotics with well-preserved renal function, no relation exists between renal plasma flow and the presence or absence of endotoxinemia.[232] In patients with the hepatorenal syndrome, attempts to correlate improvement in renal function with elimination of endotoxinemia by the administration of polymixin B have not produced conclusive results.[226,233] Therefore, although there exists an interesting association of endotoxinemia with the development of functional renal failure in cirrhosis, a causal relationship has not been demonstrated.

5.6.2. Estrogens. The liver plays a key role in the metabolism and excretion of estrogens,[234] and the estrogen–testosterone ratio and the serum estrogen levels are abnormally elevated in cirrhosis.[235] Sodium retention may be induced by estrogens through a direct renal action as well as via the stimulation of adrenal aldosterone synthesis, although the cumulative effect is only mild.[236] Therefore, the minor estrogen increases observed in the plasma of patients with Laennec's cirrhosis may contribute to sodium retention, although in view of the extreme sodium avidity often attendant to cirrhosis, their contribution to this effect may be quite small.

5.6.3. Vasoactive Intestinal Peptide. Vasoactive intestinal peptide, a hemodynamically active polypeptide synthesized in the small bowel, produces peripheral vasodilatation, pulmonary shunting, and increased cardiac output[237] and is degraded principally by the liver.[238] Circulating vasoactive intestinal peptide levels are elevated in cirrhosis.[239] To the extent that this hormone decreases peripheral vascular resistance and mean blood pressure, it might contribute to the renal retention of sodium observed in cirrhosis.

5.6.4. Prolactin. Hyperprolactinemia is a common finding in cirrhosis.[240] However, the significance of this in relation to sodium retention is obscure. Whether prolactin induces sodium retention in man, as it does in some animal species, is as yet uncertain, but the general consensus is that it does not.

5.6.5. Bilirubin. By itself, bilirubin has little effect on renal function in humans. In dogs chronic elevation of circulating bilirubin levels produces peripheral vasodilatation and secondary sodium retention.[241] The acute infusion of bile salts into the renal artery increases renal solute excretion.[242] The relevance of these observations to cirrhosis however, is not clear as neither sodium retention nor the development of functional renal failure necessarily correlates with the presence of cholestasis.

6. The Hepatorenal Syndrome

The term "hepatorenal syndrome" has long been used by physicians of various specialities to describe a clinical situation in which renal failure accompanies severe, usually preterminal, liver disease. Indeed, since there has been no widely agreed upon definition of the hepatorenal syndrome, it is difficult to obtain a clear clinical description of the syndrome and the measures required to establish the diagnosis. Recently, however, efforts have been made to formulate a definition of and a set of diagnostic criteria for the term "hepatorenal syndrome."

6.1. Definition of Hepatorenal Syndrome

An appropriate definition for hepatorenal syndrome, agreed upon by some but not all authors[243–245] is as follows: Acute renal insufficiency occurring during the course of severe liver disease in the absence of any other laboratory or clinical evidence of intrinsic acute or chronic renal disease. This definition implies that all other known forms of renal failure have been excluded. A popular synonym that we prefer is "functional renal failure of cirrhosis," which implies the absence of other causes renal disease and emphasizes that the kidneys are capable of normal function.

6.2. The Clinical Presentation of the Hepatorenal Syndrome

The clinical findings of the hepatorenal syndrome, summarized in Table I have been reviewed extensively by Conn[246] and Papper.[220,245] Typically, the patient is mildly hypotensive and oliguric and has a remarkably low urinary sodium concentration (<10 mEq/liter) and a hypertonic urine. The urinalysis may be normal or may reveal a few granular and hyaline casts, occasionally red blood cells, and low grade proteinuria. Hyponatremia, jaundice, and hepatic encephalopathy are common in patients with the hepatorenal syndrome but are not invariably present. Most patients have clinically evident ascites. The onset of their renal insufficiency may be sudden, following aggressive diuretic therapy, vomiting, paracentesis, or gastrointestinal bleeding. Alternatively, and more commonly, the hepatorenal syndrome develops quite gradually, over several days or weeks. At any point in the course of the syndrome, acute tubular necrosis may ensue, manifested by a rise in the urine sodium concentration to greater than 30–40 mEq/liter, the presence of isosthenuria, and, occasionally, the appearance of renal tubular cells and tubular

Table I. Clinical Features Typical of the Hepatorenal Syndrome

Oliguria
Low urine sodium (<10 mEq/liter)
Concentrated urine
Urinalysis—minimal abnormalities
Mild arterial hypotension
Ascites
Hyponatremia
Encephalopathy

cell casts. Subjects with the hepatorenal syndrome do not show a significant or sustained improvement of urine flow or glomerular filtration rate in response to volume expansion manuevers. Patients with renal insufficiency due to intravascular volume depletion often cannot be distinguished from those with the hepatorenal syndrome on clinical grounds alone, but, in contrast to those with hepatorenal syndrome, such patients will respond to volume expansion with improvement in their glomerular filtration rate.[41] This latter group of patients may have intractable ascites and benefit from the placement of a peritoneovenous shunt or the creation of a side-to-side portacaval shunt. The survival rate for patients with true hepatorenal syndrome is very low, although a few spontaneous recoveries have been reported.[246]

6.3. Diagnostic Criteria

Table II provides a list of the criteria required for the diagnosis of the hepatorenal syndrome, derived, in part, from those proposed recently by Bartoli.[243] The use of these criteria to make the diagnosis of the hepatorenal syndrome excludes not only prerenal causes of renal failure but also obstructive dysfunction and renal parenchymal disease. The syndrome must be progressive and associated with marked urinary concentration. The adoption of these or similar criteria by both clinicians and investigators will facilitate our eventual comprehension of the pathogenesis and therapeutic results in this poorly understood syndrome.

Table II. Diagnostic Criteria for the Hepatorenal Syndrome[a]

1. Progressive deterioration of renal function over days to weeks.
2. Absence of any known cause of renal disease.
3. Advanced hepatic disease.
4. Initially UNa < 10 mEq/l, U/P osm > 1, FENa < 1.
5. Absence of hypovolemia (CVP > 8 cm H_2O).
6. No sustained improvement following volume expansion (to CVP > 8 cm H_2O).

[a] Abbreviations: UNa, Urinary sodium concentration; U/P osm, urine to plasma osmolality ratio; FENa, fractional excretion of sodium; CVP, central venous pressure.

6.4. The Pathogenesis of the Hepatorenal Syndrome

Crucial to an understanding of the etiology of the hepatorenal syndrome is the observation that the kidneys themselves are intrinsically normal. The syndrome occurs solely due to the presence of severe hepatic disease and its associated perturbations. Thus, orthotopic liver transplantation[247] or transplantation of an hepatorenal syndrome kidney to a patient without liver disease[248] restores normal renal function.

There are no histopathologic changes in renal tissue that are characteristic of the hepatorenal syndrome.[220] However, Kanel and Peters have recently described a patency between Bowman's capsule and the adjacent proximal tubules that is present in renal tissue obtained from 71% of autopsied patients dying with the diagnosis of hepatorenal syndrome.[249] This abnormality may result from renal ischemia and is seen frequently in autopsy specimens from patients without the hepatorenal syndrome. As yet, there is no evidence that such "glomerular-tubular reflux" has either an etiologic role or any diagnostic value in the hepatorenal syndrome.

The basic pathophysiologic event in the hepatorenal syndrome is renal hypoperfusion, presumably due to marked intrinsic renal vasoconstriction.[135] When renal arteriograms are performed in patients with the hepatorenal syndrome, irregular, deficient filling of the major branches of the renal artery as well as of small arterioles within the kidney and an associated diminished cortical perfusion are clearly demonstrable.[135] Postmortem examination of the same kidneys reveals complete, regular filling of all the renal vessels with patency of the cortical vessels being reestablished. The renal vascular resistance of patients with the hepatorenal syndrome may be two- to threefold greater than that of cirrhotics with normal renal function. Similarly, the renal blood flow is depressed concomitant with the elevation of the renal vascular resistance.[40]

The factors responsible for renal vasoconstriction in cirrhosis have been reviewed in earlier sections and merit only a brief summary here. The sympathetic nervous system is activated by defective intravascular filling and, possibly, by portal hypertension and appears to be the primary effector of renal afferent vasoconstriction. Stimulation of the renin–angiotensin system is also a physiologic response to effective volume depletion and may produce renal vasoconstriction and redistribution of intrarenal blood flow. With severe hepatic dysfunction depletion of renin substrate may contribute further to the altered intrarenal hemodynamics by producing excessive afferent glomerular arteriolar constriction.

Other pathologic processes that may contribute to the reduced renal blood flow seen in the hepatorenal syndrome include an imbalance between systemic perfusion and renal perfusion induced by circulating false neurotransmitters, excessive systemic intraarterial prostaglandin production, deficient circulating bradykinin, and/or endotoxinemia. Deficient intrarenal kinin and vasodilator prostaglandin synthesis and excessive thromboxane A_2 production may be important also.

How do these etiologic factors relate to the clinical features of the hepatorenal syndrome? The onset of renal insufficiency induced by volume depletion may be primarily mediated by an acutely increased renal sympathetic nerve activity, and activation of the renin–angiotensin axis. Indeed, the decompensated cirrhotic is truly a "set-up" for this complication due to the preexisting hyperactivity of these vasoconstrictor systems. Prompt volume replacement may prevent a progressive decline of renal function, at least in part, by augmenting the renal synthesis of local vasodilators. However, for unknown reasons, in most patients this is ineffective and the hepatorenal syndrome progressively ensues. The gradual appearance of renal insufficiency in the absence of overt volume depletion is more ominous and is probably induced by many if not all of the various etiologic mechanisms discussed above. Obviously, the physician must keep all potential contributing factors in mind and act quickly to reverse any remediable abnormality, if therapy of acute renal insufficiency complicating Laennec's cirrhosis is to be successful.

7. Relationship between Sodium-Retaining Factors and Development of Hepatorenal Syndrome

It is quite evident that there is no single cause or effector of sodium retention in cirrhosis. Whereas, it is not yet clear whether vascular "underfill" or "overflow" initiates the ascitic process, the preponderance of observations suggests that defective intravascular filling is the primary process underlying the progressive sodium retention occuring in decompensated cirrhosis. Figure 7 represents an integrated view of the genesis of the various factors responsible for sodium retention in cirrhosis and emphasizes that these mechanisms, some of which occur to protect the patient from systemic hypoperfusion, may each result directly in or contribute to renal hypoperfusion. Additionally, Fig. 7 provides a broad overview of the clinical interrelationships of these pathophysiologic features of Laennec's cirrhosis.

8. Therapy of Abnormalities of Renal Function and Sodium Handling in Cirrhosis

8.1. The Medical Management of Ascites in Laennec's Cirrhosis

Having reviewed in some depth the advances in our understanding of the effects of cirrhosis on renal function, it is only appropriate to ask how these findings, largely spanning the last 10 to 15 years, have aided our approach to the therapy of ascites in cirrhosis. Suffice it to say that the standard medical management is not different in the mid-1980s than it was 15 years ago. Does this represent a failure to apply our increasing understanding of the disorder? The answer is definitely no. In contrast, this lack of any major improvement in medical therapy reflects extraordinary foresight and some

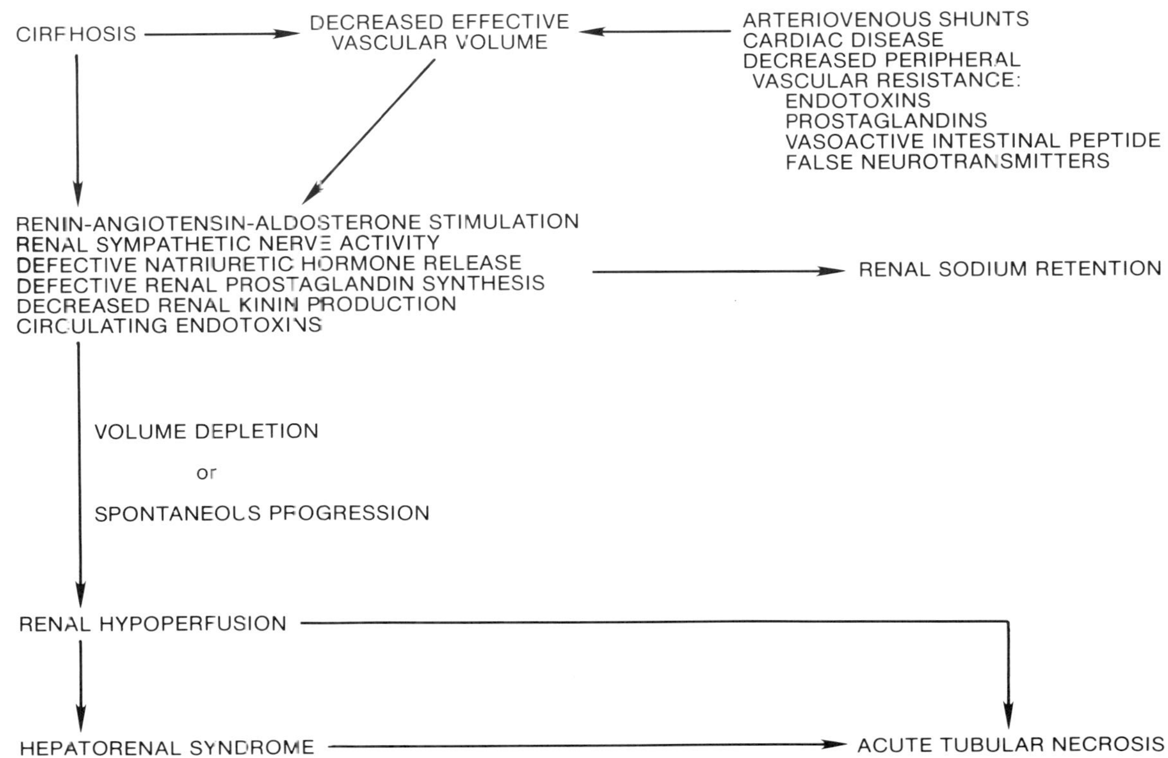

Figure 7. The relationship between the effectors of renal sodium retention in cirrhosis and the development of renal insufficiency due to the hepatorenal syndrome and acute tubular necrosis.

serendipity on the part of physicians, who, using limited data, formulated the approach developed in the early 1970s.

In an often-quoted and eloquent article published in 1972, Conn outlined his recommendations for the treatment of ascites.[250] The major constituents of his approach, listed in Table III, are hospitalization, alcohol abstention (which usually follows hospitalization), and strict dietary sodium restriction. Water restriction was not deemed necessary unless hyponatremia was present. Because Shear *et al.* demonstrated that ascitic fluid can be reabsorbed into the circulation at a maximal rate of approximately 900 ml/day,[251] a goal of 1–2 lb of weight loss daily for ascitic subjects without edema was deemed maximally safe and effective. Spironolactone was the diuretic agent of choice and was used in increasing doses as needed to reduce ascites but avoid frank hyperkalemia. Thiazide or loop diuretics were added to sprionolactone if the latter agent was ineffective alone. For patients unable to mobilize ascites on diuretic therapy or those who develop marked azotemia with diuresis, paracentesis and reinfusion of up to 2 liter of ascitic fluid was recommended.

Table III compares the approach described above with those outlined in several recent reviews.[252–254] The basic components of Conn's original approach have not been challenged. Spironolactone remains the drug of choice, not because all decompensated cirrhotics have secondary hyperaldosteronism as was once thought, but because it is a mild diuretic agent, does not produce hypokalemia, and has been shown to be more effective than furosemide alone in this clinical setting.[190] The combination of two diuretics is often necessary because the avid renal sodium reabsorption of cirrhosis occurs at many tubular sites. Reinfusion of ascites is no longer a popular approach. When a patient has been proven to be resistant to diuretics and maintains tense ascites, a trial of paracentesis may improve cardiac function.[39] However, since this procedure may also induce volume depletion it must be undertaken with extreme caution and may require concomitant systemic infusion of an isooncotic albumin solution. Patients who are deemed resistant to diuretic therapy may be candidates for placement of a peritoneovenous shunt, although this therapeutic approach is fraught with considerable hazard.[83,255]

Table III. A Comparison of the Medical Regimen Recommended by Conn over a Decade Ago with More Recent Recommendations.

Conn[250]	Recent recommendations[252–254]
Hospitalization and alcohol abstention	Hospitalization and alcohol abstention
Sodium restriction	Sodium restriction
No water restriction (unless hyponatremic)	No water restriction (unless hyponatremic)
Establish goals for weight loss	Establish goals for weight loss
Spironolactone	Spironolactone
Additional diuretics if necessary	Additional diuretics if necessary
Ascites reinfusion (resistant ascites)	Trial of paracentesis (resistant ascites)

8.2. Management of the Hepatorenal Syndrome

The treatment of the hepatorenal syndrome by virtually every measure attempted has proved futile. The most important first step is to establish the diagnosis. This requires an estimate or determination of central venous or right atrial pressure. If there is evidence for volume depletion, this must be corrected. Only if the patient is euvolemic, can the other diagnostic criteria for the hepatorenal syndrome be applied.

General supportive measures, appropriate to all patients with severe illness, should be initiated. This includes adjustment of medication dosages appropriate to the level of renal and hepatic dysfunction, preservation of ventilatory function, and correction of all electrolyte and acid–base disorders.

Dialysis, in our experience, as well as that of others,[256–258] has not been successful in prolonging patient survival. However, a brief course of dialytic therapy has occasionally been attempted, albeit unsuccessfully, for patients waiting orthotopic liver transplantation.

At the University of Pittsburgh liver transplantation has only rarely been employed for alcoholic patients due to the inability of such individuals to maintain abstinence.[259] Nonetheless, liver transplantation remains a viable therapy for the hepatorenal syndrome. In fact, the hepatorenal syndrome is a major cause of death in patients awaiting transplantation.[259]

Placement of a peritoneovenous shunt has been reported by several investigators to reverse the hepatorenal syndrome.[260–262] However, in no report has the accuracy of the diagnosis of the hepatorenal syndrome been confirmed by measurement of the patients' volume status prior to shunt placement. Because patients with hypovolemia would be expected to respond to the volume expansion induced by the shunt with an increase in glomerular filtration rate and urinary output, one cannot conclude a priori that the hepatorenal syndrome was present in such cases.

Medical therapy for the hepatorenal syndrome has included volume expansion maneuvers, infusion of pressor agents, exchange transfusion, fresh frozen plasma infusions, steroid administration, prostaglandin infusion, and antibiotic administration. None of these measures, either alone or in combination, proved to be successful. Fisher has advocated the use of branch-chain amino acids and L-dopa to improve nutrition and restore the peripheral vascular tone, thereby reversing the renal hypoperfusion of the hepatorenal syndrome.[263] However, as yet no data are available to assess the efficacy of this regimen.

The therapy of the hepatorenal syndrome, therefore, remains a difficult challenge for clinicians. Presently the best hope is that general supportive measures may prolong the patient's life sufficiently such that the hepatic dysfunction may improve spontaneously or that hepatic transplantation can be applied successfully, which in either case leads to a reversal of the renal dysfunction.

References

1. Lieber CS: Pathogenesis and early diagnosis of alcoholic liver injury. *N Engl J Med* 298:888–893, 1978.
2. Ratnoff OD, Patek AJ Jr: The natural history of Laennec's cirrhosis of the liver. An analysis of 386 cases. *Medicine* 21:207–268, 1942.
3. Flint A: Clinical report on hydroperitoneum, based on an analysis of forty-six cases. *Am J Med Sci* 45:306–339, 1863.
4. Farnsworth EB: Electrolyte partition in patients with edema of various origins. *Am J Med* 4:338–342, 1948.
5. Klingler EL Jr, Vaamonde CA, Vaamonde LS, et al: Renal function changes in cirrhosis of the liver. *Arch Int Med* 125:1010–1015, 1970.
6. Gabuzda GJ: Cirrhosis, ascites, and edema. Clinical course related to management. *Gastroenterology* 58:546–553, 1970.
7. Bosch J, Arroyo V, Rodes J, et al: Compensacion espontanea de la ascitis en la cirrhosis hepatica. *Rev Clin Esp* 133:441–446, 1973.
8. Shear L, Kleinerman J, Gabuzda GJ: Renal failure in patients with cirrhosis of the liver. I. Clinical and pathologic characteristics. *Am J Med* 39:184–198, 1965.
9. Papper S: The hepatorenal syndrome. *Clin Nephrol* 4:41–44, 1975.
10. Baldus WP, Feichter RN, Summerskill WHJ, et al: The kidney in cirrhosis. II. Disorders of renal function. *Ann Int Med* 60:366–377, 1964.
11. Baldus WP, Summerskill WHJ, Hunt JC, et al: Renal circulation in cirrhosis: Observations based on catheterization of the renal vein. *J Clin Invest* 43:1090–1097, 1964.
12. Kew MC, Varma RR, Williams HS, et al: Renal and intrarenal blood-flow in cirrhosis of the liver. *Lancet* 2:504–510, 1971.
13. Goodyer AVN, Relman AS, Lawrason FD, et al: Salt retention in cirrhosis of the liver. *J Clin Invest* 29:973–981, 1950.
14. Papper S, Belsky JL, Bleifer KH: Renal failure in Laennec's cirrhosis of the liver. I. Description of clinical and laboratory features. *Ann Int Med* 51:759–773, 1959.
15. Bosch J, Arroyo V, Betriu A, et al: Hepatic hemodynamics and the renin-angiotensin-aldosterone system in cirrhosis. *Gastroenterology* 78:92–99, 1980.
16. Arroyo V, Bosch J, Mauri M, et al: Renin, aldosterone and renal haemodynamics in cirrhosis with ascites. *Eur J Clin Invest* 9:69–73, 1979.
17. Summerskill WHJ: Hepatic failure and the kidney. *Gastroenterology* 51:94–107, 1966.
18. Eisenmenger WJ, Blondheim SH, Bongiovanni AM, et al: Electrolyte studies on patients with cirrhosis of the liver. *J Clin Invest* 29:1491–1499, 1950.
19. Naccarato R, Messa P, D'Angelo A, et al: Renal handling of sodium and water in early chronic liver disease. *Gastroenterology* 81:205–210, 1981.
20. Better OS, Massry SG: Effect of chronic bile duct obstruction on renal handling of salt and water. *J Clin Invest* 51:402–411, 1972.
21. Bank N, Aynedjian HS: A micropuncture study of renal salt and water retention in chronic bile duct obstruction. *J Clin Invest* 55:994–1002, 1975.
22. Yarger WE: Intrarenal mechanisms of salt retention after bile duct ligation in rats. *J Clin Invest* 57:408–418, 1976.
23. Lopez-Novoa JM, Santos JC, Caramelo C, et al: Mechanisms of the impaired diuretic and natriuretic responses to a sustained and moderate saline infusion in rats with experimental cirrhosis. *Hepatology* 4:419–423, 1984.
24. Schedl HP, Bartter FC: An explanation for and experimental correction of the abnormal water diuresis in cirrhosis. *J Clin Invest* 39:248–261, 1960.
25. Chiandussi L, Bartoli E, Arras S: Reabsorption of sodium in the proximal renal tubule in cirrhosis of the liver. *Gut* 19:497–503, 1978.
26. Vlahcevic ZR, Adham NF, Jick H, et al: Renal effects of acute expansion of plasma volume in cirrhosis. *N Engl J Med* 272:387–391, 1965.

27. Epstein M, Pins DS, Schneider N, et al: Determinants of deranged sodium and water homeostasis in decompensated cirrhosis. *J Lab Clin Med* 87:822–839, 1976.
28. Chaimovitz C, Szylman P, Alroy G, et al: Mechanism of increased renal tubular sodium reabsorption in cirrhosis. *Am J Med* 52:198–202, 1972.
29. Wilkinson SP, Jowett TP, Slater JDH, et al: Renal sodium retention in cirrhosis: Relation to aldosterone and nephron site. *Clin Sci* 56:169–177, 1979.
30. Rochman J, Chaimovitz C, Szylman P, et al: Tubular handling of sodium and phosphate in cirrhosis with salt retention. *Nephron* 20:95–100, 1978.
31. Epstein M, Ramachandran M, DeNunzio AG: Interrelationship of renal sodium and phosphate handling in cirrhosis. *Mineral Electrolyte Metab* 7:305–315, 1982.
32. Murray JF, Dawson AM, Sherlock S: Circulatory changes in chronic liver disease. *Am J Med* 24:358–367, 1958.
33. Lieberman FL, Reynolds TB: Plasma volume in cirrhosis of the liver: Its relation to portal hypertension, ascites, and renal failure. *J Clin Invest* 46:1297–1308, 1967.
34. Kowalski HJ, Abelmann WH: The cardiac output at rest in Laennec's cirrhosis. *J Clin Invest* 32:1025–1033, 1953.
35. Lancestremere RG, Davidson PL, Earley LE, et al: Renal failure in Laennec's cirrhosis. II. Simultaneous determination of cardiac output and renal hemodynamics. *J Clin Invest* 41:1922–1927, 1962.
36. Dal Palu C, Donaggio G, Dal Zotto I, et al: Arteriovenous shunts in cirrhotic patients studied with human serum albumin macroaggregates tagged with $I.^{131}$ *Scand J Gastroenterol* 3:425–431, 1968.
37. Kontos HA, Shapiro W, Mauck HP, et al: General and regional circulatory alterations in cirrhosis of the liver. *Am J Med* 37:526–535, 1964.
38. Limas CJ, Guiha NH, Lekagul O, et al: Impaired left ventricular function in alcoholic cirrhosis with ascites. Ineffectiveness of ouabain. *Circulation* 49:755–760, 1974.
39. Guazzi M, Polese A, Magrini F, et al: Negative influences of ascites on the cardiac function of cirrhotic patients. *Am J Med* 59:165–170, 1975.
40. Baldus WP: Etiology and management of renal failure in cirrhosis and portal hypertension. *Ann NY Acad Sci* 170:267–279, 1970.
41. Tristani FE, Cohn JN: Systemic and renal hemodynamics in oliguric hepatic failure: effect of volume expansion. *J Clin Invest* 46:1894–1906, 1967.
42. Levy M: The kidney in liver disease, in Brenner BM, Stein JH (eds): *Contemporary Issues in Nephrology*, vol 1. New York, Churchill Livingstone, 1978, pp 73–116.
43. Witte CL, Witte MH, Dumont AE: Lymph imbalance in the genesis and perpetuation of the ascites syndrome in hepatic cirrhosis. *Gastroenterology* 78:1059–1068, 1980.
44. Bredfeldt JE, Groszmann RJ. Hemodynamic aspects of portal hypertension: The effect of increased intraabdominal pressure, in Epstein M (ed): *The Kidney in Liver Disease*, ed 2. New York, Elsevier, 1983, pp 281–292.
45. Levy M: Pathophysiology of ascites formation, in Epstein M (ed): *The Kidney in Liver Disease*, ed 2. New York, Elsevier, 1983, pp 245–280.
46. Orloff MJ: Pathogenesis and surgical treatment of intractable ascites associated with alcoholic cirrhosis. *Ann NY Acad Sci* 170:213–238, 1970.
47. Orloff MJ, Snyder GB: Experimental ascites. I. Production of ascites by gradual occlusion of the hepatic veins with an internal vena cava cannula. *Surgery* 50:789–797, 1961.
48. Orloff MJ, Wall MH, Hickman EB, et al: Experimental ascites. III. Production of ascites by direct ligation of hepatic veins. *Surgery* 54:627–639, 1963.
49. Volwiler W, Grindlay JH, Bollman JL: The relation of portal vein pressure to the formation of ascites—an experimental study. *Gastroenterology* 14:40–55, 1950.
50. Piper DW: A radiographic study of the portal and hepatic venous systems in cirrhosis of the liver. *Am J Dig Dis* 6:499–510, 1961.
51. Britton RC, Shirey EK: Cineportography and dynamics of portal flow following shunt procedures. *Arch Surg* 84:25–33, 1962.

52. Madden JL, Lore JM Jr, Gerold FP, et al: The pathogenesis of ascites and a consideration of its treatment. *Surg Gynecol Obstet* 99:385–391, 1954.
53. Roth D: Pathologic anatomy of the cirrhotic liver with portal hypertension. *Am J Dig Dis* 4:721–730, 1959.
54. Dumont AE, Mulholland JH: Flow rate and composition of thoracic-duct lymph in patients with cirrhosis. *N Engl J Med* 263:471–474, 1960.
55. Orloff MJ, Ross TH, Baddeley RM, et al: Experimental ascites. VI. The effects of hepatic venous outflow obstruction and ascites on aldosterone secretion. *Surgery* 56:83–98, 1964.
56. Orloff MJ, Baddeley RM, Ross TH, et al: Regulation of aldosterone secretion by an hepatic receptor. *Surg Forum* 15:74–76, 1964.
57. Orloff MJ, Lipman CA, Noel SM, et al: Hepatic regulation of aldosterone secretion by a humoral mediator. *Surgery* 58:225–247, 1965.
58. Kostreva DR, Castaner A, Kampine JP: Reflex effects of hepatic baroreceptors on renal and cardiac sympathetic nerve activity. *Am J Physiol* 238:R390–R394, 1980.
59. Osborn JL, Holdaas H, Thames MD, et al: Renal adrenoceptor mediation of antinatriuretic and renin secretion responses to low frequency renal nerve stimulation in the dog. *Circ Res* 53:298–305, 1983.
60. Levy M: Renal function in dogs with acute selective hepatic venous outflow block. *Am J Physiol* 227:1074–1083, 1974.
61. Mitch WE, Whelton PK, Cooke CR, et al: Plasma levels and hepatic extraction of renin and aldosterone in alcoholic liver disease. *Am J Med* 66:804–810, 1979.
62. Johnson PC: Effect of venous pressure on mean capillary pressure and vascular resistance in the intestine. *Circ Res* 16:294–300, 1965.
63. Witte CL, Witte MH, Dumont AE, et al: Lymph protein in hepatic cirrhosis and experimental hepatic and portal venous hypertension. *Ann Surg* 168:567–577, 1968.
64. Witte CL, Young CC, Witte MH, et al: Observations on the origin of ascites from experimental extrahepatic portal congestion. *Ann Surg* 170:1002–1015, 1969.
65. Lennane RJ, Carey RM, Goodwin TJ, et al: A comparison of natriuresis after oral and intravenous sodium loading in sodium-depleted man: Evidence for a gastrointestinal or portal monitor of sodium intake. *Clin Sci* 49:437–440, 1975.
66. Daly JJ, Roe JW, Horrocks P: A comparison of sodium excretion following the infusion of saline into systemic and portal veins in the dog: Evidence for a hepatic role in the control of sodium excretion. *Clin Sci* 33:481–487, 1967.
67. Wilkinson SP: Fluid retention and other less severe changes in renal function, in *Kidney Disease*, vol 3. *Hepatorenal Disorders*. New York, Basel, Marcel Dekker Inc, 1982, pp 63–103.
68. Lebrec D, Kotelanski B, Cohn JN: Splanchnic hemodynamic factors in cirrhosis with refractory ascites. *J Lab Clin Med* 93:301–309, 1979.
69. Levy M: Renal function during acute graded elevation of portal venous pressure. *Am J Physiol* 227:1084–1087, 1974.
70. Anderson RJ, Cronin RE, McDonald KM, et al: Mechanisms of portal hypertension-induced alterations in renal hemodynamics, renal water excretion, and renin secretion. *J Clin Invest* 58:964–970, 1976.
71. Levy M, Wexler MJ: Renal sodium retention and ascites formation in dogs with experimental cirrhosis but without portal hypertension or increased splanchnic vascular capacity. *J Lab Clin Med* 91:520–536, 1978.
72. Gauer OH: Mechanoreceptors in the intrathoracic circulation and plasma volume control, in Epstein M (ed): *The Kidney in Liver Disease*, ed 1. New York, Elsevier, 1978, pp 3–17.
73. Thames MD: Contribution of cardiopulmonary baroreceptors to the control of the kidney. *Fed Proc* 37:1209–1213, 1978.
74. Schaffner F, Popper H: Capillarization of hepatic sinusoids in man. *Gastroenterology* 44:239–242, 1963.
75. Papper S: The role of the kidney in Laennec's cirrhosis of the liver. *Medicine* 37:299–316, 1958.

76. Bernardi M, Trevisani F, Santini C, et al: Plasma norepinephrine, weak neurotransmitters, and renin activity during active tilting in liver cirrhosis: Relationship with cardiovascular homeostasis and renal function. *Hepatology* 3:56–64, 1983.
77. Yamahiro HS, Reynolds TB: Effects of ascitic fluid infusion on sodium excretion, blood volume, and creatinine clearance in cirrhosis. *Gastroenterology* 40:497–503, 1961.
78. Vlahcevic ZR, Adham NF, Chalmers TC, et al: Intravenous therapy of massive ascites in patients with cirrhosis I. Short term comparison with diuretic treatment. *Gastroenterology* 53:211–219, 1967.
79. Eknoyan G, Martinez-Maldonado M, Yium JJ, et al: Combined ascitic-fluid and furosemide infusion in the management of ascites. *N Engl J Med* 282:713–717, 1970.
80. Barnardo DE, Summerskill WHJ, Strong CG, et al: Renal function, renin activity and endogenous vasoactive substances in cirrhosis. *Am J Dig Dis* 15:419–425, 1970.
81. Gornel DL, Lancestremere RG, Papper S, et al: Acute changes in renal excretion of water and solute in patients with Laennec's cirrhosis, reduced by the administration of the pressor amine, metaraminol. *J Clin Invest* 41:594–603, 1962.
82. Berkowitz HD, Mullen JL, Miller LD, et al: Improved renal function and inhibition of renin and aldosterone secretion following peritoneovenous (LeVeen) shunt. *Surgery* 84:120–126, 1978.
83. Blendis LM, Greig PD, Langer B, et al: The renal and hemodynamic effects of the peritoneovenous shunt for intractable hepatic ascites. *Gastroenterology* 77:250–257, 1979.
84. Greenlee HB, Stanley MM, Reinhardt GF: Intractable ascites treated with peritoneovenous shunts (LeVeen). *Arch Surgery* 116:518–524, 1981.
85. Greig PD, Blendis LM, Langer B et al: Renal and hemodynamic effects of the peritoneovenous shunt. II. Long-term effects. *Gastroenterology* 80:119–125, 1981.
86. Epstein M: Renal effects of head-out water immersion in man: Implications for an understanding of volume homeostasis. *Physiol Rev* 58:529–581, 1978.
87. Epstein M, Levinson R, Sancho J, et al: Characterization of the renin-aldosterone system in decompensated cirrhosis. *Circ Res* 41:818–829, 1977.
88. Bichet DG, Groves BM, Schrier RW: Mechanisms of improvement of water and sodium excretion by immersion in decompensated cirrhotic patients. *Kidney Int* 24:788–794, 1983.
89. Lieberman FL, Ito S, Reynolds TB: Effective plasma volume in cirrhosis with ascites. Evidence that a decreased value does not account for renal sodium retention, a spontaneous reduction in glomerular filtration rate (GFR), and a fall in GFR during drug-induced diuresis. *J Clin Invest* 48:975–981, 1969.
90. Lieberman FL, Denison EK, Reynolds TB: The relationship of plasma volume, portal hypertension, ascites, and renal sodium retention in cirrhosis: the overflow theory of ascites formation. *Ann NY Acad Sci* 170:202–212, 1970.
91. Denison EK, Lieberman FL, Reynolds TB: 9-α-fluorohydrocortisone induced ascites in alcoholic liver disease. *Gastroenterology* 61:497–503, 1971.
92. Levy M: Sodium retention and ascites formation in dogs with experimental portal cirrhosis. *Am J Physiol* 233:F572–F585, 1977.
93. Levy M, Allotey JBK: Temporal relationships between urinary salt retention and altered systemic hemodynamics in dogs with experimental cirrhosis. *J Lab Clin Med* 92:560–569, 1978.
94. Levy M: Sodium retention in dogs with cirrhosis and ascites: efferent mechanisms. *Am J Physiol* 233:F586–F592, 1977.
95. Levy M, Wexler MJ, McCaffrey C: Sodium retention in dogs with experimental cirrhosis following removal of ascites by continuous peritoneovenous shunting. *J Lab Clin Med* 94:933–946, 1979.
96. Dyrenfurth I, Stacey CH, Beck JC, et al: Aldosterone excretion in patients with cirrhosis of the liver. *Metabolism* 6:544–555, 1957.
97. Coppage WS Jr, Island DP, Cooner AE, et al: The metabolism of aldosterone in normal subjects and in patients with hepatic cirrhosis. *J Clin Invest* 41:1672–1680, 1962.

98. Rosoff L Jr, Zia P, Reynolds T, et al: Studies of renin and aldosterone in cirrhotic patients with ascites. *Gastroenterology* 69:698–705, 1975.
99. Rosoff L Jr, Williams J, Moult P, et al: Renal hemodynamics and the renin-angiotensin system in cirrhosis: relationship to sodium retention. *Dig Dis Sci* 24:25–32, 1979.
100. Saruta T, Saito I, Nakamura R, et al: Regulation of aldosterone in cirrhosis of the liver, in Epstein M (ed): *The Kidney in Liver Disease,* ed 1. New York, Elsevier, 1978, pp 271–282.
101. Wernze H, Spech HJ, Muller G: Studies on the activity of the renin-angiotensin-aldosterone system (RAAS) in patients with cirrhosis of the liver. *Klin Wschr* 56:389–397, 1978.
102. Bernardi M, Trevisani F, Santini C, et al: Aldosterone related blood volume expansion in cirrhosis before and during the early phase of ascites formation. *Gut* 24:761–766, 1983.
103. Saruta T, Kondo K, Saito I, et al: Characterization of the components of the renin-angiotensin system in cirrhosis of the liver, in Epstein M (ed): *The Kidney in Liver Disease,* ed 1. New York, Elsevier, 1978, pp 207–223.
104. Chonko AM, Bay WH, Stein JH, et al: The role of renin and aldosterone in the salt retention of edema. *Am J Med* 63:881–889, 1977.
105. Schroeder ET, Anderson GH, Goldman SH, et al: Effect of blockade of angiotensin II on blood pressure, renin and aldosterone in cirrhosis. *Kidney Int* 9:511–519, 1976.
106. Arroyo V, Bosh J, Rodes J: The renin-angiotensin system in cirrhosis: its relation to functional renal failure, in Bartoli E, Chiandussi L (eds): *Hepato-renal Syndrome.* Padova, Piccin Medical Books, 1978, pp 201–227.
107. Anderson GH Jr, Anderson T, Streeten DHP, et al: Acute effects of saralasin on plasma aldosterone in different pathophysiological conditions. *J Clin Endocrinol Metab* 50:529–536, 1980.
108. Wilkinson SP, Bernardi M, Smith IK, et al: Effect of β-adrenergic blocking drugs on the renin–aldosterone system, sodium excretion, and renal hemodynamics in cirrhosis with ascites. *Gastroenterology* 73:659–663, 1977.
109. Shohat J, Iaina A, Serban I, et al: The effect of propranolol on renal sodium handling in patients with cirrhosis. *Biomedicine* 31:128–131, 1979.
110. Wilkinson SP, Wheeler PG, Jowett TP, et al: Factors relating to aldosterone secretion rate, the excertion of aldosterone 18-glucuronide, and the plasma aldosterone concentration in cirrhosis. *Clin Endocrinol* 14:355–362, 1981.
111. Vecsei P, Dusterdieck G, Jahnecke J, et al: Secretion and turnover of aldosterone in various pathological states. *Clin Sci* 36:241–256, 1969.
112. Marson FGW: Total adrenalectomy in hepatic cirrhosis with ascites. *Lancet* 2:847–848, 1954.
113. Henley KS, Streeten DHP, Pollard HM: Hyperaldosteronism in liver disease. The treatment of refractory ascites by adrenalectomy and by the administration of spirolactones. *Gastroenterology* 38:681–689, 1960.
114. Perez-Ayuso RM, Arroyo V, Planas R, et al: Randomized comparative study of efficacy of furosemide versus spironolactone in nonazotemic cirrhosis with ascites. Relationship between the diuretic response and the activity of the renin-aldosterone system. *Gastroenterology* 84:961–968, 1983.
115. Arroyo V, Bosch J, Gaya-Beltran J, et al: Plasma renin activity and urinary sodium excretion as prognostic indicators in nonazotemic cirrhosis with ascites. *Ann Int Med* 94:198–201, 1981.
116. Peach MJ: Renin-angiotensin system: Biochemistry and mechanisms of action. *Physiol Rev* 57:313–370, 1977.
117. Reid IA, Morris BJ, Ganong WF: The renin-angiotensin system. *Ann Rev Physiol* 40:377–410, 1978.
118. Peart WS: Renin-angiotensin system. *Q J Exp Physiol* 67:401–406, 1982.
119. Navar LG, Rosivall L: Contribution of the renin-angiotensin system to the control of intrarenal hemodynamics. *Kidney Int* 24:857–868, 1984.
120. Schroeder ET, Eich RH, Smulyan H, et al: Plasma renin level of hepatic cirrhosis. Relation to functional renal failure. *Am J Med* 49:186–191, 1970
121. Wilkinson SP, Smith IK, Williams R: Changes in plasma renin activity in cirrhosis: A reap-

praisal based on studies in 67 patients and "low-renin" cirrhosis. *Hypertension* 1:125–129, 1979.

122. Berkowitz HD: Renin substrate in the hepatorenal syndrome, in Epstein M (ed): *The Kidney in Liver Disease*, ed 1. New York, Elsevier, 1978, pp 251–270.
123. Arroyo V, Planas R, Gaya J, et al: Sympathetic nervous activity, renin-angiotensin system and renal excretion of prostaglandin E_2 in cirrhosis. Relationship to functional renal failure and sodium and water excretion. *Eur J Clin Invest* 13:271–278, 1983.
124. Schweisfurth H, Wernze H: Changes of serum angiotensin I converting enzyme in patients with viral hepatitis and liver cirrhosis. *Acta Hepato-Gastroenterol* 26:207–210, 1979.
125. Kokubu T, Ueda E, Fujimoto S, et al: Plasma angiotensinase activity in liver disease. *Clin Chim Acta* 12:484–488, 1965.
126. Biron P, Baldus WP, Summerskill WHJ: Plasma angiotensinase activity in cirrhosis. *Proc Soc Exp Biol Med* 116:1074–1077, 1964.
127. Karetzky MS, Mithoefer JC: The cause of hyperventilation and arterial hypoxemia in patients with cirrhosis of the liver. *Am J Med Sci* 254:797–804, 1967.
128. Schneider EG, Davis JO, Baumber JS, et al: Renin, aldosterone, and hypertension. The hepatic metabolism of renin and aldosterone. A review with new observations on the hepatic clearance of renin. *Circ Res* 26–27, Suppl I: 1-175-I-183, 1970.
129. Wernze H, Seki A, Schneider KW, et al: Hepatische extraktion and clearance von renin bei lebercirrhosen. *Klin Wschr* 50:302–310, 1972.
130. Horky K, Rojo-Ortega JM, Rodriquez J, et al: Renin uptake and excretion by liver in the rat. *Am J Physiol* 219:387–390, 1970.
131. Barnardo DE, Strong CG, Baldus WP: Failure of the cirrhotic liver to activate renin: Evidence for a splanchnic source of renin-like activity. *J Lab Clin Med* 74:495–506, 1969.
132. Chiandussi L, Vaccarino A, Greco F, et al: Effect of drug infusion on the splanchnic circulation. I. Angiotensin infusion in normal and cirrhotic subjects. *Proc Soc Exp Biol Med* 112:324–326, 1963.
133. Segel N, Bayley TJ, Paton A, et al: The effects of synthetic vasopressin and antiogensin on the circulation in cirrhosis of the liver. *Clin Sci* 25:43–55, 1963.
134. Merkel C, Gatta A, Milani L, et al: Intrarenal blood flow, circulation time, and cortical vascular volume in patients with cirrhosis. *Scand J Gastroenterol* 16:775–780, 1981.
135. Epstein M, Berk DP, Hollenberg NK, et al: Renal failure in the patient with cirrhosis. The role of active vasoconstriction. *Am J Med* 49:175–185, 1970.
136. Stein JH, Boonjarern S, Wilson CB, et al: Alterations in intrarenal blood flow distribution. Methods of measurement and relationship to sodium balance. *Circ Res* 32–33 (Suppl I):I61–I72, 1973.
137. Wilkinson SP, Smith IK, Clarke M, et al: Intrarenal distribution of plasma flow in cirrhosis as measured by transit renography: Relationship with plasma renin activity, and sodium and water excretion. *Clin Sci* 52:469–475, 1977.
138. Carriere S: Effect of norepinephrine, isoproterenol, and adrenergic blockers upon the intrarenal distribution of blood flow. *Can J Physiol Pharmacol* 47:199–208, 1969.
139. Epstein M, Oster J: Beta-blockers and the kidney. *Mineral Electrolyte Metab* 8:237–254, 1982.
140. Carriere S, Friborg J: Intrarenal blood flow and PAH extraction during angiotension infusion. *Am J Physiol* 217:1708–1715, 1969.
141. Bumpus FM, Sen S, Smeby RR, et al: Use of angiotensin II antagonists in experimental hypertension. *Circ Res* 32–33 (Suppl I):I150–I158, 1973.
142. Tuck ML, Dluhy RG, Williams GH: A specific role for saline or the sodium ion in the regulation of renin and aldosterone secretion. *J Clin Invest* 53:988–995, 1974.
143. Churchill PC, Churchill MC, McDonald FD: Renin secretion and distal tubule Na^+ in rats. *Am J Physiol* 235:F611–F616, 1978.
144. Bernardi M, Trevisani F, Santini C, et al: Impairment of blood pressure control in patients with liver cirrhosis during tilting: study of adrenergic and renin-angiotensin systems. *Digestion* 25:124–130, 1982.

145. DiBona GF: Neurogenic regulation of renal tubular sodium reabsorption. *Am J Physiol* 233:F73–F81, 1977.
146. DiBona GF: Neural control of renal tubular sodium reabsorption in the dog. *Fed Proc* 37:1214–1217, 1978.
147. Moss NG: Renal function and renal afferent and efferent nerve activity. *Am J Physiol* 243:F425–F433, 1982.
148. Slick GL, DiBona GF, Kaloyanides GJ: Renal sympathetic nerve activity in sodium retention of acute caval constriction. *Am J Physiol* 226:925–932, 1974.
149. Slick FL, Aguilera AJ, Zambraski EJ, et al: Renal neuroadrenergic transmission. *Am J Physiol* 229:60–65, 1975.
150. Zambraski EJ, DiBona GF, Kaloyanides GJ: Effect of sympathetic blocking agents on the antinatriuresis of reflex renal nerve stimulation. *J Pharmacol Exp Ther* 198:464–472, 1976.
151. Bello-Reuss E, Colindres RE, Pastoriza-Munoz E, et al: Effects of acute unilateral renal denervation in the rat. *J Clin Invest* 56:208–217, 1975.
152. Bello-Reuss E, Trevino DL, Gottschlak CW: Effect of renal sympathetic nerve stimulation on proximal water and sodium reabsorption. *J Clin Invest* 57:1104–1107, 1976.
153. DiBona GF: The functions of the renal nerves. *Rev Physiol Biochem Pharmacol* 94:75–181, 1982.
154. Zambraski EJ, DiBona GF: Angiotensin II in antinatriuresis of low-level renal nerve stimulation. *Am J Physiol* 231:1105–1110, 1976.
155. DiBona GF, Zambraski EJ, Aguilera AJ, et al: Neurogenic control of renal tubular sodium reabsorption in the dog. A brief review and preliminary report concerning possible humoral mediation. *Circ Res* 40(Suppl I):I127–I130, 1977.
156. Wilcox CS, Aminoff MJ, Slater JDH: Sodium homeostasis in patients with autonomic failure. *Clin Sci* 53:321–328, 1977.
157. Gill JR, Bartter FC: Adrenergic nervous system in sodium metabolism. II. Effects of guanethidine on the renal response to sodium deprivation in normal man. *N Engl J Med* 275:1466–1471, 1966.
158. DiBona GF, Sawin LL: Renal nerves in renal adaptation to dietary sodium restriction. *Am J Physiol* 245:F322–F328, 1983.
159. Laragh JH, Cannon PJ, Bentzel CJ, et al: Angiotensin II, norepinephrine, and renal transport of electrolytes and water in normal man and in cirrhosis with ascites. *J Clin Invest* 42:1179–1192, 1963.
160. Joly JH, Leduc J, Bernier J, et al: Catecholamine levels in portal, hepatic, and systemic venous blood in portal hypertension. *Lancet* 2:121–123, 1967.
161. Ring-Larsen H, Hesse B, Henriksen JH, et al: Sympathetic nervous activity and renal and systemic hemodynamics in cirrhosis: Plasma norepinephrine concentration, hepatic extraction, and renal release. *Hepatology* 3:304–310, 1982.
162. Keller U, Gerber PPG, Buhler FR, et al: Role of the splanchnic bed in extracting circulating adrenaline and noradrenaline in normal subjects and in patients with cirrhosis of the liver. *Clin Sci* 67:45–49, 1984.
163. Henriksen JH, Christensen NJ, Ring-Larsen H: Noradrenaline and adrenaline concentrations in various vascular beds in patients with cirrhosis. Relation to haemodynamics. *Clin Physiol* 1:293–304, 1981.
164. Henriksen JH, Ring-Larsen H, Christensen NJ: Plasma noradrenaline in patients with liver cirrhosis in relation to ascites and treatment. *Clin Physiol* 1 (Suppl 1):66–70, 1981.
165. Folkow B, DiBona GF, Hjemdahl P, et al: Measurements of plasma norepinephrine concentrations in human primary hypertension. A word of caution on their applicability for assessing neurogenic contributions. *Hypertension* 5:399–403, 1983.
166. Kopp U, Bradley T, Hjemdahl P: Renal venous outflow and urinary excretion of norepinephrine, epinephrine, and dopamine during graded renal nerve stimulation. *Am J Physiol* 244:E52–E60, 1983.
167. Manheim P, Lecerof H, Hokfelt B: Plasma catecholamine levels in the coronary sinus, the left renal vein and peripheral vessels in healthy males at rest and during exercise. *Acta Physiol Scand* 104:364–369, 1978.

168. Gatta A, Merkel C, Grassetto M, et al: Enhanced renal sympathetic tone in liver cirrhosis: evaluation by intrarenal administration of dihydroergocristine. *Nephron* 30:364–367, 1982.
169.. Ring-Larsen H, Henriksen JH, Christensen NJ: Letter to the editor. *N Engl J Med* 308:1029, 1983.
170. Perez-Ayuso RM, Arroyo V, Camps J, et al: Renal kallikrein excretion in cirrhotics with ascites: relationship to renal hemodynamics. *Hepatology* 4:247–252, 1984.
171. Bichet DG, Van Putten VJ, Schrier RW: Potential role of increased sympathetic activity in impaired sodium and water excretion in cirrhosis. *N Engl J Med* 307:1552–1557, 1982.
172. Epstein M: Letter to the editor. *N Engl J Med* 308:1030, 1983.
173. Smith WL: Renal prostaglandin biochemistry. *Mineral Electrolyte Metab* 6:10–26, 1981.
174. Lote CJ: Renal prostaglandins and sodium excretion. *Q J Exp Physiol* 67:377–385, 1982.
175. Dunn MJ: Renal prostaglandins, in Dunn MJ (ed): *Renal Endocrinology*. Baltimore/London, Williams and Wilkins, 1983, pp 1–74.
176. Finn WF, Arendshorst WJ: Effect of prostaglandin synthetase inhibitors on renal blood flow in the rat. *Am J Physiol* 231:1541–1545, 1976.
177. Data JL, Chang LCT, Nies AS: Alteration of canine renal vascular response to hemorrhage by inhibitors of prostaglandin synthesis. *Am J Physiol* 230:940–945, 1976.
178. Blasingham MC, Nasjletti A: Differential renal effects of cyclooxygenase inhibition in sodium-replete and sodium-deprived dog. *Am J Physiol* 239:F360–F365, 1980.
179. McGiff JC, Crowshaw K, Terragno NA, et al: Renal prostaglandins: Possible regulators of the renal actions of pressor hormones. *Nature* 227:1255–1257, 1970.
180. Needleman P, Kauffman AH, Douglas JR Jr, et al: Specific stimulation and inhibition of renal prostaglandin release by angiotensin analogs. *Am J Physiol* 224:1415–1419, 1973.
181. Johnston HH, Herzog JP, Lauler DP: Effect of prostaglandin E_1 on renal hemodynamics, sodium and water excretion. *Am J Physiol* 213:939–946, 1967.
182. Shea-Donohue PT, Bolger PM, Eisner GM, et al: Effects of PGE_2 on electrolyte and fluid excretion in the canine kidney: Evidence for a direct tubular effect. *Can J Physiol Pharmacol* 57:1448–1452, 1979.
183. Stokes JB, Kokko JP: Inhibition of sodium transport by prostaglandin E_2 across the isolated perfused rabbit collecting tubule. *J Clin Invest* 59:1099–1104, 1977.
184. Dominguez JH, Pitts TO, Brown T, et al: Prostaglandin E_2 and parathyroid hormone: Comparison of their actions on the rabbit proximal tubule. *Kidney Int* 26:404–410, 1984.
185. Kirschenbaum MA, Stein JH: The effect of inhibition of prostaglandin synthesis on urinary sodium excretion in the conscious dog. *J Clin Invest* 57:517–521, 1976.
186. Epstein M, Lifschitz MD, Hoffman DS, et al: Relationship between renal prostaglandin E and renal sodium handling during water immersion in normal man. *Circ Res* 45:71–80, 1979.
187. Epstein M, Lifschitz MD: Volume status as a determinant of the influence of renal PGE on renal function. *Nephron* 25:157–159, 1980.
188. Levine SD: Renal prostaglandins in cirrhosis. *Hepatology* 3:457–459, 1983.
189. Boyer TD, Zia P, Reynolds TB: Effect of indomethacin and prostaglandin A on renal function and plasma renin activity in alcoholic liver disease. *Gastroenterology* 77:215–222, 1979.
190. Planas R, Arroyo V, Rimola A, et al: Acetysalicylic acid suppresses the renal hemodynamic effect and reduces the diuretic action of furosemide in cirrhosis with ascites. *Gastroenterology* 84:247–252, 1983.
191. Perez-Ayuso RM, Arroyo V, Camps J, et al: Evidence that renal prostaglandins are involved in renal water metabolism in cirrhosis. *Kidney Int* 26:72–80, 1984
192. Zipser RD, Hoefs JC, Speckart PF, et al: Prostaglandins: Modulators of renal function and pressor resistance in chronic liver disease. *J Clin Endocrinol Metab* 48:895–900, 1979.
193. Lianos EA, Alavi N, Tobin M, et al: Angiotensin-induced sodium excretion patterns in cirrhosis: Role of renal prostaglandins. *Kidney Int* 21:70–77, 1982.
194. Kramer HJ: Humoral and hormonal factors in the pathogenesis of sodium retention in liver cirrhosis and the hepatorenal syndrome, in Bartoli E, Chiandussi L (eds): *Hepato-renal Syndrome*. Padova, Piccin Medical Books, 1978, pp 311–343.
195. Epstein M, Lifschitz M, Ramachandran M, et al: Characterization of renal prostaglandin E

responsiveness in decompensated cirrhosis: Implications for renal sodium handling. *Clin Sci* 63:555–563, 1982.

196. Arieff AI, Chidsey CA: Renal function in cirrhosis and the effects of prostaglandin A_1. *Am J Med* 56:695–703, 1974.
197. Zussman RM, Axelrod L, Tolkoff-Rubin N: The treatment of the hepatorenal syndrome with intra-renal administration of prostaglandin E_1. *Prostaglandins* 13:819–830, 1977.
198. Zipser RD, Radvan GH, Kronborg IJ, et al: Urinary thromoboxane B_2 and prostaglandin E_2 in the hepatorenal syndrome: Evidence for increased vasoconstrictor and decreased vasodilator factors. *Gastroenterology* 84:697–703, 1983.
199. Mills IH: The renal kallikrein-kinin system and sodium excretion. *Q J Exp Physiol* 67:393–399, 1982.
200. Mayfield RK, Margolius HS: Renal kallikrein-kinin system. Relation to function and blood pressure. *Am J Nephrol* 3:145–155, 1983.
201. Wong P, Colman RW, Talamo RC, et al: Kallikrein-bradykinin system in chronic alcoholic liver disease. *Ann Int Med* 77:205–209, 1972.
202. Bagdasarian A, Lahiri B, Talamo RC, et al: Immunochemical studies of plasma kallikrein. *J Clin Invest* 54:1444–1454, 1974.
203. Wong PY, Talamo RC, Williams GH: Kallikrein-kinin and renin-angiotensin systems in functional renal failure of cirrhosis of the liver. *Gastroenterology* 73:1114–1118, 1977.
204. Greco AV, Porcelli G, Ghirlanda G, et al: L'escrezione di callicreina urinaria nella cirrosi epatica. *Minerva Med* 66:1504–1508, 1975.
205. Zipser RD, Kerlin P, Hoefs JC, et al: Renal kallikrein excretion in alcoholic cirrhosis. Relationship to other vasoactive systems. *Am J Gastroenterol* 75:183–187, 1981.
206. Perez-Ayuso RM, Arroyo V, Camps J, et al: Effect of demeclocycline on renal function and urinary prostaglandin E2 and kallikrein in hyponatremic cirrhotics. *Nephron* 36:30–37, 1984.
207. DeWardener HE: The natriuretic hormone. *Q J Exp Physiol* 67:371–376, 1982.
208. Currie MG, Geller DM, Cole BR, et al: Purification and sequence analysis of bioactive atrial peptides (atriopeptins). *Science* 223:67–69, 1984.
209. Camargo MJF, Kleinert HD, Atlas SA, et al: Ca-dependent hemodynamic and natriuretic effects of atrial extract in isolated rat kidney. *Am J Physiol* 246:F447–F456, 1984.
210. DeWardener HE: The natriuretic hormone, in Jones NF, Peters DK (eds): *Recent Advances in Renal Medicine,* vol 2. New York, Churchill Livingstone, 1982, pp 307–314.
211. Favre H: Role of the natriuretic factor in the disorders of sodium balance, in Hamburger J, Crosnier J, Grunfeld JP, et al: (eds): *Advances in Nephrology,* vol 11. Chicago, Year Book Medical Publishers, 1982, pp 3–23.
212. Epstein M, Bricker NS, Bourgoignie JJ: Presence of a natriuretic factor in urine of normal men undergoing water immersion. *Kidney Int* 13:152–158, 1978.
213. Wilkinson SP, Smith IK, Moodie H, et al: Studies on mineralocorticoid 'escape' in cirrhosis. *Clin Sci* 56:401–406, 1979.
214. August JT, Nelson DH, Thorn GW: Response of normal subjects to large amounts of aldosterone. *J Clin Invest* 37:1549–1555, 1958.
215. Buckalew VM Jr, Lancaster CD Jr: The association of a humoral sodium transport inhibitory activity with renal escape from chronic mineralocorticoid administration in the dog. *Clin Sci* 42:69–78, 1972.
216. Favre H, Hwang KH, Schmidt RW, Bricker NS, Bourgoignie JJ: An inhibitory of sodium transport in the urine of dogs with normal renal function. *J Clin Invest* 56:1302–1311, 1975.
217. Wilkinson SP, Moodie H, Alam A, Williams R: Renal retention of sodium in cirrhosis and fulminant hepatic failure. *Postgrad Med J* 51:527–531, 1975.
218. Kramer HJ: Natriuretic hormone—its possible role in fluid and electrolyte disturbances in chronic liver disease. *Postgrad Med J* 51:532–540, 1975.
219. Epstein M: Deranged sodium homeostasis in cirrhosis. *Gastroenterology* 76:622–635, 1979.
220. Papper S: Hepatorenal syndrome. *Contrib Nephrol* 23:55–74, 1980.

221. Epstein M: Pathogenesis of renal sodium handling in cirrhosis. A reappraisal. *Am J Nephrol* 3:297–309, 1983.
222. Better OS, Schrier RW: Disturbed volume homeostasis in patients with cirrhosis of the liver. *Kidney Int* 23:303–311, 1983.
223. Wilkinson SP, Gazzard BG, Arroyo V, et al: Relation of renal impairment and haemorrhagic diathesis to endotoxaemia in fulminant hepatic failure. *Lancet* 1:521–524, 1974.
224. Clemente C, Bosch J, Rodes J, et al: Functional renal failure and haemorrhagic gastritis associated with endotoxaemia in cirrhosis. *Gut* 18:556–560, 1977.
225. Tarao K, Moroi T, Nagakura Y, et al: Relationship between endotoxaemia and protein concentration of ascites in cirrhotic patients. *Gut* 20:205–210, 1979.
226. Liehr H, Grun M, Brunswig D, et al: Endotoxaemia in liver cirrhosis: treatment with polymyxin B. *Lancet* 1:810–811, 1975.
227. Wilkinson SP, Williams R: Endotoxins and renal failure in liver diseases, in Bartoli E, Chiandussi L (eds): *Hepato-renal Syndrome*. Padova, Piccin Medical Books, 1978, pp 229–255.
228. Jacob AI, Goldberg PK, Bloom N, et al: Endotoxin and bacteria in portal blood. *Gastroenterology* 72:1268–1270, 1977.
229. Nolan JP, Hare DK, McDevitt JJ, et al: In vitro studies of intestinal endotoxin absorption. I. Kinetics of absorption in the isolated everted gut sac. *Gastroenterology* 72:434–439, 1977.
230. Tarao KK, So K, Moroi T, et al: Detection of endotoxin in plasma and ascitic fluid of patients with cirrhosis: Its clinical significance. *Gastroenterology* 73:539–542, 1977.
231. Gillenwater JY, Dooley ES, Frohlich ED: Effects of endotoxin on renal function and hemodynamics. *Am J Physiol* 205:293–297, 1963.
232. Gatta A, Milani L, Merkel C, et al: Lack of correlation between endotoxaemia and renal hypoperfusion in cirrhotics without overt renal failure. *Eur J Clin Invest* 12:417–422, 1982.
233. Wilkinson SP, Moodie H, Stamatakis JD, et al: Endotoxaemia and renal failure in cirrhosis and obstructive jaundice. *Br Med J* 2:1415–1418, 1976.
234. Van Thiel D, Lester R: Editorial: Sex and alcohol. *N Engl J Med* 291:251–253, 1974.
235. Chopra IJ, Tulchinsky D, Greenway FL: Estrogen-androgen imbalance in hepatic cirrhosis. Studies in 13 male patients. *Ann Int Med* 78:198–203, 1973.
236. Christy NP, Shaver JC: Estrogens and the kidney. *Kidney Int* 6:366–376, 1974.
237. Said SI, Mutt V: Polypeptide with broad biological activity: Isolation from small intestine. *Science* 169:1217–1218, 1970.
238. Kitamura S, Yoshida T, Said SI: Vasoactive intestinal polypeptide: Inactivation in liver and potentiation in lung of anesthetized dogs. *Proc Soc Exp Biol Med* 148:25–29, 1975.
239. Hunt S, Vaamonde CA, Rattassi T, et al: Circulating levels of vasoactive intestinal polypeptide in liver disease. *Arch Int Med* 139:994–996, 1979.
240. Wernze H, Schmitz E: Plasma prolactin and prolactin release in liver cirrhosis. *Acta Hepato-Gastroenterol* 24:97–101, 1977.
241. Alon U, Berant M, Mordechovitz D, et al: Effect of isolated cholaemia on systemic haemodynamics and kidney function in conscious dogs. *Clin Sci* 63:59–64, 1982.
242. Alon U, Berant M, Mordechovitz D, et al: The effect of intrarenal infusion of bile on kidney function in the dog. *Clin Sci* 62:431–433, 1982.
243. Bartoli E: Diagnostic criteria and definition of hepato-renal syndrome, in Bartoli E, Chiandussi L (eds): *Hepato-renal Syndrome*. Padova, Piccin Medical Books, 1978, pp 73–99.
244. Wong PY, Talamo RC, Williams GH: Kallikrein-kinin and renin-angiotensin systems in functional renal failure of cirrhosis of the liver. *Gastroenterology* 73:1114–1118, 1977.
245. Papper S: Hepatorenal syndrome, in Epstein M (ed): *The Kidney in Liver Disease* (ed 2). New York, Elsevier, 1983, pp 87–106.
246. Conn HO: A rational approach to the hepatorenal syndrome. *Gastroenterology* 65:321–340, 1973.
247. Iwatsuki S, Popovtzer MM, Corman JL, et al: Recovery from the 'hepatorenal syndrome' after orthotopic liver transplantation. *N Engl J Med* 289:1155–1159, 1973.

248. Koppel MH, Coburn JW, Mims MM, et al: Transplantation of cadaveric kidneys from patients with hepatorenal syndrome. Evidence for the functional nature of renal failure in advanced liver disease. *N Engl J Med* 280:1367–1371, 1969.
249. Kanel GC, Peters RL: Glomerular tubular reflux—a morphologic renal lesion associated with the hepatorenal syndrome. *Hepatology* 4:242–246, 1984.
250. Conn HO: The rational management of ascites, in Popper H, Schaffner F (eds): *Progress in Liver Diseases,* vol 4. New York, Grune and Stratton, 1972, pp 269–288.
251. Shear L, Ching S, Gabuzda GJ: Compartmentalization of ascites and edema in patients with hepatic cirrhosis. *N Engl J Med* 282:1391–1396, 1970.
252. Wilkinson SP: Treatment of fluid retention in cirrhosis, in *Kidney Disease: Hepatorenal Disorders,* vol 3. New York and Basel, Marcel Dekker, 1982, pp 105–119.
253. Linas SL, Anderson RJ, Miller PD, et al: The rational use of diuretics in cirrhosis, in Epstein M (ed): *The Kidney in Liver Disease,* ed 2. New York, Elsevier, 1983, pp 555–567.
254. Greenberg A: Diuretic therapy in the patient with edema/ascites associated with hepatic disease, in Puschett JB, Greenberg A (eds): *The Diuretic Manual.* New York, Elsevier, 1985, pp 27–36.
255. Epstein M: Role of the peritoneovenous shunt in the management of ascites and the hepatorenal syndrome, in Epstein M (ed): *The Kidney in Liver Disease,* ed 2. New York, Elsevier, 1983, pp 583–600.
256. Perez GO, Oster JR: A critical review of the role of dialysis in the treatment of liver disease, in Epstein M (ed): *The Kidney in Liver Disease,* ed 1. New York, Elsevier, 1978, pp 325–336.
257. Ring-Larsen H, Clausen E, Ranek L: Peritoneal dialysis in hyponatremia due to liver failure. *Scand J Gastroenterol* 8:33–40, 1973.
258. Wilkinson SP, Weston MJ, Parsons V, et al: Dialysis in the treatment of renal failure in patients with liver disease. *Clin Nephrol* 8:287–292, 1977.
259. Van Thiel DH, Schade RR, Starzl TE, et al: Liver transplantation in adults. *Hepatology* 2:637–640, 1982.
260. Fullen WD: Hepatorenal syndrome: Reversal by peritoneovenous shunt. *Surgery* 82:337–341, 1977.
261. Radson TR, Parrish RM: Hepatorenal syndrome. Recovery after peritoneovenous shunt. *Arch Int Med* 137:1248–1249, 1977.
262. Wapnick S, Grosberg S, Kinner M, et al: Renal failure in ascites secondary to hepatic, renal, and pancreatic disease. Treatment with a LeVeen peritoneovenous shunt. *Arch Surg* 113:581–585, 1978.
263. Fischer JE, Bower RH: Amino acids in liver disease, in Epstein M (ed): *The Kidney in Liver Disease,* ed 2. New York, Elsevier, 1983, pp 515–534.

Index